Cybersecurity in Emerging Healthcare Systems

Other related titles:

You may also like

- PBHE044 | Singh | Medical Information Processing and Security: Techniques and applications | 2022
- PBHE035 | Tanwar | Blockchain for 5G Healthcare Applications: Security and privacy solutions | 2021
- PBHE029 | Balamurugan | Blockchain and Machine Learning for e-Healthcare Systems | 2020
- PBHE020 | Tanwar | Security and Privacy of Electronic Healthcare Records: Concepts, paradigms and solutions | 2019

We also publish a wide range of books on the following topics:
Computing and Networks
Control, Robotics and Sensors
Electrical Regulations
Electromagnetics and Radar
Energy Engineering
Healthcare Technologies
History and Management of Technology
IET Codes and Guidance
Materials, Circuits and Devices
Model Forms
Nanomaterials and Nanotechnologies
Optics, Photonics and Lasers
Production, Design and Manufacturing
Security
Telecommunications
Transportation

All books are available in print via https://shop.theiet.org or as eBooks via our Digital Library https://digital-library.theiet.org.

HEALTHCARE TECHNOLOGIES SERIES 64

IET Book Series on e-Health Technologies

Book Series Editor: Professor Joel J.P.C. Rodrigues, College of Computer Science and Technology, China University of Petroleum (East China), Qingdao, China; Senac Faculty of Ceará, Fortaleza-CE, Brazil and Instituto de Telecomunicações, Portugal
Book Series Advisor: Professor Pranjal Chandra, School of Biochemical Engineering, Indian Institute of Technology (BHU), Varanasi, India
While the demographic shifts in populations display significant socio-economic challenges, they trigger opportunities for innovations in e-Health, m-Health, precision and personalized medicine, robotics, sensing, the Internet of things, cloud computing, big data, software defined networks, and network function virtualization. Their integration is however associated with many technological, ethical, legal, social, and security issues. This book series aims to disseminate recent advances for e-health technologies to improve healthcare and people's wellbeing.

Could you be our next author?

Topics considered include intelligent e-Health systems, electronic health records, ICT-enabled personal health systems, mobile and cloud computing for e-Health, health monitoring, precision and personalized health, robotics for e-Health, security and privacy in e-Health, ambient assisted living, telemedicine, big data and IoT for e-Health, and more.
Proposals for coherently integrated international multi-authored edited or co-authored handbooks and research monographs will be considered for this book series. Each proposal will be reviewed by the book Series Editor with additional external reviews from independent reviewers.
To download our proposal form or find out more information about publishing with us, please visit https://www.theiet.org/publishing/publishing-with-iet-books/.
Please email your completed book proposal for the IET Book Series on e-Health Technologies to: Amber Thomas at athomas@theiet.org or author_support@theiet.org.

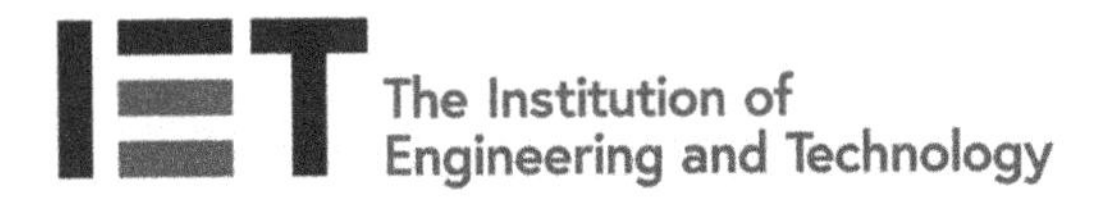

Cybersecurity in Emerging Healthcare Systems

Edited by
Agbotiname Lucky Imoize, Chandrashekhar Meshram, Joseph Bamidele Awotunde, Yousef Farhaoui and Dinh-Thuan Do

The Institution of Engineering and Technology

About the IET

This book is published by the Institution of Engineering and Technology (The IET).

We inspire, inform and influence the global engineering community to engineer a better world. As a diverse home across engineering and technology, we share knowledge that helps make better sense of the world, to accelerate innovation and solve the global challenges that matter.

The IET is a not-for-profit organisation. The surplus we make from our books is used to support activities and products for the engineering community and promote the positive role of science, engineering and technology in the world. This includes education resources and outreach, scholarships and awards, events and courses, publications, professional development and mentoring, and advocacy to governments.

To discover more about the IET please visit https://www.theiet.org/

About IET Books

The IET publishes books across many engineering and technology disciplines. Our authors and editors offer fresh perspectives from universities and industry. Within our subject areas, we have several book series steered by editorial boards made up of leading subject experts.

We peer review each book at the proposal stage to ensure the quality and relevance of our publications.

Get involved

If you are interested in becoming an author, editor, series advisor, or peer reviewer please visit https://www.theiet.org/publishing/publishing-with-iet-books/ or contact author_support@theiet.org.

Discovering our electronic content

All of our books are available online via the IET's Digital Library. Our Digital Library is the home of technical documents, eBooks, conference publications, real-life case studies and journal articles. To find out more, please visit https://digital-library.theiet.org.

In collaboration with the United Nations and the International Publishers Association, the IET is a Signatory member of the SDG Publishers Compact. The Compact aims to accelerate progress to achieve the Sustainable Development Goals (SDGs) by 2030. Signatories aspire to develop sustainable practices and act as champions of the SDGs during the Decade of Action (2020–30), publishing books and journals that will help inform, develop, and inspire action in that direction.

In line with our sustainable goals, our UK printing partner has FSC accreditation, which is reducing our environmental impact to the planet. We use a print-on-demand model to further reduce our carbon footprint.

Published by The Institution of Engineering and Technology, London, United Kingdom

The Institution of Engineering and Technology (the "**Publisher**") is registered as a Charity in England & Wales (no. 211014) and Scotland (no. SC038698).

First published 2024

The Institution of Engineering and Technology
Futures Place
Kings Way, Stevenage
Herts, SG1 2UA, United Kingdom

www.theiet.org

British Library Cataloguing in Publication Data
A catalogue record for this product is available from the British Library

ISBN 978-1-83953-951-0 (hardback)
ISBN 978-1-83953-952-7 (PDF)

Typeset in India by MPS Limited

Cover Image: Solskin/DigitalVision via Getty Images

Contents

Preface

Healthcare networks are interconnected systems that use cyber technologies for secure interaction and functionalities. The proliferation of these networks and the massive deployment of Internet of Things (IoT) devices enable remote and distributed access to cutting-edge diagnostics and medical treatment in modern healthcare systems. Consequently, new security vulnerabilities are emerging due to the increasing complexity of the healthcare architecture. Specifically, sophisticated threats to medical devices and critical infrastructure pose significant concerns owing to their potential risks to the health and safety of patients. In recent times, patients have been unnecessarily exposed to high risks from deadly attacks capable of disrupting high-end medical infrastructure, communications facilities, and services, interfering with medical devices, or compromising sensitive user data. Thus, essential cyber protection strategies and techniques must be carefully designed, which requires an active learning methodology. Developing this learning approach requires a comprehensive understanding of the complex interplay and dynamics among external threats, inside vulnerabilities, well-defined risks, and the resilience of the security system.

This book develops active and real-time surveillance and communication of cyberattacks for profiling threats to inform appropriate public policy and regulatory frameworks. The book presents cyber risk and mitigation models, considering various threats for effective policy development. Specifically, the book sheds light on how effective regulations could help guarantee medical device fidelity and trust. Additionally, the book discusses the application of artificial intelligence and machine learning to provide practical learning-based solutions to address proliferating cyberattacks in healthcare systems globally. In particular, the book focuses on the technical considerations, potential opportunities, and critical cybersecurity challenges in emerging healthcare systems. Furthermore, the book discusses the legal implications, regulatory policies and frameworks, ethical practices, prospects, and potential benefits of cybersecurity in emerging healthcare systems. Last, the book presents case studies, highlights ethical perspectives and critical lessons, and recommends designing AI-based cybersecurity architectures for secure healthcare systems. The key highlights of the book are as follows:

- Discusses critical security and privacy issues that affect all parties in the healthcare ecosystem and provide practical AI and machine learning-based solutions to solve these problems.

- Brings new insights into real-world scenarios of the deployment, applications, management, and associated benefits of robust, lightweight, secure, and efficient cybersecurity solutions in emerging healthcare systems.
- Proposes cutting-edge solutions to revamp the traditional security architecture to address the proliferating security challenges in emerging healthcare systems.

The book is structured into 22 chapters outlined as follows:

Chapter 1 gives an overview of the various aspects of cybersecurity in emerging healthcare systems. The chapter examines the significance of cybersecurity, its historical basis, prevalent threats, regulatory frameworks, and mitigation strategies. It also emphasizes the critical need for robust cybersecurity measures amidst the ongoing digital transformation in healthcare delivery and considers relevant measures to identify current cybersecurity issues in emerging healthcare systems. Additionally, the chapter highlights the importance of digitalization and technology adoption, especially the shift from paper-based records to electronic health records, emphasizing the necessity of safeguarding healthcare data throughout its lifecycle. Furthermore, the chapter examines regulatory compliance challenges and suggests tailored mitigation strategies while investigating human factors in healthcare cybersecurity. The chapter also discusses measures to protect patient data and maintain trust in healthcare systems, incorporating relevant case studies of healthcare data breaches. Finally, the chapter considers emerging trends in healthcare cybersecurity, providing recommendations for effectively securing modern healthcare systems.

Chapter 2 discusses cybersecurity in the internet of medical things (IoMT) for healthcare applications. The chapter delves into the intricate landscape of cybersecurity within the IoMT for healthcare applications. The work explores the multifaceted challenges posed by cyber threats in the healthcare sector, where the stakes are higher than ever. From safeguarding sensitive patient information to protecting the integrity of medical devices, the work dissects the evolving threat landscape and the vulnerabilities specific to the IoMT ecosystem. Moreover, the study unravels the strategies and technologies employed to fortify the defenses of healthcare systems against an ever-evolving array of cyber threats. Drawing from real-world case studies and best practices, the chapter sheds light on how cutting-edge cybersecurity measures can be seamlessly integrated into IoMT environments without compromising the agility and efficiency required for effective and efficient healthcare delivery.

Chapter 3 examines adaptive cybersecurity with a focus on AI-driven threat intelligence in healthcare systems. The chapter highlights the development and implementation of AI-driven threat intelligence platforms, which represent a paradigm shift from reactive to proactive and predictive cybersecurity models. The core of the chapter is the detailed examination of AI-driven platforms, which are designed to continuously learn from a vast array of data sources, adapt to evolving cyber threats, and predict future vulnerabilities. This involves a deep dive into the integration of various AI technologies such as machine learning algorithms for anomaly detection, natural language processing for efficient and effective threat intelligence gathering, and neural networks for advanced predictive analytics. These technologies collectively enhance the capability of healthcare systems to detect, analyze, and respond to cyber threats in real time, thereby significantly improving their security posture. Furthermore, the chapter delves into the ethical considerations and potential biases inherent in AI-driven cybersecurity solutions. It discusses the importance of maintaining a balance between enhancing security measures and protecting patient privacy, a critical concern in the healthcare sector. The ethical implications of data usage, algorithmic transparency, and the need for unbiased AI models are thoroughly examined. Through a series of illustrative case studies, the chapter demonstrates the real-world effectiveness of adaptive cybersecurity strategies in healthcare. These case studies provide insights into how various healthcare organizations have successfully implemented AI-driven solutions to combat cyber threats, highlighting the practical challenges and successes encountered. In summary, the chapter offers a comprehensive overview of the role of AI in transforming cybersecurity within healthcare. The chapter presents a balanced view of the technological advancements, ethical considerations, and practical applications of AI-driven cybersecurity, making it a valuable resource for professionals and scholars in the field of healthcare cybersecurity.

Chapter 4 presents the emerging trends in cybersecurity applications in modern healthcare systems. The study elucidates the complex challenges of integrating these robust yet often complex technologies into intricate clinical environments and workflows. The chapter offers insights into how healthcare organizations can balance improved cybersecurity with user experience, regulations, legacy systems, and resource constraints. With cyber threats growing in lockstep with healthcare digitization, the study delivers a multifaceted analysis to help medical practitioners and administrators secure critical healthcare systems. Last, the chapter provides technology leaders with a useful guide to emerging innovations for healthcare cybersecurity.

Chapter 5 discusses convolutional neural networks (CNNs) enabling the internet of medical things, emphasizing security implications, prospects, and challenges. The study buttresses the capacity of CNNs to analyze large datasets and raises concerns about data security, integrity, and availability, which are critical for retaining patient confidence and adhering to regulatory norms. Despite these impediments, CNN-enabled IoMT has the potential to significantly improve healthcare outcomes through more accurate diagnosis and predictive analytics. However, attaining these advantages requires overcoming technological hurdles such as data variety and representation, processing needs, and the interpretability of AI-driven choices. The chapter bolsters the importance of taking a balanced strategy that capitalizes on CNNs' revolutionary potential in the IoMT while thoroughly addressing the accompanying security issues.

Chapter 6 beams a laser focus on deadly cybersecurity threats in emerging healthcare systems. In particular, the chapter investigates the landscape of emerging cyber threats within the healthcare sector and presents innovative solutions to mitigate these risks. Central to the key findings is the proposal for the creation of a secure data-sharing platform tailored specifically for healthcare providers. The platform not only facilitates seamless information exchange but also integrates robust security measures to safeguard against cyberattacks. By addressing this critical research gap, the study aims to bolster the cyber security posture of the emerging healthcare system, ensuring the continuity of care and the protection of sensitive patient information in an increasingly digitized world. The chapter will benefit, not only the patient but also healthcare providers and other stakeholders in the healthcare ecosystem.

Chapter 7 explores the intricate aspects of artificial intelligence (AI) for secured cybersecurity in emerging healthcare systems. The healthcare industry rapidly adopts digital technologies to improve patient care and outcomes. However, this digital transformation has also made healthcare systems more vulnerable to cyberattacks. Artificial intelligence has the potential to enhance cybersecurity in emerging healthcare systems by providing advanced threat detection and response capabilities. The chapter explores the potential of AI in securing emerging healthcare systems against cyber threats. The current state of cybersecurity in healthcare systems and the challenges faced by emerging healthcare systems are discussed. An overview of AI and its potential applications in healthcare cybersecurity is provided. Finally, the benefits of using AI in securing emerging healthcare systems and the challenges that need to be addressed to realize the potential of AI in cybersecurity are highlighted.

Chapter 8 dissects deep-based anomalies detection in emerging healthcare systems. The study leverages the Long Short-Term Memory (LSTM) approach for performance evaluation, comparing its results with stack ensemble methods. In particular, the chapter utilizes the WUSTL Enhanced Healthcare Monitoring System (EHMS) datasets for validation, which comprises biometric and network features, totaling over 16,318 samples categorized into normal and attack categories. Additionally, the study explores the most distinctive features using the Extra Trees Classifier to minimize computational complexity and enhance abnormality detection rates using ensemble algorithms. Various evaluation metrics, including accuracy, F1-score, precision, recall, and confusion matrices, are employed. Both deep learning and stack ensemble methods demonstrate notable performance across these metrics, achieving minimal false rates. Consequently, the proposed model surpasses existing machine learning algorithms, firmly establishing its effectiveness in safeguarding the security and integrity of emerging healthcare data within the IoT ecosystem.

Chapter 9 advocates smart contracts for automated compliance in healthcare cybersecurity. The chapter delves into the innovative application of blockchain-based smart contracts in the realm of healthcare cybersecurity, presenting a comprehensive analysis of their potential to automate compliance and regulatory adherence. A key focus of the chapter is the examination of how smart contracts can be programmed to enforce compliance with stringent healthcare regulations such as HIPAA and GDPR, and this involves a critical analysis of the legal, security, and technical challenges associated with their deployment. The chapter also investigates the potential of smart contracts to streamline compliance processes, reduce administrative burdens, and minimize the risks associated with human error, thereby enhancing the efficiency and reliability of healthcare services. The comparative analysis of various blockchain platforms supporting smart contracts forms a significant part of the discussion. The analysis evaluates the platforms across multiple criteria relevant to healthcare cybersecurity, including scalability, interoperability, and financial metrics. The chapter employs the Analytic Hierarchy Process (AHP) to structure the comparison, providing a quantitative evaluation of each platform's suitability for healthcare applications. Innovative applications of smart contracts in healthcare cybersecurity are highlighted, showcasing their versatility and potential for widespread adoption. The chapter concludes with a synthesis of findings and a discussion on future directions in the application of smart contracts in healthcare cybersecurity. It reflects on the broader implications of the study and suggests areas for further research, emphasizing the need for continued development and collaboration among healthcare professionals, technologists, and legal experts.

Chapter 10 sheds light on cybersecurity computing in modern healthcare systems. The study explores the application of machine learning (ML) techniques such as K-nearest neighbors (KNN), random forest, and linear regression to address cybersecurity issues in evolving healthcare systems. The study provides a thorough analysis of the possible advantages of cybersecurity computing for enhancing healthcare systems. More significantly, the study uses machine learning-inspired algorithms to perform some data analytics on the security of data accessible in healthcare systems and includes a use case to illustrate the effectiveness of cybersecurity computing in emerging healthcare systems. Additionally, the study outlines the unique cybersecurity challenges and threats that nascent healthcare systems face, such as the abundance of networked medical devices, the complexity of healthcare information technology (IT) infrastructures, and the ever-changing landscape of threats.

Chapter 11 discusses blockchain for secured cybersecurity in emerging healthcare systems. The study looks into the use of blockchain in healthcare cybersecurity, focusing on its capacity to provide tamper-proof data storage, effective access control mechanisms, and increased transparency. Blockchain reduces the dangers of data breaches, unauthorized access, and fraudulent activities by establishing a trust-based ecosystem, increasing patient trust and confidence in digital healthcare solutions. Furthermore, the study digs into real blockchain technology deployments within healthcare systems, spanning from EHR administration to medication supply chain integrity and telemedicine platforms. Further, the chapter illustrates the benefits and drawbacks of each use case and provides real-world examples of blockchain adoption in healthcare cybersecurity. The study investigates the synergy between blockchain and developing technologies such as AI and ML for predictive threat identification and anomaly detection, in addition to blockchain. The combination of blockchain secure data storage and AI-driven cybersecurity analytics provides a proactive method for recognizing and mitigating cyber risks, boosting healthcare systems' resilience. Ethical and regulatory concerns are also addressed in the context of blockchain deployment in healthcare cybersecurity, highlighting the need to adhere to healthcare data protection standards and ethical norms while managing sensitive patient information. Finally, the chapter emphasizes the crucial importance of blockchain technology in strengthening cybersecurity in new healthcare systems.

Chapter 12 talks about the ethics of cybersecurity in emerging healthcare systems. The chapter delves into the ethics of cybersecurity in emerging healthcare systems, examining the complex relationship between ethical considerations and technological advancements. First, the chapter begins by defining evolving healthcare systems and then highlights the significance of cybersecurity in preserving trust among patients. Further, the work examines the benefits and drawbacks of integrating technology while highlighting the delicate balance that must be drawn between innovation and data security. When it comes to patient autonomy, informed consent, and responsible data sharing for investigation, ethical considerations are crucial. A thorough analysis of the legal framework is conducted, with a binocular focus on the challenges associated with enforcing cybersecurity regulations in rapidly evolving healthcare systems. More, the chapter analyses the ethical ramifications of AI and data breaches in the healthcare industry, promoting human oversight, fairness, and precautionary practices. In addition to providing a comprehensive road map for navigating this rapidly changing environment, the chapter concludes with a call to action that urges stakeholders to give ethical cybersecurity practices priority when creating and implementing new healthcare systems.

Chapter 13 examines the complex interactions between cybersecurity and ethics in modern healthcare systems. Modern healthcare systems and cutting-edge technologies have merged to bring forth a new era of opportunities to our society. However, the integration of healthcare and technology has orchestrated several issues in healthcare systems that need to be critically examined. These issues range from security and privacy to ethical concerns and dilemmas. As healthcare organizations embrace cutting-edge technologies such as artificial intelligence (AI), networked medical equipment, and the Internet of Things (IoT), the need to address ethical concerns related to the integration of cybersecurity in healthcare systems becomes more prominent. The chapter examines the complex interactions between cybersecurity and ethics within the context of functional healthcare systems. In order to navigate the complicated world of cybersecurity, the study examines the moral conundrums orchestrated by medical advancements, the necessity of preserving patient privacy, and the evolving roles that healthcare practitioners and various organizations must play to uphold ethics in modern healthcare systems.

Chapter 14 provides an exposition on securing modern insulin pumps with iCGM system with an emphasis on protecting patients from cyber threats in diabetes management. The chapter outlines the modern architecture of insulin pumps, existing vulnerabilities, threats, and risks of iCGM systems, and provides insights on security measures, mitigation, and countermeasures. The goal is to bridge the research gap by identifying current architecture and threats while highlighting necessary security mechanisms. Furthermore, the chapter provides resources of open-source datasets for further research and testing to secure iCGM systems.

Chapter 15 explores artificial intelligence and machine learning for DNS traffic anomaly detection in modern healthcare systems. The chapter aims to provide an overview of the role of AI in DNS anomaly detection and to introduce the main AI techniques used in this field. The chapter explains the multifaceted landscape of the role of artificial intelligence and machine learning in DNS traffic anomaly detection in modern healthcare systems. The chapter poses critical questions and promising avenues for future research and serves as a foundation for advancing knowledge and shaping the future of AI, DNS, and the security of modern healthcare systems.

Chapter 16 considers harnessing edge computing for real-time cybersecurity in healthcare systems. The chapter presents an in-depth exploration of the integration of edge computing with cybersecurity within healthcare systems, a critical development in the era of digital healthcare transformation. As the Internet of Medical Things (IoMT) continues to expand, generating vast amounts of data, traditional cloud-centric models are becoming increasingly insufficient. These models, while once groundbreaking, now struggle to meet the urgent demands for low-latency and high-security data processing essential in healthcare applications. Specifically, the chapter advocates for a paradigm shift toward edge computing architectures. Unlike conventional models, edge computing processes data at the network's edge, closer to where it is generated. This proximity significantly reduces response times and bandwidth usage, crucial for real-time medical data analysis and prompt decision-making in patient care. The chapter meticulously dissects the design, implementation challenges, and potential of edge-based cybersecurity frameworks. It emphasizes how these frameworks can leverage distributed data processing to enhance threat detection and mitigation, ensuring robust protection against cyber threats. In-depth case studies are presented, illustrating successful implementations of edge computing in enhancing cybersecurity in healthcare settings. These real-world examples serve as a blueprint for future implementations, demonstrating practical applications and the tangible benefits of edge computing in healthcare. Furthermore, the chapter delves into the broader implications of this technological shift. It discusses the evolving landscape of healthcare infrastructure, the need for adaptive strategies to accommodate these advanced technologies, and the role of edge computing in facilitating secure, efficient, and patient-centric healthcare services. By highlighting the synergies between edge computing and cybersecurity, the chapter underscores the critical need for healthcare systems to evolve and adapt. Last, the chapter presents edge computing not just as a technological innovation but as a strategic necessity to address modern healthcare challenges, particularly in cybersecurity and data management.

Chapter 17 focuses on enhancing healthcare data security, considering an intrusion detection system for web applications with SVM and decision tree algorithms. Improving machine learning techniques for identifying attacks on healthcare web services is the focus of the study. Reliable intrusion detection systems are essential for the protection of sensitive medical data. This research introduces a new approach to K-means clustering by fusing the strengths of the Support Vector Machine (SVM) and the Decision Tree (DT) classifiers. Tests were successful using the CIC-IDS2017 datasets. While both Support Vector Machine and Decision Tree classifiers did well, Decision Tree's 99.96% accuracy was particularly outstanding. This state-of-the-art K-Means clustering method has become the de facto standard, with an associated accuracy of 99.96%. Key findings revealed that the need to keep medical records safe extends far beyond the obvious technology advantages. Intrusion detection systems must be adaptable since cyber threats are constantly evolving.

Chapter 18 examines legal and regulatory policies for cybersecurity and information assurance in emerging healthcare systems. The healthcare sector is among the most critical and challenging domains for cybersecurity. Healthcare systems comprise numerous entities and stakeholders, such as clinics, hospitals, laboratories, pharmacies, insurance companies, patients, and medical personnel. For these institutions to deliver efficient and superior healthcare services, including diagnosis, treatment, prevention, and research, they rely on information technology and data. However, these systems and data are also vulnerable to cyberattacks, which can endanger the security and well-being of patients and healthcare providers, as well as the privacy, accuracy, and accessibility of medical records. Cyberattacks against healthcare systems can lead to several dangerous consequences, including ransomware, malware, sabotage, espionage, data breaches, identity theft, and fraud. These attacks may affect a country's general health and national security in addition to the targeted victims. As a result, it is imperative to ensure the information assurance and cybersecurity of developing healthcare systems using legislative and regulatory frameworks that take risk management, actual situations, and emerging trends into account.

Chapter 19 emphasizes federated learning (FL) for enhanced cybersecurity in modern digital healthcare systems. Federated learning, an emerging distributed and collaborative technique, appears as a potential solution to address the security and privacy challenges associated with conventional AI. By enabling the training of machine learning (ML) models on decentralized data stored across diverse wearable devices, including fitness trackers, smartwatches, implantable devices, and other IoHT devices, FL facilitates the analysis and interpretation of data while upholding the security and privacy of the participating devices and raw data. Accordingly, the chapter reviews the different FL techniques aimed at bolstering security and privacy in modern digital healthcare systems. Moreover, the study highlights the benefits and challenges of FL in healthcare and presents future research trends aimed at enhancing the cybersecurity posture of FL in modern healthcare systems.

Chapter 20 dwells on the application of directed acyclic graph (DAGs)-based blockchains for enhanced cybersecurity in the internet of medical things. Securing private medical data and guaranteeing the integrity of networked medical devices become critical challenges as the IoMT scenario changes. The chapter leverages the efficiency and resilience of DAG-based blockchains against certain attacks. The proposed access control approach is built on the decentralized and impenetrable structure of Tangle, a DAG-based consensus technique. A novel framework for access control is presented, which represents IoMT entities with DAG structures.

Directed edges encode dynamic relationships and permissions, whereas nodes represent medical equipment, healthcare providers, and patients. Blockchain-integrated smart contracts automate access decisions, guaranteeing adherence to healthcare laws and enabling real-time modifications to access rights. Security considerations encompass encryption protocols for secure communication, decentralized identity solutions for authentication, and immutable audit trails to meet regulatory requirements. To facilitate interoperability and smooth data sharing, the chapter puts a strong emphasis on integrating the access control mechanism with the current healthcare systems. The proposed solution aims to revolutionize IoMT cybersecurity by addressing the particular difficulties faced by the healthcare industry, namely security, and scalability. Furthermore, metrics like Elapsed Time vs. Number of Nodes, Access Rate vs. Number of Nodes, and Throughput vs. Number of Nodes are used to evaluate the implementation of the suggested access control, demonstrating observable improvements. The study enhances the security of developing healthcare systems amid the growth of linked medical devices and digital health technologies by providing a clear and flexible access control mechanism.

Chapter 21 captures the detection and mitigation of cyberattacks in healthcare systems. Specifically, the chapter focuses on healthcare cybersecurity and proffers ways to detect ransomware, malware, denial of service attacks, and insider threats using security information and event management (SIEM), user and entity behavior analytics (UEBA), and security onion. The authors opined that healthcare organizations are often the main target owing to the value of the patient data they own, making it critical for them to invest in robust cybersecurity measures to defend against these threats. Last, the study takes a critical look at the different methods and techniques of detecting cyber threats and provides insights and mitigation strategies. The study concludes that in the digital transformation era, healthcare systems have been exposed to a new set of challenges, chief among them being the security of delicate patient data and the potential consequences of cyberattacks.

Finally, Chapter 22 concludes the book by discussing cybersecurity concerns and risks in emerging healthcare systems. In particular, the chapter investigates a comprehensive strategy for reducing these risks in healthcare institutions by providing a thorough cybersecurity strategy that consists of risk assessments, frequent security audits, strong access controls, and data encryption. In addition, the study examines the cybersecurity challenges facing emerging healthcare systems, focusing on the vulnerabilities inherent in interconnected medical devices, electronic health records, and telehealth platforms. Further, the chapter explores the potential consequences of cyber threats, including data breaches, privacy violations, and disruptions to patient care. In conclusion, the study discusses strategies to mitigate these risks, such as implementing robust encryption protocols, adopting multi-factor authentication, and enhancing employee cybersecurity awareness through comprehensive training.

The book is an ideal reference to practitioners, industry and academic researchers, scientists, and engineers in the fields of cybersecurity, healthcare systems, healthcare technologies, artificial intelligence, smart contracts, blockchain technology, machine learning, federated learning, computing, threat intelligence, internet of medical things, cyberattacks, intrusion detection, complex healthcare data processing, healthcare ethics, medical information systems, security and privacy, and others. Also, the textbook is suitable for graduate and senior undergraduate courses in computer science, cybersecurity, healthcare systems, medical informatics, and related fields.

The editors would like to especially thank the reviewers of the original book proposal for their constructive suggestions. Special thanks to all authors of the chapters for their insightful contributions. Many thanks to the reviewers and editorial assistants at the IET for their cooperation and support.

Agbotiname Lucky Imoize
Gelsenkirchen, North Rhine-Westphalia, Germany

Chandrashekhar Meshram
Betul, Madhya Pradesh, India

Joseph Bamidele Awotunde
Ilorin, Kwara State, Nigeria

Yousef Farhaoui
Errachidia, Morocco

Dinh-Thuan Do
Alliance, Ohio, USA

About the editors

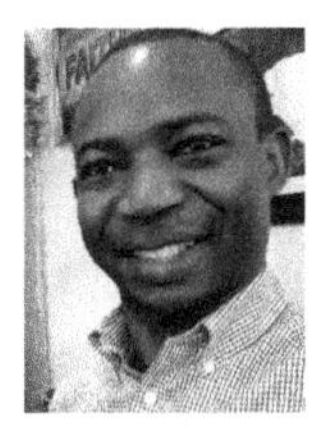

Agbotiname Lucky Imoize (senior member, IEEE) received a B.Eng. degree (Hons.) in Electrical and Electronics Engineering from Ambrose Alli University, Nigeria, in 2008 and an M.Sc. degree in Electrical and Electronics Engineering from the University of Lagos, Nigeria, in 2012. He is a lecturer in the Department of Electrical and Electronics Engineering at the University of Lagos, Nigeria. Before joining the University of Lagos, he was a lecturer at Bells University of Technology, Nigeria. He was, until recently, a research scholar at the Ruhr University Bochum, Germany, under the sponsorship of the Nigerian Petroleum Technology Development Fund (PTDF) and the German Academic Exchange Service (DAAD) through the Nigerian-German Postgraduate Program. He was awarded the Fulbright fellowship as a visiting research scholar at the Wireless@VT Laboratory, Bradley Department of Electrical and Computer Engineering, Virginia Tech., USA, where he worked under the supervision of Prof. R. Michael Buehrer from 2017 to 2018. He worked as a core network products manager at ZTE, Nigeria, and as a Network Switching Subsystem Engineer at Globacom, Nigeria. His research interests cover the fields of 6G wireless, wireless security systems, and artificial intelligence. He has co-edited 10 books and co-authored over 200 papers in peer-reviewed journals and conferences. Imoize is an active reviewer and editor for over 50 international journals and conferences. He is the Vice Chair of the IEEE Communication Society, Nigeria chapter, a Registered Engineer with the Council for the Regulation of Engineering in Nigeria, and a member of the Nigerian Society of Engineers.

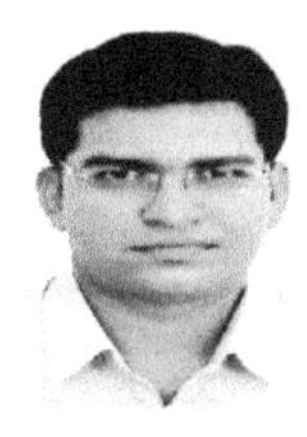

Chandrashekhar Meshram is an assistant professor in the Department of Post Graduate Studies and Research in Mathematics, Jaywanti Haksar Government Post Graduate College, Chhindwara University, Betul, India. His research interests include cryptography and its applications, neural networks, the IoT, wireless sensor networks, medical information systems, ad hoc networks, number theory, fuzzy theory, time series analysis, climate change, mathematical modeling, and chaos theory. He has published over 150 scientific articles in international journals and conferences on these research fields. In addition, he is a regular reviewer for over 60 international journals and conferences. He is a member of IAENG, WASET, CSTA, IACSIT, EAI, ILAS, SCIEI, MIR Labs, and a lifetime member of the Indian Mathematical Society and Cryptology Research Society. He received his Ph.D. degree in Mathematics from R.T.M. Nagpur University, Nagpur, India.

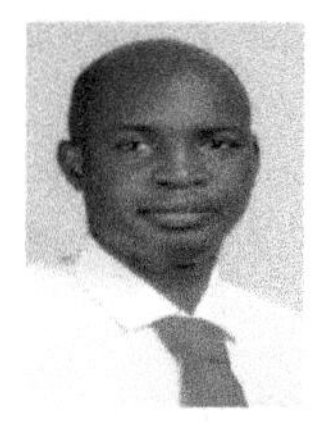

Joseph Bamidele Awotunde received a B.Sc. degree in Mathematics/Computer Science from the Federal University of Technology, Minna, Nigeria, in 2007, M.Sc. and Ph.D. degrees in Computer Science from the University of Ilorin, Ilorin, Nigeria, in 2014 and 2019, respectively. He was formerly a Lecturer with McPherson University, Nigeria. Currently, he is a Lecturer with the Computer Science Department, the University of Ilorin, Nigeria. He has authored or coauthored over 100 articles, 50 book chapters, and over 40 conference proceedings. His research interests include Information Security, Cybersecurity, Bioinformatics, Artificial Intelligence, the Internet of Medical Things, Wireless Body Sensor Networks, Telemedicine, m-Health/e-health, Medical Imaging, Software Engineering, and Biometrics. He is a member of the International Association of Engineers and Computer Scientists (IAENG), the Computer Professional Registration Council of Nigeria (CPN), and the Nigeria Computer Society (NCS).

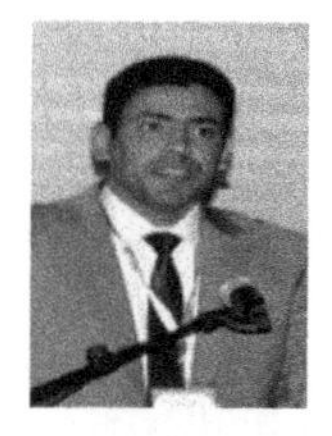

Yousef Farhaoui is a professor at the Faculty of Sciences and Techniques, Moulay Ismail University, Morocco. He is the Chair of IDMS Team, and the Director of STI laboratory. He is also the local publishing and research coordinator, Cambridge International Academics Publishing, United Kingdom. He obtained his Ph.D. in Computer Security from the Ibn Zohr University of Science. His research interests include learning, e-learning, computer security, big data analytics, and business intelligence. He is a coordinator and member of the organizing and scientific committee of several international conferences and a member of various international associations. He has authored seven books and several book chapters with Springer and IGI. He has served as a reviewer for IEEE, IET, Springer, Inderscience, and Elsevier journals. He is the Guest Editor of several journals. He has served as the General Chair, Session Chair, and Panelist in several international conferences. He is a Senior Member of IEEE, IET, ACM, and the EAI.

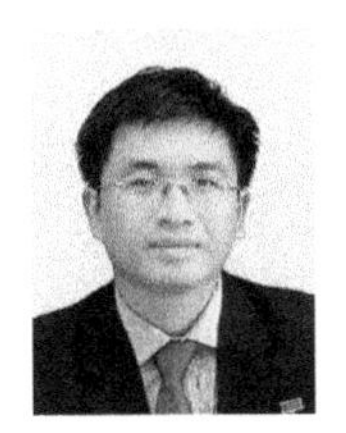

Dinh-Thuan Do is an Assistant Professor in the School of Engineering, University of Mount Union, Alliance, Ohio, USA. He was a Research Scientist at the Electrical Engineering Department, University of Colorado Denver, Denver, USA. Also, he was formerly a Research Scientist in the Department of Electrical and Computer Engineering at the University of Texas at Austin, USA. Prior to joining The University of Texas at Austin, he was an Assistant Professor at Asia University in Taiwan and a Research Assistant Professor at Ton Duc Thang University in Vietnam. His research interests include signal processing in wireless communications networks, non-orthogonal multiple access, full-duplex transmission, and reconfigurable intelligent surfaces (RIS). He received the Golden Globe Award from the Vietnam Ministry of Science and Technology in 2015 (Top ten excellent scientists nationwide). He is currently serving as an Editor of *Computer Communications*, Associate Editor of *EURASIP Journal on Wireless Communications and Networking*, Associate Editor of *Electronics*, Associate Editor of *ICT Express*, and Editor of *KSII Transactions on Internet and Information Systems*. His publications include over 100 SCIE/SCI-indexed journal articles and 40 international conference papers. In addition, he is the author of two textbooks and six book chapters. He holds a Ph.D. degree in communications engineering from the Vietnam National University (VNU-HCMC), Vietnam. He is a senior member of the IEEE.

Chapter 1

An overview of cybersecurity in emerging healthcare systems

Daniel Dauda Wisdom[1] and Olufunke Rebecca Vincent[2]

This chapter comprehensively explores various aspects of cybersecurity in healthcare. The chapter examined the significance of cybersecurity, its historical basis, prevalent threats, regulatory frameworks, and mitigation strategies. By highlighting the critical need for robust cybersecurity measures amidst the ongoing digital transformation in healthcare, the chapter considers relevant literature to identify current cybersecurity issues in emerging healthcare systems, highlighting the importance of digitalization and technology adoption, mostly the shift from paper-based records to electronic health records (EHRs), and emphasizing the necessity of safeguarding healthcare data throughout its lifecycle. Additionally, the chapter examines regulatory compliance challenges and suggests a tailored algorithm for mitigation strategies, while investigating human factors in healthcare cybersecurity. In addition, the chapter also discusses measures to protect patient data and maintain trust in healthcare systems, incorporating case studies of healthcare data breaches. Finally, the chapter considers emerging trends in healthcare cybersecurity providing recommendations for effectively securing modern healthcare systems.

Keywords: Cybersecurity; risks; healthcare; EHR; resilient systems

1.1 Introduction

Healthcare systems around the world are undergoing a profound transformation, driven by rapid technological advancements, shifting demographics, evolving patient expectations, and the need for more efficient and accessible care. This transformation has given rise to what is commonly referred to as emerging healthcare systems [1]. These systems represent a departure from traditional healthcare delivery models and are characterized by their heavy reliance on information technology, data-driven decision-making, and a *patient*-centric approach.

[1]Department of Computer Sciences, Chrisland University, Abeokuta, Ogun State, Nigeria
[2]Department of Computer Science, Federal University of Agriculture, Abeokuta, Ogun State, Nigeria

The emergence of these healthcare systems is propelled by several interconnected factors, each contributing to the growing complexity and vitality of the healthcare landscape [2]. To provide framework for our exploration of cybersecurity concerns and risks within these emerging healthcare systems, this research study will examine the key transporters behind this transformation which are as follows.

Technological Advancements: The integration of cutting-edge technologies into healthcare has redefined the possibilities of diagnosis, treatment, and patient care. Innovations such as telemedicine, wearable health devices, artificial intelligence (AI), and the Internet of Things (IoT) have become integral components of modern healthcare systems [2,3]. These technologies promise improved patient outcomes, cost efficiencies, and real-time health monitoring. Data Proliferation: Healthcare has become increasingly data-centric. Electronic health records (EHRs), genomic data, medical imaging, and patient-generated data are just a few examples of the vast data sources now available to healthcare providers. The ability to collect, analyze, and leverage this data is transforming how medical decisions are made, leading to more personalized and evidence-based care. Patients today are more informed and engaged in their healthcare decisions than ever before [4]. They expect convenient access to their health information, telehealth options, and seamless communication with their care providers. This shift toward patient-centered care is reshaping the healthcare ecosystem.

Governments and regulatory bodies worldwide are responding to the evolving healthcare landscape by enacting new laws and regulations. These include privacy laws like the General Data Protection Regulation (GDPR) and healthcare-specific regulations like the Health Insurance Portability and Accountability Act (HIPAA). Compliance with these regulations is essential for healthcare organizations to protect patient data and avoid costly penalties. The traditional boundaries of healthcare providers are perverting partnerships form between hospitals, clinics, pharmaceutical companies, tech firms, and startups [5,6]. These collaborations are fostering innovation, enabling the development of integrated care models, and expanding the reach of healthcare services. Recent global health crises, such as the COVID-19 pandemic, have accelerated the adoption of telemedicine, remote monitoring, and digital health solutions. These events have underscored the importance of resilient healthcare systems capable of responding to unexpected challenges [7].

As healthcare systems continue to evolve, they offer incredible opportunities for improving patient care, enhancing medical research, and increasing operational efficiency (see Figure 1.1). However, these advancements also bring a host of cybersecurity concerns and risks that must be addressed comprehensively to ensure the safety, privacy, and integrity of patient data and the reliability of healthcare services [8,9]. In the subsequent section, we will delve deeper into the specific cybersecurity challenges faced by emerging healthcare systems. The chapter will examine the threats, vulnerabilities, and best practices necessary to safeguard patient information, maintain the trust of healthcare stakeholders, and ensure the ongoing success of these transformative healthcare models [10,11]. The organization of this chapter is detailed in Section 1.1.2.

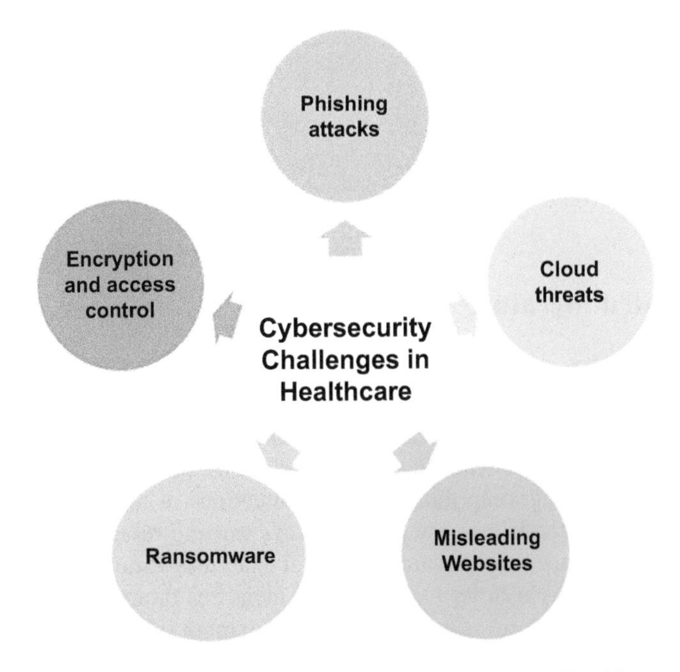

Figure 1.1 Emerging cybersecurity challenges in healthcare

1.1.1 Contributions of the chapter

This chapter offers a thorough exploration of "Cybersecurity in Emerging Healthcare Systems", with the increasing integration of technology in healthcare. By examining various dimensions of cybersecurity threats, from historical context to regulatory frameworks and emerging trends, the chapter provides valuable insights for stakeholders navigating the complex connection between healthcare and cybersecurity. It emphasizes the urgent need for robust cybersecurity measures amidst the ongoing digital revolution in healthcare, highlighting the importance of safeguarding healthcare data throughout its lifecycle. Furthermore, the chapter proposes practical mitigation strategies and discusses measures to protect patient data, addressing regulatory compliance challenges and human factors in healthcare cybersecurity. Considering research, case studies, and recommendations, the chapter equips readers with the knowledge and strategies necessary to effectively secure emerging healthcare systems, ultimately contributing to the integrity and trustworthiness of healthcare infrastructure in the digital age.

1.1.2 Chapter organization

The remaining part of this chapter is organized as follows: Section 1.2 "Related literatures," Section 1.3 "Overview of emerging healthcare systems," Section 1.4

"Importance of digitalization, technology adoption in healthcare," Section 1.5 "Growing role of data in healthcare," Section 1.6 "Transition from paper-based to electronic health records (EHRs)," Section 1.7 "Significance of cybersecurity in healthcare," Section 1.8 "Regulatory frameworks and compliance in healthcare," Section 1.9 "Technological advancements and vulnerabilities in healthcare," Section 1.10 "Data privacy and patient trust in healthcare," and finally Section 1.11 "Conclusions".

1.2 Related literature

The paper [2] presents a survey focusing on security and privacy issues in contemporary healthcare systems, encompassing attacks and defense mechanisms. Its objectives include providing an overview of existing security and privacy research in healthcare, analyzing threats and existing solutions, documenting recent attacks and defenses, and suggesting future research directions. Although it does not specify a particular methodology, the paper surveys existing research on security and privacy issues in modern healthcare systems. It examines various threats, discusses their impacts, reviews security measures, and identifies future research areas. The paper discusses security measures such as cryptographic solutions, communication protocols, and fault-tolerant design techniques. However, it lacks detailed empirical validation or implementation of proposed security measures. It suggests future research focusing on medical-centric cryptographic solutions, standard communication protocols, and fault-tolerant design techniques to enhance healthcare system security.

The study [5] examines the challenges faced by the U.S. healthcare industry in managing cybersecurity risks and proposes a roadmap for a more proactive approach to cybersecurity risk management. Through a review of existing literature and insights into the U.S. healthcare cybersecurity landscape, the study emphasizes the need for senior management involvement and a holistic cybersecurity preparedness strategy. However, it does not provide empirical findings or data analysis but rather outlines challenges and suggests improvement strategies without specific research methods. Future research could validate the proposed roadmap through case studies or surveys and explore the effectiveness of preventive measures in healthcare cybersecurity. Additionally, investigating the impact of regulatory frameworks on cybersecurity practices in the healthcare sector could offer valuable insights.

The study [7] offers a comprehensive examination of ethical issues in cybersecurity, encompassing foundational concepts, problems, and recommendations for professionals. It outlines the background of the European CANVAS project and aims to explain cybersecurity, ethics, and law while addressing problems like ethical hacking and cyber warfare. The objectives include providing recommendations for cybersecurity professionals and discussing ethical questions across sectors like business, health, and law enforcement. Drawing on contributions from experts, the book covers privacy techniques, best practices for service providers, ethical defense strategies, cybersecurity awareness in healthcare, and norms for state behavior in cyberspace. However, it lacks specific research findings or empirical data and does not explore emerging issues like cyber currencies or the role of artificial intelligence in cybersecurity, suggesting these as areas for future research.

The research [9] proposes a comprehensive approach to addressing cybersecurity vulnerabilities in medical devices by acknowledging their operational complexity, identifying technical vulnerabilities, and suggesting systemic solutions. Objectives include understanding the multifaceted nature of these vulnerabilities, identifying contributing factors, and advocating for a proactive, coordinated approach. The methodology involves reviewing factors contributing to vulnerabilities, analyzing their impact on patient safety, and examining governance and regulatory frameworks. The study emphasizes the need for embedding cybersecurity in device design, establishing accountability, and promoting awareness. However, it lacks empirical research or specific technological solutions. Future research could focus on developing algorithms or technological solutions and evaluating their effectiveness in real-world healthcare settings, alongside advocacy efforts to increase awareness.

The research [11] proposes a comprehensive strategy for mitigating cybersecurity risks in healthcare systems, with a specific focus on preventing unauthorized access to patient data. Objectives include identifying best practices, proposing an algorithm for preventing unauthorized access, and developing robust authentication and access control measures. The methodology involves an extensive literature review and the development of a Python-based algorithm. The algorithm incorporates measures such as risk assessments, multi-factor authentication, role-based access control, data encryption, software updates, incident response planning, and regular testing. The paper suggests that implementing these measures can enhance cybersecurity posture and protect patient data in healthcare organizations. However, empirical data or case studies demonstrating effectiveness are lacking, suggesting a need for future research to evaluate the proposed approach in real-world healthcare settings and to monitor and update cybersecurity measures as threats evolve.

The research [12] aims to investigate cybersecurity threats in healthcare organizations, understand stakeholder roles, and offer recommendations for enhancing cybersecurity. Objectives include identifying threats, explaining stakeholder roles, and providing policy and organizational recommendations. The methodology involves literature review, data analysis, and potential expert interviews or surveys. Results include an overview of threats, stakeholder roles, and recommendations. However, specific details about methodology and empirical data are lacking. Future research could focus on empirical studies or ongoing monitoring to assess cybersecurity practices and address emerging threats.

The research [13] proposes an investigation into cybersecurity risks intensified by pandemics, with a specific focus on the impact of the COVID-19 pandemic on healthcare industries. Objectives include understanding increased vulnerability, exploring specific threats faced, and identifying strategies to enhance cybersecurity measures. The methodology involves literature review, case study analysis, and expert insights, potentially supplemented by data collection from healthcare institutions. Results highlight heightened risks and provide examples of cyber threats and impacts. Recommendations for enhancing cybersecurity are discussed, though specific methodology, some details are missing. Future research aims to conduct empirical studies to quantify risks, monitor cybersecurity measures, and explore specific implementation strategies' effectiveness in mitigating cyber risks in healthcare settings.

The paper [14] explores converging and emerging threats to health security, focusing on challenges arising from advances in biological sciences, technology convergence, and cybersecurity risks in healthcare. Objectives include identifying and describing the new risk landscape, highlighting inadequacies in regulatory frameworks, outlining examples of converging threats, and advocating for cross-disciplinary approaches. The methodology involves a literature review, case study analysis, and expert insights. Results emphasize challenges posed by convergence, emphasizing the need for cross-disciplinary and global approaches. The study lacks empirical data and specific mitigation strategies but suggests future research directions, including new risk analysis methods, collaborative efforts, and regulatory adaptation.

The paper [15] addresses the rising cybersecurity threats within the healthcare sector, focusing on challenges posed by Electronic Medical Records (EMR) adoption, Internet of Things (IoT) devices, and the COVID-19 pandemic. It suggests measures to improve cybersecurity, including regulatory measures, software updates, data encryption, and staff training. The paper offers expert analysis and recommendations but lacks empirical research data. It emphasizes the need for regulatory bodies for IoT devices, regular updates, and encryption, without presenting empirical results. Future research could include empirical studies on cybersecurity threats' prevalence and impact, cost analysis of proposed measures, and strategies to overcome implementation barriers.

The research [16] proposes a thorough investigation into security and cybersecurity risk management within e-health systems, with a particular focus on Internet of Medical Things (IoMT) applications. Objectives include reviewing IoMT systems, assessing risk assessment methods for IoMT, and proposing a framework to enhance trust and decision-making in e-healthcare through quantified risk assessment. The methodology entails reviewing IoMT systems, analyzing risk landscapes, evaluating risk management approaches, and designing a risk quantification framework. The proposed framework involves a risk manager and orchestrator module to evaluate risks in IoMT frameworks, addressing vulnerabilities in device zones, network areas, and storage infrastructure. While specific details of the risk assessment approach are not provided, future work suggests incorporating artificial intelligence for system monitoring. This indicates a direction for further research to improve risk management effectiveness in e-health systems.

1.3 Overview of emerging healthcare systems

Emerging healthcare systems represent a shift in the paradigm of healthcare delivery, characterized by innovative approaches, technologies, and strategies aimed at improving the quality, accessibility, and efficiency of healthcare services [17]. These systems are evolving in response to a changing global landscape, which includes factors such as technological advancements, demographic shifts, rising healthcare costs, and increasing patient expectations. The key characteristics of emerging healthcare systems are as follows:

Patient-centric focus: Emerging healthcare systems prioritize the patient as the central figure in healthcare delivery. This patient-centric approach emphasizes personalized care, shared decision-making, and a focus on patient outcomes and satisfaction. Patients are encouraged to actively participate in their healthcare journey, making informed choices and having easier access to their health information [12].

Technology integration: One of the defining features of emerging healthcare systems is the extensive use of technology. EHRs, telemedicine, wearable devices, mobile health applications, and remote monitoring tools are seamlessly integrated into the healthcare workflow. These technologies facilitate real-time data sharing, remote consultations, and the ability to monitor patients' health conditions outside traditional healthcare settings [18].

Data-driven decision-making: Healthcare systems are generating vast amounts of data, and emerging systems leverage this data for informed decision-making. Advanced analytics, machine learning, and AI algorithms are employed to analyze patient data, predict health outcomes, and identify trends. Data-driven insights enhance clinical decision support, research, and population health management [19].

Interconnected care ecosystem: Emerging healthcare systems emphasize collaboration and coordination among various stakeholders within the healthcare ecosystem. This includes healthcare providers, specialists, pharmacists, social workers, and patients themselves. Interconnectedness fosters continuity of care, reduces duplication of services, and ensures that patients receive holistic and comprehensive healthcare [13,19].

Telehealth and remote care: Telehealth and remote care services are integral components of emerging healthcare systems, enabling virtual consultations, remote monitoring of chronic conditions, and timely access to healthcare professionals. These services improve healthcare access, particularly for individuals in remote or underserved areas [20].

Preventive and wellness focus: Rather than solely focusing on treating illnesses, emerging healthcare systems prioritize preventive care and wellness. Health promotion, lifestyle management, and early intervention strategies are encouraged to reduce the burden of chronic diseases and improve overall population health [21].

Regulatory and policy changes: Governments and regulatory bodies are adapting to the changes in healthcare delivery. New laws and regulations address issues such as data privacy, telemedicine licensure, and reimbursement for virtual care. These policies aim to provide a framework that supports the safe and effective operation of emerging healthcare systems [14].

Research and innovation: Emerging healthcare systems often serve as hubs for medical research and innovation. Collaborations between healthcare organizations, research institutions, and technology companies drive the development of novel treatments, therapies, and healthcare delivery methods [22].

Health equity and access: Efforts to ensure health equity and access to care for all segments of the population are central to emerging healthcare systems. These systems strive to reduce disparities in healthcare outcomes by addressing social determinants of health and improving healthcare access in underserved communities. Finally, emerging healthcare systems represent a dynamic shift in healthcare delivery models, characterized by patient-centered care, technology integration, data-driven decision-making, and a focus on prevention and wellness. These systems aim to improve the quality, accessibility, and efficiency of healthcare services while addressing the evolving needs and expectations of patients and healthcare stakeholders. However, alongside these advancements come new challenges, particularly in the realm of cybersecurity, which must be addressed to safeguard patient data and ensure the reliability of these innovative healthcare models [15].

1.4 Importance of digitalization and technology adoption in healthcare

Digitalization and the widespread adoption of technology have ushered in a transformative era in healthcare. This shift is of paramount importance and brings numerous benefits to patients, healthcare providers, and the entire healthcare ecosystem. This section delves into the key reasons highlighting the significance of digitalization and technology adoption in healthcare respectively as follows, namely [23],

1. **Enhanced patient care and outcomes**: Digital health records and data analytics enable healthcare providers to make informed, evidence-based decisions. Patient data is readily available, helping in accurate diagnoses, treatment planning, and the prediction of health trends.

   Wearable devices and telehealth technologies allow continuous monitoring of patients' health, especially those with chronic conditions. This facilitates early intervention, reduces hospital readmissions, and improves overall health outcomes [1,24].
2. **Improved efficiency and streamlined processes:** Digitalization minimizes paperwork, automates administrative tasks, and streamlines billing and insurance processes. This not only saves time but also reduces errors and lowers administrative costs. Electronic communication tools facilitate seamless communication among healthcare providers, improving care coordination and reducing delays in treatment [25].
3. **Enhanced patient experience:** Technology enables remote consultations, offering patients greater flexibility and convenience in accessing healthcare

services. This is especially valuable for individuals in remote areas or those with mobility issues.

Online appointment scheduling: Digital platforms allow patients to schedule appointments, access test results, and communicate with healthcare providers at their convenience, enhancing patient satisfaction [26,27].

4. **Personalized medicine**: Advances in genomics and personalized medicine use a patient's genetic information to tailor treatments and therapies. This approach increases treatment efficacy and reduces adverse effects. Algorithms can predict patient health risks, allowing early interventions and preventive measures to be put in place, ultimately reducing the burden of chronic diseases [28].
5. **Research and innovation**: Digitalization enables the aggregation and analysis of large datasets, accelerating medical research and drug discovery. Researchers can access comprehensive patient records and real-world data for clinical studies. The digital health sector has seen the emergence of innovative startups that develop apps, wearable devices, and telemedicine platforms, fostering a culture of continuous innovation [29].
6. **Healthcare accessibility**: Virtual healthcare visits and consultations transcend geographical barriers, improving access to healthcare services, especially in rural or underserved areas.

   Digitalization facilitates the sharing of patient data across different healthcare organizations and systems, ensuring that patient information is accessible when needed [30].
7. **Cost savings**: Early detection and intervention made possible through technology can reduce the costs associated with treating advanced diseases.

   Streamlined processes and reduced administrative overhead lead to cost savings for healthcare providers [31].
8. **Data security and privacy**: While technology adoption presents security challenges, it also drives advancements in healthcare cybersecurity to protect patient data and maintain trust.

Finally, the importance of digitalization and technology adoption in healthcare cannot be overstated. These advancements have the potential to revolutionize healthcare delivery, enhance patient care, improve outcomes, and drive efficiencies across the healthcare system. However, they also necessitate careful consideration of data privacy and cybersecurity measures to ensure the secure and responsible use of technology in healthcare [31,32].

1.5 Growing role of data in healthcare

The healthcare industry is undergoing a significant transformation, largely driven by the exponential growth and utilization of data. Data has emerged as a powerful tool that is revolutionizing healthcare in numerous ways, fundamentally changing how healthcare is delivered, managed, and improved [33]. This section discusses the growing role of data in healthcare and its far-reaching implications as follows:

1. Data-driven decision-making: Healthcare providers increasingly rely on data-driven clinical decision support systems that provide real-time information, best practice guidelines, and predictive analytics. This assists in making more accurate diagnoses and treatment decisions, ultimately improving patient outcomes [34].
2. Electronic Health Records (EHRs): EHRs centralize patient data, including medical history, test results, treatment plans, and medications. This accessibility ensures that healthcare providers have a complete picture of a patient's health, leading to safer and more coordinated care.

   The ability to share EHR data among different healthcare organizations enhances care continuity and reduces duplication of tests and procedures [35].
3. Telemedicine and remote monitoring: Telehealth technologies enable remote patient monitoring through wearable devices and mobile apps. These devices collect vital health data, allowing healthcare providers to monitor patients' conditions in real time, intervene when necessary, and reduce hospital readmissions [36].
4. Population health management: Data analytics can identify population health trends, helping healthcare organizations allocate resources efficiently and implement targeted interventions to improve the health of specific communities or patient groups.

   Data analytics can identify individuals at higher risk for certain conditions, allowing for proactive outreach and preventive care strategies [37].
5. Precision medicine: Genomic data and molecular profiling enable precision medicine approaches. By analyzing an individual's genetic makeup and biomarkers, healthcare providers can tailor treatment plans and therapies to maximize effectiveness while minimizing side effects [33,38].
6. Drug discovery and development: Pharmaceutical companies use big data analytics to analyze vast datasets, accelerating drug discovery and development processes. This has the potential to bring new treatments to market more quickly and efficiently [39].
7. Healthcare operations and efficiency: Healthcare administrators use data to optimize resource allocation, staffing, and capacity planning, ensuring that healthcare facilities operate efficiently.

   Streamlining administrative processes with data-driven solutions reduces paperwork, billing errors, and administrative overhead [2,40].
8. Research and Clinical Trials: Real-world data from EHRs and patient records can be leveraged in clinical trials and research studies, providing a more comprehensive view of treatment effectiveness and safety.
9. Healthcare Policy and Decision-Making: Policymakers use healthcare data to make informed decisions about healthcare regulations, funding, and public health initiatives [4,41].
10. Predictive Analytics: Predictive analytics can forecast patient health risks, allowing healthcare providers to intervene early, prevent complications, and reduce healthcare costs.

While the growing role of data in healthcare presents numerous opportunities and benefits, it also comes with challenges, such as data security, privacy concerns, and the need for robust data governance. Addressing these challenges is crucial to harness the full potential of data-driven healthcare and ensure that patient information is handled responsibly and securely. Overall, data-driven healthcare has the potential to improve patient care, drive efficiencies, and contribute to advancements in medical research and treatment [2,42].

1.5.1 How healthcare data is collected, stored, and shared

Healthcare data is a critical component of modern healthcare systems, and its effective collection, storage, and sharing are essential for providing quality patient care, conducting medical research, and managing healthcare operations [43]. The process of healthcare data management involves various technologies, standards, and protocols to ensure the integrity, security, and accessibility of this valuable information. This section explores how healthcare data is collected, stored, and shared as follows:

1. Data collection: Healthcare data is primarily generated during patient encounters with healthcare providers. This includes information collected during physical examinations, medical history interviews, diagnostic tests, and treatments.

   EHRs are a central repository for healthcare data. They capture patient information in digital formats, making it easier to record and access data across different healthcare settings.

   Patients increasingly use wearable devices and Internet of Things (IoT) devices that collect health-related data, such as heart rate, activity levels, and sleep patterns. This data can be integrated into EHRs for a more comprehensive view of a patient's health [44].

   Telehealth visits and remote monitoring solutions enable healthcare providers to collect data remotely, including video consultations, vital signs, and patient-reported outcomes.

   Data from laboratory tests, imaging studies (e.g., X-rays, MRIs), and medical devices (e.g., ECG machines) are crucial for diagnosing and monitoring medical conditions.
2. Data storage as EHRs serves as the primary storage system for healthcare data. They are secure, digital repositories that store patient demographics, medical histories, diagnoses, treatment plans, and more [45].

   Health information exchange (HIE): These systems allow the sharing of patient data among different healthcare organizations. They ensure that relevant patient information is available to authorized providers across various care settings while adhering to privacy and security standards.

   Cloud-based storage: Many healthcare organizations opt for cloud-based storage solutions for scalability, accessibility, and disaster recovery. Cloud providers offer secure and compliant healthcare data storage options.

Data warehouses: Data warehouses are used to store large volumes of healthcare data for analysis and research purposes. They consolidate data from various sources and allow for complex queries and reporting [46].

Backup and disaster recovery: Robust backup and disaster recovery systems ensure data integrity and availability, even in the event of system failures or disasters.

3. Data sharing: Healthcare data must adhere to interoperability standards like HL7 (Health Level Seven) and Fast Healthcare Interoperability Resources (FHIR) to facilitate seamless data exchange between different EHR systems and healthcare entities [1,47].

HIE networks enable healthcare providers, laboratories, and other authorized entities to share patient data securely, ensuring that relevant information is available at the point of care.

Patients have the right to access their healthcare data, and many healthcare organizations offer patient portals or secure online platforms for patients to view and download their records.

De-identified or anonymized healthcare data is often shared with researchers and public health organizations to advance medical knowledge, conduct clinical trials, and monitor population health trends.

Data sharing in healthcare must adhere to strict security and privacy regulations, such as HIPAA in the United States and GDPR in Europe, to protect patient confidentiality and data integrity [48].

Patient's informed consent and authorization are essential for sharing their healthcare data. Healthcare organizations must have processes in place to obtain and manage these permissions. Effective data collection, storage, and sharing in healthcare are critical not only for improving patient care but also for advancing medical research, reducing healthcare costs, and supporting public health initiatives. It is essential for healthcare organizations to prioritize data security, privacy, and interoperability to ensure the responsible use of healthcare data for the benefit of patients and society as a whole [49].

1.6 Transition from paper-based to Electronic Health Records (EHRs)

The transition from paper-based medical records to EHRs has been a transformative journey in the healthcare industry. This shift represents a fundamental change in the way healthcare data is collected, stored, and managed [50]. Let us delve into the key aspects and implications of this transition:

1. Efficiency and accessibility: Traditionally, healthcare data was documented on paper, leading to cumbersome and time-consuming record-keeping processes. Accessing patient information required physically locating and retrieving paper records, leading to delays in care [51].

EHRs have revolutionized the efficiency and accessibility of patient data. Healthcare providers can instantly access patient records, view historical data, and make informed decisions at the point of care. This leads to improved patient safety and reduced administrative overhead.

2. Data accuracy and legibility: Illegible handwriting and manual data entry errors were common problems with paper records, potentially resulting in medical errors and compromised patient safety [52].

   EHRs eliminate illegible handwriting issues and minimize data entry errors. Structured data entry and validation checks help ensure data accuracy and completeness.
3. Comprehensive patient profiles: Patient information in paper records is often fragmented across different departments and healthcare facilities, making it challenging to compile a complete patient profile.

   EHRs consolidate patient data from various sources into a single, comprehensive electronic record. This allows healthcare providers to have a holistic view of a patient's medical history, diagnoses, medications, and test results [53].
4. Interoperability and information exchange: Sharing paper records between healthcare organizations or during patient referrals is slow, cumbersome, and prone to errors.

   EHR systems support interoperability standards, enabling the secure and seamless exchange of patient data between different healthcare entities, and enhancing care coordination and continuity.
5. Remote access and telemedicine: Paper records cannot support remote access or telemedicine, limiting healthcare delivery options.

   EHRs facilitate remote access to patient data, making telemedicine and virtual consultations feasible. This is especially valuable in rural or underserved areas [54].
6. Data security and privacy: Physical paper records are vulnerable to theft, loss, and unauthorized access. Protecting patient privacy is challenging with paper records.

   EHRs employ robust security measures, including user authentication, encryption, and audit trails, to protect patient data. Strict access controls and compliance with data privacy regulations, such as HIPAA, ensure patient confidentiality [55].
7. Research and analytics: Analyzing and extracting insights from paper records is labor-intensive and limited in scope.

   EHRs enable data analytics, allowing healthcare organizations to conduct research, track healthcare trends, and improve clinical outcomes by leveraging vast datasets.
8. Environmental impact: The extensive use of paper records contributes to deforestation and environmental harm [56].

Transitioning to EHRs aligns with sustainability goals, as it reduces paper usage and minimizes the environmental footprint of healthcare operations.

While the transition to EHRs offers numerous benefits, it is not without challenges. These include initial implementation costs, staff training, interoperability issues, and concerns about data security and privacy. However, the overall shift toward EHRs represents a significant step forward in improving patient care, healthcare efficiency, and data management in the modern healthcare landscape [57].

1.7 Significance of cybersecurity in healthcare

Cybersecurity in healthcare is of paramount importance due to the sensitive nature of patient data and the potential consequences of unauthorized access or breaches. As the healthcare industry increasingly adopts digital technologies to improve patient care and streamline operations, the need for robust cybersecurity measures becomes even more critical [58]. Some key aspects highlighting the significance of cybersecurity in healthcare are as follows:

1. Protection of patient data: Healthcare organizations store vast amounts of sensitive patient information, including personal details, medical history, and financial data. Cybersecurity measures are essential to safeguard this information and protect patient privacy.
2. Compliance with regulations: Various regulations, such as the Health Insurance Portability and Accountability Act (HIPAA) in the United States, mandate strict security standards for protecting patient information. Compliance with these regulations is not only a legal requirement but also crucial for maintaining the trust of patients [59].
3. Prevention of data breaches: Data breaches in healthcare can have severe consequences, including identity theft, fraud, and unauthorized access to medical records. Cybersecurity measures help prevent and mitigate the impact of data breaches by implementing encryption, access controls, and monitoring systems.
4. Maintaining trust and reputation: Patients trust healthcare providers with their most personal information. A data breach can erode this trust and damage the reputation of the healthcare organization. Demonstrating a commitment to cybersecurity is vital for maintaining the confidence of patients and stakeholders.
5. Ensuring continuity of care: Cyberattacks, such as ransomware, can disrupt healthcare operations, affecting patient care and safety. Robust cybersecurity measures help ensure the continuity of care by preventing disruptions and maintaining access to critical healthcare systems [60].
6. Integration of emerging technologies: The healthcare industry is increasingly adopting emerging technologies like telemedicine, Internet of Things (IoT) devices, and EHRs. These technologies offer numerous benefits but also introduce new vulnerabilities, making cybersecurity crucial for their safe and effective implementation [61].

1.7.1 Historical examples

1. Anthem (2015): Anthem, one of the largest health insurance companies in the United States, suffered a massive data breach in 2015, exposing personal information of nearly 78.8 million individuals. The breach included names,

social security numbers, and medical IDs. Anthem agreed to pay a settlement of $16 million as a result of the incident [1,61].

2. Equifax breach (2017): While not specific to healthcare, the Equifax breach highlighted the broader issue of cybersecurity vulnerabilities. The breach exposed sensitive information, including social security numbers, of millions of individuals. Given the interconnected nature of data, breaches in other sectors can indirectly impact healthcare.
3. WannaCry ransomware attack (2017): The WannaCry ransomware attack affected numerous organizations worldwide, including healthcare institutions. The attack disrupted hospital operations, leading to canceled appointments and delayed treatments. This incident underscored the vulnerability of healthcare systems to cyber threats. These historical examples emphasize the real and immediate consequences of inadequate cybersecurity measures in the healthcare sector. As technology continues to evolve, healthcare organizations must prioritize cybersecurity to protect patient data, maintain trust, and ensure the integrity of healthcare services [3,62].

1.7.2 Common cybersecurity threats in healthcare

An overview of common cybersecurity threats in healthcare is as follows (Figure 1.2):

1. Ransomware attacks: Ransomware is a type of malware that encrypts files or systems, rendering them inaccessible until a ransom is paid. Healthcare organizations are often targeted due to the critical nature of patient data, and the attackers may threaten to publish or permanently delete the data unless the ransom is paid [63].
2. Phishing attacks: Phishing involves fraudulent attempts to obtain sensitive information, such as usernames, passwords, and financial details, by posing as a trustworthy entity. In healthcare, phishing attacks can target employees to gain access to confidential patient information or compromise the integrity of systems [64].

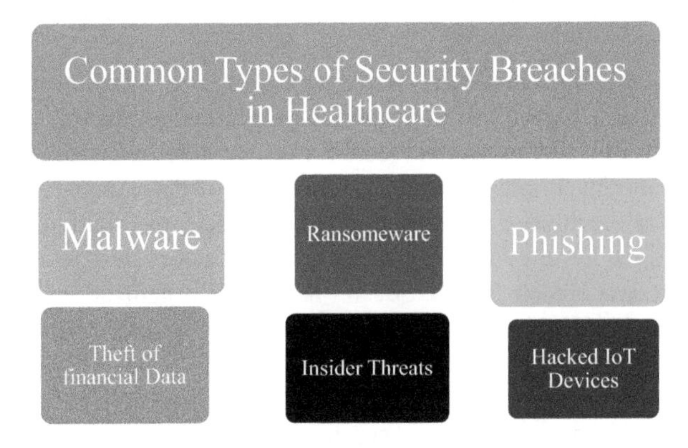

Figure 1.2 Common cybersecurity threats in healthcare

3. Insider threats: Insider threats arise when individuals within an organization intentionally or unintentionally compromise security. This can include employees, contractors, or other trusted entities who misuse their access to sensitive information. Insider threats may involve data theft, sabotage, or accidental disclosure of confidential data.
4. Malware and viruses: Malicious software (malware) and viruses can infect healthcare systems, compromising the confidentiality and integrity of patient data. Malware can be introduced through malicious downloads, email attachments, or compromised external devices [65].
5. Denial-of-service (DoS) attacks: DoS attacks aim to overwhelm a healthcare organization's network or system, causing a disruption in services. This can lead to delayed or denied access to critical patient information, impacting the delivery of healthcare services.
6. Internet of Things (IoT) vulnerabilities: The increasing use of IoT devices in healthcare, such as medical devices and wearables, introduces new cybersecurity challenges [14]. These devices may have vulnerabilities that, if exploited, could compromise patient data or disrupt healthcare operations.

1.7.3 Examples of recent cybersecurity incidents in healthcare

1. Universal Health Services (UHS) ransomware attack (2020): UHS, a large healthcare system in the United States, experienced a ransomware attack that affected its systems nationwide. The attack disrupted hospital operations, leading to the temporary shutdown of IT systems. Patient care was impacted, and the incident highlighted the vulnerability of healthcare institutions to ransomware threats [66].
2. Magellan Health phishing incident (2020): Magellan Health, a healthcare company specializing in managing behavioral health services, fell victim to a phishing attack. The incident exposed sensitive information, including personal and health details, of employees and plan members. Phishing remains a prevalent threat targeting healthcare organizations and their employees.
3. Blackbaud data breach (2020): While not exclusively a healthcare incident, the Blackbaud data breach had implications for healthcare institutions. Blackbaud, a provider of fundraising and donor management software, experienced a ransomware attack that led to the compromise of data, including donor information for healthcare organizations. This incident highlighted the interconnected nature of cybersecurity risks across sectors [67].
4. Accellion data breach (2021): Several healthcare organizations were impacted by a data breach involving the Accellion file transfer service. Attackers exploited vulnerabilities in the software, leading to unauthorized access and exposure of sensitive data. This incident underscored the importance of securing third-party services and applications used in the healthcare ecosystem. These examples demonstrate the ongoing and evolving nature of cybersecurity

threats in the healthcare sector. As technology continues to advance, healthcare organizations must remain vigilant in implementing robust cybersecurity measures to protect patient data and ensure the uninterrupted delivery of healthcare services [68].

1.8 Regulatory frameworks and compliance in healthcare

1. Health Insurance Portability and Accountability Act (HIPAA): HIPAA, enacted in the United States, sets standards for the protection of sensitive patient information, known as Protected Health Information (PHI). The Privacy Rule regulates the use and disclosure of PHI, while the Security Rule establishes safeguards for the protection of electronic PHI (ePHI). HIPAA compliance is crucial for healthcare organizations to ensure the confidentiality, integrity, and availability of patient information [16,24].
2. General Data Protection Regulation (GDPR): GDPR is a comprehensive data protection regulation applicable to European Union (EU) member states. Although not specific to healthcare, it has implications for organizations that process personal data, including health-related information. GDPR emphasizes the principles of data minimization, purpose limitation, and the need for explicit consent. Healthcare organizations dealing with EU residents' data must ensure GDPR compliance to protect individuals' privacy rights [40,61].

1.8.1 Compliance challenges

1. Complexity and evolving nature of regulations: HIPAA and GDPR are complex regulations with specific requirements that healthcare organizations must navigate. The evolving nature of technology and healthcare practices poses challenges in maintaining compliance with these regulations, as organizations need to adapt their security measures accordingly [55].
2. Third-party vendor management: Healthcare organizations often engage third-party vendors for various services, such as cloud storage, data analytics, or software solutions. Ensuring that these vendors comply with regulations and adequately protect patient data introduces challenges in terms of oversight, contractual agreements, and risk management.
3. Interoperability and data sharing: The healthcare industry is moving towards greater interoperability to improve patient care. However, sharing patient data across different systems and entities raises challenges in maintaining compliance with privacy and security regulations. Healthcare organizations must find a balance between data sharing for clinical purposes and protecting patient privacy.
4. Cybersecurity threats: The increasing sophistication of cyber threats, such as ransomware and phishing attacks, poses a constant challenge to healthcare cybersecurity. Organizations must continuously update their security measures

to stay ahead of evolving threats and ensure compliance with regulations that mandate robust security practices [15].

1.8.2 Consequences of lack of compliance for healthcare organizations

1. Legal and financial penalties: Non-compliance with regulations like HIPAA and GDPR can result in significant legal and financial consequences. Fines and penalties may be imposed for breaches, and the costs associated with legal actions, investigations, and potential settlements can be substantial [3].
2. Reputation damage: Data breaches and non-compliance incidents can severely damage the reputation of healthcare organizations. Loss of trust from patients, partners, and the public may lead to a decline in patient engagement, partnerships, and overall business success.
3. Operational disruptions: Investigations and remediation efforts following a compliance breach can lead to operational disruptions. Healthcare organizations may face temporary shutdowns, interruptions in patient care, and financial losses during the recovery period [7].
4. Loss of business opportunities: Non-compliance with data protection regulations may hinder collaboration with other organizations, especially in an era where data sharing is crucial for research and healthcare advancements. Loss of compliance may limit a healthcare organization's participation in collaborative initiatives and partnerships. To navigate these challenges and mitigate risks, healthcare organizations need to establish comprehensive compliance programs. This includes conducting regular risk assessments, implementing robust security measures, providing ongoing staff training, and staying abreast of changes in regulatory requirements. By prioritizing compliance, healthcare organizations can protect patient data, maintain trust, and avoid the detrimental consequences associated with non-compliance [9].

1.9 Technological advancements and vulnerabilities in healthcare

1. Telemedicine: Telemedicine involves the use of technology to deliver healthcare services remotely. It includes video consultations, remote monitoring, and digital communication between healthcare providers and patients. Telemedicine has gained significant traction, providing increased accessibility to healthcare services, especially in remote or underserved areas [1].
2. Internet of Things (IoT) devices: IoT devices in healthcare include wearables, smart medical devices, and sensors that collect and transmit data. These devices play a crucial role in remote patient monitoring, real-time health data collection, and improving overall patient outcomes. IoT technology enables healthcare professionals to gather data for diagnosis, treatment, and preventive care [10,11].

1.9.1 Potential cybersecurity vulnerabilities

The technological advancements and vulnerabilities in healthcare are presented in Figure 1.3:

1. Data privacy concerns: Telemedicine platforms handle sensitive patient information during virtual consultations. The transmission and storage of this data raise concerns about data privacy. Unauthorized access to telemedicine sessions or the interception of patient data during transmission can compromise patient confidentiality [17].
2. Insecure communication channels: The use of insecure communication channels in telemedicine, such as unencrypted video conferencing tools, may expose patient data to interception by malicious actors. Ensuring end-to-end encryption and secure communication protocols is essential to protect the integrity and confidentiality of patient information.
3. Device security in IoT: Many IoT devices in healthcare, such as medical wearables and connected medical devices, may have security vulnerabilities. Inadequate security measures can make these devices susceptible to hacking, potentially leading to unauthorized access to patient data or manipulation of device functionality [12].
4. Lack of standardization: The lack of standardized security protocols across telemedicine platforms and IoT devices can create vulnerabilities. Inconsistencies in security measures may result in gaps that attackers can exploit. Standardization and adherence to security best practices are crucial for minimizing vulnerabilities [18].

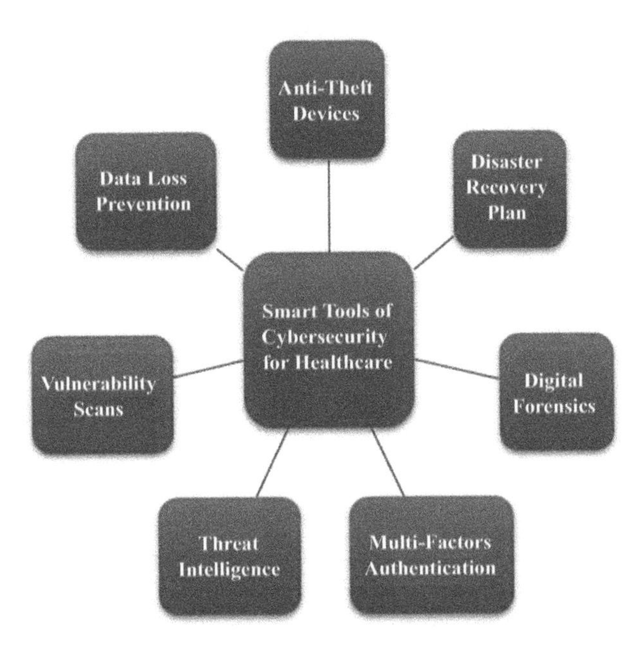

Figure 1.3 Technological advancements and vulnerabilities in healthcare

5. Integration challenges: Integrating new technologies into existing healthcare systems can introduce vulnerabilities if not done securely. Incompatibility between systems, improper configuration, and gaps in the integration process may create opportunities for cyber threats.
6. Authentication and authorization issues: Ensuring proper authentication and authorization mechanisms is crucial in both telemedicine and IoT environments. Weak or compromised credentials can lead to unauthorized access to healthcare systems, patient data, or control of connected devices.
7. Ransomware threats: Telemedicine platforms and IoT devices are potential targets for ransomware attacks. The disruption of telemedicine services or control over connected medical devices through ransomware can have severe consequences for patient care and safety [65].
8. Regulatory compliance challenges: Meeting regulatory requirements for cybersecurity, such as those outlined in HIPAA or GDPR, can be challenging when implementing new technologies. Failure to address compliance issues can result in legal consequences and compromise patient data security [1,3].

1.9.2 Mitigation strategies

1. Encryption and secure communication protocols: Implementing end-to-end encryption and secure communication protocols ensures the confidentiality of patient data during telemedicine sessions and data transmission [9].
2. Regular security audits and assessments: Conducting regular security audits and assessments of telemedicine platforms and IoT devices helps identify vulnerabilities and ensures that security measures are up-to-date.
3. Standardization of security protocols: Industry-wide efforts to standardize security protocols for telemedicine and IoT devices can contribute to a more secure healthcare ecosystem. Adhering to recognized standards helps establish a baseline for cybersecurity measures [17].
4. User education and training: Educating healthcare professionals, patients, and users about cybersecurity best practices is essential. This includes guidance on secure usage of telemedicine platforms and awareness of potential risks associated with IoT devices.
5. Multi-factor authentication: Implementing multi-factor authentication adds an extra layer of security by requiring users to provide multiple forms of identification, reducing the risk of unauthorized access [12].
6. Collaboration with cybersecurity experts: Healthcare organizations should collaborate with cybersecurity experts to assess and enhance the security posture of their telemedicine platforms and IoT devices. Regular consultation with experts helps identify and address emerging threats.

As healthcare continues to embrace technological advancements, it is crucial to prioritize cybersecurity to ensure the integrity, confidentiality, and availability of patient data. A proactive and comprehensive approach to cybersecurity is essential in mitigating potential vulnerabilities associated with emerging healthcare technologies [18].

1.9.3 Human factors in healthcare cybersecurity

Human factors play a significant role in healthcare cybersecurity, as the actions and behaviors of healthcare staff can either contribute to or mitigate cybersecurity risks. Understanding the human element is crucial for developing effective strategies to safeguard sensitive patient data [19]. Sources of cyberthreats in healthcare are given in Figure 1.4. Some key aspects to consider are as follows:

1. Role of healthcare staff in cybersecurity risks such as **phishing and social engineering**: Healthcare staff can be targets of phishing attacks, where malicious actors use deceptive emails or messages to trick individuals into divulging sensitive information or clicking on malicious links. Social engineering tactics exploit human psychology to manipulate individuals into taking actions that compromise security.

   Weak passwords and authentication practices: Poor password management, such as using weak passwords or sharing credentials, can lead to unauthorized access. Healthcare staff may inadvertently compromise security by not adhering to strong password policies or failing to implement multi-factor authentication [13].

   Insider threats: Human factors contribute to insider threats, where employees intentionally or unintentionally compromise security. This can include individuals mishandling patient data, accessing information beyond their roles, or falling victim to external coercion.

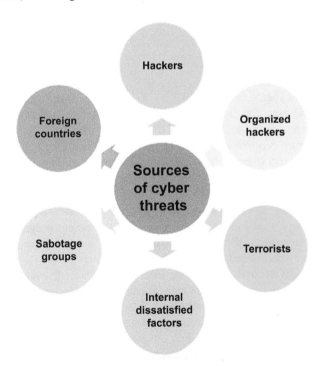

Figure 1.4 Sources of cyberthreats in healthcare

Lack of security awareness: Limited awareness of cybersecurity best practices and potential threats can make healthcare staff more susceptible to cyberattacks. This lack of awareness may result in unintentional actions that expose vulnerabilities [20].

Device and data handling practices: Healthcare professionals may use personal devices for work, share information insecurely, or fail to follow protocols for secure data handling. Such practices can expose patient data to unauthorized access.

2. Training and awareness programs to mitigate human-related risks: Healthcare organizations should implement regular and comprehensive cybersecurity training programs for all staff members. Training should cover topics such as recognizing phishing attempts, creating strong passwords, and understanding the importance of secure data handling [21].

Simulated phishing exercises: Conducting simulated phishing exercises helps healthcare staff recognize and respond to phishing attempts in a controlled environment. These exercises can provide valuable insights into areas that require additional training and reinforcement.

Role-based training: Tailoring training programs based on job roles helps address specific cybersecurity concerns relevant to each staff member's responsibilities. For example, administrative staff may focus on data entry security, while clinicians may prioritize patient data protection during telemedicine sessions [14].

Regular updates on emerging threats: Cyber threats evolve, and healthcare staff need to stay informed about the latest trends and tactics used by cybercriminals. Regular updates on emerging threats and cybersecurity trends can empower staff to recognize and respond to new risks effectively.

Clear policies and guidelines: Healthcare organizations should establish clear and accessible cybersecurity policies and guidelines. These documents should outline expectations for secure behavior, data handling procedures, and consequences for non-compliance [22].

Encouraging reporting of security incidents: Creating a culture where staff feel comfortable reporting potential security incidents, such as phishing attempts or suspicious activities, is crucial. Prompt reporting allows organizations to respond swiftly and mitigate potential risks.

Incorporating cybersecurity into professional development: Integrate cybersecurity topics into ongoing professional development programs for healthcare staff. This ensures that cybersecurity remains a priority as staff members advance in their careers and take on new responsibilities [15].

User-friendly security measures: Implementing user-friendly security measures, such as secure but convenient authentication methods, reduces the likelihood of staff circumventing security protocols due to inconvenience. By addressing human factors through targeted training, awareness programs, and ongoing education, healthcare organizations can strengthen their cybersecurity posture. Combining technical safeguards with a human-centric approach creates a more resilient defense against cyber threats in the healthcare sector [23,31].

1.9.4 Incident response and cybersecurity resilience in healthcare

Incident response in healthcare involves the coordinated effort to detect, respond to, and recover from cybersecurity incidents. A robust incident response plan is crucial for minimizing the impact of security breaches [16]. Here are key strategies for responding to cybersecurity incidents in healthcare:

1. **Preparation:** Develop and regularly update an incident response plan that outlines roles, responsibilities, and procedures for responding to cybersecurity incidents. Ensure that the plan is tailored to the specific needs of the healthcare organization. Conduct regular training and simulations to familiarize staff with the incident response plan. This helps ensure a prompt and effective response in the event of an actual incident [24].
2. **Detection and analysis:** Implement monitoring systems and intrusion detection tools to promptly identify unusual or suspicious activities. Continuous monitoring helps detect potential incidents early in their life-cycle. Establish a Security Information and Event Management (SIEM) system to aggregate and analyze security logs, enabling rapid detection, and analysis of potential threats.
3. **Containment and eradication:** Upon detecting a cybersecurity incident, initiate containment measures to prevent the further spread of the threat. This may involve isolating affected systems or restricting access to compromised areas. Work to eradicate the root cause of the incident. This may include removing malware, closing vulnerabilities, or patching systems to prevent a similar incident from occurring in the future [6,7].
4. **Communication:** Establish clear communication channels both internally and externally. Ensure that key stakeholders, including senior management, legal, and regulatory bodies, are informed promptly and regularly throughout the incident response process. Prepare templates for communication messages that can be quickly customized based on the nature and severity of the incident.
5. **Investigation:** Conduct a thorough investigation to understand the scope, impact, and methods used in the incident. This includes forensic analysis to gather evidence and identify the extent of data compromise. Collaborate with law enforcement, if necessary, and maintain a chain of custody for evidence collected during the investigation [22].
6. **Recovery:** Develop a recovery plan to restore affected systems and services to normal operation. Prioritize critical systems and services to minimize disruptions in patient care. Implement lessons learned from the incident to strengthen cybersecurity measures and prevent similar incidents in the future.
7. **Post-incident review:** Conduct a comprehensive post-incident review to evaluate the effectiveness of the incident response process. Identify areas for improvement, update the incident response plan, and incorporate lessons learned into future training programs [25].

1.9.5 Cybersecurity resilience in healthcare

Building cybersecurity resilience in healthcare involves adopting a proactive and adaptive approach to mitigate the impact of cyberattacks and ensure the continuity of healthcare operations [36]. Some strategies to enhance cybersecurity resilience are as follows:

1. **Risk assessment and management:** Conduct regular risk assessments to identify vulnerabilities and prioritize cybersecurity efforts. Develop a risk management strategy that aligns with the organization's goals and regulatory requirements.
2. **Backup and recovery planning:** Implement regular data backups and ensure the availability of backup systems. This enables the rapid restoration of critical data and services in the event of a cyber incident, such as a ransomware attack [27].
3. **Continuous monitoring:** Establish continuous monitoring systems to detect and respond to cybersecurity threats in real-time. Use automated tools to identify anomalies and potential security incidents promptly.
4. **Adaptive security measures:** Implement adaptive security measures that can evolve to address emerging threats. Stay informed about the latest cybersecurity trends and update security controls accordingly [28].
5. **Collaboration and information sharing:** Foster collaboration within the healthcare industry to share threat intelligence and best practices. Participate in information-sharing platforms and collaborate with other organizations to enhance collective cybersecurity defenses.
6. **Third-party risk management:** Assess and manage the cybersecurity risks associated with third-party vendors and partners. Ensure that external entities handling sensitive patient data adhere to robust cybersecurity practices [29].
7. **Employee training and awareness:** Provide ongoing training and awareness programs for healthcare staff to enhance their cybersecurity knowledge and promote a security-conscious culture. Informed and vigilant employees are key to preventing and mitigating cyber threats.
8. **Regulatory compliance:** Stay current with regulatory requirements, such as HIPAA, and ensure ongoing compliance. Adherence to regulatory standards helps maintain a baseline level of cybersecurity resilience and avoids potential legal consequences [30].
9. **Incident response exercises:** Conduct regular incident response exercises to test the organization's readiness and resilience. Simulate different types of cyber incidents to evaluate the effectiveness of response processes and identify areas for improvement.
10. **Cybersecurity insurance:** Consider cybersecurity insurance as part of the overall risk management strategy. Cybersecurity insurance can provide financial protection and resources to support recovery efforts in the aftermath of a cyber incident [31,46].

By combining effective incident response strategies with proactive measures to enhance cybersecurity resilience, healthcare organizations can significantly reduce the impact of cyber threats and ensure the continuous delivery of critical healthcare services. Regular evaluation and adaptation of cybersecurity practices are essential in an ever-evolving threat landscape [29].

1.10 Data privacy and patient trust in healthcare

Patient trust is fundamental to the success of healthcare systems. When individuals seek medical care, they entrust healthcare providers with sensitive personal information, including medical history and other private details. Trust is crucial for open communication between patients and healthcare professionals, leading to better health outcomes. Maintaining patient trust is directly tied to respecting and protecting the privacy of their data [34].

1.10.1 Measures to protect patient data and maintain trust

Essential measures are taken in order to protect patient data and trust, which are as follows:

1. **Compliance with data protection regulations**: Adherence to data protection regulations, such as HIPAA in the United States or GDPR in the European Union, is essential. These regulations mandate strict standards for the protection and privacy of patient data. Compliance demonstrates a commitment to safeguarding patient information and can enhance trust [28].
2. **Transparent communication:** Transparent communication about how patient data is collected, stored, and used is vital for building and maintaining trust. Healthcare organizations should provide clear and easily understandable privacy policies to inform patients about data practices [41].
3. **Consent mechanisms:** Implement robust consent mechanisms that allow patients to understand and control how their data is used. Clearly explain the purposes for which data will be used and obtain explicit consent before collecting and sharing patient information.
4. **Secure data storage and transmission:** Utilize secure and encrypted systems for storing and transmitting patient data. This includes implementing encryption for EHRs, securing communication channels, and regularly updating security protocols to address emerging threats.
5. **Access controls and authentication:** Implement access controls and strong authentication mechanisms to ensure that only authorized personnel have access to patient data. Role-based access should be enforced to restrict access to sensitive information based on job responsibilities [42].
6. **Data minimization:** Practice data minimization by collecting only the necessary information required for patient care. Avoid unnecessary data retention, and periodically review and delete outdated or irrelevant patient information to reduce the risk of unauthorized access.
7. **Employee training and awareness:** Provide comprehensive training to healthcare staff on the importance of patient privacy and data protection.

Employees should be aware of security best practices, recognize potential threats, and understand their role in maintaining patient trust [66].

8. **Incident response and breach notification:** Establish a robust incident response plan to promptly address and mitigate data breaches. In the event of a breach, promptly notify affected individuals and regulatory authorities in accordance with legal requirements. Transparent communication during a data breach is crucial for maintaining trust.
9. **Regular security audits and assessments:** Conduct regular security audits and assessments to identify vulnerabilities and weaknesses in data protection measures. Periodic assessments help ensure that security controls remain effective against evolving threats.
10. **Patient education:** Educate patients about the steps taken to protect their data and empower them to actively participate in their data privacy. Providing information on how patients can securely access their health information and control data sharing settings fosters transparency and trust [67].
11. **Ethical data use practices:** Establish and adhere to ethical data use practices. This includes using patient data for legitimate and necessary purposes, avoiding discriminatory practices, and ensuring that data is not exploited for unauthorized commercial gain.
12. **Continuous improvement:** Embrace a culture of continuous improvement in data privacy practices. Regularly review and update policies, procedures, and technologies to address emerging threats and adhere to evolving best practices.

By prioritizing data privacy and implementing robust measures to protect patient information, healthcare organizations can build and maintain patient trust. A trustful relationship between healthcare providers and patients is not only critical for individual care but also contributes to the overall success and effectiveness of healthcare systems [26,68].

1.10.2 Case studies of healthcare data breaches

Case study 1: Anthem Incorporated data breach (2015): Anthem Incorporated, one of the largest health insurance companies in the United States, suffered a massive data breach in 2015. Approximately 78.8 million individuals were affected, and the breach exposed sensitive information, including names, dates of birth, Social Security numbers, and medical IDs [51].

Impact: The breach had severe consequences for affected individuals, including the increased risk of identity theft and fraud. Anthem agreed to pay a settlement of $16 million as a result of the breach.

Lessons learned and best practices: Encryption: Implement robust encryption for sensitive data to protect it from unauthorized access, even if a breach occurs. Regular security audits: Conduct regular security audits and assessments to identify vulnerabilities and weaknesses in the security infrastructure. Incident response plan: Have a well-defined incident response plan in place to facilitate a swift and coordinated response to data breaches [52].

Case study 2: Equifax data breach (2017): While not specific to healthcare, the Equifax data breach had implications for individuals in various sectors, including healthcare. The breach exposed personal information, including Social Security numbers, of approximately 147 million people.

Impact: The compromise of sensitive personal information had widespread consequences, leading to increased risks of identity theft and financial fraud [53].

Lessons learned and best practices: Third-party risk management: Assess and manage the cybersecurity risks associated with third-party vendors, emphasizing the need for secure data handling practices. Regular software patching: Keep software and systems up-to-date with the latest security patches to address known vulnerabilities. Data minimization: Practice data minimization by collecting only the necessary information and regularly reviewing and deleting outdated or irrelevant data [54].

Case study 3: WannaCry ransomware attack (2017): The WannaCry ransomware attack affected numerous organizations worldwide, including healthcare institutions. The attack exploited vulnerabilities in outdated versions of Microsoft Windows operating systems.

Impact: The attack disrupted hospital operations, leading to canceled appointments and delayed treatments. The incident underscored the vulnerability of healthcare systems to ransomware threats [55].

Lessons learned and best practices: Timely software updates: Ensure timely software updates and patch management to address known vulnerabilities and protect against ransomware attacks. Regular training: Conduct regular cybersecurity training for staff to raise awareness about the risks of phishing and other social engineering tactics. Backup and recovery planning: Implement regular data backups and recovery planning to minimize the impact of ransomware attacks and facilitate the restoration of critical systems [56].

Case study 4: Accellion data breach (2021): Several healthcare organizations were impacted by a data breach involving the Accellion file transfer service. Attackers exploited vulnerabilities in the software, leading to unauthorized access and exposure of sensitive data [57].

Impact: The breach highlighted the challenges of securing third-party services and applications in the healthcare ecosystem.

Lessons learned and best practices: Third-party vendor security: Conduct thorough security assessments of third-party vendors and ensure they adhere to robust cybersecurity practices. Incident response planning: Have a well-documented incident response plan that includes procedures for handling breaches involving third-party services. Continuous monitoring: Implement continuous monitoring systems to detect and respond to cybersecurity threats in real-time. These case studies emphasize the complexity and evolving nature of cybersecurity challenges in the healthcare sector. Lessons learned from these incidents include the importance of encryption, regular security audits, incident response planning, third-party risk management, timely software updates, and continuous monitoring. Healthcare organizations can enhance their cybersecurity posture by adopting these best practices and staying vigilant in the face of evolving cyber threats [2,25].

1.10.3 Emerging trends in healthcare cybersecurity

The trends in healthcare cybersecurity is given in Figure 1.5. These are described briefly as follows:

1. AI-powered threat detection: Artificial Intelligence (AI) is being increasingly utilized in healthcare cybersecurity for advanced threat detection and response. Machine learning algorithms can analyze patterns, detect anomalies, and identify potential security threats in real-time. **Early detection:** AI algorithms can detect subtle signs of cyber threats before they escalate, allowing for early intervention. **Automation:** AI enables automated threat response, reducing the time between detection and mitigation. **Adaptive defense:** Machine learning models can adapt to evolving cyber threats, providing a dynamic defense mechanism [1,4].

   Challenges: Cybercriminals may also leverage AI to create more sophisticated attacks. **Data privacy concerns:** The use of AI often involves analyzing large datasets, raising concerns about patient data privacy.
2. Blockchain for data security: Blockchain, a decentralized and tamper-proof ledger, is gaining attention for its potential in enhancing data security and integrity in healthcare. **Immutable records:** Once data is added to the blockchain, it becomes nearly impossible to alter, ensuring data integrity. **Decentralization:** The distributed nature of blockchain reduces the risk of a single point of failure, enhancing resilience against cyber-attacks. **Secure data sharing:** Blockchain can facilitate secure and transparent sharing of healthcare data among authorized parties [3,7].

   Challenges: Blockchain networks may face challenges in handling the scale of healthcare data transactions. **Interoperability:** Achieving interoperability

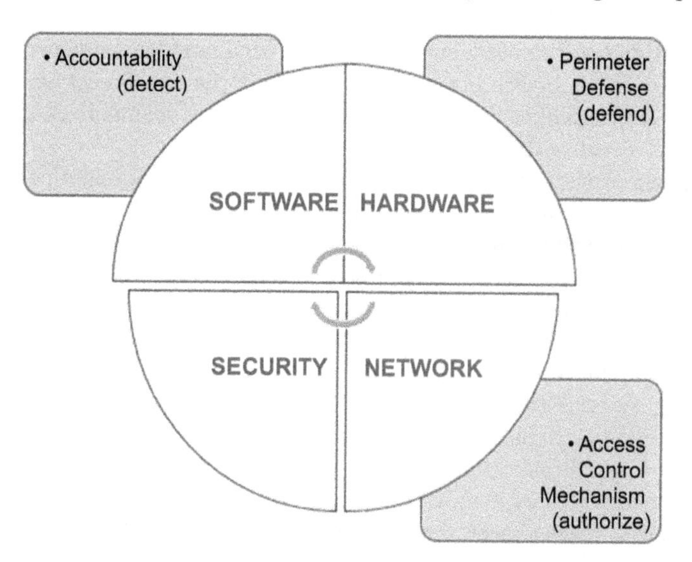

Figure 1.5 Trends in healthcare cybersecurity

with existing healthcare systems and standards can be complex. **Regulatory uncertainties:** Regulatory frameworks for blockchain in healthcare are still evolving.

3. Zero Trust security model: The Zero Trust model assumes that no user or system, whether inside or outside the network, should be trusted by default. Verification is required from everyone trying to access resources.

   Benefits: By requiring authentication at every step, the attack surface is minimized, making it harder for malicious actors to move laterally within the network. **Continuous monitoring:** Continuous monitoring of user and device behavior helps identify abnormal activities. **Adaptive security:** The model adapts to changes in the network and user behavior, providing dynamic security [12,26].

   Challenges: Implementing a Zero Trust model can be complex, requiring careful planning and integration with existing systems. **User experience:** Striking a balance between security and a seamless user experience is challenging.
4. Cloud security posture management (CSPM): As healthcare organizations increasingly leverage cloud services, CSPM tools are gaining importance. These tools help ensure that cloud environments are configured securely. **Visibility:** CSPM tools provide visibility into cloud infrastructure, helping organizations identify and address security misconfigurations. **Compliance monitoring:** Ensures compliance with regulatory standards by continuously monitoring cloud configurations. **Automated remediation:** Automated remediation features help address security issues promptly [5,6].

   Complexity: Managing security across diverse cloud environments can be complex.

   Integration: Ensuring seamless integration with existing security tools and practices is crucial.
5. Internet of Medical Things (IoMT) Security: the proliferation of connected medical devices poses new challenges for healthcare cybersecurity. Securing the IoMT involves protecting networked medical devices from cyber threats. **Improved patient care:** IoMT devices contribute to improved patient care through real-time monitoring and data analysis. **Operational efficiency:** Connected devices enhance operational efficiency in healthcare settings [15,46].

Vulnerabilities: IoMT devices may have security vulnerabilities that can be exploited.

Device management: The sheer number and diversity of IoMT devices make effective management and security challenging.

Interoperability: Ensuring interoperability and standardized security measures across different IoMT devices is a complex task. These emerging trends in healthcare cybersecurity reflect the industry's ongoing efforts to adapt to evolving cyber threats. While these technologies offer significant benefits, their implementation also comes with challenges that need to be carefully addressed. As healthcare organizations navigate these trends, a comprehensive and proactive approach to cybersecurity remains essential to safeguard patient data and ensure the integrity of healthcare systems [1,16].

1.10.4 Proposed algorithm: cybersecurity concerns and risks in emerging healthcare systems

1. Define scope and objectives
2. Gather background information
3. Identify key components
4. Assess threat landscape
5. Evaluate vulnerabilities
6. Conduct risk assessment
7. Propose mitigation strategies
8. Consider human factors
9. Establish an incident response plan
10. Ensure regulatory compliance
11. Continuous monitoring and improvement
12. Document findings and recommendations
13. Review and validation
14. Implementation and monitoring

1. **Define scope and objectives**: Identify the scope of the cybersecurity analysis within emerging healthcare systems. Define the objectives of the algorithm, such as identifying vulnerabilities, assessing risks, and proposing mitigation strategies.
2. **Gather background information**: Collect relevant literature, reports, and case studies related to cybersecurity concerns in emerging healthcare systems. Review regulatory frameworks and compliance requirements specific to healthcare data security.
3. **Identify key components**: Break down the emerging healthcare system into its key components, including EHRs, medical devices, data storage systems, communication networks, etc.
4. **Assess Threat Landscape**: Analyze common cybersecurity threats facing healthcare systems, such as malware attacks, ransomware, insider threats, and phishing scams. Consider the potential impact of these threats on patient safety, confidentiality, and data integrity.
5. **Evaluate vulnerabilities**: Identify potential vulnerabilities within each component of the healthcare system, considering factors such as outdated software, inadequate encryption, and weak access controls. Prioritize vulnerabilities based on their likelihood and potential impact.
6. **Conduct risk assessment**: Evaluate the likelihood and potential impact of cybersecurity threats exploiting identified vulnerabilities. Use risk assessment techniques such as qualitative and quantitative analysis to prioritize risks.
7. **Propose mitigation strategies**: Develop mitigation strategies tailored to address identified vulnerabilities and mitigate high-risk threats. Consider measures such as implementing robust access controls, regularly updating software patches, conducting security awareness training for staff, and encrypting sensitive data.

8. **Consider human factors**: Recognize the role of human factors in cybersecurity, including employee negligence, malicious insider threats, and social engineering attacks. Incorporate strategies to address human factors, such as establishing clear security policies, fostering a culture of cybersecurity awareness, and implementing user authentication measures.
9. **Establish an incident response plan**: Develop an incident response plan outlining procedure for detecting, responding to, and recovering from cybersecurity incidents. Assign roles and responsibilities within the incident response team and establish communication channels for reporting and escalating incidents.
10. **Ensure regulatory compliance**: Ensure compliance with relevant regulatory frameworks such as HIPAA, GDPR, and other industry-specific standards. Implement measures to maintain audit trails, conduct regular security assessments, and report data breaches as required by regulations.
11. **Continuous monitoring and improvement**: Implement mechanisms for continuous monitoring of cybersecurity controls and threat intelligence. Regularly review and update cybersecurity policies, procedures, and mitigation strategies based on emerging threats and evolving regulatory requirements.
12. **Document findings and recommendations**: Document the findings of the cybersecurity analysis, including identified vulnerabilities, risk assessment results, mitigation strategies, and incident response procedures. Provide recommendations for securing emerging healthcare systems based on the analysis conducted.
13. **Review and validation:** Review the algorithm outputs with relevant stakeholders, including IT security professionals, healthcare administrators, and regulatory compliance officers. Validate the effectiveness of proposed mitigation strategies through testing and simulation exercises.
14. **Implementation and monitoring**: Implement the recommended mitigation strategies within the healthcare system. Monitor the effectiveness of implemented controls and periodically reassess cybersecurity risks to ensure ongoing protection of healthcare data.

1.10.5 Recommendations for securing emerging healthcare systems

Healthcare organizations face evolving cybersecurity challenges as they integrate emerging technologies into their systems. Adopting a proactive and collaborative approach is essential to strengthen the overall cybersecurity posture [1,7,14,16]. Section 1.10.6 presents practical recommendations to enhance security in emerging healthcare systems.

1.10.6 Recommendations

The precise recommendations for securing emerging healthcare systems are as follows:

1. Risk assessment and security by design: Conduct thorough risk assessments for new technologies and integrate security measures into their development lifecycle.
2. Collaboration and information sharing: Participate in industry-specific information-sharing platforms, foster public-private partnerships, and conduct joint incident response drills [3,10].
3. Data encryption and privacy measures: Implement end-to-end encryption, practice data minimization, and communicate privacy policies to patients.
4. Employee training and awareness: Conduct regular cybersecurity training programs, and simulated phishing exercises, and foster a reporting culture.
5. Continuous monitoring and incident response: Implement SIEM, develop incident response plans, and conduct post-incident reviews.
6. Regulatory compliance and audits: Conduct regular security audits, stay informed about regulatory updates, and ensure third-party vendors comply with regulations.
7. Cloud security and third-party risk management: Implement Cloud Security Posture Management (CSPM), conduct thorough risk assessments for third-party vendors, and encrypt data in transit and at rest [46,51].
8. Cybersecurity guidelines for emerging technologies: As healthcare systems integrate Artificial Intelligence (AI), the Internet of Things (IoT), and other emerging technologies, understanding the specific risks associated with each is crucial. These recommendations aim to address the multifaceted nature of cybersecurity in healthcare and emphasize collaboration, proactive measures, and continuous improvement to safeguard patient data effectively [68].

1.11 Conclusion

The proposed chapter examines various dimensions of cybersecurity in healthcare, exploring its importance, historical context, prevalent threats, regulatory frameworks, and mitigation strategies. The study outlines the critical need for robust cybersecurity measures amidst the digital revolution in healthcare. Drawing from related literature, the chapter contextualizes the current state of cybersecurity concerns within emerging healthcare systems, providing a foundation for subsequent discussions. An overview of emerging healthcare systems highlights the significance of digitalization and technology adoption, emphasizing the growing reliance on data-driven approaches. The transition from paper-based to EHRs exemplifies this shift and highlights the imperative of safeguarding healthcare data throughout its lifecycle. The chapter investigates the significance of cybersecurity in healthcare, supported by historical examples and insights into common cybersecurity threats and recent incidents. Regulatory frameworks and compliance challenges within healthcare organizations are explored, alongside potential consequences for non-compliance, underscoring the importance of adherence to industry standards. Technological advancements in healthcare are compared with vulnerabilities, prompting the proposal of mitigation strategies tailored to address identified risks. Human factors in healthcare cybersecurity, such as employee negligence and insider threats, are scrutinized, along with the establishment of incident response mechanisms and cybersecurity resilience. Amidst concerns about data privacy and patient trust, the chapter discusses measures to protect patient data and uphold trust in healthcare systems, supplemented by case studies of healthcare data breaches. Emerging trends in healthcare cybersecurity inform recommendations for securing emerging healthcare systems effectively.

Acknowledgments

The authors wish to appreciate the reviewers and Chief Editor, who took their time to constructively review this chapter, which has significantly improved the research study. However, the research was not funded.

References

[1] Vijayakumar, K. P., Pradeep, K., Balasundaram, A., and Prusty, M. R. (2023). Enhanced Cyber Attack Detection Process for Internet of Health Things (IoHT) Devices Using Deep Neural Network. *Processes*, 2023, 11(4), 1072.

[2] Newaz, A. I., Sikder, A. K., Rahman, M. A., and Uluagac, A. S. (2021). A Survey on Security and Privacy Issues in Modern Healthcare Systems: Attacks and Defenses. *ACM Transactions on Computational Healthcare*, 2(3), 27. https://doi.org/10.1145/3453176.

[3] Ahmad, M. A., Wisdom, D. D., and Isaac, S. (2020). An Empirical Analysis of Cybercrime Trends and Its Impact on Moral Decadence Among Secondary School Level Students in Nigeria. *In The 26th iSTEAMS Bespoke Multidisciplinary Conference*, Accra, Ghana.

[4] Telo, J. (2017). AI for Enhanced Healthcare Security: An Investigation of Anomaly Detection, Predictive Analytics, Access Control, Threat Intelligence, and Incident Response. *Journal of Advanced Analytics in Healthcare Management*, 1(1), 21–37.

[5] Abraham, C., Chatterjee, D., and Sims, R. R. (2019). *Muddling through cybersecurity: Insights from the U.S. healthcare industry*. Business Horizons. Advanced online publication. https://doi.org/10.1016/j.bushor.2019.03.010.

[6] Gudu, E. B., Wisdom, D. D., Gudu, G. J., Ahmad, M. A., Isaac, S., and Akinyemi, A. E. (2021). *Data science for Covid-19 (Mathematical Recipe for Curbing Coronavirus (Covid-19) Transmission Dynamics)*, Elsevier Book Chapter 28, 2021: pp. 527–545. https://doi.org/10.1016%2FB978-0-12-824536-1.00013-7.

[7] Christen, M., Gordijn, B., and Loi, M. (2020). *The Ethics of Cybersecurity. The International Library of Ethics, Law and Technology*, Springer, 21. https://doi.org/10.1007/978-3-030-29053-5_1.

[8] Wisdom, D. D., Vincent, O. R., Igulu, K., *et al.* (2023). *Cybersecurity in the Industry 4.0 and 5.0.* Taylor and Francis.

[9] Williams, P. A. H., and Woodward, A. J. (2015). Cybersecurity Vulnerabilities in Medical Devices: A Complex Environment and Multifaceted Problem. *Medical Devices: Evidence and Research*, Taylor and Francis, 8, 305–316. https://doi.org/10.2147/MDER.S50048.

[10] Gudu, E. B., Wisdom, D. D., Ahmed, M. A, Akinyemi, A.E., Isaac, S., and Dazi, A. J. (2021). Mathematical Model for the Spread and Control of Ebola Virus by Quarantine Techniques, *Annals. Journal of Computer Science Series*, 19(1), 81–87.

[11] Wisdom, D. D., Ajayi E. A., Arinze U. C., Idris, H., Bello, U. M., and Aladesote O. I. (2021). An Optimized TWIN Battery Resource Management Scheme in Wireless Networks, Lecture Notes in Networks, Vol. 217, *Proceedings of Sixth International Congress on Information and Communication Technology*, Springer Nature, 2021: pp. 73–95.

[12] Bhuyan, S. S., Kabir, U. Y., Escareno, J. M., *et al.* (2020). Transforming Healthcare Cybersecurity from Reactive to Proactive: Current Status and Future Recommendations. *Journal of Medical Systems*, 44(98). https://doi.org/10.1007/s10916-019-1507-y.

[13] Williams, C. M., Chaturvedi, R., and Chakravarthy, K. (2020). Cybersecurity Risks in a Pandemic. *Journal of Medical Internet Research*, 22(9), e23692. https://doi.org/10.2196/23692.

[14] MacIntyre, C. R., Engells, T. E., Scotch, M., *et al.* (2018). Converging and Emerging Threats to Health Security. *Environment Systems and Decisions*, 38(2), 198–207. https://doi.org/10.1007/s10669-017-9667-0.

[15] Cartwright, A. J. (2023). The Elephant in the Room: Cybersecurity in Healthcare. *Journal of Clinical Monitoring and Computing*, 37(10), 1123–1132. https://doi.org/10.1007/s10877-023-01013-5.

[16] Ksibi, S., Jaidi, F., and Bouhoula, A. (2023). A Comprehensive Study of Security and Cyber-security Risk Management within e-Health Systems: Synthesis, Analysis and a Novel Quantified Approach. *Mobile Networks and Applications*, 28(1), 107–127. https://doi.org/10.1007/s11036-022-02042-1.

[17] Jabarulla, M. Y., and Lee, H.-N. (2021). A Blockchain and Artificial Intelligence-Based, Patient-Centric Healthcare System for Combating the COVID-19 Pandemic: Opportunities and Applications. *Healthcare*, 9, 1019. https://doi.org/10.3390/healthcare9081019.

[18] Gudu, E. B., Wisdom, D. D., Hyacinth, E. A., *et al.* (2023). Transmission Dynamics of COVID-19 Virus Disease. In *Artificial Intelligence in Biomedical and Modern Healthcare Informatics*, Elsevier, 2023.

[19] Imoize, A. L., Gbadega, P. A., Obakhena, H. I., Irabor, D. O., Kavitha, K. V. N., and Chakraborty, C. (2022). Artificial Intelligence-enabled Internet of Medical Things for COVID-19 Pandemic Data Management. In *Explainable Artificial Intelligence in Medical Decision Support Systems* (pp. 357–380). (Vol. 50). Web of Science. https://covidwho-2323747., doi:10.1049/PBHE050E_ch13.

[20] Kavitha, S., Bora, A., Naved, M., Raj, K. B., and Nadh Singh, B. R. (2021). An Internet of Things For Data Security In Cloud Using Artificial Intelligence. *International Journal of Grid and Distributed Computing*, 14(1), 1257–1275.

[21] Ahsan, M., Nygard, K. E., Gomes, R., Chowdhury, M. M., Rifat, N., and Connolly, J. F. (2022). Cybersecurity Threats and Their Mitigation Approaches Using Machine Learning—A Review.

[22] Isaac, S., Wisdom, D.D., Ahmed, M.A. and Arinze, U.C. (2020). Battery-Life Management with an Efficient Sleep-Mode Power Saving Scheme (BM-ESPSS) in IEEE 802.16e Networks, *International Journal of Mechatronics, Electrical and Computer Technology (JMEC)*, 7(2), 2020.

[23] Li, B., Wu, Y., Song, J., Lu, R., Li, T., and Zhao, L. (2021). DeepFed: Federated Deep Learning for Intrusion Detection in Industrial Cyber–Physical Systems. *IEEE Transactions on Industrial Informatics*, 17(8), 5658–5667. DOI:10.1109/TII.2021.3060480.

[24] Naseem, M., Akhund, R., Arshad, H., and Ibrahim, M. T. (2020). Exploring the Potential of Artificial Intelligence and Machine Learning to Combat COVID-19 and Existing Opportunities for LMIC: A Scoping Review. *Journal of Primary Care & Community Health*, 11, 1–11. DOI:10.1177/2150132720963634. https://journals.sagepub.com/home/jpc.

[25] Radoglou-Grammatikis, P., Rompolos, K., Sarigiannidis, P., *et al.* (2022). Modeling, Detecting, and Mitigating Threats Against Industrial Healthcare Systems: A Combined Software Defined Networking and Reinforcement Learning Approach. *IEEE Transactions on Industrial Informatics*, 18(3), 2022.

[26] Meshram, C., Imoize, A. L., Aljaedi, A., Alharbi, A. R., Jamal, S. S., and Barve, S. K. (2021). An Efficient Electronic Cash System Based on Certificateless Group Signcryption Scheme Using Conformable Chaotic Maps. *Sensors*, 21(21), 7039. https://doi.org/10.3390/s21217039.

[27] Wisdom, D. D., Saidu, I., Tambuwal, A. Y., Ahmad, M. A, Isaac, S., and Farouk, N. An Efficient Sleep- Window-Based Power Saving Scheme (ESPSS) in IEEE 802.16e Networks, *15th International Conference on Electronics Computer and Computation ICECCO* 2019.

[28] Imoize, A. L., Irabor, D. O., Peter, G., and Chakraborty, C. (2022). Blockchain technology for secure COVID-19 pandemic data handling. In *Smart Health Technologies for the COVID-19 Pandemic: Internet of Medical Things Perspectives* (pp. 141–179). DOI:10.1049/PBHE042E_ch6. University of Lagos, University of KwaZulu-Natal, Birla Institute of Technology, Mesra.

[29] Imoize, L., Hemanth, J., Do, D.-T., and Sur, S. N. (Eds.). (2022). *Explainable Artificial Intelligence in Medical Decision Support Systems*. Institution of Engineering and Technology. https://doi.org/10.1049/PBHE050E.

[30] Ramasamy, L. K., Khan K. P. F., Imoize, A. L., Ogbebor, J. O., Kadry, S., and Rho, S. (2021). Blockchain-Based Wireless Sensor Networks for Malicious Node Detection: A Survey. *IEEE Access*, 9, 128765–128785. https://doi.org/10.1109/ACCESS.2021.3111923.

[31] Awotunde, J. B., Imoize, A. L., Ayoade, O. B., *et al.* (2022). An Enhanced Hyper-parameter Optimization of a Convolutional Neural Network Model for Leukemia Cancer Diagnosis in an Artificial Intelligence and Blockchain Technology Smart Healthcare System. *Sensors*, 22(24), 9689. https://doi.org/10.3390/s22249689.

[32] Wisdom, D. D., Isaac, S., Ahmed, M. A., Farouk, N., Magami, S., and Elijah, Y. (2020). An Improved Battery-Life Power Saving Scheme (IBPSS) in IEEE 802.16e Networks. *International Journal of Information Processing and Communication (IJIPC)*, 8(2), April.

[33] Rufai, A. T., Dukor, K. F., Ageh, O. M., and Imoize, A. L. (2022). XAI Robot-Assisted Surgeries in Future Medical Decision Support Systems. In L. Imoize, J. Hemanth, D.-T. Do, and S. N. Sur (Eds.), *Explainable Artificial Intelligence in Medical Decision Support Systems* (pp. 167–195). Institution of Engineering and Technology. https://doi.org/10.1049/PBHE050E_ch6.

[34] Sei, Y., Ohsuga, A., and Imoize, A. L. (2022). Statistical Test with Differential Privacy for Medical Decision Support Systems. In L. Imoize, J. Hemanth, D.-T. Do, and S. N. Sur (Eds.), *Explainable Artificial Intelligence in Medical Decision Support Systems* (pp. 401–433). Institution of Engineering and Technology. https://doi.org/10.1049/PBHE050E_ch15.

[35] Ayoade, O. B., Oladele, T. O., Imoize, A. L., *et al.* (2022). Explainable Artificial Intelligence (XAI) in Medical Decision Systems (MDSSs): Healthcare Systems Perspective. In L. Imoize, J. Hemanth, D.-T. Do, and S. N. Sur (Eds.), *Explainable Artificial Intelligence in Medical Decision Support Systems* (pp. 1–43). Institution of Engineering and Technology. https://doi.org/10.1049/PBHE050E_ch1.

[36] Kumar, R. L., Wang, Y., Poongodi, T., and Imoize, A. L. (2021). *Internet of Things, Artificial Intelligence and Blockchain Technology*. Cham: Springer International Publishing. https://doi.org/10.1007/978-3-030-74150-1.

[37] Abikoye, O. C., Oladipupo, E. T., Imoize, A. L., Awotunde, J. B., Lee, C.-C., and Li, C.-T. (2023). Securing Critical User Information over the Internet of Medical Things Platforms Using a Hybrid Cryptography Scheme. *Future Internet*, 15(3), 99. https://doi.org/10.3390/fi15030099.

[38] Wisdom, D. D., Farouk, N., Ahmed, M. A., Isaac, S., Idris, H., and Hassan, J. B. (2020). An Enhanced Power Saving Scheme (EPSS) in IEEE 802.16e Networks. *International Journal of Information Processing and Communication (IJIPC)*, 8(2).

[39] Oyebiyi, O. G., Abayomi-Alli, A., Arogundade, O. T., Qazi, A., Imoize, A. L., and Awotunde, J. B. (2023). A Systematic Literature Review on Human Ear Biometrics: Approaches, Algorithms, and Trend in the Last Decade. *Information*, 14(3), 192. https://doi.org/10.3390/info14030192.

[40] Eneh, A. H., Wisdom, D. D., Wisdom, D. D., Arinze, U. C., Philibus, E., and Philibus, E. (2022). An Optimized Database Management System. *In Proceedings of the LASUSTECH 30th Multidisciplinary Innovation Conference* 2020, Series 30 Vol-2 (p. 25). Lagos, Nigeria. DOI:10.22624/AIMS/iSTEAMS/LASUSTECH2022V30P25.

[41] Wisdom, D. D., Christian, A. U., Igulu, K., Hyacinth, E. A., Odunayo, O. E. and Umar, B. (2023). Industrial IoT Security Infrastructure and Threats. In A. Prasad, T. P. Singh, and S. D. Sharma (Eds.), *Communication technologies in IoT and Their Security Challenges: Present and Future. Springer Nature.*

[42] Kavitha, K.V. N., Ashok, S., Imoize, A. L., *et al.* (2022). On the Use of Wavelet Domain and Machine Learning for the Analysis of Epileptic Seizure Detection from EEG Signals. *Journal of Healthcare Engineering*, 2022, 1–16. https://doi.org/10.1155/2022/8928021.

[43] Wisdom, D. D., Vincent, O. R., Igulu, K. T., *et al.* (2023). Mitigating Cyber Threats in Healthcare Systems: The Role of Artificial Intelligence and Machine Learning. *Artificial Intelligence and Blockchain Technology in Modern Telehealth Systems, Institute of Engineering and Technology (IET)*, 2023.

[44] Igulu, K. T., Wisdom, D. D., Arowolo, M. O., and Singh, T. P., (2023). Computational Intelligence in Big Data Analytics. *CI-Industry-4.0: Computational Intelligence in Industry 4.0 and 5.0 Applications. Taylor and Francis group.*

[45] Wisdom, D. D., Vincent, O. R., Oduntan, O. O., Igulu, K., and Garba, A. B., (2022). Enhanced Cybersecurity Framework for 5G-Integrated Oil and Gas Industry. *COMPUTOLOGY: Journal of Applied Computer Science and Intelligent Technologies*, 2(1), 8–22. Publisher: Journal Press India.

[46] Alhasan, S., Akinyemi, A. E., and Wisdom, D. D. (2020). A Comparative Performance Study of Machine Learning Algorithms for Efficient Data Mining Management of Intrusion Detection Systems. *International Journal of Engineering Applied Sciences and Technology*, 5(6), 85–110. ISSN 2455-2143.

[47] Wisdom, D. D., Vincent, O. R., Igulu, K. T., *et al.* (2023). *Cyber-threats in Healthcare Systems: The Role and Application of Artificial Intelligence and Machine Learning*, Nova Science Publishers, USA. 2023.

[48] Van der Giessen, E., Schultz, P. A., Bertin, N., *et al.* (2020). Roadmap on Multiscale Materials Modeling. *Modeling and Simulation in Materials Science and Engineering*, 28(4), 043001. https://doi.org/10.1088/1361-651X/ab7150.

[49] Wisdom, D. D., Vincent, O. R., Abayomi-Alli, A., Olusegun, F., Ayetuoma, I.O., and Baba, G. A. (2024). Security Measures in Computational Modeling and Simulations, In *CRC Computational* Taylor and Francis.

[50] Vincent, O., Folorunso, O., and Akinde, A. (2009). On Consolidation Model in e-Bill Presentment and Payment. *Information Management & Computer Security*, *17*(3), 234–247.

[51] Isabona, J., Imoize, A. L., Ojo, S., *et al.* (2022). Development of a Multilayer Perceptron Neural Network for Optimal Predictive Modeling in Urban Microcellular Radio Environments. *MDPI.* https://doi.org/10.3390/app12115713.

[52] Wisdom, D. D., Christian, A. U., Hyacinth, E. A., Esther, O. O., Igulu, K., and Garba, A. B. (2022). IoT Devices Battery Life Energy Management Scheme. *Computology: Journal of Applied Computer Science and Intelligent Technologies*, 2(2), 1–13. https://doi.org/10.17492/computology.v2i2.2201.

[53] Folorunso, O., Ogunde, A. O., Vincent, R. O., and Salako, O. (2010). Data Mining for Business Intelligence in Distribution Chain Analytics. *International Journal of the Computer, the Internet and Management, 18*(1), 15–26..

[54] Wisdom, D. D., Igulu, K., Esther, O. O., Baba, G. A., Ahmad, A., and Sidi, A. (2021). A Review of Best Practices and Methods of Mitigating Cybersecurity Risks in Healthcare Systems and a Newly Proposed Algorithm. *Computology: Journal of Applied Computer Science and Intelligent Technologies*, 1 (2), 27–36. DOI:10.17492/computology.v1i2.2104.

[55] Olaleye, T. O., and Vincent, O. R. (2020). A Predictive Model for Students Performance and Risk Level Indicators Using Machine Learning. In *2020 International Conference in Mathematics, Computer Engineering and Computer Science (ICMCECS)* (pp. 1–7). IEEE.

[56] Nubi, O. J., and Vincent, O. R. (2020). Virtual Reality: A Pedagogical Model for Simulation-Based Learning. *In 2020 International Conference in Mathematics, Computer Engineering and Computer Science (ICMCECS)* (pp. 1–6). IEEE.

[57] Wisdom, D. D., Singh, T. P., Igulu, K. T., and Choudhary, R. (2023). ChatGPT and its Impact on Human-Computer Interaction: A Comprehension. *In Proceedings of the 4th International Conference on Computational Intelligence & Internet of Things (ICCIIoT).* Springer PROMS. 4–6, 2023. The Faculty of ICT, University of Malta, Msida, Malta.

[58] Lawal, O. M., Vincent, O. R., Agboola, A. A. A., and Folorunso, O. (2021). An Improved Hybrid Scheme for e-Payment Security Using Elliptic Curve Cryptography. *International Journal of Information Technology, 13*, 139–153.

[59] Wisdom, D. D., Tambuwal, A. Y., Mohammed, A., Audu, A., Soroyewun, M. B., and Isaac, S. (2019). A Delay Aware Power Saving Scheme (DAPSS-BT) Based on Load on Traffic in IEEE 802.16e WiMAX Networks, *Institute of Electrical and Electronic Engineers Conference IEEE, Ahmadu Bello University Zaria*, Kaduna State, Nigeria.

[60] Ajose, S. O., and Imoize, A. L. (2013). Propagation Measurements and Modelling at 1800MHz in Lagos, Nigeria. *International Journal of Wireless and Mobile Computing*, 6(2). Department of Electrical and Electronics Engineering, University of Lagos, Akoka-Lagos, Nigeria.

[61] Imoize, A. L., Balas, V. E., Solanki, V. K., Lee, C. C., and Obaidat, M. S. (Eds.). (2023). *Handbook of Security and Privacy of AI-Enabled Healthcare Systems and Internet of Medical Things* (1st ed.). CRC Press. DOI:10.1201/9781003370321.

[62] Awotunde, J. B., Folorunso, S. O., Imoize, A. L., *et al.* (2023). An Ensemble Tree-Based Model for Intrusion Detection in Industrial Internet of Things networks. *Applied Sciences*, 13(4), 2479. https://doi.org/10.3390/app13042479.

[63] Meshram, C., Ibrahim, R. W., Meshram, S. G., Jamal, S. S., and Imoize, A. L. (2022). An Efficient Authentication with Key Agreement Procedure Using Mittag–Leffler–Chebyshev Summation Chaotic Map under the Multi-server Architecture. *Springer Journal of Supercomputing*, 78, 4938–4959.

[64] Oladipupo, E. T., Abikoye, O. C., Imoize, A. L., *et al.* (2023). An Efficient Authenticated Elliptic Curve Cryptography Scheme for Multicore Wireless Sensor Networks. *IEEE Access*, 11, 1306–1323. doi:10.1109/ACCESS.2022.3233632.

[65] Wisdom, D. D., Ajayi, E. A., Akindayo, S. O., Yanah, Y. M., Kwaido, E., and Shehu, S. A. (2019). An Efficient Automated Revenue Generation Database Management System. *Annals Journal of Computer Science Series*, 17(2), 201–215.

[66] Jelić, L. (2024). Cybersecurity, Data Protection, and Artificial Intelligence in Medical Devices. In: Badnjević, A., Cifrek, M., Magjarević, R., and Džemić, Z. (eds.), *Inspection of Medical Devices*. Series in Biomedical Engineering. Cham: Springer Nature: pp. 417–445. https://doi.org/10.1007/978-3-031-43444-0_17.

[67] Jakka, G., Yathiraju, N., and Ansari, M. F. (2022). Artificial Intelligence in Terms of Spotting Malware and Delivering Cyber Risk Management. *Journal of Positive School Psychology*, 6(3), 6156–6165.

[68] Van der Schaar, M., Alaa, A. M., Floto, A., *et al.* (2021). How Artificial Intelligence and Machine Learning Can Help Healthcare Systems Respond to COVID-19. *Machine Learning*, 110(1), 1–14. https://doi.org/10.1007/s10994-020-05928-x.

Chapter 2

Cybersecurity in the Internet of Medical Things for healthcare applications

Hawau I. Olagunju[1], Emmanuel Alozie[1], Agbotiname Lucky Imoize[2], Nasir Faruk[1,3], Salisu Garba[4] and Bashir Abdullahi Baba[5]

In the era of digital healthcare transformation, the integration of the Internet of Medical Things (IoMT) has ushered in unprecedented opportunities for enhanced patient care and medical advancements. However, this connectivity comes with the looming specter of cybersecurity threats that could compromise patient data and, in some cases, even endanger lives. This chapter delves into the intricate landscape of cybersecurity within the IoMT for healthcare applications. We explore the multifaceted challenges posed by cyber threats in the healthcare sector, where the stakes are higher than ever. From safeguarding sensitive patient information to protecting the integrity of medical devices, we dissect the evolving threat landscape and the vulnerabilities specific to the IoMT ecosystem. Moreover, we unravel the strategies and technologies employed to fortify the defenses of healthcare systems against an ever-evolving array of cyber threats. Drawing from real-world case studies and best practices, we shed light on how cutting-edge cybersecurity measures can be seamlessly integrated into IoMT environments without compromising the agility and efficiency required for modern healthcare.

Keywords: IoMT; cybersecurity; cyberattacks; healthcare; blockchain; artificial intelligence

2.1 Introduction

The Internet of Things (IoT) is a novel technology that enables the seamless connectivity of various physical devices, sensors, software, and objects, facilitating

[1]Department of Information Technology, Sule Lamido University, Nigeria
[2]Department of Electrical and Electronics Engineering, Faculty of Engineering, University of Lagos, Nigeria
[3]Directorate of Information Technology, Sule Lamido University, Nigeria
[4]Department of Software Engineering, Sule Lamido University, Nigeria
[5]Department of Cybersecurity, Sule Lamido University, Nigeria

interaction without human intervention [1,2]. It entails the interconnection of smart devices physically and logically to a dedicated cloud network, aiming for consistent smart coordination, intelligent monitoring, and scalable operational administration [3]. These devices, operable remotely across existing network infrastructure, present opportunities for seamless scalability, leading to more direct integration into computer-based systems, thereby enhancing efficiency and accuracy. This network of smart things finds applications in diverse sectors such as transportation, industry, agriculture, smart homes, education, smart cities, the military, and notably, healthcare [4,5]. The healthcare sector has transformed significantly with the introduction of the Internet of Medical Things (IoMT).

The IoMT, essentially a network connecting medical devices and individuals through wireless communication, is an emerging technology designed to enhance the quality of patient care by enabling personalized e-health services unrestricted by time and location [2,6,7]. This medical innovation contributes to increased patient convenience, cost-effective healthcare treatments, improved medical therapies, and more personalized care. The proliferation of wearable devices further fuels the growth of IoMT, offering benefits such as continuous monitoring of vitals and health parameters. IoMT devices enable remote, real-time patient condition monitoring, with captured data analyzed and transmitted to cloud data storage or medical data centers for further processing and storage, catering to various stakeholders like physicians, medical staff, caregivers, and insurance providers [8–10]. IoMT applications encompass solutions tailored for remote health monitoring, emergency patient care, healthcare management, monitoring elderly patients, clinical decision support systems, wireless capsule endoscopy, etc.

While the integration of physical things in the IoMT environment to the Internet allows for remote access and monitoring, it also introduces vulnerabilities due to the rapidly evolving IoMT threat landscape [8,11]. Intruders may exploit the IoMT network, risking the overall security and privacy of devices and patients. As the volume of data that is handled and generated by IoMT devices grows exponentially, it will eventually lead to greater exposure to confidential medical data [8,12]. Thus, despite the numerous advantages of IoMT, it faces significant challenges, with one of the most prominent being cybersecurity threats and attacks. Cybersecurity, as a safeguarding mechanism, aims to protect computer systems, networks, and information from potential disruption or unauthorized activities. While literature extensively addresses the security and privacy issues of IoMT, the cybersecurity aspect remains relatively unexplored. This chapter thus aims to fill this gap by exploring the cybersecurity issues of IoMT based on its architecture with the aim of not only uncovering the potential vulnerabilities but also reviewing the various solutions and countermeasures to defend against cyber threats and attacks.

2.1.1 Key contributions

- An extensive review of related works on cybersecurity and privacy within the IoMT for healthcare applications.

- An outlook into IoMT including its architecture, communication protocols, and use cases.
- The security requirement of IoMT for healthcare applications is presented and reviewed.
- A review of the cybersecurity threats and attacks in IoMT for healthcare applications.
- A review of the innovative cyberattack countermeasures proffered to defend against the various threats and attacks in the IoMT network is provided.
- Various emerging technologies to strengthen IoMT security are presented and reviewed.
- Critical lessons learned from the chapter are identified and elaborated.

2.1.2 Chapter organization

The remaining part of this chapter is organized as follows: Section 2.2 presents the review of previous review work on the cybersecurity, security, and privacy challenges in IoMT. Section 2.3 presents an overview of the IoMT, its architecture, and use cases. Section 2.4 briefly introduces the security requirements for the Internet of Medical Things for Healthcare Applications. Section 2.5 discusses cybersecurity for the Internet of Medical Things for Healthcare Applications. Section 2.6 presents the emerging Technologies for Securing IoMT. Section 2.7 highlights countermeasures for the Internet of Medical Things for Healthcare Applications, and Section 2.8 discusses the lessons learned from the review. Finally, Section 2.9 concludes the chapter and provides recommendations for further research directions.

2.2 Review of related works

This section presents an extensive review of related works and further presents the limitations of these works.

Security and privacy are two major concerns in the healthcare system, particularly when it comes to the Internet of Things (IoT). Several research works have explored security risks, threats, and attacks. Sun *et al.* [13] conducted an extensive survey on the security and privacy of IoMT-enabled healthcare systems, discussing security and privacy challenges and requirements from the data level to the medical server level of IoMT-based healthcare systems. Additionally, the work presented the potential of utilizing biometrics and its applications to secure IoMT healthcare systems. The conclusion was made that although several security schemes have been developed for IoMT devices to protect medical devices, wearable and implantable devices tend to be built with very limited resources due to size and power constraints, and they may not have sufficient resources to implement those schemes.

The security and privacy issues of Medical IoT (MIoT) were reviewed in [8], where various threats and attacks such as eavesdropping, man-in-the-middle attacks, tag cloning, Denial of Service (DoS), replay attacks, etc., were discussed and classified based on the architectural layers of MIoT, including the perception, network, and application layers. Different countermeasures were also identified and discussed, such as data encryption, data auditing, and IoT healthcare policies. The security and privacy challenges of IoT in healthcare systems were also investigated in [12], where critical findings revealed that most threats occur due to unauthorized access to data, data breaches, and impersonation. Furthermore, the device layer, one of the five layers of the IoT healthcare application architecture, is the most vulnerable.

Similarly, the security and privacy challenges with IoT in healthcare were reviewed in [3] where four critical points were obtained, one of which is the countermeasures that can be utilized to defend against threats and attacks in IoT for healthcare. The countermeasures include Absolute Data Confidentiality (ADC), Dynamic Information-Integrity (DII), and Reliable Authorized-Accessibility (RAA). Several other authors also explored and reviewed the security and privacy issues of IoT in healthcare such as [2,4,14–20], however, one common limitation of these research works is that most of them did not consider the cybersecurity aspects of these security and privacy issues of IoMT.

With this, Thomasian *et al.* [11] reviewed cybersecurity in the IoMT; however, they aimed to analyze the robustness of existing policy measures in securing IoMT technologies. Emphasis was given to the regulatory ecosystem in the United States (US), which included regulatory frameworks for the industry, public-private partnerships, and transparency initiatives. Conclusions were drawn that additional regulatory guidance is required to mitigate risks associated with IoMT devices. Furthermore, the authors concluded that there is a need for interventions to promote awareness and limit these security risks around IoMT devices, as novel attacks and threats are emerging with the advancement of the cyber world.

Similarly, Bhukya *et al.* [21] investigated the cybersecurity issues of the Internet of Medical Vehicles (IoMV), which was derived from IoT, IoV, and IoMT. Findings from the review showed that IoMV has security risks from a variety of sophisticated cyberattacks as devices communicate with different networks, endangering the onboard patient's life. Hence, there is a great need to implement robust cybersecurity measures. However, the research did not fully or thoroughly cover all the security aspects of the IoMV system. The roles of cybersecurity, Artificial Intelligence (AI), and Blockchain (BC) technologies in the IoMT were reviewed in [22], where it was noted that most of the reviewed studies have used lightweight algorithms that reduce energy and resource consumption but are more expensive.

Furthermore, AI, BC, and cybersecurity techniques face challenges in making IoMT infrastructure for healthcare applications, such as security, privacy, latency, energy, availability, integrity, and scalability. Blockchain-assisted cybersecurity for IoMT in the healthcare industry was proposed and developed in [23], utilizing a conventional in-depth approach and blockchain to create a procedure for collecting medical information from the IoMT and integrated devices. Experimental results showed that the proposed system has a high-security rate of 99.8% and the lowest latency rate of 4.3% compared to traditional approaches. Furthermore, the reliability of the proposed system gives the highest rate of 99.4%. Table 2.1 summarizes the limitations of related works based on various sections explored in this chapter,

Table 2.1 Comparison between the related works

Reference	IoMT architecture	IoMT communication protocols	IoMT use cases	IoMT cybersecurity requirements	Cyberattacks in IoMT	Emerging technology for IoMT security	Countermeasures for IoMT cyberattacks
[13]	✓	×	×	✓	×	✓	×
[8]	✓	×	×	✓	×	×	×
[12]	×	×	×	×	×	×	×
[3]	×	×	×	×	×	×	×
[14]	×	×	×	×	×	×	×
[4]	×	×	×	×	×	×	×
[15]	×	×	✓	×	×	×	×
[16]	✓	×	×	✓	×	×	×
[17]	✓	×	×	✓	×	×	×
[18]	✓	×	×	×	×	×	×
[19]	✓	✓	×	✓	×	✓	×
[2]	×	×	×	×	×	×	×
[11]	×	×	✓	✓	×	×	×
[21]	✓	×	×	×	✓	✓	×
[22]	×	×	×	×	✓	✓	✓
[23]	✓	×	×	×	✓	✓	×
This chapter	✓	✓	✓	✓	✓	✓	✓

encompassing the IoMT architecture, communication protocols in IoMT, use cases of IoMT, cybersecurity requirements, cyberattacks in IoMT, emerging technologies for IoMT security, and countermeasures against IoMT cyberattacks.

From Table 2.1, it is evident that while there have been extensive studies addressing the security and privacy concerns of the IoMT, encompassing considerations of IoMT architecture, some use cases, and innovative countermeasures, a critical gap exists regarding the cybersecurity aspects of IoMT. Specifically, only a few researches considered the cybersecurity aspects of IoMT, incorporating explorations of emerging technologies like artificial intelligence and blockchain to strengthen IoMT systems against diverse cyber threats. This chapter, thus, aims to fill these gaps by providing an overview of cybersecurity in IoMT for healthcare applications.

2.3 Overview of the Internet of Medical Things (IoMT)

IoMT is the combination of several devices in the medical sector for the collection, transfer, analysis, and management of patients' data. Initially, health-related information will be gathered from the individual's body through intelligent sensors incorporated into smart wearables or implanted devices, which are interconnected through Body Sensor Networks (BSN) or Wireless Sensor Networks (WSN) [24]. Subsequently, this collected data will be transmitted via the internet to the subsequent stage, focusing on prediction and analysis. Once the medical data is received, an appropriate data transformation and interpretation technique, based on Artificial Intelligence (AI), can be applied for analysis. In instances of severe issues, healthcare professionals or other medical services can be contacted with the assistance of intelligent AI-based applications on smartphones. For less critical situations, individuals can implement self-preventive measures [25,26].

2.3.1 IoMT architecture

The IoMT infrastructure consists mainly of the application layer, network layer, and perception layer which are mostly utilized as seen in various research works that have been done such as in [27] where it was stated that the three major layers an IoMT infrastructure should consist of are the perception layer, network layer, and application layer. Similarly, the study [28] identified the application layer, network layer, and perception layer as part of the three-layered architecture of IoT for IoMT.

Other reviews also proposed different and more layers in the IoMT architecture including the four-layer and five-layer architecture such as in [29], where the infrastructure was said to consist of three major layers namely: things layer, fog layer, and cloud layer. The study [5] stated that the IoMT architecture consists of four layers which are the environment-awareness layer, gateway layer, cloud layer, and function layer. Similarly, a four-layer architecture, namely: the device layer, communication network layer, IoT platform layer, and application layer was also proposed in [24].

The architecture of the IoMT is illustrated in Figure 2.1, comprising five major layers. The first layer, known as the perception layer, serves as the initial tier that

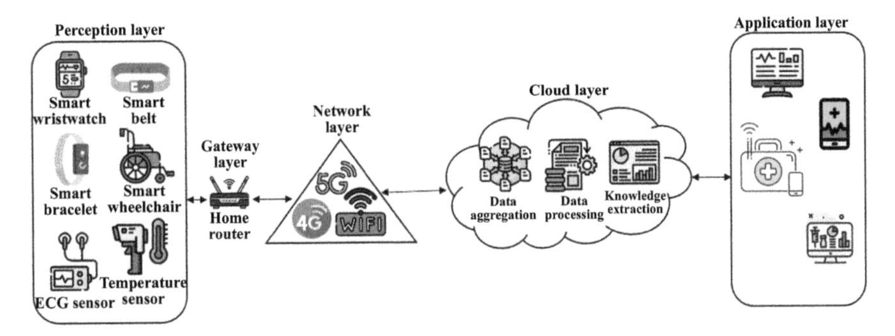

Figure 2.1 IoMT architecture

accommodates all IoMT sensors and devices. Following this, the second layer, identified as the gateway layer, houses the gateway router responsible for routing signals from IoMT devices or sensors to the cloud via the internet. This communication is facilitated through various wireless and mobile network technologies, including 4G, 5G, and Wi-Fi, situated at the network layer. The fourth layer, referred to as the cloud layer, undertakes data aggregation and processing, leading to knowledge extraction. The knowledge extracted from the cloud layer is then presented in the application layer, the fifth layer. This layer comprises end-user devices that enable the remote monitoring of vital readings and activities of the user.

2.3.1.1 Application layer

This is the topmost layer of the architecture that corresponds to the session and application layer of the OSI model. This layer provides application and data control services and plays a crucial role in facilitating communication, data exchange, and interaction between medical devices, wearables, and healthcare systems within the IoMT. It also encompasses a range of healthcare applications that leverage data collected from sensors, wearables, and other medical devices to provide valuable insights, support clinical decision-making, and enhance patient care [30].

2.3.1.2 Network layer

This is responsible for the communication, interconnection, and transport of data packets among devices through the network [30]. It includes technologies such as wireless communication protocols, networking solutions, and internet connectivity for medical applications. It also ensures efficient and secure transmission of health-related data, enabling real-time monitoring, data collection, and analysis.

2.3.1.3 Perception layer

This is the lowest layer closest to the hardware Medium Access Control and it is where the signal measurement and transmission takes place [30]. This layer is responsible for the acquisition of medical data from patients' bodies through sensors concatenated into smart wearables or implanted devices. This layer is very crucial for gathering real-time information about the patient's health status.

2.3.1.4 Gateway layer

This is the intermediary layer that houses the gateway router responsible for routing signals from IoMT devices or sensors to the cloud via the internet [5].

2.3.1.5 Cloud layer

This layer plays a crucial role in securely storing extensive medical data and effective management of health records from a wide patient base, ensuring universal access to electronic records. Authorized healthcare professionals can promptly access relevant information for diagnosis and treatment [31].

2.3.2 IoMT communication protocols

Communication protocols play a critical role in facilitating seamless and secure data exchange in IoMT which contains a variety of devices and systems that communicate with each other to collect, transmit, and analyze data for improved patient care, diagnostics, and overall healthcare management [32]. Figure 2.2 presents the various IoMT communication protocols which are further discussed in this section.

1. **Bluetooth low energy (BLE):** is a wireless technology designed for short-range communication in healthcare applications, emphasizing low power consumption. Operating in the 2.4 GHz ISM band, BLE's range of 10 m suits close proximity scenarios, making it optimal for wearable health devices like trackers and sensors. Its energy efficiency is crucial for battery-powered devices, enabling periodic or continuous data transmission without rapid battery depletion [32]. BLE supports sensor networks in healthcare settings,

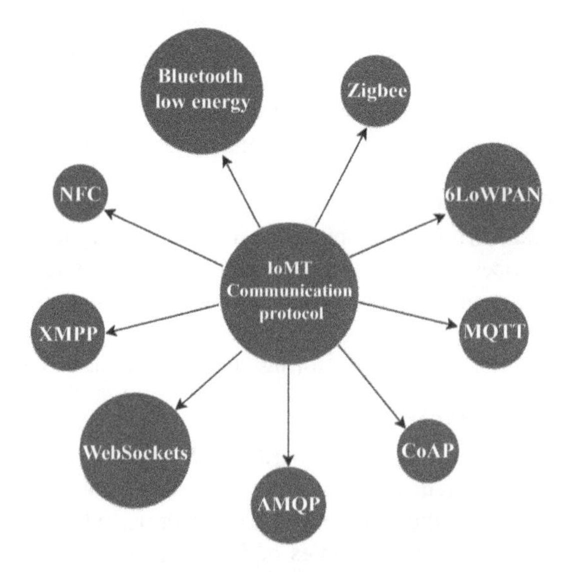

Figure 2.2 IoMT communication protocols

facilitating wireless communication between devices and central monitoring systems [33]. Its standardization ensures interoperability among diverse healthcare devices, and security features protect sensitive patient data, while real-time data transmission supports applications like continuous health monitoring and emergency alerts.

2. **Zigbee:** is a wireless communication protocol useful for low-power, short-range communication in diverse applications, including home health in IoMT. Its optimization for low-power operation is crucial for battery-operated devices, ensuring extended reliability without frequent replacements. Operating in the 2.4 GHz frequency band, Zigbee supports short-range communication, making it suitable for confined home environments [34]. Its key feature, mesh networking, enhances communication reliability and extends the range, forming a robust network for health monitoring devices. Zigbee's applications in home health monitoring include facilitating communication between devices and a central hub and forming scalable networks that can evolve with additional devices. With security features, interoperability based on open standards, and cost-effective implementation, Zigbee stands as a suitable choice for building energy-efficient and reliable home health monitoring systems [35].
3. **IPv6 over low-power wireless personal area networks (6LoWPAN):** serves as a communication protocol that enables the use of IPv6 over low-power, wireless networks in IoMT. This protocol is specifically designed to facilitate efficient and lightweight communication for devices with limited power resources, making it well-suited for applications in healthcare where energy efficiency is crucial. By allowing the integration of IPv6, 6LoWPAN ensures compatibility with existing internet protocols while addressing the constraints of low-power devices in IoMT networks, contributing to the seamless connectivity and communication of medical devices [36].
4. **Message queuing telemetry transport (MQTT):** is a lightweight and efficient protocol designed for real-time communication between devices and servers. Known for its simplicity and low overhead, MQTT excels in scenarios where low bandwidth and reliable communication are paramount. Its publish-subscribe architecture facilitates seamless data exchange, making it a preferred choice for IoT applications, including those within the healthcare sector, where real-time data updates and efficient communication between devices and servers are crucial for monitoring and decision-making processes [37].
5. **Constrained application protocol (CoAP):** is a communication protocol that provides a lightweight and efficient method for constrained devices utilizing the RESTful principles, such as those with limited processing power or energy resources, to exchange information in IoMT applications [38]. By focusing on simplicity and resource efficiency, CoAP facilitates seamless and standardized communication, ensuring optimal performance in healthcare settings where devices may have constraints on processing capability and power consumption [39].
6. **Advanced message queuing protocol (AMQP):** is a messaging protocol designed for efficient and secure message exchange, allowing devices to communicate asynchronously in a distributed system. By providing a

standardized way for devices to exchange messages, AMQP ensures reliable and resilient communication, making it well-suited for IoMT applications where timely and secure data transfer is crucial for effective healthcare management [40].

7. **WebSockets:** is a communication protocol that enables bidirectional, full-duplex communication over a single, long-lived connection, making them ideal for real-time updates in various applications [41]. This protocol establishes a continuous channel between devices and servers, allowing them to send and receive data in real-time without the need for repeated connections and also supports instantaneous updates and alerts, making them suitable for applications such as remote patient monitoring and timely communication of critical information between medical devices and centralized systems.
8. **Extensible messaging and presence protocol (XMPP):** is a communication protocol that supports real-time messaging and collaboration among healthcare professionals in the IoMT. By providing a secure and extensible framework, XMPP facilitates instant messaging, presence detection, and collaborative efforts. This protocol is particularly beneficial for enabling timely communication and information sharing among healthcare teams, contributing to efficient collaboration and decision-making in dynamic medical environments [40].
9. **Near field communication (NFC):** is a communication protocol utilized in the IoMT for short-range wireless communication between devices. NFC enables secure and efficient data exchange by bringing devices close together. In healthcare applications, NFC can be employed for tasks such as patient identification, access control to medical facilities, or the transfer of small sets of data between medical devices, contributing to streamlined and secure interactions within IoMT [42].

The choice of communication protocols in IoMT depends on factors such as device capabilities, power constraints, data transfer requirements, and the specific needs of the healthcare application. It is crucial to select a combination of protocols that provide the necessary features while ensuring interoperability, security, and efficiency in healthcare data exchange. Nevertheless, technologies like Wi-Fi, LoRa, SigFox, or cellular (5G) can also serve as complements or substitutes.

2.3.3 IoMT use cases

This section presents the different IoMT use cases considering various aspects of healthcare applications. Figure 2.3 illustrates these different IoMT use cases.

2.3.3.1 Remote patient monitoring

Remote Patient Monitoring (RPM) stands as a transformative application within the IoMT, revolutionizing healthcare delivery by introducing real-time and remote monitoring capabilities. This facet of IoMT leverages a spectrum of interconnected medical devices and sensors to continually observe and collect critical patient data, such as vital signs and health metrics, from a distance. Through this continuous surveillance, healthcare providers gain the ability to track patients' well-being

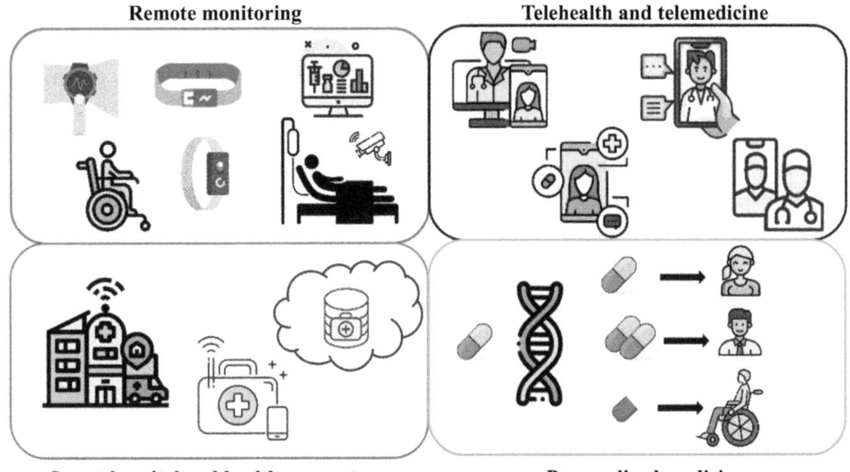

Figure 2.3 IoMT use cases

remotely, offering an unprecedented level of visibility into their health status [43,44]. The significance of RPM becomes particularly evident in the context of managing chronic conditions. IoMT facilitates the seamless monitoring of patients with long-term health issues, allowing healthcare professionals to keep a watchful eye on key indicators without the need for frequent in-person visits. This proactive approach enables early detection of abnormalities or deviations from baseline health parameters. The remote nature of patient monitoring not only enhances the efficiency of healthcare delivery but also empowers providers to intervene promptly and make informed decisions, contributing to more effective and personalized care strategies [45,46]. In essence, RPM exemplifies how IoMT applications are reshaping healthcare practices, promoting preventive care, and fostering a more patient-centric approach to medical management.

2.3.3.2 Telehealth and Telemedicine

Telehealth and Telemedicine, in healthcare delivery, provide an innovative approach to medical consultations as they facilitate virtual healthcare consultations, breaking down geographical barriers and enabling patients to connect with healthcare professionals from the convenience of their homes. Through this technology, individuals can access medical expertise without the need for physical presence, fostering a more accessible and flexible healthcare landscape [47]. This capability is especially crucial for individuals in remote areas where access to healthcare facilities may be limited. IoMT-driven Telehealth bridges the gap, ensuring that even those in geographically isolated regions can receive timely medical consultations and advice. Moreover, during global health crises, such as pandemics, where physical distancing is imperative, Telehealth becomes an indispensable tool [48]. IoMT facilitates the seamless exchange of medical information, allowing healthcare providers to remotely assess and diagnose patients while minimizing the risk of viral transmission. This not only ensures continuity of care but also plays a vital role in reducing the strain on healthcare systems during periods of heightened demand.

2.3.3.3 Smart Hospitals and healthcare systems

Smart Hospitals leverage IoMT to create interconnected networks of medical devices, sensors, and systems, fostering an environment where data-driven insights contribute to enhanced decision-making [25,49]. IoMT's impact on Smart Hospitals is particularly pronounced in optimizing resource utilization. Through real-time monitoring and analysis, IoMT allows healthcare administrators to gain a comprehensive understanding of resource allocation and consumption patterns. This enables proactive decision-making to ensure that resources such as medical equipment, staff, and beds are utilized optimally, minimizing inefficiencies and enhancing overall operational efficiency [50,51]. IoMT's contribution extends to improving patient flow within the hospital. By leveraging data on patient movement, bed occupancy, and treatment progress, healthcare providers can streamline processes, reduce wait times, and ensure a more fluid and patient-centric healthcare experience [13].

2.3.3.4 Personalized medicine

In the context of personalized medicine, this granular patient data becomes instrumental. Healthcare providers can leverage this wealth of information to tailor treatment plans with an unprecedented level of precision. Instead of employing generalized approaches, personalized medicine enables healthcare professionals to consider an individual's unique genetic makeup, lifestyle factors, and real-time health data [52]. This tailored approach not only enhances the effectiveness of medical interventions but also minimizes potential side effects, leading to more targeted and optimized healthcare strategies. IoMT, in this capacity, emerges as a key enabler in the realization of personalized medicine, fostering a healthcare landscape where treatments are finely tuned to the specific needs of each patient [44].

2.4 Cybersecurity requirements for the IoMT for healthcare applications

This section provides an overview of technical system requirements related to cybersecurity IoMT for healthcare applications.

Cybersecurity requirements for IoMT consist of several conventional security requirements to ensure the security and privacy of clinical data and systems through two main segments as shown in Figure 2.4. First, the CIA triad ensures the data security for IoMT through confidentiality, integrity, and availability. Second is the non-CIA which unlike the first consists of seven main features which include authentication, authorization, accountability, privacy, auditing, and non-repudiation [1,53]. Although privacy was categorized under the non-CIA triad, it is sometimes used interchangeably with confidentiality [54].

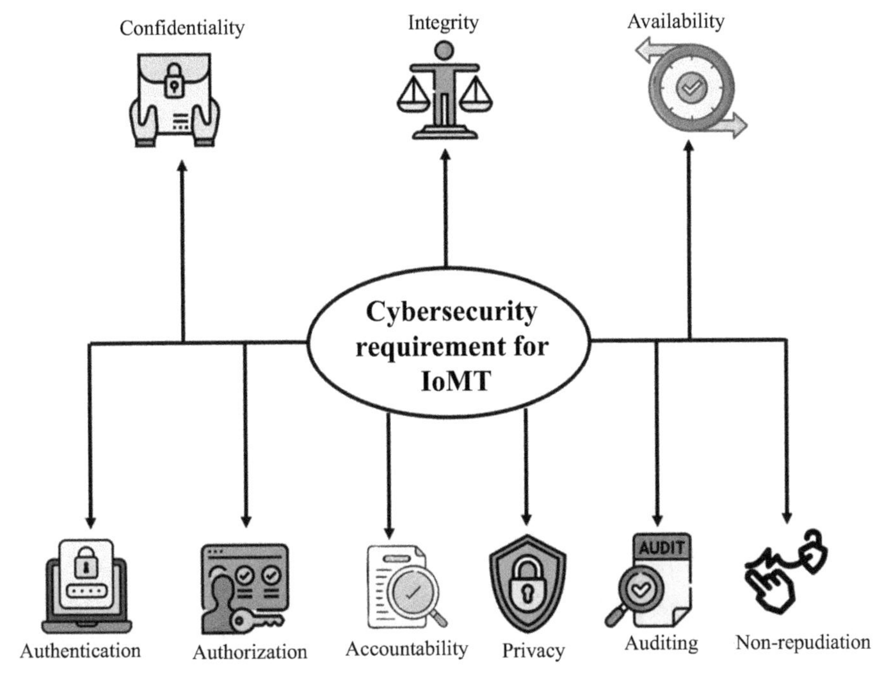

Figure 2.4 Cybersecurity requirements for IoMT for healthcare applications

2.4.1 Confidentiality/privacy

Confidentiality or privacy is a crucial aspect of securing sensitive patient information in IoMT applications, encompassing interconnected medical devices, wearables, and sensors [17]. The data exchanged in this ecosystem often includes highly personal and confidential details about a patient's health. Interception, often considered a primary attack vector, involves attackers intercepting communications between devices (e.g., wearables, sensors, or medical devices) and servers or clouds [55]. Notably, eavesdropping, either active or passive eavesdropping, is a common example of an interception attack. To ensure confidentiality, various measures are recommended in the literature. These include implementing strong authentication methods and access controls [56–58], conducting penetration testing and vulnerability assessments [59,60], and employing end-to-end encryption during the transmission of sensitive medical data to prevent unauthorized access [61]. Additionally, compliance with industry-specific privacy regulations, standards, and continuous security awareness training for healthcare professionals and users are integral components of a comprehensive approach to reinforce confidentiality measures within the IoMT landscape.

2.4.2 Integrity

Integrity refers to the assurance that data and information transmitted or stored remain accurate, unaltered, and trustworthy throughout its lifecycle [58]. It is another crucial aspect of securing sensitive patient information as it directly influences the reliability of medical diagnoses, treatment plans, and patient outcomes. A breach in data integrity could lead to severe consequences, including misdiagnoses, incorrect treatment decisions, or unauthorized access to sensitive patient information [13,62]. Modification and fabrication attacks are the two major threats to integrity [63]. A modification attack refers to the unauthorized alterations or changes made to data during its transmission or storage to manipulate information, thus compromising its integrity. A fabrication attack, on the other hand, involves the creation and insertion of counterfeit or fictitious data into a system with the intent to deceive or disrupt normal operations. Maintaining the integrity of clinical data in IoMT both during transmission and storage can be achieved by implementing mechanisms such as tamper-evident technologies, cryptographic techniques, and secure data transmission protocols [63]. Furthermore, similar to ensuring confidentiality, adherence to regulations, guidelines, and standards can further enhance the overall data reliability and effectiveness of IoMT-enabled healthcare applications, fostering a secure and resilient healthcare infrastructure.

2.4.3 Availability

Availability is another cybersecurity requirement within the CIA triad, and it involves safeguarding against disruptions caused by cyberattacks, system failures, or unforeseen events. In healthcare, where timely access to critical information can be a matter of life and death, ensuring the continuous availability of IoMT systems is paramount. The interruption attack, such as Denial of Service (DoS), is a major threat to availability [11,64]. To achieve robust availability in IoMT for healthcare applications, various measures are implemented. Redundancy mechanisms, such as backup systems and failover capabilities, are crucial for maintaining continuous operation even in the face of hardware failures or cyber incidents. Additionally, real-time monitoring and proactive threat detection help identify potential issues before they escalate, allowing for timely intervention. Robust data backup and recovery strategies ensure that critical healthcare data remains accessible, even in the aftermath of security incidents.

2.4.4 Authentication

Authentication is a fundamental cybersecurity requirement, however within the non-CIA triad [1,53]. It plays a crucial role in verifying the identity of users, devices, and entities accessing sensitive healthcare data. Given the sensitive nature of medical information and the potential consequences of unauthorized access or tampering, robust authentication mechanisms are essential to ensure the confidentiality and integrity of patient data. Proper authentication protocols help establish trust in the IoMT system, preventing unauthorized individuals or malicious entities from gaining access to patient records, treatment plans, or other critical healthcare information. A Man-in-the-Middle (MitM) is one of the major threats to authentication, wherein the attacker controls and monitors the communication between two legitimate parties while altering the transmitted data [64]. Other examples of attacks on authentication include brute force attacks, masquerading attacks, replay attacks, cracking attacks, dictionary attacks, rainbow table attacks, session hijacking attacks, and birthday attacks [64]. Authentication measures can include multi-factor authentication, biometric verification, and secure access controls. Implementing strong authentication mechanisms not only protects individual patient data but also upholds the overall integrity and trustworthiness of the IoMT infrastructure.

2.4.5 Authorization

Authorization refers to the process of granting or denying access to specific resources or functionalities within a network or system. It is a fundamental mechanism to ensure that only authorized individuals, devices, or entities have the right to access and manipulate sensitive medical data and connected devices [1,6,65]. In healthcare, where the confidentiality and integrity of patient information are paramount, robust authorization mechanisms play a crucial role in safeguarding against unauthorized access, data breaches, and potential malicious activities. It involves the implementation of access control policies, defining who or what can access specific resources and under what circumstances [19,66]. This encompasses user authentication, device validation, and the assignment of appropriate privileges based on roles and responsibilities. For example, healthcare professionals may have different levels of access to patient records based on their roles, and devices such as medical sensors may be granted specific permissions to interact with the healthcare network.

2.4.6 Accountability

Accountability is a crucial element in preserving the integrity, confidentiality, and availability of sensitive data, particularly clinical data. Traceability, a key component of accountability, enables the tracking and attribution of actions to specific entities or devices, essential for investigating security incidents and identifying the sources of breaches [19]. This traceability not only discourages malicious actors but also fosters a culture of responsible use, instilling confidence among healthcare providers and patients regarding the security of IoMT systems. Social engineering and malware attacks are the two major attacks on authorization [6,67,68]. Moreover, accountability in IoMT extends beyond individual devices to encompass the entire ecosystem, involving manufacturers, healthcare providers, regulatory bodies, and end-users. Manufacturers are accountable for designing and producing secure devices, implementing robust security measures, and providing updates to address emerging threats [69]. Healthcare providers bear the responsibility of implementing and maintaining secure networks, employing encryption methods, and ensuring the confidentiality of patient information. Regulatory bodies play a pivotal role in holding all stakeholders accountable through the establishment and enforcement of cybersecurity standards and regulations.

2.4.7 Auditing

Auditing serves as a critical cybersecurity requirement for IoMT in healthcare applications, ensuring the integrity, confidentiality, and availability of sensitive clinical data. Given the diverse and interconnected nature of IoMT devices, ranging from medical sensors to smart healthcare devices, establishing a robust auditing framework becomes imperative. This framework involves continuous monitoring, examination of system activities, and tracking of user interactions and data transactions to promptly detect and respond to security incidents [1,70]. Adopting a proactive approach, auditing allows healthcare organizations to identify potential vulnerabilities, unauthorized access, or anomalous behavior indicative of cyber threats [6]. Beyond enhancing security, auditing assists organizations in demonstrating compliance with regulations by maintaining detailed records of security events. In the event of a security breach, audit logs prove invaluable for forensic analysis, enabling organizations to trace the breach's source, understand its impact, and implement necessary corrective measures. Integrating auditing as a fundamental cybersecurity requirement strengthens IoMT environments, fortifying their overall security posture and mitigating the evolving threat landscape in the healthcare sector.

2.4.8 Non-repudiation

Non-repudiation is another crucial cybersecurity requirement for the IoMT that ensures the integrity and accountability of digital communications within healthcare systems [1,6]. Non-repudiation implies that a sender of information, such as a medical device or system, cannot deny the authenticity of the transmitted data or the fact that they initiated the communication [54,71]. For example, when a medical device records patient data or when a healthcare professional accesses electronic health records, non-repudiation ensures that the origin and authenticity of these actions cannot be denied. This cybersecurity measure is particularly vital in healthcare settings, where accurate and unambiguous records of patient data, treatment decisions, and device interactions are paramount. Non-repudiation safeguards against disputes or denial of involvement in a particular action, providing a verifiable trail of communication that can be relied upon for legal and regulatory purposes. In the IoMT landscape, where the potential consequences of information tampering or false claims could be severe, non-repudiation mechanisms contribute to the establishment of trust, accountability, and the overall security posture of connected medical devices and systems.

2.5 Cyberattacks in the IoMT for healthcare applications

The terms "*cyber threat*" and "*cyberattacks*" are related to the field of cybersecurity, but they represent different stages in the lifecycle of a potential security incident. A cyber threat is a general term used to describe any potential or actual malicious activity or occurrence that may exploit vulnerabilities in a computer system or network. A cyberattack, on the other hand, is a specific, deliberate, and purposeful action or series of actions carried out by cybercriminals or threat actors with the intent to compromise the confidentiality, integrity, or availability of information systems, data, or networks. Essentially, cyberattacks are the actual execution or implementation of a cyber threat. This section presents and discusses these different cyberattacks in IoMT for healthcare applications [72], these include the following.

2.5.1 Malware attacks

Malware, in the context of IoMT, refers to any malicious software designed to infiltrate, disrupt, or damage medical devices and systems connected to the internet. The diverse range of medical devices within IoMT, including wearables, implantable devices, and connected medical equipment, creates a broad attack surface for malware [73]. Common methods for malware attacks encompass worms, computer viruses, ransomware, harmful mobile code, Trojan horses, rootkits, or other code-based entities with malicious intent that effectively infiltrate a system [6,64]. These malicious programs can compromise the functionality of medical devices, leading to potentially life-threatening consequences for patients. For instance, malware may target the software controlling drug infusion pumps or manipulate the readings of vital signs monitoring devices, endangering patient safety and disrupting critical healthcare operations. The unique challenges posed by malware in IoMT include the need for real-time data processing and transmission, making rapid detection and response crucial. Furthermore, the interconnected nature of IoMT devices allows malware to propagate swiftly through the network, potentially compromising an entire healthcare system [74]. Essentially, the consequences of malware attacks on the IoMT extend beyond data breaches, reaching the potential compromise of patient well-being. This emphasizes the need for a comprehensive and proactive cybersecurity approach to mitigate these risks.

2.5.2 Man-in-the-middle (MitM) attacks

In an IoMT environment, where devices such as medical sensors, wearables, and monitoring systems communicate seamlessly to collect and transmit patient data, MitM attacks involve an unauthorized entity intercepting and potentially altering the information exchanged [72]. For example, an attacker could position themselves between a medical device and the central monitoring system, as shown in Figure 2.5, intercepting sensitive patient data such as vital signs or treatment information.

By doing so, the attacker gains unauthorized access to confidential medical information, jeopardizing patient privacy and the integrity of healthcare data. The consequences of MitM attacks in IoMT extend beyond data interception. Attackers can manipulate the transmitted data, leading to false readings or deceptive information sent to healthcare providers [64]. This not only compromises the accuracy of medical diagnoses and treatment decisions but also poses severe risks to patient safety.

2.5.3 Traffic analysis attacks

A traffic analysis attack, a form of passive attack, involves the meticulous monitoring and examination of communication traffic among medical devices, sensors,

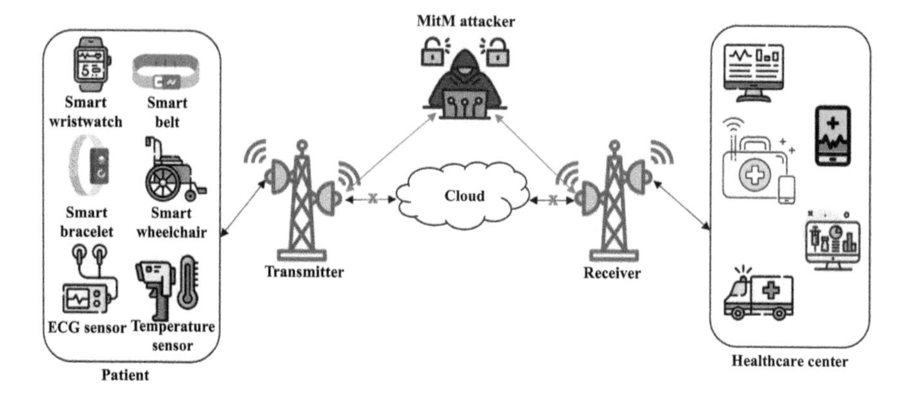

Figure 2.5 Man-in-the-middle attack on IoMT systems

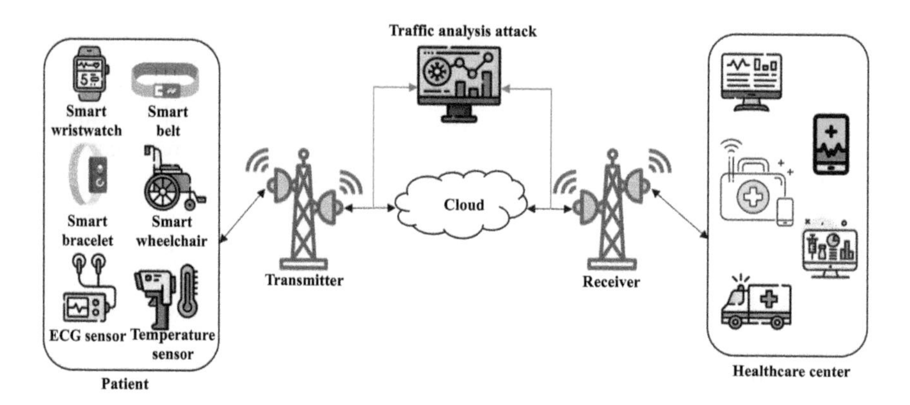

Figure 2.6 Traffic analysis attack

and healthcare systems [6]. Unlike traditional cyber threats, these attacks aim to extract sensitive information without directly intercepting the actual content of the transmitted data as shown in Figure 2.6.

Adversaries employ techniques that scrutinize the timing, frequency, and size of data packets, allowing them to deduce patterns related to patient activities, treatment routines, and specific medical conditions [72,75]. The potential consequences of these attacks in IoMT are severe, posing risks such as compromising patient privacy, enabling unauthorized medical interventions, or manipulating health records. Beyond privacy breaches, these attacks impact the integrity and reliability of medical data [64]. Attackers may manipulate or disrupt communication patterns between medical devices, leading to potential misinformation in healthcare decision-making processes. Furthermore, the insights gained through traffic analysis can be leveraged for more advanced cyber threats, including targeted attacks and social engineering schemes.

2.5.4 Ransomware attacks

Ransomware attacks, a subset of malware attacks, represent a prominent cyber threat in IoMT, wherein malicious actors exploit specific vulnerabilities, such as outdated software or inadequate access controls, to gain unauthorized entry into critical healthcare infrastructure [64]. Once infiltrated, assailants encrypt vital medical data or disable access to essential medical devices, demanding a ransom for their release. Given the unique and critical nature of healthcare data, IoMT becomes an attractive target for ransomware perpetrators, as compromised systems often house sensitive patient records, treatment plans, and other life-saving information [72]. The effects of a successful ransomware attack on IoMT are severe, potentially disrupting patient care, compromising sensitive medical information, and causing extensive financial losses to healthcare institutions. Attackers frequently target vulnerabilities in connected medical devices and exploit weak cybersecurity protocols within healthcare networks, emphasizing the importance of robust security measures to safeguard critical medical data [76]. The aftermath of such attacks extends beyond immediate financial losses, encompassing recovery expenses, legal consequences, regulatory fines, and a significant erosion of public trust in the ability of healthcare systems to secure crucial medical information.

2.5.5 Denial-of-service (DoS) attacks

As previously highlighted, DoS attacks pose a significant threat to the availability of IoMT systems. In a DoS attack, malicious actors flood a system with an overwhelming volume of traffic, rendering it unresponsive or completely unavailable [6,65,72], as shown in Figure 2.7.

This assault can result in disruptions to essential medical services, affecting real-time patient monitoring, the seamless transmission of crucial health data, and the overall operational efficiency of IoMT-enabled healthcare solutions [64]. The effects of a successful DoS attack in a medical context are severe, potentially jeopardizing patient safety and hindering the timely delivery of healthcare

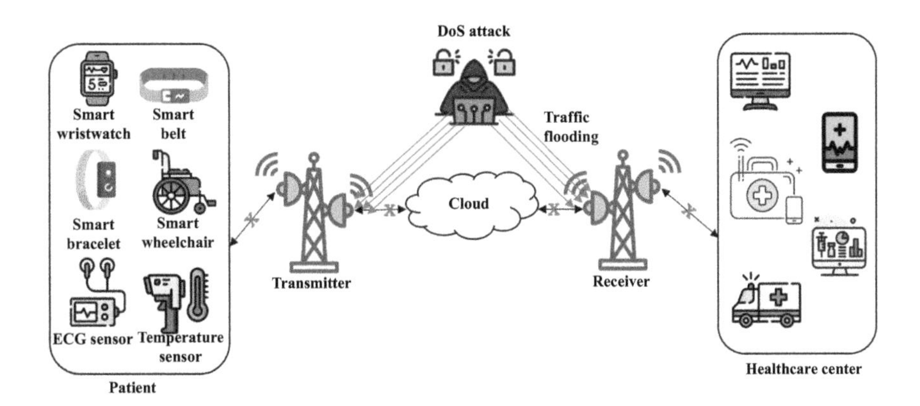

Figure 2.7 Denial-of-service (DoS) attack

services [65]. DoS attacks may take various forms, including bandwidth depletion, resource exhaustion, or exploitation of communication protocols. Attackers may employ tactics such as flooding the network with excessive traffic, exploiting vulnerabilities in medical devices, or manipulating communication protocols to deplete resources and disrupt the normal functioning of the interconnected medical system.

2.5.6 Social engineering attacks

Social engineering attacks represent a significant cybersecurity attack on IoMT, employing manipulative techniques to exploit human behavior and gain unauthorized access to sensitive medical data and connected devices [77]. Techniques such as phishing, pretexting, and baiting are frequently utilized to deceive healthcare professionals or individuals, leading them to disclose confidential information, inadvertently download malware, or compromise the integrity of medical devices [78]. The two major types of social engineering attacks include reverse engineering and error debugging attacks [64]. The success of social engineering attacks relies on the exploitation of trust, often involving the impersonation of trusted entities within the healthcare environment. Infiltrating IoMT through social engineering not only jeopardizes patient privacy but also poses risks to the integrity of medical data, potentially leading to misdiagnoses, unauthorized access to medical records, or even tampering with treatment plans.

2.5.7 Identity spoofing attacks

In an identity spoofing attack, malicious entities attempt to gain unauthorized access to IoMT devices or networks by impersonating a legitimate user, device, or system [72]. This could involve the use of stolen credentials, fake authentication tokens, or other deceptive means to trick the IoMT system into believing that the attacker is a trusted entity. Once successful, the attacker may exploit this false identity to manipulate or access sensitive medical information, disrupt healthcare operations, or even introduce malicious software into the IoMT network [75]. The consequences of identity spoofing attacks on IoMT can be severe, as they compromise the trustworthiness of the entire healthcare infrastructure. Patient confidentiality is jeopardized, potentially leading to unauthorized access to medical records, unauthorized control of medical devices, and interference with critical healthcare processes.

2.6 Countermeasures for IoMT cyberattacks in healthcare applications

Securing and safeguarding sensitive patient data is paramount in IoMT to ensure the integrity of medical devices, and prevent cyberattacks that could compromise patient safety. Several methods have been proposed in the literature to protect against cyberattacks, below are the countermeasures to enhance the cybersecurity of IoMT.

2.6.1 Network segmentation

Network segmentation is a cybersecurity strategy that isolates critical healthcare systems and devices from broader networks, this approach creates distinct segments, minimizing the attack surface and mitigating the risk of lateral movement by malicious actors. In the event of a security breach, network segmentation acts as a containment measure, confining the impact within specific segments and safeguarding sensitive medical data and critical infrastructure [8].

2.6.2 Strong authentication and access controls

This can safeguard sensitive medical data and maintain the integrity of IoMT networks Implementing strong authentication measures such as multi-factor authentication is crucial for securing IoMT devices and systems. This ensures that only authorized individuals have access, thereby enhancing the overall security of the system. Strict access controls based on the principle of least privilege further limit user permissions, minimizing the risk of unauthorized access or potential breaches [79].

2.6.3 Encryption

Encryption employs algorithms to encode sensitive information, ensuring the confidentiality and integrity of patient data. End-to-end encryption safeguards information both during transmission and storage, thwarting potential breaches. By converting data into unreadable code, unauthorized access becomes challenging, bolstering the security of healthcare systems. This technology plays a crucial role in maintaining the privacy of patient information and securing communication channels between medical devices [79].

2.6.4 Jamming solution

To mitigate jamming attacks that can disrupt services and communication between medical devices and healthcare professionals, it is imperative to implement security measures such as deploying backup computational medical devices and servers. This ensures uninterrupted availability and minimal loss of critical patient health updates. Implementing security measures such as the deployment of backup computational medical devices and servers for uninterrupted availability is highly imperative. Additionally, incorporating measures like channel surfing, spatial retreat, and priority messages can enhance defense against wireless denial-of-service attacks in the IoMT domain [64].

2.6.5 Intrusion detection system (IDS)

Intrusion Detection System (IDS) serves as the primary means for identifying attacks within IoMT systems. There are various types of IDS applicable in this context, including Host-based IDS (HIDS) and Network-based IDS (NIDS). HIDS is connected to specific IoMT devices to oversee potential malicious activities, while NIDS monitors the network traffic of multiple IoMT devices to identify any suspicious behavior. Safeguarding IoMT systems and networks involves the

Table 2.2 Cyberattacks and corresponding countermeasures with descriptions

Ref.	Cyberattacks	Countermeasures	Description
[8]	Malware attacks and denial-of-service (DoS) attacks	Network segmentation	Minimizes attack surface, mitigates lateral movement risks, and acts as a containment measure during security breaches
[79]	Identity spoofing attacks and social engineering attacks	Strong authentication and access controls	Implements multi-factor authentication and strict access controls to safeguard sensitive medical data and maintain IoMT network integrity
[79]	Man-in-the-middle (MitM) attacks, traffic analysis attacks, and ransomware attacks.	Encryption	Utilizes algorithms to encode sensitive information, ensuring confidentiality and integrity of patient data
[64]	Denial-of-service (DoS) attacks	Jamming solution	Addresses the risks of jamming attacks that disrupt services and communication between medical devices
[64]	Ransomware attacks, and malware attacks	Intrusion detection system (IDS)	Serves as the primary means for identifying attacks within IoMT systems

implementation of IDS to promptly detect abnormal activities, allowing timely intervention and appropriate actions to prevent any incidents [64].

By implementing a combination of these countermeasures, healthcare organizations can enhance the resilience of their IoMT infrastructure and better protect against cyber threats. Given the evolving nature of cybersecurity risks, continuous monitoring, adaptation, and collaboration within the healthcare industry are crucial to staying ahead of potential threats. Table 2.2 provides an overview of various cyberattacks along with their corresponding countermeasures, accompanied by concise descriptions of these preventative measures. Although these countermeasures can be used alone for these attacks, a combination of two or more countermeasures would be stronger and more effective.

2.7 Emerging technologies for IoMT security

IoMT is transforming healthcare with its interconnected devices, facilitating remote monitoring, personalized medicine, and efficient healthcare delivery. However, the proliferation of IoMT also introduces security challenges, necessitating the adoption of emerging technologies to fortify the cybersecurity landscape [80]. Below are some of the key emerging technologies contributing to IoMT security:

2.7.1 Blockchain

Blockchain offers a decentralized and tamper-resistant system [81]. By utilizing a secure and immutable ledger for health data, Blockchain enhances data integrity and protects against unauthorized access. Its decentralized nature, coupled with cryptographic features, ensures that health records are resistant to tampering, providing a robust layer of security for sensitive patient information [82,83]. Additionally, the introduction of smart contracts in Blockchain enables automated and enforceable security protocols, allowing for streamlined access management and enhancing data privacy within complex healthcare ecosystems. While challenges such as scalability and regulatory considerations exist, the potential of Blockchain in bolstering IoMT security showcases a proactive approach to fortifying interconnected medical devices and fostering trust among stakeholders [84–86].

2.7.2 Artificial Intelligence

Artificial Intelligence (AI) is playing a pivotal role in enhancing the security of the IoMT. With IoMT's intricate network of medical devices and vast health data, AI brings advanced capabilities to address security challenges effectively [87–90]. One key application is in threat detection and anomaly identification, where machine learning algorithms analyze patterns in data to establish baseline behavior [91,92]. This proactive approach allows AI systems to detect deviations and potential security threats, enabling early intervention and minimizing the risk of unauthorized access or data compromise [93,94]. Additionally, AI contributes to authentication and access control through advanced biometric techniques, ensuring that only authorized personnel have access to medical devices. The use of AI-driven behavioral analytics further enhances security by continuously assessing user behavior for any signs of suspicious activities. Furthermore, AI is instrumental in securing health data within IoMT. Advanced encryption algorithms, often powered by AI, provide robust protection for data both in transit and at rest. This ensures the confidentiality and privacy of sensitive medical information. While the integration of AI in IoMT security holds immense promise, addressing challenges such as interpretability and ethical considerations is crucial [95–97]. Nevertheless, AI stands as a key enabler in fortifying IoMT's security infrastructure, providing advanced capabilities for threat detection, authentication, and data encryption to uphold the integrity and confidentiality of medical information.

2.7.3 Software defined network (SDN)

SDN provides centralized control and programmability, enabling enhanced network segmentation. This segmentation isolates different categories of medical devices, reducing the risk of lateral movement by potential threats [98,99]. SDN's dynamic and adaptive security policies enable real-time adjustments based on evolving threats, ensuring a proactive response to security incidents. Furthermore, SDN contributes to improved visibility and monitoring of network traffic, allowing for timely detection of anomalies and potential security threats [99]. While challenges like interoperability need consideration, SDN's application in IoMT security demonstrates its potential to create a flexible and adaptive framework, elevating the overall cybersecurity posture in healthcare environments [100,101].

2.7.4 Big Data

Big Data analytics plays a crucial role in anomaly detection and predictive analytics. By employing advanced algorithms, it can sift through massive datasets to identify patterns and anomalies, enabling the early detection of potential security threats within the IoMT ecosystem. Additionally, Big Data analytics contributes to contextual understanding by correlating diverse data sources, facilitating a comprehensive view of the security landscape, and enhancing incident response in near real-time [102,103]. While challenges like data privacy and interoperability persist, the application of Big Data analytics in IoMT security underscores its potential to harness data insights and fortify the overall cybersecurity posture in healthcare environments.

2.8 Lessons learned

This section highlights and discusses the salient lessons learned from the chapter, which can be used to guide further research in cybersecurity in IoMT.

2.8.1 Lesson 1: IoMT has revolutionized the modern healthcare system

The introduction of IoMT, as discussed in this chapter, marks a transformative era for the modern healthcare system. This interconnected network has significantly improved patient care through remote monitoring, real-time data analysis, and personalized treatment plans. Continuous monitoring of vital signs enables healthcare providers to detect anomalies early, facilitating timely interventions and preventive measures. This not only enhances care quality but also boosts overall healthcare system efficiency, alleviating the burden on hospitals and promoting a more proactive, patient-centric approach. Furthermore, IoMT has demonstrated its ability to streamline healthcare processes and enhance communication among healthcare professionals. The seamless exchange of information between medical devices, electronic health records, and healthcare practitioners has enhanced collaboration and decision-making. For instance, wearable devices and smart medical equipment can transmit real-time data to healthcare providers, enabling them to make informed decisions promptly. Thus, there is a need for further advancement of this technology which will result in the enhancement of the overall healthcare systems.

2.8.2 Lesson 2: IoMT system is vulnerable to several cyber threats and attacks

While IoMT systems offer numerous advantages in the healthcare sector, their interconnected nature also exposes them to potential cyber threats and attacks. This creates opportunities for malicious actors to exploit vulnerabilities, compromising the integrity, confidentiality, and availability of sensitive health data. Cyber adversaries may exploit these interconnected devices to gain unauthorized access, manipulate patient data, or disrupt critical healthcare services. IoMT systems are susceptible to various types of cyberattacks, including malware, ransomware, and identity theft. This inherent vulnerability underscores the critical necessity for implementing robust cybersecurity measures. Ensuring the security of sensitive medical data is paramount to safeguarding the overall integrity and functionality of IoMT systems, reinforcing the need for proactive cybersecurity strategies in the healthcare industry.

2.8.3 Lesson 3: IoMT system security can be enhanced with emerging technologies

The increasing integration of connected devices in healthcare necessitates a proactive approach to address vulnerabilities associated with interconnected technologies. Emerging technologies such as AI, SDN, Big Data, and blockchain have demonstrated their effectiveness in bolstering the security of IoMT systems. AI, for example, proves valuable in real-time threat detection and anomaly identification within medical networks, serving as a proactive defense against potential cyber threats. SDN contributes to improved visibility and monitoring of network traffic, facilitating timely detection of anomalies and potential security threats. Additionally, blockchain technology ensures data integrity and transparency, safeguarding the immutability of medical records and transactions to mitigate the risk of unauthorized access or tampering. To further strengthen the security of IoMT systems, there is a need for continued integration and enhancement of these emerging technologies. This collaborative approach aims to fortify defenses against potential security threats and attacks on IoMT systems, ultimately safeguarding the integrity and confidentiality of healthcare data.

2.8.4 Lesson 4: Collaborative governance and standardization are crucial for IoMT security

As the IoMT network involves a multitude of stakeholders, including healthcare providers, technology developers, regulatory bodies, and end-users, a cohesive and standardized approach to security is paramount. Collaborative governance involves the joint efforts of various stakeholders, including healthcare providers, technology developers, regulatory bodies, and cybersecurity experts, to establish comprehensive security protocols. This collaborative approach fosters a shared understanding of potential threats and vulnerabilities, allowing for the development of standardized security measures that can be universally applied across the IoMT ecosystem. By leveraging the collective expertise of diverse stakeholders, collaborative governance enhances the adaptability and effectiveness of security frameworks, ensuring that they remain agile in addressing emerging challenges and technological advancements. Industry-wide standards foster interoperability, facilitating seamless communication and integration within the IoMT infrastructure while maintaining robust security. Standardization simplifies regulatory compliance and audits, streamlining processes for manufacturers and healthcare organizations. Adherence to standardized security practices enhances transparency and accountability, instilling confidence among end-users, healthcare professionals, and regulators.

2.8.5 Lesson 5: Continuous education and training are essential for IoMT security

As previously mentioned, the IoMT network involves numerous stakeholders, providing opportunities for cyber attackers to exploit vulnerabilities. Unauthorized access stands out as the most common threat to the IoMT network, with attackers employing tactics like social engineering to manipulate human behavior and gain entry to sensitive medical data and connected devices. To address this, there is a critical need for ongoing education, training, and security awareness campaigns for all stakeholders. These initiatives play a vital role in ensuring and maintaining the security measures of IoMT devices, fortifying the entire ecosystem against potential cyber threats.

2.9 Conclusion and future scope

The integration of IoMT in healthcare presents unparalleled opportunities for improved patient care and medical advancements. However, the increased connectivity also introduces substantial cybersecurity challenges that threaten patient data and, in severe cases, lives. This chapter has explored the complex cybersecurity landscape within the IoMT for healthcare applications, scrutinizing the evolving threat landscape and vulnerabilities specific to this ecosystem. Additionally, it has delved into the strategies and technologies employed to bolster the defenses of healthcare systems against a diverse array of cyber threats. Continuous awareness training for healthcare staff is imperative to ensure vigilance against evolving cyber threats. Regular updates on cybersecurity best practices, including recognizing phishing attempts and adhering to secure password policies, to significantly mitigate the risk of human error as a common entry point for cyberattacks are further recommended. Future work or research can focus on utilizing emerging technologies for securing and enhancing the use of IoMT in healthcare organizations.

References

[1] Nasiri, S.; Sadoughi, F.; Tadayon, M.; Dehnad, A. Security Requirements of Internet of Things-Based Healthcare System: A Survey Study. *Acta Inform. Medica* 2019, *27*, 253, doi:10.5455/aim.2019.27.253-258.

[2] Kagita, M.K.; Thilakarathne, N.; Gadekallu, T.R.; Maddikunta, P.K.R. A Review on Security and Privacy of Internet of Medical Things. In *Intelligent Internet of Things for Healthcare and Industry*; Springer, 2022; pp. 171–187.

[3] Chukwu, N.P.; Edeagu, S.; Chijindu, V.; *et al.* Challenges of Security and Privacy with IoT in Healthcare: An Overview. In Proceedings of the International Conference on Technological Innovation for Holistic Sustainable Development; Nsukka, Nigeria, 2022; pp. 98–104.

[4] Raj, H.; Kumar, M.; Kumar, P.; Singh, A.; Verma, O.P. Issues and Challenges Related to Privacy and Security in Healthcare Using IoT, Fog, and Cloud Computing. In *Advanced Healthcare Systems*; Wiley, 2022; pp. 21–32.

[5] Huang, C.; Wang, J.; Wang, S.; Zhang, Y. Internet of Medical Things: A Systematic Review. *Neurocomputing* 2023, *557*, 126719, doi:10.1016/j.neucom.2023.126719.

[6] Papaioannou, M.; Karageorgou, M.; Mantas, G.; *et al.* A Survey on Security Threats and Countermeasures in Internet of Medical Things (IoMT). *Trans. Emerg. Telecommun. Technol.* 2022, *33*, e4049.

[7] Khaled, A.E. Internet of Medical Things (IoMT): Overview, Taxonomies, and Classifications. *J. Comput. Commun.* 2022, *10*, 64–89, doi:10.4236/jcc.2022.108005.

[8] Elhoseny, M.; Thilakarathne, N.N.; Alghamdi, M.I.; *et al.* Security and Privacy Issues in Medical Internet of Things: Overview, Countermeasures, Challenges and Future Directions. *Sustainability* 2021, *13*, 11645, doi:10.3390/su132111645.

[9] Jacqulyn, V.; Thiruchelvi, R.; Rajakumari, K. Internet of Medical Things (IoMT) – Medical Applications and It's Cyber Security. In *Applications of Artificial Intelligence and Machine Learning in Healthcare*; Technoarete Publishing, 2022.

[10] Vishnu, S.; Ramson, S.R.J.; Jegan, R. Internet of Medical Things (IoMT)-An Overview. In *Proceedings of the 2020 5th International Conference on Devices, Circuits and Systems (ICDCS)*; IEEE, 2020; pp. 101–104.

[11] Thomasian, N.M.; Adashi, E.Y. Cybersecurity in the Internet of Medical Things. *Heal. Policy Technol.* 2021, *10*, 100549, doi:10.1016/j.hlpt.2021.100549.

[12] Amaraweera, S.P.; Halgamuge, M.N. Internet of Things in the Healthcare Sector: Overview of Security and Privacy Issues. In *Security, Privacy and Trust in the IoT Environment*; Springer International Publishing: Cham, 2019; pp. 153–179.

[13] Sun, Y.; Lo, F.P.-W.; Lo, B. Security and Privacy for the Internet of Medical Things Enabled Healthcare Systems: A Survey. *IEEE Access* 2019, *7*, 183339–183355, doi:10.1109/ACCESS.2019.2960617.

[14] Abounassar, E.M.; El-Kafrawy, P.; Abd El-Latif, A.A. Security and Interoperability Issues with Internet of Things (IoT) in Healthcare Industry: A Survey. In *Studies in Big Data*; Abd El-Latif, A.A., Abd-El-Atty, B., Venegas-Andraca, S.E., Mazurczyk, W., Gupta, B.B., Eds.; Springer International Publishing: Cham, 2022; Vol. 95, pp. 159–189.

[15] Awotunde, J.B.; Jimoh, R.G.; Folorunso, S.O.; Adeniyi, E.A.; Abiodun, K. M.; Banjo, O.O. Privacy and Security Concerns in IoT-Based Healthcare Systems. In *Internet of Things*; Springer, 2021; pp. 105–134.

[16] Sun, W.; Cai, Z.; Li, Y.; Liu, F.; Fang, S.; Wang, G. Security and Privacy in the Medical Internet of Things: A Review. *Secur. Commun. Networks* 2018, *2018*, 1–9, doi:10.1155/2018/5978636.

[17] Butpheng, C.; Yeh, K.-H.; Xiong, H. Security and Privacy in IoT-Cloud-Based e-Health Systems—A Comprehensive Review. *Symmetry (Basel).* 2020, *12*, 1191, doi:10.3390/sym12071191.

[18] Kamalov, F.; Pourghebleh, B.; Gheisari, M.; Liu, Y.; Moussa, S. Internet of Medical Things Privacy and Security: Challenges, Solutions, and Future Trends from a New Perspective. *Sustainability* 2023, *15*, 3317, doi:10.3390/su15043317.

[19] Hireche, R.; Mansouri, H.; Pathan, A.-S.K. Security and Privacy Management in Internet of Medical Things (IoMT): A Synthesis. *J. Cybersecurity Priv.* 2022, *2*, 640–661, doi:10.3390/jcp2030033.

[20] Pothuganti, K. Security Challenges in Internet of Things and Artificial Intelligence in Healthcare Applications. *J. Res. Dev.* 2021, *16*, 77–81.

[21] Bhukya, C.; Thakur, P.; Mudhivarthi, B.; Singh, G. Cybersecurity in Internet of Medical Vehicles: State-of-the-Art Analysis, Research Challenges and Future Perspectives. *Sensors* 2023, *23*, 8107, doi:10.3390/s23198107.

[22] Ameen, A.H.; Mohammed, M.A.; Rashid, A.N. Dimensions of Artificial Intelligence Techniques, Blockchain, and Cyber Security in the Internet of Medical Things: Opportunities, Challenges, and Future Directions. *J. Intell. Syst.* 2023, *32*, doi:10.1515/jisys-2022-0267.

[23] Alkatheiri, M.S.; Alghamdi, A.S. Blockchain-Assisted Cybersecurity for the Internet of Medical Things in the Healthcare Industry. *Electronics* 2023, *12*, 1801, doi:10.3390/electronics12081801.

[24] Mohd Aman, A.H.; Hassan, W.H.; Sameen, S.; Attarbashi, Z.S.; Alizadeh, M.; Latiff, L.A. IoMT amid COVID-19 Pandemic: Application, Architecture, Technology, and Security. *J. Netw. Comput. Appl.* 2021, *174*, 102886, doi:10.1016/j.jnca.2020.102886.

[25] Srivastava, J.; Routray, S.; Ahmad, S.; Waris, M.M. Internet of Medical Things (IoMT)-Based Smart Healthcare System: Trends and Progress. *Comput. Intell. Neurosci.* 2022, *2022*, doi:10.1155/2022/7218113.

[26] Bharati, S.; Podder, P.; Mondal, M.R.H.; Paul, P.K. Applications and Challenges of Cloud Integrated IoMT. *Stud. Syst. Decis. Control* 2021, *311*, 67–85, doi:10.1007/978-3-030-55833-8_4.

[27] Dilibal, C. Development of Edge-IoMT Computing Architecture for Smart Healthcare Monitoring Platform. In *Proceedings of the 4th International Symposium on Multidisciplinary Studies and Innovative Technologies, ISMSIT 2020 – Proceedings*; IEEE, 2020; pp. 1–4.

[28] Askar, N.A.; Habbal, A.; Mohammed, A.H.; Sajat, M.S.; Yusupov, Z.; Kodirov, D. Architecture, Protocols, and Applications of the Internet of Medical Things (IoMT). *J. Commun* 2022, *17*, 900–918.

[29] Razdan, S.; Sharma, S. Internet of Medical Things (IoMT): Overview, Emerging Technologies, and Case Studies. *IETE Tech. Rev. (Institution Electron. Telecommun. Eng. India)* 2022, *39*, 775–788, doi:10.1080/02564602.2021.1927863.

[30] Koutras, D.; Stergiopoulos, G.; Dasaklis, T.; Kotzanikolaou, P.; Glynos, D.; Douligeris, C. Security in IoMT Communications: A Survey. *Sensors (Switzerland)* 2020, *20*, 1–49, doi:10.3390/s20174828.

[31] Zaydi, H.; Bakkoury, Z. Holistic Data Processing: Designing the Intelligent Edge-to-Cloud Pathway for IoMT. *Int. J. Math. Comput. Sci.* 2024, *19*, 261–277.

[32] Pushpalatha, N.; Anbarasu, P.; Venkatesh, A. Communication Protocols for IoMT-Based Healthcare Systems. In *Cognitive Computing for Internet of Medical Things*; Chapman and Hall/CRC, 2022; pp. 59–75.

[33] Zubair, M.; Ghubaish, A.; Unal, D.; *et al.* Secure Bluetooth Communication in Smart Healthcare Systems: A Novel Community Dataset and Intrusion Detection System. *Sensors* 2022, *22*, 8280, doi:10.3390/s22218280.

[34] Ma, S.C.; Alkhaleefah, M.; Chang, Y.L.; *et al.* Inter-Multilevel Super-Orthogonal Space–Time Coding Scheme for Reliable ZigBee-Based IoMT Communications. *Sensors* 2022, *22*, 2695, doi:10.3390/s22072695.

[35] Martinez, C.J.; Galmes, S. Analysis of the Primary Attacks on IoMT Internet of Medical Things Communications Protocols. In *Proceedings of the 2022 IEEE World AI IoT Congress, AIIoT 2022*; IEEE, 2022; pp. 708–714.

[36] Palve, A.; Patel, H. Towards Securing Real Time Data in IoMT Environment. In Proceedings of the Proceedings - 2018 8th International Conference on Communication Systems and Network Technologies, CSNT 2018; IEEE, 2018; pp. 113–119.

[37] Mubdir, B.A.; Bayram, H.M.A. Adopting MQTT for a Multi Protocols IoMT System. *Int. J. Electr. Comput. Eng.* 2022, *12*, 834–844, doi:10.11591/ijece.v12i1.pp834-844.

[38] Das, K.; Dutta, T.L.; Ray, K.; *et al.* Performances of M2M Protocols in Internet of Medical Things. In Proceedings of the 2023 IEEE International Conference on Communications Workshops: Sustainable Communications for Renaissance, ICC Workshops 2023; IEEE, 2023; pp. 1289–1294.

[39] Zorkany, M.; Fahmy, K.; Yahya, A. Performance Evaluation of IoT Messaging Protocol Implementation for E-Health Systems. *Int. J. Adv. Comput. Sci. Appl.* 2019, *10*, 412–419, doi:10.14569/IJACSA.2019.0101157.

[40] Islam, M.M.; Nooruddin, S.; Karray, F.; Muhammad, G. Internet of Things: Device Capabilities, Architectures, Protocols, and Smart Applications in Healthcare Domain. *IEEE Internet Things J.* 2023, *10*, 3611–3641, doi:10.1109/JIOT.2022.3228795.

[41] Guo, R.; Zhou, X. The Design and Implementation of a Subway Monitoring System. In *Proceedings of the Academic Journal of Science and Technology*; 2022; Vol. 3, pp. 167–169.

[42] Al-Sarawi, S.; Anbar, M.; Alieyan, K.; Alzubaidi, M. Internet of Things (IoT) Communication Protocols: Review. In Proceedings of the ICIT 2017 – 8th International Conference on Information Technology, Proceedings; IEEE, 2017; pp. 685–690.

[43] Wijayarathne, S.N. Cyber Security Threats & Mitigations in the Healthcare Sector.

[44] Ejiyi, C.; Qin, Z.; Ejiyi, M.B.; *et al.* The Internet of Medical Things in Healthcare Management: A Review. *J. Digit. Heal.* 2023, 30–62, doi:10.55976/jdh.22023116330-62.

[45] Polu, S.K. IoMT Based Smart Health Care Monitoring System. *CEUR Workshop Proc.* 2019, *2544*, 58–64.

[46] Al Shorman, O.; Al Shorman, B.; Al-Khassaweneh, M.; Alkahtani, F. A Review of Internet of Medical Things (IoMT)-Based Remote Health Monitoring through Wearable Sensors: A Case Study for Diabetic Patients. *Indones. J. Electr. Eng. Comput. Sci.* 2020, *20*, 414–422, doi:10.11591/ijeecs.v20.i1.pp414-422.

[47] Mohamed, W.; Abdellatif, M.M. Telemedicine: An IoT Application for Healthcare Systems. In Proceedings of the ACM International Conference Proceeding Series; 2019; pp. 173–177.

[48] Shah, V.; Khang, A. Internet of Medical Things (IoMT) Driving the Digital Transformation of the Healthcare Sector. In *Data-Centric AI Solutions and Emerging Technologies in the Healthcare Ecosystem*; CRC Press, 2023; pp. 15–26.

[49] Dwivedi, R.; Mehrotra, D.; Chandra, S. Potential of Internet of Medical Things (IoMT) Applications in Building a Smart Healthcare System: A Systematic Review. *J. Oral Biol. Craniofacial Res.* 2022, *12*, 302–318.

[50] Awotunde, J.B.; Folorunso, S.O.; Ajagbe, S.A.; Garg, J.; Ajamu, G.J. AiIoMT: IoMT-Based System-Enabled Artificial Intelligence for Enhanced Smart Healthcare Systems. *Mach. Learn. Crit. Internet Med. Things Appl. Use Cases* 2022, 229–254, doi:10.1007/978-3-030-80928-7_10.

[51] Khan, M.F.; Ghazal, T.M.; Said, R.A.; *et al.* An IoMT-Enabled Smart Healthcare Model to Monitor Elderly People Using Machine Learning Technique. *Comput. Intell. Neurosci.* 2021, *2021*.

[52] Bajeh, A.O.; Abikoye, O.C.; Mojeed, H.A.; *et al.* Application of Computational Intelligence Models in IoMT Big Data for Heart Disease Diagnosis in Personalized Health Care. In *Intelligent IoT Systems in Personalized Health Care*; Elsevier, 2020; pp. 177–206.

[53] Jiang, L. IoT Sensors for Smart Health Devices and Data Security in Healthcare. *J. Biomed. Sustain. Healthc. Appl.* 2021, 105–112, doi:10.53759/0088/JBSHA202101013.

[54] Bhushan, B.; Kumar, A.; Agarwal, A.K.; Kumar, A.; Bhattacharya, P.; Kumar, A. Towards a Secure and Sustainable Internet of Medical Things (IoMT): Requirements, Design Challenges, Security Techniques, and Future Trends. *Sustainability* 2023, *15*, 6177, doi:10.3390/su15076177.

[55] Williams, P.; Dutta, I.K.; Daoud, H.; Bayoumi, M. A Survey on Security in Internet of Things with a Focus on the Impact of Emerging Technologies. *Internet of Things* 2022, *19*, 100564, doi:10.1016/j.iot.2022.100564.

[56] Alsaeed, N.; Nadeem, F. Authentication in the Internet of Medical Things: Taxonomy, Review, and Open Issues. *Appl. Sci.* 2022, *12*, 7487, doi:10.3390/app12157487.

[57] Mawgoud, A.A.; Karadawy, A.I.; Tawfik, B.S. A Secure Authentication Technique in Internet of Medical Things through Machine Learning. *arXiv Prepr. arXiv1912.12143* 2019, doi:10.6084/m9.figshare.13311479.v2.

[58] Newaz, A.I.; Sikder, A.K.; Rahman, M.A.; Uluagac, A.S. A Survey on Security and Privacy Issues in Modern Healthcare Systems. *ACM Trans. Comput. Healthc.* 2021, *2*, 1–44, doi:10.1145/3453176.

[59] Alsubaei, F.; Abuhussein, A.; Shandilya, V.; Shiva, S. IoMT-SAF: Internet of Medical Things Security Assessment Framework. *Internet of Things* 2019, *8*, 100123, doi:10.1016/j.iot.2019.100123.

[60] Fatima, A.; Khan, T.A.; Abdellatif, T.M.; *et al.* Impact and Research Challenges of Penetrating Testing and Vulnerability Assessment on Network Threat. In *Proceedings of the 2023 International Conference on Business Analytics for Technology and Security (ICBATS)*; IEEE, 2023; pp. 1–8.

[61] Bilal, M.A.; Hameed, S. Comparative Analysis of Encryption Techniques for Sharing Data in IoMT Devices. *Am. J. Comput. Sci. Inf. Technol* 2020, *8*, 46, doi:10.36648/2349-3917.8.1.46.

[62] Hatzivasilis, G.; Soultatos, O.; Ioannidis, S.; Verikoukis, C.; Demetriou, G.; Tsatsoulis, C. Review of Security and Privacy for the Internet of Medical Things (IoMT). In *Proceedings of the 2019 15th International Conference on Distributed Computing in Sensor Systems (DCOSS)*; IEEE, 2019; pp. 457–464.

[63] Herrmann, D.; Pridöhl, H. Basic Concepts and Models of Cybersecurity. In *International Library of Ethics, Law and Technology*; Springer International Publishing, 2020; Vol. 21, pp. 11–44.

[64] Yaacoub, J.P.A.; Noura, M.; Noura, H.N.; *et al.* Securing Internet of Medical Things Systems: Limitations, Issues and Recommendations. *Futur. Gener. Comput. Syst.* 2020, *105*, 581–606, doi:10.1016/j.future.2019.12.028.

[65] Ahmed, S.F.; Alam, M.S. Bin; Afrin, S.; Rafa, S.J.; Rafa, N.; Gandomi, A. H. Insights into Internet of Medical Things (IoMT): Data Fusion, Security Issues and Potential Solutions. *Inf. Fusion* 2024, *102*, 102060, doi:10.1016/j.inffus.2023.102060.

[66] Liu, Y.; Ju, F.; Zhang, Q.; *et al.* Overview of Internet of Medical Things Security Based on Blockchain Access Control. *J. Database Manag.* 2023, *34*, 1–20, doi:10.4018/JDM.321545.

[67] Rains, T. *Cybersecurity Threats, Malware Trends, and Strategies: Mitigate Exploits, Malware, Phishing, and Other Social Engineering Attacks*; Packt Publishing Ltd, 2020.

[68] Salahdine, F.; Kaabouch, N. Social Engineering Attacks: A Survey. *Futur. Internet* 2019, *11*, 89, doi:10.3390/fi11040089.

[69] Gumiel Quintana, J.Á.; Mabe Álvarez, J.; Jiménez Verde, J.; Barruetabeña Pujana, J. A Holistic Approach on Automotive Cybersecurity for Suppliers. *Veh. 2023 Twelfth Int. Conf. Adv. Veh. Syst. Technol. Appl.* 2023, 47–53.

[70] Nadir, I.; Ahmad, Z.; Mahmood, H.; *et al.* An Auditing Framework for Vulnerability Analysis of IoT System. In *Proceedings of the 2019 IEEE European Symposium on Security and Privacy Workshops (EuroS&PW)*; IEEE, 2019; pp. 39–47.

[71] Hireche, R.; Mansouri, H.; Pathan, A.-S.K. Fault Tolerance and Security Management in IoMT. In *Towards a Wireless Connected World:*

Achievements and New Technologies; Pathan, A.-S.K., Ed.; Springer International Publishing: Cham, 2022; pp. 65–104.

[72] Allouzi, M.A.; Khan, J.I. Identifying and Modeling Security Threats for IoMT Edge Network Using Markov Chain and Common Vulnerability Scoring System (CVSS). *arXiv Prepr. arXiv2104.11580* 2021.

[73] Bates, J.A. Cyber Threats That Lurk in the Internet of Medical Things (IoMT) 2020.

[74] Wazid, M.; Das, A.K.; Rodrigues, J.J.P.C.; Shetty, S.; Park, Y. IoMT Malware Detection Approaches: Analysis and Research Challenges. *IEEE Access* 2019, *7*, 182459–182476, doi:10.1109/ACCESS.2019.2960412.

[75] Jan, S.U.; Ali, S.; Abbasi, I.A.; Mosleh, M.A.A.; Alsanad, A.; Khattak, H. Secure Patient Authentication Framework in the Healthcare System Using Wireless Medical Sensor Networks. *J. Healthc. Eng.* 2021, *2021*, 1–20, doi:10.1155/2021/9954089.

[76] Kioskli, K.; Fotis, T.; Mouratidis, H. The Landscape of Cybersecurity Vulnerabilities and Challenges in Healthcare: Security Standards and Paradigm Shift Recommendations. In Proceedings of the Proceedings of the 16th International Conference on Availability, Reliability and Security; ACM: New York, August 2021; pp. 1–9.

[77] Wang, Z.; Zhu, H.; Sun, L. Social Engineering in Cybersecurity: Effect Mechanisms, Human Vulnerabilities and Attack Methods. *IEEE Access* 2021, *9*, 11895–11910, doi:10.1109/ACCESS.2021.3051633.

[78] Mahanta, K.; Maringanti, H.B. Social Engineering Attacks and Countermeasures. In *Perspectives on Ethical Hacking and Penetration Testing*; IGI Global, 2023; pp. 307–337.

[79] Hasan, M.K.; Ghazal, T.M.; Saeed, R.A.; *et al.* A Review on Security Threats, Vulnerabilities, and Counter Measures of 5G Enabled Internet-of-Medical-Things. *IET Commun.* 2022, *16*, 421–432.

[80] Rizk, D.; Rizk, R.; Hsu, S. Applied Layered-Security Model to IoMT. In Proceedings of the 2019 IEEE International Conference on Intelligence and Security Informatics, ISI 2019; IEEE, 2019; p. 227.

[81] Alozie, E.; Imoize, A.L.; Olagunju, H.I.; Faruk, N. Introduction to Emerging Security and Privacy Schemes for Dense 6G Wireless Communication Networks. In *Security and Privacy Schemes for Dense 6G Wireless Communication Networks*; 2023; pp. 1–29.

[82] Adavoudi Jolfaei, A.; Aghili, S.F.; Singelee, D. A Survey on Blockchain-Based IoMT Systems: Towards Scalability. *IEEE Access* 2021, *9*, 148948–148975, doi:10.1109/ACCESS.2021.3117662.

[83] Almalki, J.; Al Shehri, W.; Mehmood, R.; *et al.* Enabling Blockchain with IoMT Devices for Healthcare. *Inf.* 2022, *13*, 448, doi:10.3390/info13100448.

[84] Dilawar, N.; Rizwan, M.; Ahmad, F.; Akram, S. Blockchain: Securing Internet of Medical Things (IoMT). *Int. J. Adv. Comput. Sci. Appl.* 2019, *10*, 82–89, doi:10.14569/IJACSA.2019.0100110.

[85] Girardi, F.; De Gennaro, G.; Colizzi, L.; Convertini, N. Improving the Healthcare Effectiveness: The Possible Role of EHR, IoMT and Blockchain. *Electron*. 2020, *9*, 884, doi:10.3390/electronics9060884.

[86] Xiong, H.; Jin, C.; Alazab, M.; *et al.* On the Design of Blockchain-Based ECDSA With Fault-Tolerant Batch Verification Protocol for Blockchain-Enabled IoMT. *IEEE J. Biomed. Heal. Informatics* 2022, *26*, 1977–1986, doi:10.1109/JBHI.2021.3112693.

[87] Manickam, P.; Mariappan, S.A.; Murugesan, S.M.; *et al.* Artificial Intelligence (AI) and Internet of Medical Things (IoMT) Assisted Biomedical Systems for Intelligent Healthcare. *Biosensors* 2022, *12*, 562, doi:10.3390/bios12080562.

[88] Awotunde, J.B.; Imoize, A.L.; Jimoh, R.G.; *et al.* AIoMT Enabling Real-Time Monitoring of Healthcare Systems Security and Privacy Considerations. *Handb. Secur. Priv. AI-Enabled Healthc. Syst. Internet Med. Things* 2023, 97–133, doi:10.1201/9781003370321-5.

[89] Rufai, A.U.; Fasina, E.P.; Uwadia, C.O.; Rufai, A.T.; Imoize, A.L. Cyberattacks against Artificial Intelligence-Enabled Internet of Medical Things. In *Handbook of Security and Privacy of AI-Enabled Healthcare Systems and Internet of Medical Things*; CRC Press, 2023; pp. 191–216.

[90] Rufai, A.T.; Rufai, A.U.; Imoize, A.L. Application of AIoMT in Medical Robotics. In *Handbook of Security and Privacy of AI-Enabled Healthcare Systems and Internet of Medical Things*; CRC Press, 2023; pp. 335–364.

[91] Sei, Y.; Ohsuga, A.; Onesimu, J.A.; Imoize, A.L. Local Differential Privacy for Artificial Intelligence of Medical Things. In *Handbook of Security and Privacy of AI-Enabled Healthcare Systems and Internet of Medical Things*; CRC Press, 2023; pp. 241–270.

[92] Wang, X.; Wang, Y.; Javaheri, Z.; Almutairi, L.; Moghadamnejad, N.; Younes, O.S. Federated Deep Learning for Anomaly Detection in the Internet of Things. *Comput. Electr. Eng.* 2023, *108*, doi:10.1016/j.compeleceng.2023.108651.

[93] Villegas-Ch, W.; Govea, J.; Jaramillo-Alcazar, A. IoT Anomaly Detection to Strengthen Cybersecurity in the Critical Infrastructure of Smart Cities. *Appl. Sci.* 2023, *13*, 10977, doi:10.3390/app131910977.

[94] Venkatesh, A.N. Reimagining the Future of Healthcare Industry through Internet of Medical Things (IoMT), Artificial Intelligence (AI), Machine Learning (ML), Big Data, Mobile Apps and Advanced Sensors. *Int. J. Eng. Adv. Technol.* 2019, *9*, 3014–3019, doi:10.35940/ijeat.A1412.109119.

[95] Abdulraheem, M.; Adeniyi, E.A.; Awotunde, J.B.; *et al.* Artificial Intelligence of Medical Things for Medical Information Systems Privacy and Security. In *Handbook of Security and Privacy of AI-Enabled Healthcare Systems and Internet of Medical Things*; CRC Press, 2024; pp. 63–96.

[96] Iguoba, V.A.; Imoize, A.L. AIoMT Training, Testing, and Validation. In *Handbook of Security and Privacy of AI-Enabled Healthcare Systems and Internet of Medical Things*; CRC Press, 2024; pp. 394–410.

[97] Edmund, A.N.; Alabi, C.A.; Tooki, O.O.; Imoize, A.L.; Salka, T.D. Artificial Intelligence-Assisted Internet of Medical Things Enabling Medical

Image Processing. In *Handbook of Security and Privacy of AI-Enabled Healthcare Systems and Internet of Medical Things*; CRC Press, 2023; pp. 309–334.

[98] Cicioglu, M.; Calhan, A. A Multiprotocol Controller Deployment in SDN-Based IoMT Architecture. *IEEE Internet Things J.* 2022, *9*, 20833–20840, doi:10.1109/JIOT.2022.3175669.

[99] Liaqat, S.; Akhunzada, A.; Shaikh, F.S.; Giannetsos, A.; Jan, M.A. SDN Orchestration to Combat Evolving Cyber Threats in Internet of Medical Things (IoMT). *Comput. Commun.* 2020, *160*, 697–705, doi:10.1016/j.comcom.2020.07.006.

[100] Khan, S.; Akhunzada, A. A Hybrid DL-Driven Intelligent SDN-Enabled Malware Detection Framework for Internet of Medical Things (IoMT). *Comput. Commun.* 2021, *170*, 209–216, doi:10.1016/j.comcom.2021.01.013.

[101] Haseeb, K.; Ahmad, I.; Awan, I.I.; Lloret, J.; Bosch, I. A Machine Learning SDN-Enabled Big Data Model for IoMT Systems. *Electronics* 2021, *10*, 2228.

[102] Syed, L.; Jabeen, S.; S., M.; Alsaeedi, A. Smart Healthcare Framework for Ambient Assisted Living Using IoMT and Big Data Analytics Techniques. *Futur. Gener. Comput. Syst.* 2019, *101*, 136–151, doi:10.1016/j.future.2019.06.004.

[103] Hamid, S.; Bawany, N.Z.; Sodhro, A.H.; Lakhan, A.; Ahmed, S. A Systematic Review and IoMT Based Big Data Framework for COVID-19 Prevention and Detection. *Electron.* 2022, *11*, 2777, doi:10.3390/electronics11172777.

Chapter 3

Adaptive cybersecurity: AI-driven threat intelligence in healthcare systems

Oleksandr Kuznetsov[1,2,3], Emanuele Frontoni[1,4], Natalia Kryvinska[5], Dmytro Prokopovych-Tkachenko[6] and Boris Khruskov[6]

This chapter provides an exploration of adaptive cybersecurity strategies in healthcare, focusing on the integration and impact of Artificial Intelligence (AI). In an era where cyber threats are increasingly dynamic and sophisticated, traditional defensive measures in healthcare cybersecurity are often found lacking. This chapter addresses this gap by highlighting the development and implementation of AI-driven threat intelligence platforms, which represent a paradigm shift from reactive to proactive and predictive cybersecurity models. The core of the chapter is the detailed examination of AI-driven platforms, which are designed to continuously learn from a vast array of data sources, adapt to evolving cyber threats, and predict future vulnerabilities. This involves a deep dive into the integration of various AI technologies such as machine learning algorithms for anomaly detection, natural language processing for efficient and effective threat intelligence gathering, and neural networks for advanced predictive analytics. These technologies collectively enhance the capability of healthcare systems to detect, analyze, and respond to cyber threats in real-time, thereby significantly improving their security posture. Furthermore, the chapter delves into the ethical considerations and potential biases inherent in AI-driven cybersecurity solutions. It discusses the importance of maintaining a balance between enhancing security measures and protecting patient privacy, a critical concern in the healthcare sector. The ethical implications of data usage, algorithmic transparency, and the need for unbiased AI models are thoroughly examined.

[1]Department of Political Sciences, Communication and International Relations, University of Macerata, Italy
[2]Department of Information and Communication Systems Security, V. N. Karazin Kharkiv National University, Ukraine
[3]Faculty of Engineering, eCampus University, Italy
[4]Department of Information Engineering, Marche Polytechnic University, Italy
[5]Department of Information Management and Business Systems, University of Comenius, Slovakia
[6]Department of Cyber Security and Information Technology, University of Customs and Finance, Ukraine

Through a series of illustrative case studies, the chapter demonstrates the real-world effectiveness of adaptive cybersecurity strategies in healthcare. These case studies provide insights into how various healthcare organizations have successfully implemented AI-driven solutions to combat cyber threats, highlighting the practical challenges and successes encountered. In summary, this chapter offers a comprehensive overview of the role of AI in transforming cybersecurity within healthcare. It presents a balanced view of the technological advancements, ethical considerations, and practical applications of AI-driven cybersecurity, making it a valuable resource for professionals and scholars in the field of healthcare cybersecurity.

Keywords: Adaptive cybersecurity; artificial intelligence; threat intelligence; machine learning; healthcare systems; predictive analytics

3.1 Introduction

The realm of healthcare has undergone a profound transformation in the digital age, with advancements in technology bringing about significant improvements in patient care and data management [1]. However, this digitalization has also introduced complex challenges in cybersecurity, making healthcare systems increasingly vulnerable to cyber threats [2]. The protection of sensitive patient data and healthcare infrastructure from these threats is paramount, necessitating innovative and effective cybersecurity strategies [3].

This chapter delves into the critical role of Artificial Intelligence (AI) in enhancing cybersecurity within the healthcare sector. AI, with its advanced analytical capabilities and adaptability, presents a promising solution to the complex and evolving nature of cyber threats. The focus of this chapter is to provide a comprehensive overview of how AI technologies are being integrated into healthcare cybersecurity, enhancing the security and efficiency of systems, particularly in managing and protecting Electronic Health Records (EHRs).

Through a series of case studies and a detailed statistical analysis of recent cybersecurity threats, this chapter offers insights into the practical applications, challenges, and successes of AI-driven cybersecurity solutions in various healthcare settings. We explore the transformative impact of AI in detecting and mitigating cyber threats, highlighting the advancements AI brings compared to traditional cybersecurity methods.

Furthermore, we make a significant contribution to the field by detailing the architecture and functioning of AI-Driven Threat Intelligence Platforms. This includes an in-depth analysis of how different AI components such as machine learning (ML), Natural Language Processing (NLP), and neural networks are integrated within these platforms to provide a dynamic and effective defense against cyber threats.

In essence, this chapter aims to provide a thorough understanding of the current state of AI implementation in healthcare cybersecurity, the nature of cyber threats faced by the healthcare sector, and the potential of AI-driven solutions in addressing these challenges. Our exploration into this domain is intended to serve as both an academic resource and a practical guide for healthcare organizations looking to enhance their cybersecurity measures in an increasingly digital world.

3.1.1 Key contributions of the chapter

The following are the significant contributions of this chapter:

(i) In-depth analysis of AI-driven threat intelligence platforms: This chapter provides a comprehensive examination of AI-driven threat intelligence platforms in healthcare cybersecurity, detailing their architecture, functioning, and integration of various AI technologies.
(ii) Evaluation of the role of AI in healthcare cybersecurity: It evaluates the role of AI technologies, such as ML, NLP, and neural networks, in enhancing the security and efficiency of healthcare systems, particularly in managing and protecting Electronic Health Records (EHRs).
(iii) Ethical and regulatory considerations: The chapter addresses the critical ethical and regulatory aspects of implementing AI in healthcare cybersecurity, discussing the balance between technological advancement and the protection of patient privacy.
(iv) Comparative analysis and case studies: Through comparative analysis and a series of case studies, the chapter demonstrates the effectiveness of AI-driven cybersecurity solutions compared to traditional methods, providing real-world insights into their application in various healthcare settings.
(v) Statistical analysis of cybersecurity threats: It presents a detailed statistical analysis of recent cybersecurity threats in healthcare, offering insights into the types of breaches, locations of breached information, and distribution of threats across different states.

3.1.2 Novelty and contribution

The novel contribution of this chapter lies in its holistic examination of AI-driven threat intelligence platforms specifically tailored for healthcare cybersecurity. It uniquely synthesizes the architectural intricacies of these platforms with practical applications, bridging the gap between theoretical AI models and their real-world implications in healthcare. Additionally, this chapter stands out in its comprehensive approach, combining in-depth case studies, ethical considerations, and a robust statistical analysis of recent cybersecurity threats, thereby offering a multifaceted perspective on the integration of AI in healthcare cybersecurity.

3.1.3 Chapter organization

Section 3.2 presents the related work and research methodology, including a historical overview of cybersecurity evolution in healthcare and a literature gap analysis focusing on AI-driven threat intelligence platforms.

Section 3.3 discusses the research findings on AI-driven threat intelligence platforms, detailing their architecture and the role of ML, NLP, and neural networks in predictive threat analysis.

Section 3.4 explores the ethical and regulatory aspects in AI-driven healthcare cybersecurity, highlighting the challenges and considerations in implementing AI technologies.

Section 3.5 provides a comprehensive analysis of AI implementation and cybersecurity threats in healthcare, including an overview of AI applications, a statistical analysis of cybersecurity threats, and a comparative analysis of AI-driven and traditional methods.

Section 3.6 explores the research findings and contributions, highlighting the importance of the insights and analyses provided in this chapter for advancing healthcare cybersecurity.

Section 3.7 concludes the chapter, summarizing the key findings and implications for future research and practice in AI-driven healthcare cybersecurity.

3.2 Related work and research methodology

In this section, we embark on a comprehensive exploration of the existing literature and research in the field of cybersecurity, particularly within the healthcare sector. This review not only contextualizes our study within the broader academic discourse but also highlights the progression and pivotal shifts that have shaped the current state of cybersecurity in healthcare. At the end of the section, we also review the research methodology of our study

3.2.1 Historical perspective: overview of cybersecurity evolution in healthcare

The evolution of cybersecurity in healthcare is a narrative marked by rapid technological advancements, growing digital threats, and an ever-increasing reliance on EHRs and connected medical devices. This historical perspective provides a lens through which we can understand the current challenges and anticipate future trends in healthcare cybersecurity.

Early stages of healthcare cybersecurity:

- Initial digitalization (late 20th century) [4]: The inception of cybersecurity in healthcare coincided with the digitalization of medical records and the introduction of basic IT systems. Early cybersecurity measures were rudimentary, primarily focused on preventing unauthorized access to patient data.
- HIPAA implementation (1996) [5]: The Health Insurance Portability and Accountability Act (HIPAA) represented a significant milestone in healthcare cybersecurity in the United States. HIPAA established national standards for the protection of patient health information, catalyzing a more structured approach to data security.

The 21st century: a new era of challenges and innovations:

- Rise of EHRs [6,7]: The widespread adoption of EHRs in the early 21st century transformed healthcare delivery but also introduced new vulnerabilities.

Cybersecurity efforts had to evolve to protect these digital records from breaches and cyberattacks.

- Increasing connectivity and telemedicine [8]: The advent of telemedicine and the increasing connectivity of healthcare systems with wearable technologies and IoT devices expanded the cybersecurity landscape. This era saw the emergence of more sophisticated cyber threats, including ransomware and phishing attacks targeting healthcare institutions.
- Regulatory evolution [9,10]: In response to these emerging threats, regulatory frameworks continued to evolve. The introduction of additional guidelines and standards, such as the Health Information Technology for Economic and Clinical Health (HITECH) Act, underscored the growing importance of cybersecurity in healthcare.

Current landscape and emerging Trends:

- Advanced cyber threats [3,11]: Today, healthcare systems face advanced cyber threats like state-sponsored attacks, sophisticated ransomware, and AI-driven cyberattacks. These threats have necessitated the adoption of more advanced cybersecurity measures, including AI and ML-based solutions.
- Data privacy and patient trust [12,13]: As healthcare data becomes increasingly digitized, maintaining patient trust through robust data privacy and security measures has become paramount.
- Integration of advanced technologies [14,15]: The integration of blockchain, cloud computing, and advanced encryption methods are current trends shaping the future of healthcare cybersecurity.

In summary, the historical evolution of cybersecurity in healthcare reflects a trajectory from basic data protection to a complex, multi-faceted discipline that now encompasses advanced technological solutions and comprehensive regulatory frameworks. This progression underscores the critical role of cybersecurity in safeguarding patient data and the integrity of healthcare systems in an increasingly digital world.

3.2.2 Literature gap analysis: AI-driven threat intelligence platforms

The burgeoning field of AI-driven threat intelligence in healthcare cybersecurity has been the subject of extensive research [11,16]. However, a thorough analysis of existing literature reveals several gaps that this chapter aims to address, particularly in the context of AI-driven threat intelligence platforms [17,18].

Identified gaps in existing literature:

1. Comprehensive architectural understanding: While existing studies discuss various aspects of AI in cybersecurity, there is a noticeable lack of comprehensive literature that delves into the detailed architecture of AI-driven threat intelligence platforms. This includes a granular exploration of how different AI components (like ML, NLP, and neural networks) integrate and function cohesively within these platforms.

2. Real-world application and case studies: There is a scarcity of literature that connects theoretical AI models to practical, real-world applications in healthcare cybersecurity. Detailed case studies demonstrating the implementation and effectiveness of these AI-driven systems in actual healthcare settings are limited.
3. Ethical and regulatory considerations: While some studies touch upon the ethical implications of AI in cybersecurity, there is a gap in literature that specifically addresses the ethical and regulatory challenges of implementing AI-driven platforms in healthcare, considering the sensitivity of health data and patient privacy.
4. Adaptability and evolution of AI systems: Existing research often fails to adequately address the adaptability and evolutionary aspects of AI systems in response to the dynamic nature of cyber threats. Literature that explores how these systems evolve over time, learning from new data and threats, is sparse.
5. Integration challenges with healthcare IT infrastructure: There is a lack of detailed exploration of the challenges and best practices in integrating AI-driven threat intelligence platforms with existing healthcare IT infrastructure, a critical aspect for the successful deployment of these systems.

How this chapter addresses these gaps:

- Detailed architectural analysis: This chapter provides an in-depth analysis of the architecture of AI-driven threat intelligence platforms, elucidating how various AI components are integrated and function in unison within these systems.
- Real-world implementation and case studies: We bridge the gap between theory and practice by including comprehensive case studies that demonstrate the practical application and effectiveness of AI-driven threat intelligence platforms in healthcare cybersecurity.
- Focus on ethical and regulatory aspects: The chapter delves into the ethical considerations and regulatory compliance issues specific to the deployment of AI-driven systems in healthcare, providing insights into navigating these complex aspects.
- Adaptability and evolutionary perspective: We address the adaptability of AI-driven systems, discussing how they can evolve and learn from new data and threats, thereby remaining effective against an ever-changing threat landscape.
- Integration with healthcare IT systems: The chapter also focuses on the integration challenges and outlines best practices for embedding AI-driven threat intelligence platforms within existing healthcare IT infrastructures.

In summary, this chapter aims to fill the identified gaps in the literature by providing a comprehensive, practical, and ethically informed perspective on AI-driven threat intelligence platforms in healthcare cybersecurity. This contribution not only advances academic understanding but also offers valuable insights for practitioners in the field.

3.2.3 Research methodology

In this section, we focus on the research methodologies that underpin our study of AI-driven cybersecurity in healthcare. This segment is dedicated to outlining the systematic approaches employed in our research. It encompasses the data collection methods, analytical frameworks, and algorithmic models used to evaluate the effectiveness of AI in cybersecurity within the healthcare sector.

Our research methodology is structured to provide a comprehensive understanding of AI-driven cybersecurity solutions. It includes:

- Data collection: Gathering data from various case studies, academic journals, and cybersecurity reports to understand the current landscape of AI in healthcare cybersecurity.
- Algorithm analysis: Examining the specific AI algorithms and ML models used in cybersecurity platforms, focusing on their design, functionality, and adaptability.
- Quantitative analysis: Utilizing statistical methods to analyze the data collected, assessing the effectiveness of AI solutions in real-world scenarios.

3.3 Research findings: AI-driven threat intelligence platforms

This section presents the findings of our research, focusing on the architecture and functionality of AI-Driven Threat Intelligence Platforms in healthcare cybersecurity. It provides an in-depth analysis of how these platforms are designed, their operational mechanisms, and their impact on healthcare cybersecurity.

3.3.1 AI-driven threat intelligence platforms

AI-driven threat intelligence platforms represent a paradigm shift in cybersecurity, moving from reactive to proactive and predictive security models. These platforms harness the power of AI to analyze, predict, and respond to cyber threats in real-time [9,16]. The core of these platforms lies in their ability to continuously learn and adapt, making them particularly suited for the dynamic and complex landscape of healthcare cybersecurity.

Figure 3.1 represents a comprehensive cybersecurity platform architecture, emphasizing a systematic approach to data-driven threat detection and response. It integrates data collection, ML analysis, threat intelligence feeds, and real-time monitoring, culminating in predictive analytics and proactive response mechanisms. This system exemplifies a dynamic, feedback-driven model, ensuring continuous adaptation and improvement in cybersecurity measures.

1. Data collection and aggregation: The platform begins with the collection of vast amounts of data from various sources, including network traffic, logs, and external threat feeds. This data is aggregated and normalized to form a comprehensive dataset for analysis.
2. Machine learning and analysis: At the heart of the platform is a suite of ML algorithms. These algorithms are trained on both historical and real-time data to identify patterns and anomalies indicative of potential threats. Techniques

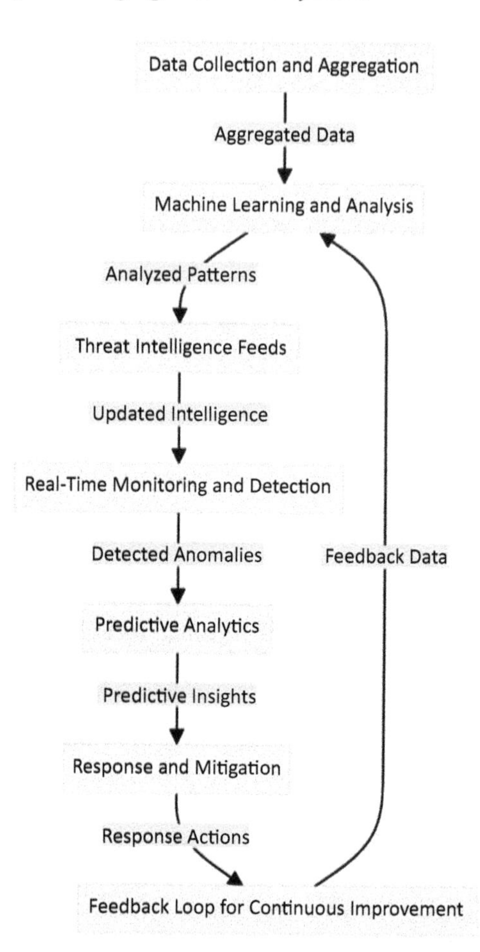

Figure 3.1 Architecture and functioning of AI-driven threat intelligence platforms

such as supervised and unsupervised learning, along with deep learning models, are employed to enhance detection accuracy.

3. Threat intelligence feeds: Integration with external threat intelligence feeds is crucial. These feeds provide information on new and emerging threats, ensuring the platform is updated with the latest threat landscape.
4. Real-time monitoring and detection: The platform continuously monitors network activity. Using the trained ML models, it can detect anomalies and potential threats in real-time, often before they manifest into actual attacks.
5. Predictive analytics: Leveraging predictive analytics, the platform can forecast potential future threats based on current trends and historical data. This predictive capability allows healthcare organizations to prepare and mitigate risks proactively.

6. Response and mitigation: Upon detection of a threat, the platform can initiate predefined response protocols. These may include alerts, automatic containment measures, and informing cybersecurity teams for further investigation.
7. Feedback loop for continuous improvement: A feedback mechanism is integral to the platform. Information from resolved threats and false positives is fed back into the system, allowing the ML models to learn and improve over time.

Figure 3.1 presents a detailed architecture of an AI-driven cybersecurity platform, showcasing the integration of various components such as data collection, ML analysis, and threat intelligence feeds. It visually represents the flow from data aggregation to real-time monitoring and predictive analytics, illustrating the comprehensive approach to proactive cybersecurity in healthcare.

Figure 3.2 visually summarizes the key features and benefits of AI-driven cybersecurity platforms, such as adaptability, efficiency, and predictive capabilities. It provides a clear representation of how these platforms enhance threat detection and response, and how they can be customized and scaled to meet diverse healthcare organizational needs.

- Adaptability: The platform's ability to learn and adapt to new threats makes it highly effective against evolving cyber threats in healthcare.
- Speed and efficiency: AI-driven analysis enables rapid detection and response, a critical factor in minimizing the impact of cyber incidents.
- Predictive capabilities: Predicting future threats allows healthcare organizations to be proactive rather than reactive in their cybersecurity approach.
- Customization and scalability: The platform can be customized to the specific needs of a healthcare organization and scaled as per the changing data environment and threat landscape.

Figure 3.3 focuses on the challenges and considerations in implementing an AI-driven cybersecurity platform in healthcare. It covers the importance of data privacy and security compliance, the need for seamless integration with existing

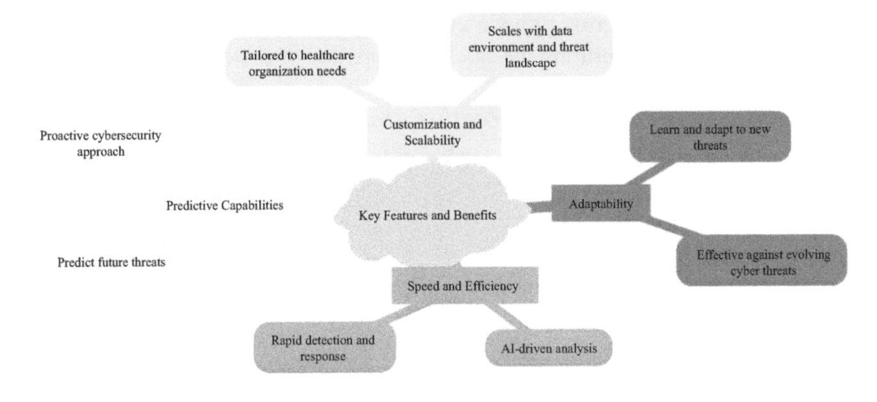

Figure 3.2 Key features and benefits

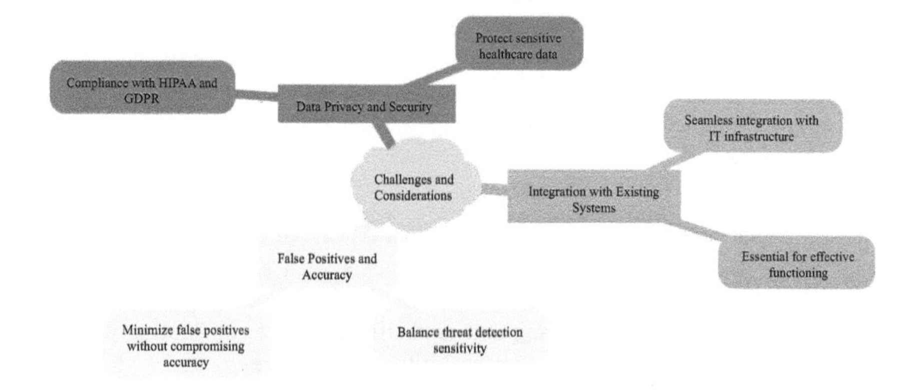

Figure 3.3 Challenges and considerations

systems, and the balance between minimizing false positives and maintaining accuracy in threat detection:

- Data privacy and security: Ensuring the privacy and security of sensitive healthcare data is paramount. The platform must comply with regulations like HIPAA and GDPR.
- Integration with existing systems: Seamless integration with existing healthcare IT infrastructure is essential for the effective functioning of the platform.
- False positives and accuracy: Balancing the sensitivity of threat detection to minimize false positives without compromising on accuracy is a critical challenge.

Figure 3.3 outlines the primary challenges in implementing AI-driven cybersecurity in healthcare, including data privacy concerns, integration complexities, and the balance required in threat detection accuracy. It visually emphasizes the critical aspects that need to be addressed for successful implementation.

In conclusion, AI-driven threat intelligence platforms offer a sophisticated and dynamic approach to cybersecurity in healthcare systems. By leveraging advanced AI technologies, these platforms provide enhanced protection against an ever-evolving cyber threat landscape, ensuring the safety and privacy of critical healthcare data.

3.3.2 Machine learning algorithms for anomaly detection

ML algorithms play a pivotal role in the realm of AI-driven cybersecurity, particularly in anomaly detection. Anomaly detection is crucial in identifying unusual patterns or behaviors that may signify a cyber threat, such as a data breach or a malware attack. In healthcare systems, where the security and privacy of sensitive data are paramount, the effective use of ML algorithms can significantly enhance the robustness of cybersecurity measures.

Types of ML algorithms used in anomaly detection (Table 3.1):

1. Supervised learning algorithms: These algorithms require labeled training data to learn and make predictions. In the context of cybersecurity, they are trained

Table 3.1 Machine learning algorithms in anomaly detection

Algorithm type	Algorithm	Data requirement	Application	Advantages	Challenges	Use cases
Supervised Learning	Logistic Regression	Labeled data	Binary classification	Simple, interpretable	Limited to linear relationships	Identifying binary anomalies (normal/abnormal)
	Support Vector Machines (SVM)	Labeled data	Complex pattern detection	Effective in high-dimensional spaces	Computationally intensive	Classifying complex cyber threats
	Decision Trees and Random Forests	Labeled data	Multi-class classification	Easy to interpret, handles non-linear data	Prone to overfitting	Classifying different types of cyber threats
Unsupervised Learning	K-Means Clustering	Unlabeled data	Pattern recognition	Simple, efficient	Assumes spherical clusters	Grouping data to identify patterns
	Autoencoders	Unlabeled data	Data reconstruction	Efficient in dimensionality reduction	Requires large datasets	Identifying deviations in data patterns
	Principal Component Analysis (PCA)	Unlabeled data	Data reduction	Reduces data complexity	Loss of information	Simplifying data for outlier detection
Semi-Supervised Learning	-	Labeled and unlabeled data	Various	Balances supervision and exploration	Complex model training	Scenarios with limited labeled data
Deep Learning	Convolutional Neural Networks (CNNs)	Large datasets	Image and pattern analysis	High accuracy, handles complex data	Requires extensive training data	Advanced threat detection in complex data
	Recurrent Neural Networks (RNNs)	Large datasets	Sequential data analysis	Effective in time-series data	Prone to vanishing gradient problem	Analyzing time-dependent cyber threats

with data labeled as "normal" and "anomalous" to detect known types of attacks. Common supervised learning algorithms include:

- Logistic regression: Used for binary classification of data into normal and anomalous.
- Support vector machines (SVM): Effective in high-dimensional spaces, SVMs are used for detecting more complex anomalies.
- Decision trees and random forests: These algorithms are known for their interpretability and are used to identify and classify different types of cyber threats.

2. Unsupervised learning algorithms: These algorithms are used when the training data is not labeled. They are adept at detecting unknown or new types of cyber threats by identifying outliers or unusual patterns in data. Key unsupervised learning algorithms include:
   - K-means clustering: This algorithm groups data into clusters to identify patterns and anomalies.
   - Autoencoders: A type of neural network used to encode and decode data, effectively identifying anomalies by reconstructing input data and detecting deviations.
   - Principal component analysis (PCA): PCA reduces the dimensionality of data, making it easier to identify outliers.
3. Semi-supervised learning algorithms: These algorithms use a small amount of labeled data along with a large amount of unlabeled data. This approach is beneficial in scenarios where obtaining labeled data is costly or impractical.
4. Deep learning algorithms: A subset of ML, deep learning algorithms, particularly neural networks, are increasingly being used for anomaly detection due to their ability to process and learn from large volumes of data. Convolutional Neural Networks (CNNs) and Recurrent Neural Networks (RNNs) are examples of deep learning models used in complex anomaly detection scenarios.

Table 3.1 provides a comprehensive overview of the ML algorithms used in anomaly detection, particularly in the context of cybersecurity in healthcare systems. Each algorithm type and specific algorithm has its unique characteristics, making them suitable for different aspects of anomaly detection.

- Supervised learning algorithms are ideal for scenarios where historical data is available to train the model. They are particularly effective in environments where the types of anomalies are known and can be labeled.
- Unsupervised learning algorithms excel in situations where anomalies are not known beforehand or the data is not labeled. They are adept at identifying unusual patterns or outliers in the data.
- Semi-supervised learning offers a middle ground, utilizing both labeled and unlabeled data, which can be particularly useful in healthcare settings where acquiring large amounts of labeled data can be challenging.
- Deep learning algorithms are powerful tools for complex anomaly detection tasks. They are capable of handling large volumes of data and can identify intricate patterns that other algorithms might miss.

Each algorithm comes with its own set of advantages and challenges, and the choice of algorithm depends on the specific requirements of the cybersecurity task, such as the nature of the data, the complexity of the patterns to be detected, and the computational resources available.

Implementation challenges and considerations (Table 3.2):

- Data quality and quantity: The effectiveness of ML algorithms heavily depends on the quality and quantity of the data. In healthcare, ensuring data integrity while complying with privacy regulations is crucial.
- Model training and tuning: Selecting the right algorithm and tuning its parameters for optimal performance requires expertise and experimentation.
- Real-time processing: The ability to process and analyze data in real-time is essential for timely threat detection.
- Interpretability and explainability: Understanding the decision-making process of ML models is important, especially in a sensitive field like healthcare. Models should be interpretable to ensure trust and accountability.

Table 3.2 Implementation challenges and considerations in ML anomaly detection

Challenge	**Description**	**Impact on anomaly detection**	**Mitigation strategies**	**Tools and technologies**	**Key considerations**
Data Quality and Quantity	Ensuring high-quality and sufficient data for training	Essential for model accuracy	Data preprocessing and augmentation	Data cleaning tools, Big Data platforms	Balancing data privacy with data needs
Model Training and Tuning	Selecting and optimizing ML models	Directly affects performance	Cross-validation, hyperparameter tuning	ML frameworks like TensorFlow, Scikit-learn	Understanding model complexity and resource requirements
Real-Time Processing	Analyzing data as it is generated	Crucial for timely detection	Stream processing, efficient algorithms	Stream processing tools like Apache Kafka, Spark Streaming	Balancing speed with accuracy
Interpretability and Explainability	Understanding model decisions and logic	Important for trust and accountability	Use of interpretable models, feature importance analysis	Tools like LIME, SHAP	Ensuring model transparency and user trust
Adaptability	Keeping the model relevant to evolving threats	Key to long-term effectiveness	Continuous learning, model retraining	Automated ML platforms, continuous integration tools	Regular updates and monitoring of model performance

- Adaptability: Cyber threats are constantly evolving; thus, ML models must be adaptable and regularly updated to recognize new types of anomalies.

Table 3.2 provides an in-depth look at the various challenges encountered when implementing ML algorithms for anomaly detection, particularly in the context of cybersecurity in healthcare systems.

- Data quality and quantity: The foundation of any ML model is data. Ensuring that the data is of high quality and in sufficient quantity is crucial for the accuracy of anomaly detection. This challenge can be mitigated through careful data preprocessing and augmentation, using tools specifically designed for data cleaning and big data platforms.
- Model training and tuning: The effectiveness of ML models heavily depends on proper training and tuning. This involves selecting the right model and optimizing its parameters, which can be achieved through techniques like cross-validation and hyperparameter tuning, using ML frameworks such as TensorFlow or Scikit-learn.
- Real-time processing: The ability to process and analyze data in real-time is essential for timely threat detection. This can be addressed by employing stream processing techniques and efficient algorithms, with tools like Apache Kafka and Spark Streaming.
- Interpretability and explainability are critical in sectors like healthcare, where ML models must be accurate and interpretable. This means understanding how and why a model makes certain decisions, which can be facilitated by using interpretable models and tools like LIME or SHAP.
- Adaptability: Cyber threats are constantly evolving, and ML models need to keep pace. This involves continuous learning and regular model retraining, which can be managed through automated ML platforms and continuous integration tools.

Each of these challenges requires careful consideration and a balanced approach to ensure that the ML models used in anomaly detection are not only effective but also reliable, transparent, and adaptable to the ever-changing landscape of cybersecurity threats.

In summary, ML algorithms are integral to the development of sophisticated anomaly detection systems in healthcare cybersecurity. Their ability to learn from data and identify patterns makes them invaluable in detecting both known and unknown threats, thereby fortifying the security posture of healthcare organizations against a wide array of cyber threats.

3.3.3 Natural Language Processing (NLP) for threat intelligence gathering

Natural Language Processing (NLP), a branch of AI, has become increasingly pivotal in enhancing cybersecurity, particularly in the domain of threat intelligence gathering. NLP enables the automated analysis and interpretation of human

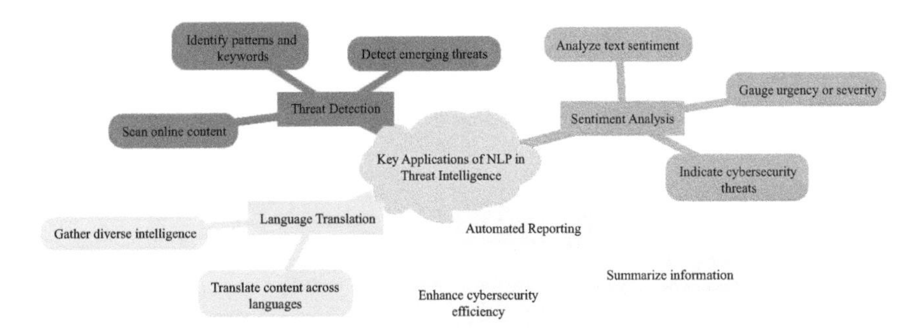

Figure 3.4 Key applications of NLP in threat intelligence

language, a capability that is instrumental in processing and understanding vast amounts of unstructured data prevalent in the cybersecurity landscape.

NLP technologies are adept at extracting meaningful information from various sources such as social media, news reports, blogs, and technical articles, which often contain early indicators of cyber threats and vulnerabilities. By analyzing this data, NLP systems can identify potential threats and provide actionable intelligence to cybersecurity teams.

Key applications of NLP in threat intelligence (Figure 3.4):

1. Threat detection: NLP algorithms can scan through extensive online content to detect emerging threats, such as new malware or phishing campaigns, by identifying relevant patterns and keywords.
2. Sentiment analysis: By analyzing the sentiment of texts, NLP can gauge the urgency or severity of a threat. For instance, a sudden spike in negative sentiments on tech forums could indicate a new cybersecurity threat.
3. Automated reporting: NLP can automate the generation of threat intelligence reports by summarizing relevant information gathered from various sources, thus enhancing the efficiency of the cybersecurity team.
4. Language translation: NLP facilitates the translation of content across different languages, enabling the gathering of threat intelligence from diverse geographical and linguistic sources.

Figure 3.4 illustrates the diverse applications of NLP in cybersecurity, highlighting its role in threat detection, sentiment analysis, and automated reporting. Figure 3.4 helps in understanding how NLP contributes to enhancing threat intelligence in the cybersecurity landscape.

Overall, Figure 3.4 offers a detailed look at the diverse applications of NLP in enhancing threat intelligence, emphasizing its importance in the cybersecurity landscape.

Challenges in implementing NLP for cybersecurity (Figure 3.5):

- Contextual understanding: One of the primary challenges for NLP in cybersecurity is understanding the context. Cybersecurity-related texts often contain

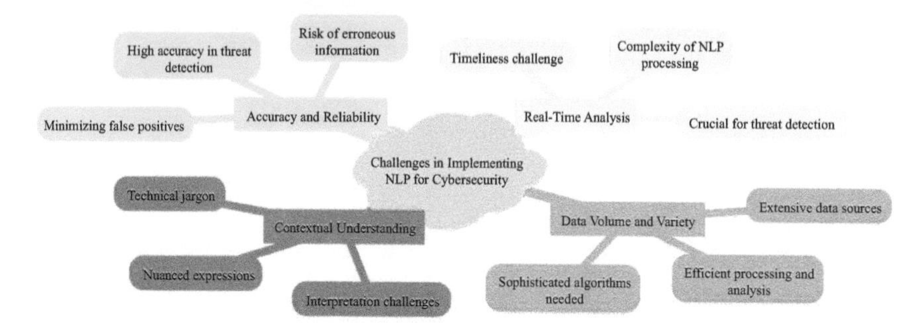

Figure 3.5 Challenges in implementing NLP for cybersecurity

technical jargon and nuanced expressions that can be challenging for NLP systems to interpret accurately.

- Data volume and variety: The sheer volume and variety of data sources can be overwhelming, requiring sophisticated NLP algorithms capable of efficient processing and analysis.
- Real-time analysis: The capability to analyze data in real-time is crucial for timely threat detection, posing a significant challenge given the complexity of NLP processing.
- Accuracy and reliability: Ensuring high accuracy in threat detection and minimizing false positives is critical, as erroneous information can lead to misguided responses.

Figure 3.5 provides a visual representation of the challenges faced when implementing NLP in cybersecurity, such as contextual understanding and data volume management. It underscores the complexities involved in leveraging NLP for enhanced cybersecurity in healthcare.

The future of NLP in cybersecurity looks promising with advancements in AI and ML. The integration of NLP with other AI technologies like ML and deep learning is expected to enhance its capabilities further. Additionally, the development of more sophisticated algorithms for context understanding and sentiment analysis will significantly improve the accuracy and reliability of NLP in threat intelligence gathering.

In conclusion, NLP stands as a powerful tool in the arsenal of cybersecurity, offering significant advantages in the realm of threat intelligence. Its ability to process and analyze large volumes of unstructured data makes it an invaluable asset in the early detection and response to cyber threats, particularly in the dynamic and data-intensive environment of healthcare systems.

3.3.4 Neural networks and predictive analytics in predictive threat analysis

Neural networks, a subset of ML characterized by their ability to learn and model complex patterns, have become a cornerstone in the field of predictive analytics, especially in the context of cybersecurity threat analysis. Their application in predictive threat analysis is a testament to the evolving landscape of cybersecurity, where proactive measures are increasingly paramount.

Neural networks, resembling the structure and function of the human brain, use layers of interconnected nodes to process and analyze data. In cybersecurity, these networks, trained on extensive datasets, are adept at recognizing patterns indicative of potential cyber threats.

Applications of neural networks in predictive threat analysis:

1. Anomaly detection: Neural networks excel in identifying deviations from normal behavior, which is crucial in detecting sophisticated cyber threats that traditional methods might miss.
2. Pattern recognition: They are adept at recognizing complex patterns within large datasets, a capability that is instrumental in identifying subtle indicators of cyber threats.
3. Predictive modeling: Neural networks can forecast future cybersecurity threats based on historical data, allowing organizations to prepare and implement preemptive measures.
4. Behavioral analysis: By analyzing user behavior patterns, neural networks can detect unusual activities that might signify a security breach or insider threat.

Challenges in implementing neural networks for cybersecurity:

- Data sensitivity and privacy: In healthcare systems, the data used for training neural networks often contain sensitive information, necessitating stringent privacy and security measures.
- Complexity and resource intensity: Neural networks, especially deep learning models, are computationally intensive and require significant resources for training and operation.
- Model interpretability: The "black box" nature of neural networks poses a challenge in understanding how these models arrive at certain conclusions, which is critical in a cybersecurity context.
- Dynamic threat landscape: The constantly evolving nature of cyber threats requires neural networks to be continually updated and retrained to remain effective.

The integration of neural networks in cybersecurity is witnessing rapid advancements, driven by the increasing computational power and the development of more sophisticated algorithms. Future prospects include (Figure 3.6):

- Enhanced deep learning models: The development of more advanced deep learning models that can process larger datasets more efficiently and with greater accuracy.
- Improved interpretability: Efforts are being made to make neural network models more interpretable and transparent, which is crucial for their acceptance and trustworthiness in critical sectors like healthcare.
- Real-time processing capabilities: Advancements in hardware and software are enabling faster processing capabilities, allowing neural networks to analyze data in real-time, a critical requirement for timely threat detection.

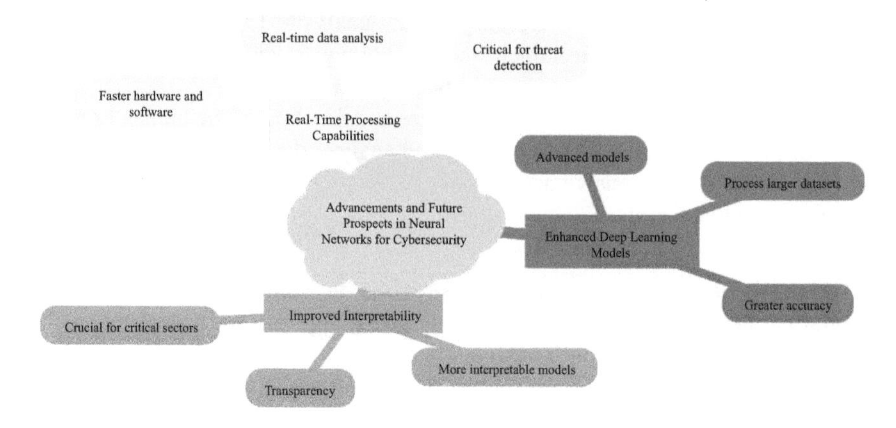

Figure 3.6 Advancements and future prospects in neural networks for cybersecurity

Figure 3.6 illustrates the key areas of advancement and future prospects in neural networks for cybersecurity. It highlights the development of enhanced deep learning models, the importance of improved interpretability, and the need for real-time processing capabilities, underscoring the evolving landscape of neural network applications in cybersecurity.

In summary, neural networks represent a significant advancement in the field of predictive threat analysis in cybersecurity. Their ability to learn from data and identify complex patterns offers a proactive approach to cybersecurity, essential in the dynamic and sensitive environment of healthcare systems. As these technologies continue to evolve, they hold the promise of significantly enhancing the capability to predict and mitigate cyber threats effectively.

3.4 Ethical and regulatory aspects in AI-driven healthcare cybersecurity

The integration of AI in healthcare cybersecurity, while offering significant benefits, also brings forth a range of ethical and regulatory considerations. This section explores these aspects, focusing on the implications of employing AI-driven technologies in the sensitive domain of healthcare data protection.

Figure 3.7 outlines three critical areas of ethical concern:

1. Data privacy and confidentiality:
   - This branch addresses the handling of sensitive patient data, emphasizing the need for strict confidentiality.
   - It highlights the risks associated with data misuse and the potential for unintended biases in AI algorithms.
   - The ethical implications of infringing on patient privacy are also considered, underscoring the importance of safeguarding personal health information.

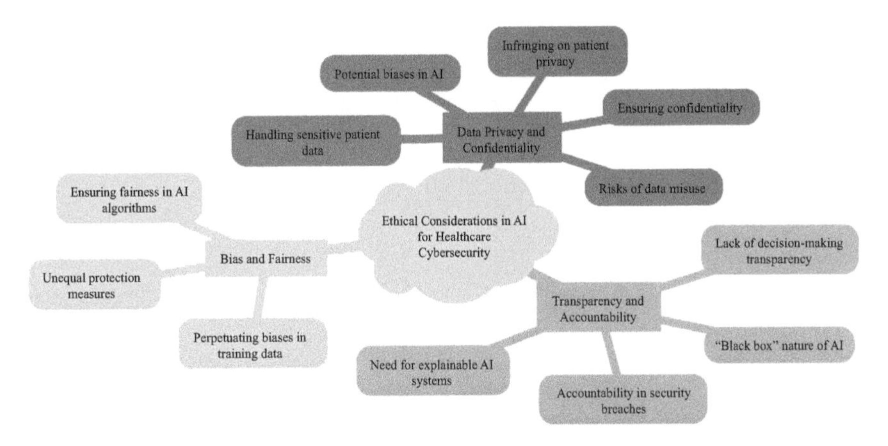

Figure 3.7 Ethical considerations

2. Transparency and accountability:
   - This segment focuses on the "black box" nature of some AI systems, which can obscure the decision-making process.
   - The opaque decision-making process in AI systems raises concerns about accountability, especially in cases of security breaches or misuse of data.
   - The diagram points to the necessity for developing AI systems that are not only effective but also transparent and explainable.
3. Bias and fairness:
   - This area delves into the issue of biases that AI algorithms might inadvertently perpetuate, based on the data they are trained on.
   - It highlights the potential for unequal protection measures across different patient groups, which could arise from these biases.
   - Ensuring fairness in AI algorithms and avoiding bias is presented as an ethical imperative in the development and implementation of AI in healthcare cybersecurity.

Figure 3.7 outlines three critical areas of ethical concern in AI-driven cybersecurity, including data privacy, algorithmic transparency, and bias. Figure 3.7 visually emphasizes the ethical dimensions that must be considered in the deployment of AI technologies in healthcare cybersecurity.

Figure 3.8 details three key areas of regulatory focus:

1. Compliance with healthcare regulations:
   - This branch emphasizes the necessity for AI-driven cybersecurity solutions in healthcare to adhere to existing regulations like the Health Insurance Portability and Accountability Act (HIPAA) in the United States and the General Data Protection Regulation (GDPR) in the European Union.
   - It highlights the importance of these regulations in setting the framework for data protection, privacy, and security in healthcare.

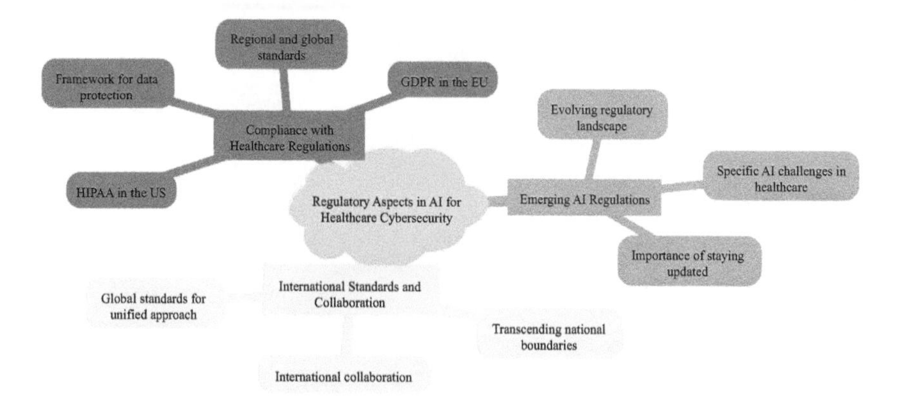

Figure 3.8 Regulatory aspects

- The compliance extends to various regional and global standards, ensuring a comprehensive approach to safeguarding sensitive patient data.

2. Emerging AI regulations:
   - As AI technology continues to evolve, so does the regulatory landscape. This segment addresses the development of new regulations and guidelines specifically tailored to the challenges posed by AI in healthcare.
   - The diagram underscores the importance for healthcare organizations to stay updated with these changes to ensure ongoing compliance.
   - It points to the dynamic nature of AI regulation and the need for adaptive strategies in response to these emerging guidelines.
3. International standards and collaboration:
   - Given that cybersecurity threats often cross national boundaries, this area stresses the significance of international collaboration and adherence to global standards.
   - The diagram suggests that developing and following international guidelines for AI in cybersecurity can help harmonize efforts and ensure a unified approach to data protection.
   - It highlights the role of global cooperation in establishing and maintaining robust cybersecurity measures in the healthcare sector.

Figure 3.8 provides a visual overview of the regulatory landscape surrounding AI-driven cybersecurity in healthcare. It illustrates the key regulations and standards that govern the use of AI in protecting patient data and maintaining system integrity.

To effectively navigate these ethical and regulatory challenges, healthcare organizations should:

- Implement robust data governance frameworks to ensure data privacy and ethical use of AI.

- Engage in transparent and open communication with stakeholders about how AI is used in cybersecurity efforts.
- Invest in developing and using AI systems that are explainable and accountable.
- Regularly review and update AI algorithms to avoid biases and ensure fairness.
- Stay informed about evolving regulations and standards in AI and cybersecurity, and ensure compliance.

In conclusion, while AI-driven approaches in healthcare cybersecurity offer transformative potential, they must be implemented with a keen awareness of the associated ethical and regulatory challenges. Balancing the benefits of AI with responsible and compliant use is key to harnessing its full potential in protecting healthcare data.

3.5 Comprehensive analysis of AI implementation and cybersecurity threats in healthcare

This section presents a holistic examination of the role of AI in enhancing cybersecurity within the healthcare sector, coupled with a detailed statistical analysis of various cybersecurity threats. The integration of AI in healthcare cybersecurity is a critical step toward addressing the increasing complexity and frequency of cyber threats. By examining real-world case studies and analyzing recent data on cybersecurity breaches, this section aims to provide a comprehensive understanding of the current landscape and the effectiveness of AI-driven solutions in mitigating these risks.

We explore several case studies that demonstrate the practical application of AI in healthcare cybersecurity. These include collaborations between renowned healthcare institutions and AI technology providers, such as Johns Hopkins Hospital with Protenus, MIT CSAIL with Beth Israel Deaconess Medical Center, and Swope Health Services with Darktrace. Each case study offers insights into how AI-driven platforms are being utilized to enhance data privacy, streamline EHRs, and bolster network security. The successes and challenges highlighted in these case studies provide valuable lessons on the implementation and impact of AI in healthcare cybersecurity.

Following the case studies, we delve into a statistical analysis of cybersecurity threats in healthcare, based on data from the U.S. Department of Health & Human Services—Office for Civil Rights. This analysis includes the categorization of breaches by type, location of breached information, covered entity type, and a state-wise distribution of reported threats. The findings reveal significant trends and patterns in cybersecurity breaches, such as the predominance of hacking/IT incidents and the vulnerability of network servers and email systems. This analysis not only highlights the areas most susceptible to cyber threats but also underscores the necessity for robust and adaptive cybersecurity measures, particularly in the digital domain.

3.5.1 Overview of AI implementation in healthcare cybersecurity

This section delves into the integration of AI in cybersecurity within the healthcare sector, focusing on the application of AI technologies to enhance security and efficiency. The case studies presented here offer a comprehensive view of the practical applications, challenges, and successes of AI-driven cybersecurity solutions in various healthcare settings, with a particular emphasis on AI-Driven Threat Intelligence Platforms.

- Johns Hopkins and Protenus: AI-Driven Privacy Analytics [19]. Johns Hopkins Hospital, in collaboration with Protenus, implemented an AI-driven platform for privacy analytics, a quintessential example of an AI-Driven Threat Intelligence Platform. The designed system monitors every access to patient data, significantly boosting the hospital's capability in detecting and responding to privacy violations and potential data breaches. The AI model, trained on diverse datasets, effectively distinguished between normal and anomalous access patterns. The implementation led to a dramatic reduction in investigation time and a significant decrease in the false-positive rate of alerts. This case study exemplifies the precision and efficiency of AI systems in safeguarding patient data and highlights the potential of AI in transforming healthcare cybersecurity.
- MIT CSAIL and Beth Israel Deaconess Medical Center: MedKnowts [20]. The collaboration between MIT's CSAIL and Beth Israel Deaconess Medical Center resulted in "MedKnowts," an AI-powered system aimed at improving the usability and efficiency of EHRs. MedKnowts integrates advanced information retrieval with intuitive note-taking capabilities, streamlining the documentation process for healthcare professionals. The system's integration of NLP and structured data intake made it easier for medical staff to record and retrieve patient information. The high system usability scale score indicates its effectiveness in enhancing the EHR experience, showcasing how AI can optimize healthcare data management and security.
- Swope Health Services and Darktrace: Network Security Enhancement [21]. Swope Health Services partnered with Darktrace to enhance its cybersecurity infrastructure. Darktrace's AI technology provided crucial insights into the network infrastructure, enabling better internal visibility and threat detection. The AI system's proficiency in identifying unusual network patterns underscored the importance of AI in providing comprehensive network security for large healthcare organizations. This case study highlights the role of AI in enhancing network security and protecting sensitive medical information.
- Cylance's Healthcare Clients: Proactive Cyber Threat Mitigation [21]. Cylance has been instrumental in providing AI-driven cybersecurity solutions to various healthcare organizations. Their approach, using ML algorithms to preemptively identify and neutralize cyber threats, demonstrates the proactive capabilities of AI in cybersecurity. The continuous learning aspect of the AI

system enhances its ability to detect sophisticated cyberattacks, underscoring the evolving nature of AI-driven threat intelligence platforms in healthcare.

- ClearDATA and Benson Area Medical Center: EHR System Optimization [21]. The collaboration between ClearDATA and Benson Area Medical Center aimed at optimizing the center's Electronic Health Record system using AI algorithms. These algorithms, trained on large datasets of patient and provider data, identified potential security threats and ensured compliance with healthcare regulations. The implementation led to increased productivity for healthcare providers and reduced operational costs, highlighting the potential of AI in optimizing EHR systems for both security and efficiency.
- IBM and United Family Healthcare: Enhanced Threat Management [22]. United Family Healthcare implemented IBM Security QRadar SIEM to enhance its cybersecurity capabilities. The system allowed team members to effectively manage and investigate prioritized threats, even with limited formal security training. IBM's ML add-ons provided real-time alerts on potential insider threats and monitored sensitive patient data flow, illustrating the effectiveness of AI in centralized threat management and regulatory compliance.
- CyncHealth: Achieving High Standards in Data Protection [23]. CyncHealth's achievements in obtaining SOC 2 Type 2 and HITRUST Certifications demonstrate their commitment to maintaining high standards of data protection and information security. These certifications highlight the importance of robust cybersecurity measures, particularly in health information exchanges. CyncHealth's success in cybersecurity standards showcases how AI and advanced security protocols can enhance data protection in healthcare.

These case studies collectively illustrate the transformative impact of AI in healthcare cybersecurity. They demonstrate how AI-driven solutions, particularly AI-Driven Threat Intelligence Platforms, are invaluable in enhancing EHR systems, providing comprehensive network security, and ensuring regulatory compliance, thereby safeguarding sensitive healthcare data against an ever-evolving landscape of cyber threats.

3.5.2 *Statistical analysis of cybersecurity threats in healthcare*

This section presents a comprehensive statistical analysis of various cybersecurity threats in the healthcare sector, utilizing data from the U.S. Department of Health & Human Services—Office for Civil Rights [24]. The analysis is based on reported breaches within the last 24 months and offers insights into the types of breaches, locations of breached information, covered entity types, and the distribution of threats across different states.

The first dataset categorizes the breaches by their type (Figure 3.9).

This frequency diagram visually represents the distribution of different types of cybersecurity breaches, such as hacking incidents and unauthorized access.

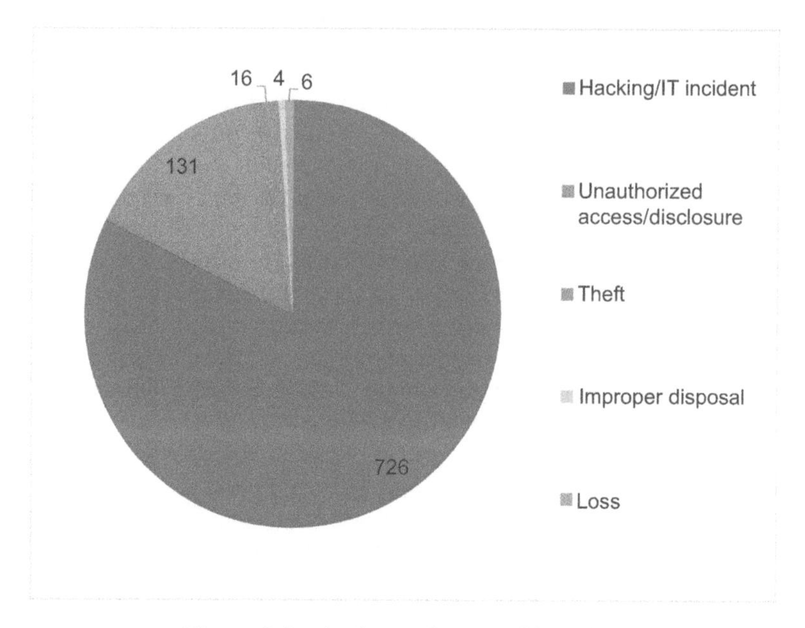

Figure 3.9 Analysis of types of breaches

Figure 3.9 helps in understanding the prevalence of various breach types in the healthcare sector.

The overwhelming majority of breaches are due to Hacking/IT Incidents, indicating a significant vulnerability in digital infrastructure. This underscores the critical need for robust cybersecurity measures, particularly against sophisticated cyberattacks. Unauthorized access/disclosure also forms a substantial portion, highlighting the importance of internal security protocols and employee training to prevent data breaches.

The second dataset focuses on where the breached information was located (Figure 3.10).

Figure 3.10 offers a frequency diagram that illustrates where breached information is most commonly found, such as network servers and emails. This visual representation aids in identifying the most vulnerable points in healthcare cybersecurity.

Network servers and email are the most common locations for breached information, suggesting that digital platforms are the primary targets for cyberattacks. This data highlights the necessity for enhanced security protocols for network servers and email systems. The presence of breaches in paper/films and portable devices also indicates the need for comprehensive security strategies covering both digital and physical data.

The third dataset categorizes the breaches by the type of covered entity (Figure 3.11).

This figure presents a frequency diagram of the types of entities most affected by cybersecurity breaches, including healthcare providers and business associates.

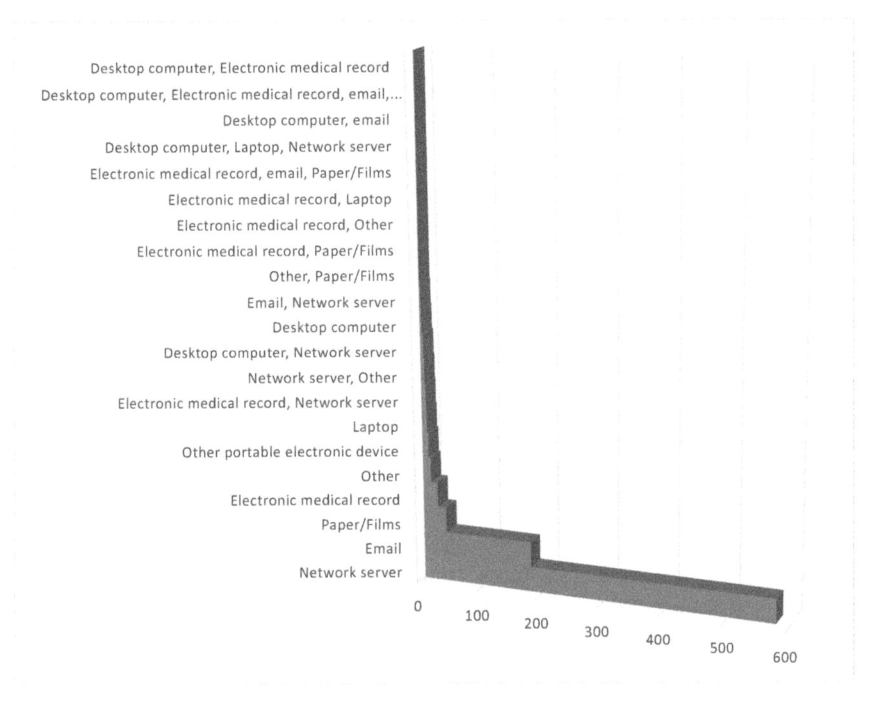

Figure 3.10 Analysis of location of breached information

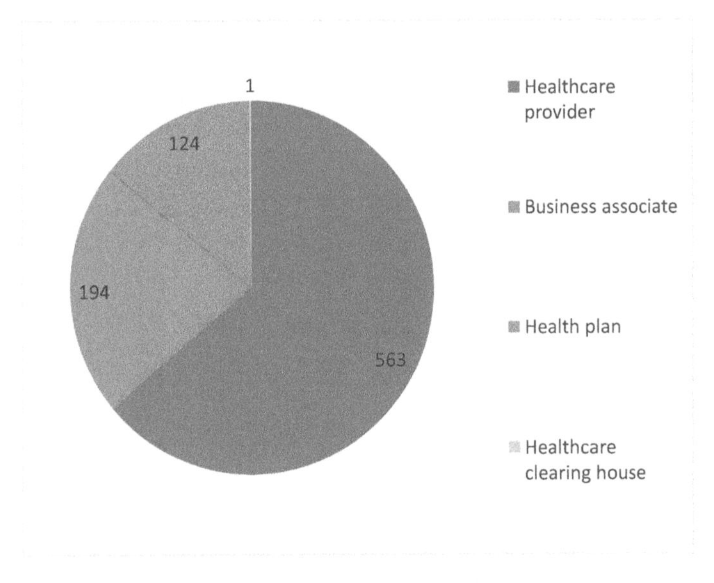

Figure 3.11 Analysis of covered entity type

Figure 3.11 visually underscores which entities in the healthcare sector are most at risk.

Healthcare providers are the most affected entity, which is not surprising given their direct involvement in patient care and data handling. Business associates and health plans also represent significant portions, emphasizing the need for stringent cybersecurity measures across all entities involved in healthcare.

The fourth dataset provides a state-wise distribution of reported threats (Figure 3.12):

- The highest number of breaches are reported in states like NY, TX, IL, CA, and MA.
- Other states follow with varying numbers of reported breaches.

Figure 3.12 provides a frequency diagram showing the distribution of cybersecurity threats across different states. This visual representation is crucial for understanding the geographical spread of cyber threats in the healthcare sector.

The distribution of breaches across states indicates that cybersecurity threats are a nationwide concern. States with larger populations and more healthcare facilities, like New York and Texas, naturally report more incidents. This geographic distribution underscores the need for a unified national strategy for healthcare cybersecurity, while also catering to state-specific needs.

This statistical analysis reveals critical insights into the cybersecurity landscape in healthcare. The predominance of digital breaches, particularly through hacking and IT incidents, highlights an urgent need for advanced cybersecurity solutions, including AI-driven threat intelligence platforms. These platforms can significantly contribute to detecting and mitigating such threats, especially in network servers and email systems, which are the most common breach locations.

Furthermore, the analysis underscores the importance of a holistic approach to cybersecurity, encompassing both digital and physical data protection across various healthcare entities. Tailored strategies are required to address the specific

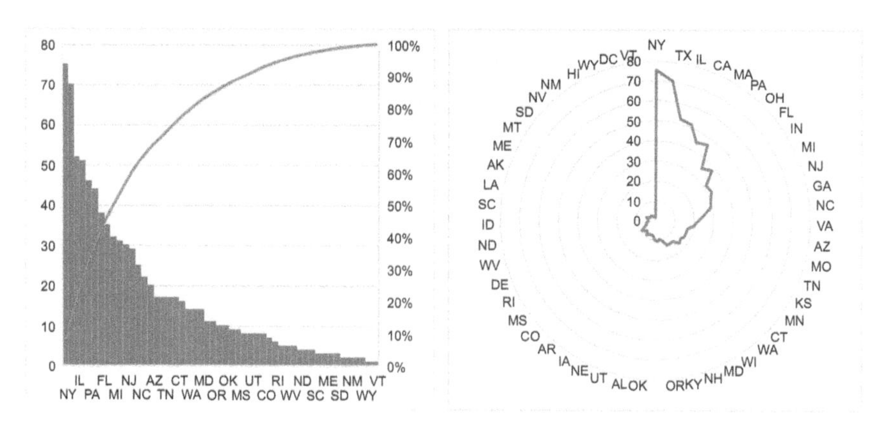

Figure 3.12 State-wise distribution of identified threats

needs of different states, considering their unique healthcare infrastructures and patient populations.

In conclusion, this analysis not only provides a clear picture of the current state of cybersecurity threats in healthcare but also reinforces the importance of integrating advanced AI-driven solutions to enhance the security and integrity of healthcare systems nationwide.

3.5.3 Comparative analysis: AI-driven approach vs. existing methods in healthcare cybersecurity

In this subsection, we conduct a comparative analysis between the proposed AI-driven approach to cybersecurity in healthcare and the existing traditional methods. This comparison aims to highlight the advancements and improvements brought about by AI technologies and to underscore the areas where AI significantly outperforms conventional cybersecurity strategies.

Traditional methods in healthcare cybersecurity primarily involve rule-based systems, regular software updates, firewalls, antivirus software, and manual monitoring. These methods focus on establishing a defensive perimeter to prevent unauthorized access and rely heavily on human intervention for threat detection and response.

AI-driven cybersecurity, on the other hand, incorporates advanced technologies such as ML algorithms, NLP, and neural networks. These technologies enable proactive threat detection, real-time data analysis, predictive threat modeling, and automated response mechanisms.

Table 3.3 provides a clear comparison between traditional and AI-driven cybersecurity methods in healthcare. While traditional methods offer simplicity and are well-established, they fall short in addressing the evolving and sophisticated nature

Table 3.3 Comparative analysis of traditional vs. AI-driven cybersecurity methods

Aspect	**Method**	**Description**	**Advantages**	**Limitations**
Threat Detection and Response	Traditional Methods	Rule-based systems, manual monitoring	Familiarity and simplicity	Ineffective against new/sophisticated attacks
	AI-Driven Approach	ML for pattern recognition	Detects unknown threats, faster response	Requires initial training and data
Scalability and Adaptability	Traditional Methods	Manual updates and adjustments	Established procedures	Time-consuming, not adaptive
	AI-Driven Approach	Continuous learning, adaptable algorithms	Scales with organization, adapts to new threats	Higher initial investment
Efficiency and Accuracy	Traditional Methods	Predefined rules, human intervention	Effective for known threats	High false-positive rates

(Continues)

Table 3.3 (*Continued*)

Aspect	Method	Description	Advantages	Limitations
	AI-Driven Approach	Automated detection, reduced false positives	Higher accuracy, operational efficiency	Depends on data quality and algorithms
Data Analysis Capabilities	Traditional Methods	Limited data handling	Suitable for smaller datasets	Misses critical insights in large data
	AI-Driven Approach	Handles large and unstructured data	Comprehensive insights, informed decisions	Requires advanced data processing capabilities
Cost and Resource Utilization	Traditional Methods	Frequent manual interventions	Lower initial cost	Higher long-term costs
	AI-Driven Approach	Automation, reduced manpower requirements	Cost-effective in the long run	Initial setup and training costs
Compliance and Reporting	Traditional Methods	Manual compliance processes	Direct control over processes	Time-consuming, error-prone
	AI-Driven Approach	Automated compliance monitoring and reporting	Accurate, consistent compliance	Requires alignment with regulatory standards

of cyber threats. AI-driven approaches, conversely, bring advanced capabilities like predictive analytics, real-time threat detection, and automated compliance management, making them more effective in the current cybersecurity landscape.

The AI-driven approach, despite requiring a higher initial investment and reliance on data quality, offers significant long-term benefits in terms of efficiency, accuracy, and cost-effectiveness. This makes it a more sustainable and forward-looking solution for healthcare cybersecurity challenges.

In conclusion, the shift toward AI-driven cybersecurity methods is a strategic move for healthcare organizations to enhance their defense mechanisms against an increasingly complex array of cyber threats.

3.6 Discussion of research findings and contributions

This section discusses the results of our research into the implementation of AI in healthcare cybersecurity and the statistical analysis of cybersecurity threats. We also highlight our significant contribution to the development and description of the architecture and functioning of AI-Driven Threat Intelligence Platforms:

- AI implementation in healthcare cybersecurity: The case studies reviewed demonstrate the effective integration of AI in various aspects of healthcare cybersecurity. These practical examples show the ability of AI to improve data privacy, enhance the efficiency of Electronic Health Record systems, and strengthen network security. The success of AI-driven platforms in reducing investigation times, lowering false-positive rates, and enhancing user experience in EHR systems underscores the transformative impact of AI in healthcare cybersecurity.

- Statistical analysis of cybersecurity threats: The analysis reveals a high prevalence of hacking/IT incidents, indicating a critical need for advanced security measures to protect against digital threats. The vulnerability of network servers and email systems to breaches highlights the importance of focusing cybersecurity efforts on these areas. The distribution of breaches across various states and entity types emphasizes the need for a comprehensive and adaptable cybersecurity strategy nationwide.

Our research makes a significant contribution to the field of AI-driven threat intelligence platforms in healthcare cybersecurity:

- Architecture and functioning: We provide a detailed description of the architecture of AI-driven threat intelligence platforms, elucidating how different AI components are integrated and function together. This includes the use of ML for anomaly detection, NLP for threat intelligence gathering, and neural networks for predictive analytics. Our analysis offers insights into the adaptability of these systems, highlighting their ability to evolve and learn from new data and threats.
- Practical implications: By presenting real-world case studies, we bridge the gap between theoretical AI models and their practical applications in healthcare cybersecurity. This not only demonstrates the effectiveness of AI-driven platforms but also provides a roadmap for their implementation in various healthcare settings. Our discussion on the integration challenges and best practices offers valuable guidance for healthcare organizations looking to adopt AI-driven cybersecurity solutions.
- Advancing the field: Our comprehensive analysis of existing cybersecurity threats and AI-driven solutions contributes to the ongoing discourse in the field. It provides a foundation for future research and development in AI-driven cybersecurity strategies. The comparative analysis between traditional methods and AI-driven approaches highlights the advancements brought about by AI technologies, encouraging their wider adoption in healthcare cybersecurity.

The findings from our research underscore the critical role of AI in enhancing healthcare cybersecurity. Our contribution to the understanding of AI-driven threat intelligence platforms, particularly in terms of their architecture and functioning, represents a significant advancement in this field. As cyber threats continue to evolve, the need for innovative and adaptive solutions like AI-driven platforms becomes increasingly paramount. Our research not only contributes to the academic understanding of these technologies but also serves as a practical guide for their implementation in safeguarding healthcare data.

3.7 Conclusion

In conclusion, our comprehensive investigation into the integration of AI in healthcare cybersecurity, coupled with a statistical analysis of recent cybersecurity threats, provides a nuanced understanding of the current landscape and the critical role of AI-driven solutions. The case studies and comparative analyses presented in this research highlight the transformative impact of AI technologies in enhancing data privacy, improving the efficiency of EHRs, and strengthening network security across various healthcare settings.

Our contribution to the development and description of the architecture and functioning of AI-Driven Threat Intelligence Platforms marks an advancement in this field. By elucidating the integration of ML, NLP, and neural networks within these platforms, we have outlined a roadmap for their effective implementation and adaptation in response to the evolving cybersecurity threats.

The findings from our research underscore the necessity for healthcare organizations to adopt advanced, AI-driven cybersecurity strategies to combat the increasing sophistication of cyber threats. As the digital landscape continues to evolve, the importance of innovative and adaptable solutions like AI-driven platforms becomes ever more paramount. Our research not only contributes to the academic discourse in this field but also serves as a practical guide for healthcare organizations seeking to enhance their cybersecurity measures and safeguard sensitive healthcare data against the ever-changing backdrop of cyber threats.

Finally, this chapter not only provides a thorough understanding of AI-driven cybersecurity in healthcare but also sets a foundation for future advancements in this field. Looking ahead, the scope for further research includes exploring the integration of emerging AI technologies, such as quantum computing and advanced predictive analytics, to enhance cybersecurity measures. Additionally, future studies could focus on developing more robust AI algorithms that are capable of adapting to the rapidly evolving landscape of cyber threats while ensuring compliance with evolving global data protection regulations.

Acknowledgment

- This project has received funding from the European Union's Horizon 2020 research and innovation program under the Marie Skłodowska-Curie grant agreement No. 101007820 – TRUST.
- This publication reflects only the author's view and the REA is not responsible for any use that may be made of the information it contains.

References

[1] P. Tao, N. Liu, and C. Dong, "Research progress of MIoT and digital healthcare in the new era," *Clinical eHealth*, 2023, doi:10.1016/j.ceh.2023.11.004.

[2] M. Javaid, A. Haleem, R. P. Singh, and R. Suman, "Towards insighting cybersecurity for healthcare domains: A comprehensive review of recent practices and trends," *Cyber Security and Applications*, vol. 1, p. 100016, 2023, doi:10.1016/j.csa.2023.100016.

[3] N. U. I. Hossain, S. Rahman, and S. A. Liza, "Cyber-susiliency index: A comprehensive resiliency-sustainability-cybersecurity index for healthcare supply chain networks," *Decision Analytics Journal*, vol. 9, p. 100319, 2023, doi:10.1016/j.dajour.2023.100319.

[4] C. Gong and V. Ribiere, "Chapter 1 - A historical outline of digital transformation," in *Digital Transformation in Healthcare in Post-Covid-19 Times*, M. D. Lytras, A. A. Housawi, and B. S. Alsaywid, (Eds.), in *Next Generation Technology Driven Personalized Medicine and Smart Healthcare.* Academic Press, 2023, pp. 3–25. doi:10.1016/B978-0-323-98353-2.00016-2.

[5] A. R. Iossifova and S. Meyer-Goldstein, "Impact of standards adoption on healthcare transaction performance: The case of HIPAA," *International Journal of Production Economics*, vol. 141, no. 1, pp. 277–285, 2013, doi:10.1016/j.ijpe.2012.08.002.

[6] J. Huang, Y. Y. Wong, W. S. Pang, *et al.*, "Usage of electronic health record (eHR) viewer among healthcare professionals (HCProfs): A territory-wide study of 3972 participants," *International Journal of Medical Informatics*, vol. 177, p. 105137, 2023, doi:10.1016/j.ijmedinf.2023.105137.

[7] E. Kim, S. M. Rubinstein, K. T. Nead, A. P. Wojcieszynski, P. E. Gabriel, and J. L. Warner, "The evolving use of electronic health records (EHR) for research," *Seminars in Radiation Oncology*, vol. 29, no. 4, pp. 354–361, 2019, doi:10.1016/j.semradonc.2019.05.010.

[8] A. Haleem, M. Javaid, R. P. Singh, and R. Suman, "Telemedicine for healthcare: Capabilities, features, barriers, and applications," *Sensors International*, vol. 2, p. 100117, 2021, doi:10.1016/j.sintl.2021.100117.

[9] S. Hansen and A. J. Baroody, "Beyond the boundaries of care: Electronic health records and the changing practices of healthcare," *Information and Organization*, vol. 33, no. 3, p. 100477, 2023, doi:10.1016/j.infoandorg.2023.100477.

[10] P. Mccaffrey, "Chapter 1 - The healthcare IT landscape," in *An Introduction to Healthcare Informatics*, P. Mccaffrey, (Ed.), Academic Press, 2020, pp. 3–15. doi:10.1016/B978-0-12-814915-7.00001-6.

[11] W. S. Admass, Y. Y. Munaye, and A. A. Diro, "Cyber security: State of the art, challenges and future directions," *Cyber Security and Applications*, vol. 2, p. 100031, 2024, doi:10.1016/j.csa.2023.100031.

[12] S. Mikuletič, S. Vrhovec, B. Skela-Savič, and B. Žvanut, "Security and privacy oriented information security culture (ISC): Explaining unauthorized access to healthcare data by nursing employees," *Computers & Security*, vol. 136, p. 103489, 2024, doi:10.1016/j.cose.2023.103489.

[13] F. Yan, N. Li, A. M. Iliyasu, A. S. Salama, and K. Hirota, "Insights into security and privacy issues in smart healthcare systems based on medical

images," *Journal of Information Security and Applications*, vol. 78, p. 103621, 2023, doi:10.1016/j.jisa.2023.103621.

[14] S. Qamar, "Federated convolutional model with cyber blockchain in medical image encryption using Multiple Rossler lightweight Logistic sine mapping," *Computers and Electrical Engineering*, vol. 110, p. 108883, 2023, doi:10.1016/j.compeleceng.2023.108883.

[15] S. Shukla, S. Thakur, S. Hussain, J. G. Breslin, and S. M. Jameel, "Identification and authentication in healthcare Internet-of-Things using integrated fog computing based blockchain model," *Internet of Things*, vol. 15, p. 100422, 2021, doi:10.1016/j.iot.2021.100422.

[16] A. G. Sreedevi, T. Nitya Harshitha, V. Sugumaran, and P. Shankar, "Application of cognitive computing in healthcare, cybersecurity, big data and IoT: A literature review," *Information Processing & Management*, vol. 59, no. 2, p. 102888, 2022, doi:10.1016/j.ipm.2022.102888.

[17] B. Coutinho, J. Ferreira, I. Yevseyeva, and V. Basto-Fernandes, "Integrated cybersecurity methodology and supporting tools for healthcare operational information systems," *Computers & Security*, vol. 129, p. 103189, 2023, doi:10.1016/j.cose.2023.103189.

[18] S. Tarikere, I. Donner, and D. Woods, "Diagnosing a healthcare cybersecurity crisis: The impact of IoMT advancements and 5G," *Business Horizons*, vol. 64, no. 6, pp. 799–807, 2021, doi:10.1016/j.bushor.2021.07.015.

[19] "Improving Healthcare Data Security with AI." Accessed: Dec. 11, 2023. [Online]. Available: https://www.healthcatalyst.com/insights/improving-healthcare-data-security-with-ai

[20] "AI Improves Electronic Health Record (EHR) Systems | Psychology Today." Accessed: Dec. 11, 2023. [Online]. Available: https://www.psychologytoday.com/us/blog/the-future-brain/202110/ai-improves-electronic-health-record-ehr-systems

[21] "Cybersecurity in Healthcare – Comparing 5 AI-Based Vendor Offerings | Emerj Artificial Intelligence Research." Accessed: Dec. 11, 2023. [Online]. Available: https://emerj.com/ai-application-comparisons/cybersecurity-healthcare-comparing-5-ai-based-vendor-offerings/

[22] "United Family Healthcare (UFH) | IBM." Accessed: Dec. 11, 2023. [Online]. Available: https://www.ibm.com/case-studies/united-family-healthcare

[23] D. Raths, "HIE CyncHealth Beefs Up Cybersecurity with SOC 2, HITRUST Certifications," Healthcare Innovation. Accessed: Dec. 11, 2023. [Online]. Available: https://www.hcinnovationgroup.com/cybersecurity/frameworks/news/53066961/hie-cynchealth-beefs-up-cybersecurity-with-soc-2-hitrust-certifications

[24] "U.S. Department of Health & Human Services - Office for Civil Rights." Accessed: Nov. 12, 2023. [Online]. Available: https://ocrportal.hhs.gov/ocr/breach/breach_report.jsf#

Chapter 4

Emerging trends in cybersecurity applications in healthcare systems

Kassim Kalinaki[1,2], *Rufai Yusuf Zakari*[3] *and Wasswa Shafik*[4]

As healthcare organizations rapidly adopt connected technologies and amass troves of sensitive patient data, they have become prime targets for increasingly sophisticated cyberattacks. This comprehensive study investigates the growing synergy between cybersecurity and healthcare in an era of heightened digitalization and cyber threats. It underscores the alarming vulnerabilities introduced by digitization across patient care, medical facilities, and administrative systems. Through real-world case analyses, it delineates the mounting risks of disruptive intrusions, privacy violations, and systemic compromises that jeopardize patient safety and public health. Accordingly, the study surveys cutting-edge technologies poised to harden healthcare cybersecurity. It examines the potential of artificial intelligence and ML to predict, detect, and autonomously respond to threats. The viability of blockchain, quantum computing, and zero trust frameworks in strengthening data protection and identity management are analyzed. The critical importance of security awareness training and actionable threat intelligence is also explored. Moreover, the study elucidates the complex challenges of integrating these robust yet often complex technologies into intricate clinical environments and workflows. It offers insights into how healthcare organizations can balance improved cybersecurity with user experience, regulations, legacy systems, and resource constraints. With cyber threats growing in lockstep with healthcare digitization, this study delivers a multifaceted analysis to help medical practitioners and administrators secure critical healthcare systems. It provides technology leaders a guide to emerging innovations for healthcare cybersecurity. Policymakers and regulators will benefit from its scrutiny of existing gaps.

Keywords: Healthcare systems; electronic health records; security; privacy; artificial intelligence; cyber threat intelligence

[1]Department of Computer Science, Islamic University in Uganda (IUIU), Uganda
[2]Department of Computer Science, Borderline Research Laboratory, Uganda
[3]School of Digital Science, Universiti Brunei Darussalam Jalan Tungku Link, Brunei
[4]Department of Computer Engineering, Dig Connectivity Research Laboratory, Uganda

4.1 Introduction

In the age of rapid technological advancement, the interplay between healthcare and cybersecurity has emerged as a crucial focus, necessitating thorough exploration to confront challenges arising from the swiftly evolving digital terrain [1,2]. The healthcare sector, holding highly sensitive patient information, is a prime target for cyber threats, ranging from financially motivated malicious actors to state-sponsored entities engaged in espionage. Patient records, such as medical histories, diagnostic details, and personally identifiable information (PII), serve as invaluable assets in the hands of cybercriminals [3,4]. The compromise of such data directly jeopardizes individual privacy and erodes the trust between patients and healthcare providers, undermining the fundamental basis of effective healthcare delivery.

The backbone of modern healthcare delivery lies in healthcare infrastructure, which includes interconnected medical devices, Electronic Health Records (EHRs), and communication systems [5]. These systems' escalating digitization and interconnectivity expand the attack surfaces, exposing vulnerabilities exploitable by cyber adversaries. The repercussions of a successful cyberattack on healthcare infrastructure extend beyond data breaches, encompassing disruptions to patient care, compromised medical procedures, and, in extreme cases, threats to patient safety [3,6].

Consequently, the imperative of establishing robust cybersecurity practices in healthcare systems is underscored by the evolving tactics employed by cyber threats [7]. Ransomware attacks, in particular, have evolved into sophisticated and targeted operations, often paralyzing healthcare institutions and demanding substantial ransoms for critical data release [8].

Moreover, Advanced Persistent Threats (APTs) and data breaches have become more targeted and intricately planned, posing significant challenges to the traditionally risk-averse healthcare industry [9,10]. Cyber adversaries, ranging from individual hackers to organized criminal groups, increasingly target healthcare institutions, recognizing the intrinsic value of sensitive patient data and potential disruptions to critical healthcare services [11]. The financial implications of such attacks are staggering. Still, their potential impact on patient care and public health is even more profound, as was noticed in the recent SolarWinds cyberattack [12]. Moreover, the intricate relationship between healthcare and cybersecurity transcends technological considerations, involving legal, ethical, and regulatory dimensions that necessitate careful navigation [13].

Addressing these challenges requires healthcare systems to adopt a proactive and multifaceted approach to cybersecurity involving advanced encryption protocols, robust access controls, and continuous monitoring of network activities. Regular cybersecurity audits and penetration testing can identify vulnerabilities before exploitation, contributing to developing a resilient cybersecurity posture [3]. Additionally, the integration of Artificial Intelligence (AI) and machine learning (ML) in cybersecurity practices enhances the ability to detect and respond to evolving threats in real time, as these technologies can analyze vast amounts of data, identify patterns indicative of malicious activities, and enable a rapid response to mitigate potential risks [1,14].

Collaboration among healthcare organizations, cybersecurity experts, and regulatory bodies is crucial to establishing a unified front against cyber threats. Information sharing about emerging threats, best practices, and lessons learned from past incidents can collectively elevate the cybersecurity posture of the entire healthcare sector [15]. In summary, the urgency to establish and maintain robust cybersecurity practices in the healthcare domain is paramount, driven by the sensitive nature of patient information and the vulnerability of healthcare infrastructure. This study aims to provide a comprehensive review of emerging cybersecurity trends and applications in the healthcare sector, fortifying existing cybersecurity measures and enabling the healthcare sector to navigate the evolving threat landscape, ensuring the integrity of patient data and the uninterrupted delivery of quality healthcare services.

4.1.1 Chapter contributions

- A comprehensive analysis of the vulnerabilities emerging when healthcare institutions embrace digital technologies underscores the potential repercussions of cyberattacks on healthcare institutions, patients, and the broader healthcare ecosystem.
- An extensive discussion of the various emerging cybersecurity trends and solutions in healthcare, encompassing AI-powered techniques, Blockchain technology, ZTAs, security awareness and training, cyber threat intelligence, and quantum computing
- Highlight the different challenges resulting from embracing emerging cybersecurity applications in healthcare systems.

4.1.2 Chapter organization

After the introduction in Section 4.1, the rest of the chapter is structured as follows: Section 4.2 details the various emerging cybersecurity trends in fortifying healthcare systems. Section 4.3 discusses the challenges of adopting emerging cybersecurity trends including a summary of solutions, highlighting examples. Section 4.4 highlights the lessons learned, and Section 4.5 concludes the chapter.

4.2 Emerging trends in cybersecurity applications in healthcare systems

This section details the selected identified emerging trends demonstrating the existing techniques and their applications in healthcare systems, including ML, AI, blockchain technologies, and zero trust architecture (ZTA). They are depicted in Figure 4.1.

4.2.1 Machine learning and Artificial Intelligence

The application of AI-driven techniques in healthcare security is extensively examined, particularly in threat detection, anomaly identification, and predictive

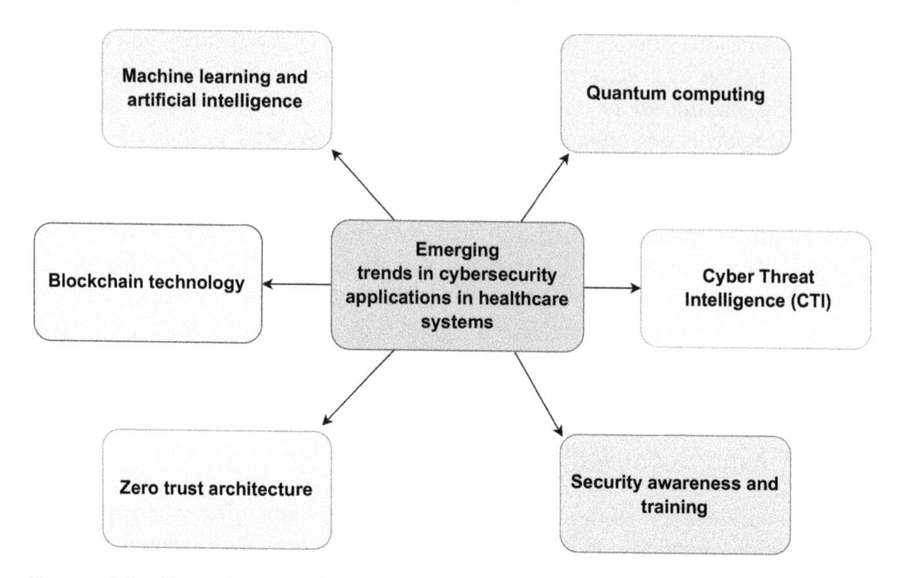

Figure 4.1 Emerging trends in cybersecurity applications in healthcare systems

analysis. Particular focus is placed on implementing precise algorithms and models and their effectiveness in identifying and reducing cyber threats in healthcare systems, as illustrated below.

4.2.1.1 Anomaly detection and behavioral analysis

AI-enabled algorithms have demonstrated a vital role in detecting abnormalities and inconsistencies in healthcare system data. Baseline behaviors and patterns are established to identify aberrant activity that could potentially indicate a cyber threat [16]. These systems employ unsupervised learning methods to assess user access patterns, device actions, and network traffic consistently. These technologies promptly identify potential security breaches and autonomously adjust to changing threats, improving the system's capacity to detect and counter cyberattacks [17].

4.2.1.2 Predictive analytics for threat intelligence

This is achieved by evaluating extensive volumes of historical and real-time data [18]. Through analyzing trends, vulnerabilities, and historical attack patterns, these systems offer significant information to security teams, enabling them to strengthen defenses and proactively avoid prospective breaches [19]. They accomplish this by actively finding and resolving vulnerabilities in the system, enabling healthcare businesses to remain ahead of cyber threats.

4.2.1.3 Cyberattack detection and response

AI-driven solutions in the healthcare sector employ constant surveillance of network traffic, device actions, and system records to identify and counteract cyber assaults promptly. By utilizing supervised and unsupervised learning techniques,

ML algorithms can distinguish between regular and harmful actions, facilitating prompt reactions to incidents; Arctic Wolf, as illustrated, demonstrated the top 15 cybercrimes that happened to healthcare in the United States [1]. Autonomous systems can autonomously isolate compromised systems, notify security personnel, and implement preventive measures to limit the consequences of a cyberattack. This helps to reduce the disruption to healthcare services and safeguard confidential patient information [20].

4.2.1.4 Enhanced authentication and access control

These advanced technologies enhance authentication processes in healthcare systems by analyzing user behavior, biometric data, and contextual information. These systems employ supervised learning models to constantly adjust and acquire knowledge from fresh data, resulting in enhanced and flexible authentication procedures, like data breach prevention [21,22]. These systems detect irregular user activity, such as atypical login times or locations, and initiate additional verification measures to ensure access security. By implementing adaptive access restrictions that rely on ongoing ML analysis, illegal access attempts can be prevented, safeguarding patient information from unauthorized individuals [23].

4.2.1.5 Vulnerability management and patching automation

These technologies aid in vulnerability management by examining system vulnerabilities and ranking them according to their potential danger to healthcare systems. These solutions streamline the detection of vulnerabilities and the implementation of necessary updates or corrections [24]. These systems employ machine learning algorithms to prioritize vulnerabilities based on their criticality and possible impact. This approach optimizes the allocation of resources for patching. By adopting this proactive approach, healthcare companies can effectively anticipate and tackle weaknesses, minimizing the time they are susceptible to potential cyber threats.

4.2.1.6 Real-time threat intelligence and adaptive defense

Cybersecurity systems that utilize existing technologies consistently collect and analyze data on potential threats from several sources. These systems use natural language processing (NLP) and ML to analyze extensive quantities of real-time threat data, detecting emerging threats and attack patterns [14,25]. These technologies possess the ability to independently adjust their protection systems in response to the changing threat of the environment. Engaging in ongoing education enhances their capacity to identify and thwart novel and intricate cyber assaults, thereby offering proactive protection for healthcare systems.

4.2.2 Blockchain technology

Blockchain technology provides the capacity to safeguard patient records and improve data reliability in the healthcare sector. It specifically emphasizes its ability to reduce data breaches and facilitate secure data sharing, real-world instances of blockchain implementations in the healthcare sector, specifically focusing on the secure administration of patient data.

4.2.2.1 Secure health data exchange

Blockchain provides secure and decentralized health data transmission across multiple healthcare providers while respecting patient privacy. The system creates an immutable and easily verifiable record where cryptographic means logs every transaction as a block, securely connected to the preceding one. The unchangeable record guarantees the authenticity of patient data, preventing any illegal modifications or unauthorized access [26]. Patients maintain authority over their data via cryptographic keys, enabling them to authorize or withdraw access to specified entities, promoting confidence and confidentiality in data exchange.

4.2.2.2 Protected electronic health records

Blockchain ensures the security of EHRs by establishing a decentralized and encrypted ledger. Confidential data, including patient records, diagnoses, treatment histories, and other sensitive information, are distributed and kept on various nodes inside the network. This distributed storage method mitigates a singular vulnerability, diminishing the likelihood of data breaches [27]. Furthermore, the utilization of consensus techniques guarantees that any alterations to the records necessitate validation by the network, ensuring the data's accuracy and dependability.

4.2.2.3 Supply chain integrity and drug traceability

Blockchain improves the reliability of the pharmaceutical supply chain by offering visibility and the capacity to track the movement of products. The blockchain records every step involved in medicine manufacturing, distribution, and delivery [28]. This establishes unchangeable goods and enables interested parties to confirm the genuineness of medications, thwart the production of fake goods, and monitor the transportation of pharmaceuticals from producer to recipient, diminishing the likelihood of deceitful or compromised drugs infiltrating the system.

4.2.2.4 Identity management and authentication

Blockchain technology enhances identity management and authentication procedures in the healthcare sector. The technology offers a decentralized approach to managing patient IDs and authentication credentials. The patients' identifying information is encrypted and securely maintained on the blockchain, eliminating the necessity for centralized systems susceptible to breaches. In addition, authentication methods that utilize blockchain technology, such as digital signatures or biometric data saved on the blockchain, provide high security and unchangeable identity verification [29]. This helps to minimize the chances of identity theft and unauthorized entry into healthcare systems.

4.2.2.5 Immutable audit trails and compliance

The unchangeable ledger of blockchain ensures that all interactions with healthcare data are recorded transparently and auditable. This capability is beneficial in guaranteeing adherence to rigorous requirements, for example, the Health Insurance Portability and Accountability Act. All instances of accessing or altering patient records are consistently documented, creating an immutable record of the actions taken [30]. This feature facilitates the demonstration of compliance during audits and investigations, making the process more efficient and assuring responsibility throughout the healthcare system.

4.2.2.6 Tamper-resistant clinical trials and research data

The tamper-resistant nature of blockchain guarantees the integrity and security of clinical trial data and research outcomes. Storing trial data on a blockchain network ensures the integrity of records by preventing any tampering or illegal modifications due to the immutability of the data. The transparency and dependability of data fosters trust among stakeholders, such as regulatory agencies, researchers, and participants [31]. Additionally, it accelerates verifying and confirming trial findings, improving the reliability of medical research conclusions. The capacity of blockchain to securely trace and authenticate data from multiple origins enhances data integrity, enabling the advancement of more precise and dependable medical treatments and interventions [32]. As a result, it enhances healthcare systems' overall reliability and protection by defending crucial research data against possible breaches or manipulations.

4.2.2.7 Research and clinical trials integrity

Blockchain guarantees the authenticity and openness of data utilized in medical research and clinical trials. Storing research data on a decentralized ledger ensures its immunity against tampering. This ensures the integrity of study findings and trial results, preventing any modification or falsification of data [29]. Moreover, it facilitates the streamlined and protected exchange of research data between institutions, promoting cooperation while safeguarding intellectual assets and guaranteeing the precision of research results, a critical factor in advancing medical knowledge and innovation.

4.2.2.8 Decentralized identity and access management

Blockchain enables decentralized identification solutions, allowing patients to control their healthcare identities securely. Individuals can manage healthy data access by authorizing cryptographic keys on the blockchain. This decentralized strategy diminishes dependence on centralized databases susceptible to breaches at a single location [31]. Furthermore, it simplifies the process of managing access for healthcare providers, enabling them to retrieve pertinent patient information securely when granted permission, enhancing care coordination while upholding rigorous data security and privacy standards.

4.2.3 Zero trust architecture

This explores the concept of a "zero trust architecture" (ZTA) security approach, highlighting its increasing significance in healthcare systems, and delves into the thorough examination of the utilization of ZTA to verify identities and safeguard network access, with the added benefit of reducing risks posed by insiders.

4.2.3.1 Micro-segmentation for access control

ZTA utilizes micro-segmentation to partition the network into smaller, distinct portions. The granular method employed here limits lateral mobility within the network by restricting access to specific resources according to the concept of least privilege. This entails dividing patient data, systems, and equipment into separate segments in healthcare, permitting only authorized individuals to access the required information [33]. ZTA, with the implementation of stringent access controls and uniform security rules across segments, minimizes the potential for unauthorized access or data breaches by reducing the attack surface.

4.2.3.2 Continuous authentication and monitoring

ZTA employs ongoing authentication procedures to verify user identities and device integrity prior to authorizing access to resources. Healthcare systems utilize multifactor authentication, behavioral analytics, and ML to authenticate the legitimacy of users and devices consistently. This method guarantees that access privileges are adaptively modified according to instantaneous evaluations of user conduct, device conditions, and contextual data [21]. As a result, it effectively blocks unwanted access attempts and quickly identifies and addresses suspicious behaviors, improving the overall security level.

4.2.3.3 Application-centric security

ZTA places high importance on securing apps by specifically safeguarding applications and their data rather than just depending on network boundaries [19]. This method ensures the protection of vital healthcare apps and confidential data by implementing security controls and encryption at the application level. ZTA effectively reduces the likelihood of data breaches and unauthorized access to healthcare data by directly integrating robust authentication and encryption measures into the applications [33]. This ensures that the data remains secure, even if there are breaches in the system's perimeter.

4.2.3.4 Policy-based access control and least privilege

ZTA utilizes access controls based on policies to enforce the notion of granting the minimum necessary privileges. Access determinations are influenced by contextual variables such as user authentication, device condition, geographical position, and conduct [30]. In healthcare, this entails providing access exclusively to authorized individuals for particular purposes and durations. ZTA consistently assesses access requests based on specified criteria, guaranteeing that users and devices possess the necessary level of access needed to carry out their activities [31]. This strategy mitigates the potential for insider attacks, inadvertent data disclosure, or compromised devices gaining access to critical healthcare information.

4.2.3.5 Dynamic risk assessment and adaptive controls

ZTA employs dynamic risk assessment methods that continuously evaluate the risk status of individuals, devices, and apps that contact healthcare systems. ZTA employs real-time threat intelligence, behavioral analytics, and ML algorithms to adjust security settings in response to changing threats and contextual risk factors. For example, suppose a user or device exhibits anomalous behavior or faces a possible danger. In that case, ZTA promptly modifies access privileges or implements supplementary security measures in real-time [32]. This adaptable strategy guarantees that security measures align with the existing risk landscape, reducing the effects of developing threats and vulnerabilities within healthcare networks.

4.2.3.6 Secure remote access and secure connectivity

Within the healthcare industry, which is experiencing a growing presence of remote access and telemedicine, ZTA places significant importance on ensuring safe connectivity and implementing controls for remote access. ZTA frameworks use robust security mechanisms such as zero-trust VPNs and secure access service edge* (SASE) solutions to guarantee that remote users and devices are held to the same rigorous security standards as on-site systems [34]. ZTA ensures a constant security stance by confirming identities, validating the trustworthiness of devices, and encrypting data flow independent of the user's location. This safeguards patient data and healthcare systems from potential dangers from remote connections.

4.2.3.7 Continuous monitoring and incident response

ZTA prioritizes the ongoing surveillance of network traffic, user actions, and device patterns in healthcare systems. This method examines network telemetry, logs, and user activities to identify irregularities and possible security risks. ZTA frameworks utilize sophisticated analytics and ML techniques to detect deviations from typical behavior and rapidly initiate incident response methods [33]. Continuous monitoring guarantees a proactive security approach, allowing healthcare companies to promptly address and reduce security issues before they worsen, reducing the consequences on patient data and essential infrastructure.

4.2.3.8 Integration of security automation and orchestration

ZTA frameworks in the healthcare industry incorporate security automation and orchestration to optimize security procedures and response measures. ZTA minimizes the need for manual intervention and decreases response times by automating basic security operations, including threat detection, validation, and containment. Security orchestration coordinates and integrates different security tools and systems to achieve a unified and coordinated response to security occurrences [35]. This method improves the effectiveness of incident response and guarantees the uniform implementation of security policies throughout the healthcare environment, thereby preserving a solid security position.

4.2.4 Security awareness and training

As healthcare organizations increasingly rely on digital technologies to streamline operations and enhance patient care, a well-informed and vigilant workforce

*https://www.barracuda.com/products/network-protection

becomes paramount. This section explores the constituents of effective security training programs, highlighting the importance of comprehensive knowledge about cyber threats, social engineering tactics, and optimal strategies for maintaining a secure environment.

4.2.4.1 Comprehensive knowledge of cyber threats

Healthcare personnel should possess an in-depth understanding of various cyber threats that pose risks to the organization. This includes malware, ransomware, phishing attacks, and other malicious activities prevalent in the healthcare sector. For instance, a training module could consist of case studies on recent cyberattacks in the healthcare industry, analyzing how specific malware infiltrated systems, or detailing the impact of a successful phishing campaign. Real-life examples enhance awareness and provide practical insights into the tactics employed by cybercriminals [36].

4.2.4.2 Social engineering tactics

To fortify defenses against social engineering, healthcare training programs should focus on educating professionals about various manipulation tactics cybercriminals use, including phishing emails, pretexting, and impersonation [37]. Simulated phishing exercises can be integrated into the training, allowing employees to receive mock phishing emails and testing their ability to discern potential threats. These hands-on exercises serve to reinforce the importance of skepticism and vigilance when interacting with digital communications.

4.2.4.3 Optimal strategies for maintaining a secure environment

Equipping healthcare personnel with the knowledge to implement optimal security strategies is crucial. Training workshops can cover topics such as creating strong and unique passwords and demonstrations of multifactor authentication implementation. Real-world scenarios demonstrating the consequences of lax security practices can underscore the workforce's collective responsibility in maintaining a secure environment [36,37].

4.2.4.4 Incident response training

In addition to preventive measures, healthcare personnel must be well-prepared to handle cybersecurity incidents effectively. Incident response training can include tabletop exercises simulating various cybersecurity incidents, such as ransomware attacks or data breaches. Through these simulations, participants can practice response strategies in a controlled environment, honing their skills in containment, investigation, and recovery [37].

4.2.4.5 Continuous monitoring and updating

Training programs should emphasize the significance of continuous monitoring and staying updated on the latest cybersecurity trends. Regularly scheduled webinars or newsletters can provide ongoing updates on emerging threats and best practices.

This approach ensures that healthcare personnel remain informed and reinforces the dynamic nature of cybersecurity, fostering a proactive attitude toward security awareness [36].

4.2.5 Cyber threat intelligence (CTI)

Cyber threat intelligence is a proactive approach to cybersecurity that involves gathering, analyzing, and applying information about potential threats and vulnerabilities to enhance an organization's defenses [38]. In healthcare, where sensitive patient data and critical infrastructure are at stake, the proactive use of CTI is crucial in preventing and mitigating cyber threats. CTI allows healthcare professionals to stay ahead of these threats by continuously monitoring and analyzing emerging trends in the cyber threat landscape [39].

4.2.5.1 Successful threat intelligence sharing initiatives

Collaboration and information sharing are crucial components of effective CTI implementation. Several successful initiatives showcase the power of shared intelligence in bolstering cybersecurity within healthcare systems. While not exclusive to healthcare, the Multi-State Information Sharing and Analysis Center (MS-ISAC) is a notable example of cross-sector collaboration. Healthcare organizations benefit from its threat intelligence sharing platform, which facilitates real-time information exchange [40]. This shared intelligence helps healthcare entities preemptively respond to threats that may have implications beyond the healthcare sector. Dedicated specifically to the healthcare industry, the Health Information Sharing and Analysis Center (H-ISAC) focuses on providing a secure platform for sharing cyber threat intelligence [41]. Healthcare organizations can gain insights into industry-specific threats, tactics, and vulnerabilities through this collaborative effort, allowing them to fortify their defenses accordingly.

4.2.6 Quantum computing

Due to its unparalleled processing power, quantum computing introduces a new frontier in the ongoing battle against cyber threats. Its integration into healthcare cybersecurity marks a paradigm shift in safeguarding sensitive medical data [42]. One of the critical aspects of quantum computing lies in its ability to break conventional encryption algorithms currently employed to secure sensitive healthcare information. The sheer computational prowess of quantum computers renders traditional cryptographic methods vulnerable. Therefore, integrating quantum-resistant cryptographic techniques becomes imperative to fortify healthcare systems against potential breaches. In addition to its disruptive impact on conventional encryption, quantum computing offers a unique opportunity to enhance data protection by developing quantum-safe encryption. Quantum key distribution (QKD) is a prime example, leveraging the principles of quantum mechanics to create unbreakable cryptographic keys. Implementing QKD ensures that data transmission remains secure, even in the face of quantum-powered decryption attempts [43]. As the quantum computing paradigm evolves, there is a pressing need to anticipate potential threats and adopt quantum-resistant security solutions. Proactive preparations involve staying abreast of advancements in quantum computing and collaborating with experts in the field to fortify existing cybersecurity infrastructures.

4.3 Challenges of adopting emerging technologies in healthcare systems

This section discusses the challenges of adopting cutting-edge cybersecurity technologies in healthcare systems.

4.3.1 Increased attack surface

The pervasive connectivity in healthcare systems expands the attack surface, making them more vulnerable to cyber threats. For instance, integrating IoT devices, such as medical wearables and smart infusion pumps, introduces additional points of access that malicious actors may exploit [1]. The proliferation of connected healthcare devices has expanded the attack surface, exemplified by the 2021 Accellion data breach affecting healthcare organizations [44]. Cybercriminals exploited vulnerabilities in a file transfer system, underscoring the urgency for robust security protocols to safeguard against evolving threats. Hence, ensuring robust security protocols becomes imperative to protect against potential breaches.

4.3.2 Sophisticated cyberattacks

Cyber adversaries employ increasingly sophisticated methodologies, including ransomware, phishing, and zero-day exploits, posing formidable threats to healthcare data integrity [45–47]. The deployment of advanced attack vectors underscores the imperative for heightened cybersecurity measures and continuous vigilance. Sophisticated cyber threats, such as ransomware attacks like WannaCry in 2017, impacted numerous hospitals globally [48]. Recent instances, like the SolarWinds supply chain attack in 2020, demonstrate the sophistication of cyberattacks targeting healthcare systems [12]. The incident compromised several organizations, emphasizing the need for advanced cybersecurity measures, constant threat monitoring, and adaptive defense strategies.

4.3.3 Data privacy and compliance

Adherence to data protection regulations, like the Health Insurance Portability and Accountability Act (HIPAA) and General Data Protection Regulation (GDPR), is critical to maintaining patient trust. The recent surge in ransomware attacks, such as the 2021 attack on Ireland's Health Service Executive, underscores the crucial importance of refined policy formulation to balance compliance with robust cybersecurity [49,50]. Moreover, the ongoing evolution of cybersecurity threats is exemplified by the 2021 Microsoft Exchange Server vulnerabilities [51]. Healthcare organizations adapting to such dynamics, alongside continuous updates to regulations like HIPAA and GDPR, demonstrate the need for an agile cybersecurity strategy to navigate the evolving threat landscape effectively.

4.3.4 Insider threats

The susceptibility of healthcare systems to insider threats, whether inadvertent or deliberate, accentuates the importance of stringent access controls and continuous monitoring. Figure 4.2 depicts the different motivations of insider attacks in any organization including healthcare facilities. Mitigating such risks requires continuous employee education, behavioral analytics, and vigilant privileged access management [52].

4.3.5 Legacy systems and interoperability

The persistence of legacy infrastructure within healthcare environments, like outdated EHR systems, presents challenges concerning security vulnerabilities and interoperability [53,54]. Transitioning to secure alternatives is exemplified by the UK's National Health Service (NHS), which faced cybersecurity challenges due to outdated systems during the WannaCry attack [55]. Striking a balance between technological advancement and operational continuity is crucial.

4.3.6 Human factor

The human element remains a substantial vulnerability in healthcare cybersecurity, necessitating emphasis on comprehensive training programs addressing social engineering and best security practices. Human vulnerabilities in cybersecurity are

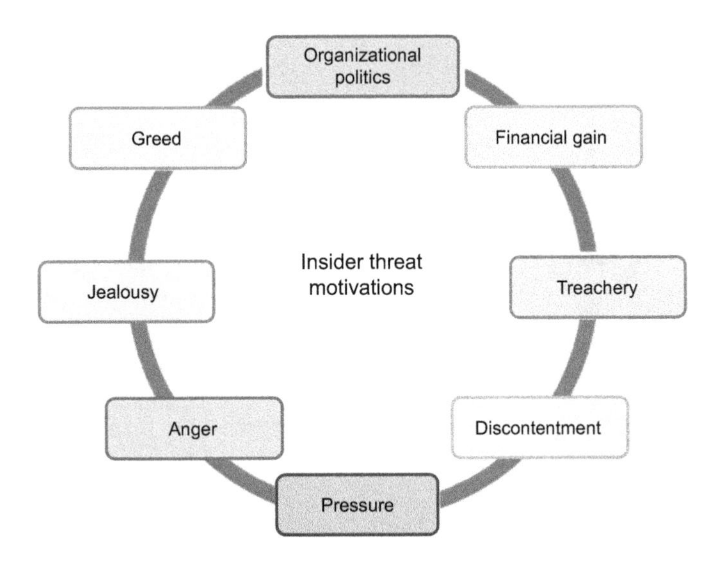
Organizational politics
Financial gain
Treachery
Discontentment
Pressure
Anger
Jealousy
Greed
Insider threat motivations

Figure 4.2 Insider threat motivations

evident in healthcare professionals falling victim to phishing attacks [56]. A well-known example is the 2015 Anthem breach, where a phishing email compromised employee credentials [57]. Comprehensive training programs emphasizing social engineering awareness are essential to mitigate these risks.

4.3.7 Supply chain risks

The intricate supply chain ecosystem inherent to healthcare introduces vulnerabilities stemming from third-party vendors [58]. Third-party vendors in the healthcare supply chain introduce vulnerabilities, as seen in the 2020 Blackbaud data breach affecting healthcare organizations [59]. Robust supply chain risk management involves vetting vendors, contractual cybersecurity stipulations, and continuous monitoring to ensure the security of the entire ecosystem. Figure 4.3 illustrates a supply chain attack scenario, applicable to entities including healthcare facilities.

4.3.8 Incident response and recovery

The evolving threat landscape underscores the imperative of a well-defined incident response and recovery strategy. The 2020 Universal Health Services cyber-attack showcased the significance of preemptive planning, regular drills, and continuous refinement of response protocols to mitigate the impact of cybersecurity incidents on healthcare services [60].

Table 4.1 summarizes the challenges of adopting cutting-edge cybersecurity technologies in healthcare systems along with proposed solutions.

In conclusion, the challenges faced by healthcare systems in adapting to emerging trends in cybersecurity applications are both multifaceted and pressing.

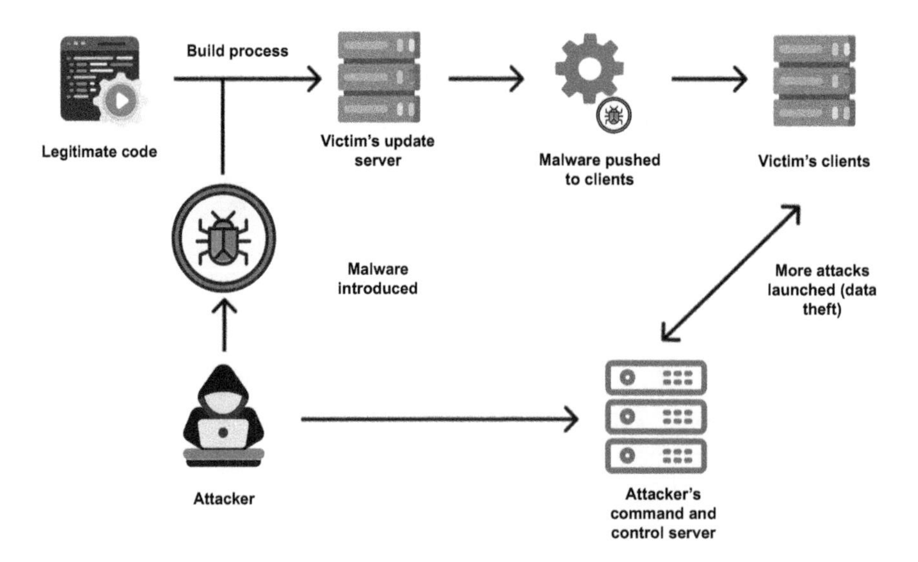

Figure 4.3 Supply chain attack scenario

Table 4.1 Summary of the challenges of adopting cutting-edge cybersecurity technologies in healthcare systems along with proposed solutions

Challenge	Summary of the solutions
Increased attack surface	Ensure robust security protocols to protect against potential breaches
Sophisticated cyberattacks	Implement advanced cybersecurity measures, ensure constant threat monitoring, and deploy adaptive defense strategies
Data privacy and compliance	Provide continuous updates to regulations like HIPAA and GDPR, and deploy agile cybersecurity strategies
Insider threats	Ensure continuous employee education, adopt behavioral analytics, and deploy vigilant privileged access management
Legacy systems and interoperability	Strike a balance between technological advancement and operational continuity
Human factor	Comprehensive training programs emphasizing social engineering awareness are essential to mitigate these risks
Supply chain risks	Ensure robust supply chain risk management through vetting vendors, contractual cybersecurity stipulations, and continuous monitoring to ensure the security of the entire ecosystem
Incident response and recovery	Ensure preemptive planning, perform regular drills, and continuous refinement of response protocols to mitigate the impact of cybersecurity incidents on healthcare services

Recent examples underscore the urgency of addressing these challenges to safeguard sensitive medical data, ensure the continuity of healthcare services, and maintain the trust of patients and stakeholders. As technology continues to advance, the healthcare sector must fortify its cybersecurity posture to ensure the confidentiality, integrity, and availability of patient data and uphold the trust placed in healthcare systems by individuals and society at large.

4.4 Lessons learned

This chapter imparts profound insights into the dynamic intersection of healthcare and cybersecurity. For instance, the integration of ML and AI emerges as a groundbreaking approach, equipping healthcare systems with advanced tools for real-time threat identification, predictive analysis, anomaly detection, cyberattack detection and response, improved authentication and access control, and vulnerability management and patching automation. With its decentralized and immutable nature, blockchain technology emerges as a beacon for secure data management, offering a promising solution to the perpetual concerns of data privacy and compliance within the healthcare domain. Moreover, it improves supply chain integrity and drug traceability, guarantees tamper-resistant clinical trials and research data, and is vital for identity management and authentication. As highlighted in the chapter, ZTA underscores a paradigm shift by emphasizing continuous verification, monitoring, incident response, and stringent access controls, mitigating the risks associated with unauthorized access.

The chapter further emphasizes the critical role of Security Awareness and Training, recognizing that a cyber-resilient healthcare workforce is pivotal in preventing inadvertent human errors that may lead to security breaches. The strategic integration of Cyber Threat Intelligence stands out as a proactive measure, empowering healthcare organizations to anticipate and respond effectively to increasingly sophisticated cyber threats. However, the challenges outlined in the chapter reveal the complexity of adopting these innovative technologies. Managing the increased attack surface from integrating these technologies demands a comprehensive understanding of vulnerabilities and effective mitigation strategies. Balancing the adoption of emerging technologies with stringent data privacy regulations and compliance standards poses a delicate challenge, requiring a careful navigation of legal and ethical considerations.

Moreover, the chapter highlights the multifaceted challenge of addressing legacy systems and ensuring interoperability, reflecting the coexistence of traditional infrastructure with cutting-edge solutions. Acknowledging the human factor in cybersecurity, the imperative for continuous training and awareness programs is underscored to mitigate risks associated with human error. Robust incident response and recovery plans are recognized as indispensable, ensuring a swift and effective response during a security breach. Additionally, the chapter sheds light on the importance of navigating supply chain risks, emphasizing the need for healthcare organizations to scrutinize the security practices of third-party vendors and partners.

In conclusion, the lessons derived from this chapter extend beyond the adoption of emerging technologies in healthcare cybersecurity. They encompass a comprehensive understanding of the interconnected challenges, demanding a holistic and adaptive approach to fortify healthcare systems against the evolving threat landscape. The chapter serves as a guide for professionals and policymakers. It acts as a call to action, urging stakeholders to collaboratively address these challenges for a more resilient and secure future in healthcare cybersecurity.

4.5 Conclusion

In conclusion, the exploration of emerging trends in cybersecurity applications within healthcare systems has shed light on the dynamic landscape of challenges and solutions facing the industry. The analysis began by unveiling the vulnerabilities inherent in the transition toward digitized healthcare, emphasizing the profound consequences of cyber threats on patients, healthcare institutions, and the broader ecosystem. The subsequent in-depth examination of evolving cybersecurity trends revealed a multifaceted approach to fortifying healthcare systems. From harnessing the power of AI to leveraging blockchain technology, implementing ZTAs, promoting security awareness and training, embracing cyber threat intelligence, and even considering the implications of quantum computing, the chapter navigated through a diverse array of cutting-edge solutions. However, the narrative did not shy away from the complexities of integrating these innovations into healthcare systems. Challenges such as increased attack surfaces, sophisticated cyberattacks, data privacy and compliance concerns, insider threats, reliance on legacy systems, interoperability issues, the human factor, supply chain risks, and incident response and recovery strategies were meticulously explored. This chapter serves as a comprehensive guide as the healthcare sector stands at the crossroads of technological advancement and cybersecurity imperatives. It underscores the urgency of addressing vulnerabilities and provides insights into the intricate balance required to successfully adopt emerging technologies. Moving forward, healthcare practitioners, policymakers, and cybersecurity experts must collaborate to navigate these challenges, ensuring the resilience of healthcare systems against the ever-evolving landscape of cyber threats. The journey toward a secure and technologically advanced healthcare future demands continual vigilance, adaptive strategies, and a collective commitment to safeguarding the well-being of patients and the integrity of healthcare institutions.

References

[1] K. Kalinaki, M. Fahadi, A. A. Alli, W. Shafik, M. Yasin, and N. Mutwalibi, "Artificial Intelligence of Internet of Medical Things (AIoMT) in Smart Cities: A Review of Cybersecurity for Smart Healthcare," in *Handbook of Security and Privacy of AI-Enabled Healthcare Systems and Internet of Medical Things*, 1st edn. Boca Raton, FL: CRC Press, 2023, pp. 271–292. doi: 10.1201/9781003370321-11.

[2] A. A. Alli, K. Kassim, N. Mutwalibi, H. Hamid, and L. Ibrahim, "Secure Fog-Cloud of Things: Architectures, Opportunities and Challenges," in *Secure Edge Computing*, 1st edn, M. Ahmed and P. Haskell-Dowland, (Eds.), CRC Press, Boca Raton, FL, 2021, pp. 3–20. doi:10.1201/9781003028635-2.

[3] A. Alabdulatif, N. N. Thilakarathne, and K. Kalinaki, "A Novel Cloud Enabled Access Control Model for Preserving the Security and Privacy of Medical Big Data," *Electronics (Basel)*, vol. 12, no. 12, p. 2646, 2023, doi:10.3390/electronics12122646.

[4] M. Chemisto, T. J. Gutu, K. Kalinaki, *et al.*, "Artificial Intelligence for Improved Maternal Healthcare: A Systematic Literature Review," *2023 IEEE AFRICON*, pp. 1–6, 2023, doi:10.1109/AFRICON55910.2023.10293674.

[5] K. E. Fahim, K. Kalinaki, and W. Shafik, "Electronic Devices in the Artificial Intelligence of the Internet of Medical Things (AIoMT)," in *Handbook of Security and Privacy of AI-Enabled Healthcare Systems and Internet of Medical Things*, 1st edn. Boca Raton, FL: CRC Press, 2023, pp. 41–62. doi:10.1201/9781003370321-3.

[6] M. Abdulraheem, E. A. Adeniyi, J. B. Awotunde, *et al.*, "Artificial Intelligence of Medical Things for Medical Information Systems Privacy and Security," *Handbook of Security and Privacy of AI-Enabled Healthcare Systems and Internet of Medical Things*, pp. 63–96, 2023, doi:10.1201/9781003370321-4.

[7] K. Kalinaki, N. N. Thilakarathne, H. R. Mubarak, O. A. Malik, and M. Abdullatif, "Cybersafe Capabilities and Utilities for Smart Cities," in *Cybersecurity for Smart Cities*. Cham: Springer, 2023, pp. 71–86. doi:10.1007/978-3-031-24946-4_6.

[8] A. Mukhopadhyay and S. Jain, "A Framework for Cyber-risk Insurance against Ransomware: A Mixed-Method Approach," *International Journal of Information Management*, vol. 74, p. 102724, 2024, doi:10.1016/J.IJINFOMGT.2023.102724.

[9] S. Papastergiou, H. Mouratidis, and E. M. Kalogeraki, "Handling of Advanced Persistent Threats and Complex Incidents in Healthcare, Transportation and Energy ICT Infrastructures," *Evolving Systems*, vol. 12, no. 1, pp. 91–108, 2021, doi:10.1007/S12530-020-09335-4.

[10] A. U. Rufai, E. P. Fasina, C. O. Uwadia, A. T. Rufai, and A. L. Imoize, "Cyberattacks against Artificial Intelligence- Enabled Internet of Medical Things," *Handbook of Security and Privacy of AI-Enabled Healthcare Systems and Internet of Medical Things*, pp. 191–216, 2023, doi:10.1201/9781003370321-8.

[11] W. Shafik and K. Kalinaki, "Smart City Ecosystem: An Exploration of Requirements, Architecture, Applications, Security, and Emerging Motivations," in *Handbook of Research on Network-Enabled IoT Applications for Smart City Services*. Hershey, PA: IGI Global, 2023, pp. 75–98. doi:10.4018/979-8-3693-0744-1.CH005.

[12] D. P. F. Möller, "Ransomware Attacks and Scenarios: Cost Factors and Loss of Reputation," *Advances in Information Security*, vol. 103, pp. 273–303, 2023, doi:10.1007/978-3-031-26845-8_6.

[13] R. A. Wessel and T. Nascimento Heim, "The Various Dimensions of Cyberthreats: (In)consistencies in the Global Regulation of Cybersecurity," *Anales de Derecho*, vol. 40, pp. 40–65, 2023, doi:10.6018/analesderecho.546921.

[14] J. B. Awotunde, A. L. Imoize, R. G. Jimoh, *et al.*, "AIoMT Enabling Real-Time Monitoring of Healthcare Systems Security and Privacy Considerations," *Handbook of Security and Privacy of AI-Enabled Healthcare Systems and Internet of Medical Things*, pp. 97–133, 2023, doi:10.1201/9781003370321-5.

[15] M. Javaid, A. Haleem, R. P. Singh, and R. Suman, "Towards Insighting Cybersecurity for Healthcare Domains: A Comprehensive Review of Recent Practices and Trends," *Cyber Security and Applications*, vol. 1, p. 100016, 2023, doi:10.1016/J.CSA.2023.100016.

[16] L. M. Halman and M. J. F. Alenazi, "Threshold-Based Software-Defined Networking (SDN) Solution for Healthcare Systems against Intrusion Attacks," *Computer Modeling in Engineering & Sciences*, vol. 138, no. 2, pp. 1469–1483, 2024, doi:10.32604/cmes.2023.028077.

[17] P. B. Dash, M. R. Senapati, H. S. Behera, J. Nayak, and S. Vimal, "Self-adaptive Memetic Firefly Algorithm and CatBoost-based Security

Framework for IoT Healthcare Environment," *J Eng Math*, vol. 144, no. 1, pp. 1–29, 2024, doi:10.1007/S10665-023-10309-Z.

[18] K. Kalinaki, U. Yahya, O. A. Malik, and D. T. C. Lai, "A Review of Big Data Analytics and Artificial Intelligence in Industry 5.0 for Smart Decision-Making," in *Human-Centered Approaches in Industry 5.0: Human-Machine Interaction, Virtual Reality Training, and Customer Sentiment Analysis*, 2023, pp. 24–47. doi:10.4018/979-8-3693-2647-3.ch002.

[19] R. Chhabra and S. Singh, "E-Healthcare and Society 5.0," in *Artificial Intelligence and Society 5.0: Issues, Opportunities, and Challenges*. New York: Taylor & Francis Group, 2024, p. 133.

[20] W. Shafik, "Cyber Security Perspectives in Public Spaces: Drone Case Study," in *Handbook of Research on Cybersecurity Risk in Contemporary Business Systems*. Hershey, PA: IGI Global, 2023, pp. 79–97. doi:10.4018/978-1-6684-7207-1.ch004.

[21] A. S. Nadhan and I. Jeena Jacob, "Enhancing Healthcare Security in the Digital Era: Safeguarding Medical Images with Lightweight Cryptographic Techniques in IoT Healthcare Applications," *Biomed Signal Process Control*, vol. 88, p. 105511, 2024, doi:10.1016/J.BSPC.2023.105511.

[22] A. N. Edmund, C. A. Alabi, O. O. Tooki, A. L. Imoize, and T. D. Salka, "Artificial Intelligence-Assisted Internet of Medical Things Enabling Medical Image Processing," in *Handbook of Security and Privacy of AI-Enabled Healthcare Systems and Internet of Medical Things*. Boca Raton, FL: CRC Press, 2023, pp. 309–334, doi:10.1201/9781003370321-13.

[23] A. Habbal, M. K. Ali, and M. A. Abuzaraida, "Artificial Intelligence Trust, Risk and Security Management (AI TRiSM): Frameworks, Applications, Challenges and Future Research Directions," *Expert Systems with Applications*, vol. 240, p. 122442, 2024, doi:10.1016/J.ESWA.2023.122442.

[24] D. Bansal, M. Bhatia, A. Atrey, and A. K. Yadav, "Perspective of Cybersecurity and Ethical Hacking with Vulnerability Assessment and Exploitation Tools," in *Big Data Analytics Framework for Smart Grids*. Boca Raton, FL: CRC Press, 2023, pp. 98–111. doi:10.1201/9781032665399-6.

[25] M. Mohammadzad, J. Karimpour, and F. Mahan, "Cyber Attacker's Next Action Prediction on Dynamic Real-time Behavior Model," *Computers and Electrical Engineering*, vol. 113, p. 109031, 2024, doi:10.1016/J.COMPELECENG.2023.109031.

[26] J. Pool, S. Akhlaghpour, F. Fatehi, and A. Burton-Jones, "A Systematic Analysis of Failures in Protecting Personal Health Data: A Scoping Review," *International Journal of Information Management*, vol. 74, p. 102719, 2024, doi:10.1016/J.IJINFOMGT.2023.102719.

[27] C. Xu, Z. Chan, L. Zhu, R. Lu, Y. Guan, and K. Sharif, "Efficient and Privacy-Preserving Similar Electronic Medical Records Query for Large-scale eHealthcare Systems," *Computer Standards & Interfaces*, vol. 87, p. 103746, 2024, doi:10.1016/J.CSI.2023.103746.

[28] A. Sayal, J. Jha, and C. N, "Blockchain: A Digital Breakthrough in Healthcare," in *Blockchain for Healthcare 4.0*, CRC Press, Boca Raton, FL, 2023, pp. 1–25. doi:10.1201/9781003408246-1.

[29] M. Grichi and F. Jaafar, "Demystifying the Digital Identity Challenges and the Blockchain Role," in *Blockchain and Artificial Intelligence-Based Solution to Enhance the Privacy in Digital Identity and IoT*. Boca Raton, FL: CRC Press, 2023, pp. 9–24. doi:10.1201/9781003227656-3.

[30] H. Bansal, D. Gupta, and D. Anand, "Blockchain and Artificial Intelligence in Telemedicine and Remote Patient Monitoring," in *Handbook on Augmenting Telehealth Services*. Boca Raton, FL: CRC Press, 2023, pp. 279–294. doi:10.1201/9781003346289-17.

[31] S. Sajid, R. E. Lawrence, H. C. Galfalvy, *et al.*, "Intramuscular Ketamine vs. Midazolam for Rapid Risk-reduction in Suicidal, Depressed Emergency Patients: Clinical Trial Design and Rationale," *Journal of Affective Disorders Reports*, vol. 15, p. 100690, 2024, doi:10.1016/J.JADR.2023.100690.

[32] T. Rai, R. Malviya, N. Kaushik, and P. K. Sharma, "Blockchain in Tracing and Securing Medical Supplies," in *Blockchain for Healthcare 4.0*, CRC Press, 2023, Boca Raton, FL, pp. 185–198. doi:10.1201/9781003408246-9.

[33] A. Diro, L. Zhou, A. Saini, S. Kaisar, and P. C. Hiep, "Leveraging Zero Knowledge Proofs for Blockchain-based Identity Sharing: A Survey of Advancements, Challenges and Opportunities," *Journal of Information Security and Applications*, vol. 80, p. 103678, 2024, doi:10.1016/J.JISA.2023.103678.

[34] W. A. N. A. Al-Nbhany, A. T. Zahary, and A. A. Al-Shargabi, "Blockchain-IoT Healthcare Applications and Trends: A Review," *IEEE Access*, vol. 12, pp. 4178–4212, 2024, doi:10.1109/ACCESS.2023.3349187.

[35] C. Lee, J. Kim, H. Ko, and B. Yoo, "Addressing IoT Storage Constraints: A Hybrid Architecture for Decentralized Data Storage and Centralized Management," *Internet of Things*, vol. 25, p. 101014, 2024, doi:10.1016/J.IOT.2023.101014.

[36] F. Frati, G. Darau, N. Salamanos, *et al.*, "Cybersecurity Training and Healthcare: The AERAS Approach," *International Journal of Information Security*, vol. 23, pp. 1527–1539, 2024, doi:10.1007/s10207-023-00802-y.

[37] N. Jerry-Egemba, "Safe and Sound: Strengthening Cybersecurity in Healthcare through Robust Staff Educational Programs," *Healthcare Management Forum*, vol. 37, no. 1, pp. 21–25, 2024, doi:10.1177/08404704231194577.

[38] S. Saeed, S. A. Suayyid, M. S. Al-Ghamdi, H. Al-Muhaisen, and A. M. Almuhaideb, "A Systematic Literature Review on Cyber Threat Intelligence for Organizational Cybersecurity Resilience," *Sensors* 2023, vol. 23, no. 16, p. 7273, 2023, doi:10.3390/S23167273.

[39] M. Sills, P. Ranade, and S. Mittal, "Cybersecurity Threat Intelligence Augmentation and Embedding Improvement – A Healthcare Usecase," *Proceedings – 2020 IEEE International Conference on Intelligence and Security Informatics, ISI 2020*, 2020, doi:10.1109/ISI49825.2020.9280482.

[40] MS-ISAC, "MS-ISAC." Accessed: Jan. 10, 2024. [Online]. Available: https://www.cisecurity.org/ms-isac
[41] Health-ISAC, "Health-ISAC – Health Information Sharing and Analysis Center." Accessed: Jan. 10, 2024. [Online]. Available: https://h-isac.org/
[42] S. K. Palvadi, "Exploring the Potential of Quantum Computing in AI, Medical Advancements, and Cyber Security," in *Quantum Innovations at the Nexus of Biomedical Intelligence*. Hershey, PA: IGI Global, 2024, pp. 58–77. doi:10.4018/979-8-3693-1479-1.ch004.
[43] V. Zapatero, T. van Leent, R. Arnon-Friedman, *et al.*, "Advances in Device-independent Quantum Key Distribution," *npj Quantum Information*, vol. 9, no. 1, pp. 1–11, 2023, doi:10.1038/s41534-023-00684-x.
[44] J. Allen, "Accellion Data Breach: What Happened & Who Was Impacted?" Accessed: Jan. 10, 2024. [Online]. Available: https://purplesec.us/accellion-data-breach-explained/
[45] A. L. Imoize, V. E. Balas, V. K. Solanki, C.-C. Lee, and M. S. Obaidat, *Handbook of Security and Privacy of AI-Enabled Healthcare Systems and Internet of Medical Things*. Boca Raton, FL: CRC Press, 2023.
[46] M. Ahmed and P. Haskell-Dowland, *Secure Edge Computing: Applications, Techniques and Challenges.* 2021. Accessed: Jan. 18, 2024. [Online]. Available: https://www.routledge.com/Secure-Edge-Computing-Applications-Techniques-and-Challenges/Ahmed-Haskell-Dowland/p/book/9780367464141
[47] M. Ahmed and P. Haskell-Dowland, *Cybersecurity for Smart Cities*. Cham: Springer International Publishing, 2023. doi:10.1007/978-3-031-24946-4.
[48] S. Jimo, T. Abdullah, and A. Jamal, "IoE Security Risk Analysis in a Modern Hospital Ecosystem," in *Advanced Sciences and Technologies for Security Applications*. Cham: Springer, 2023, pp. 451–467, doi:10.1007/978-3-031-20160-8_26.
[49] P. Daly, "Writing on a Curved Surface' The Operational Response to the Cyber-attack on the Irish Health Service," *Médecine de Catastrophe – Urgences Collectives*, vol. 6, no. 4, pp. 275–277, 2022, doi:10.1016/J.PXUR.2022.10.002.
[50] L. S. van Boven, R.W. Kusters, D. Tin, *et al.*, "Hacking Acute Care: A Qualitative Study on the Health Care Impacts of Ransomware Attacks Against Hospitals," *Ann Emerg Med*, vol. 83, no. 1, pp. 46–56, 2024, doi:10.1016/J.ANNEMERGMED.2023.04.025.
[51] A. M. Pitney, S. Penrod, M. Foraker, and S. Bhunia, "A Systematic Review of 2021 Microsoft Exchange Data Breach Exploiting Multiple Vulnerabilities," in *2022 7th International Conference on Smart and Sustainable Technologies (SpliTech)*, IEEE, 2022, pp. 1–6. doi:10.23919/SpliTech55088.2022.9854268.
[52] D. N. Burrell, C. Nobles, A. Cusak, *et al.*, "Cybersecurity and Cyberbiosecurity Insider Threat Risk Management," in *Handbook of Research on Cybersecurity Risk in Contemporary Business Systems*. Hershey, PA: IGI Global, 2023, pp. 121–136. doi:10.4018/978-1-6684-7207-1.ch006.

[53] B. Kelly, C. Quinn, A. Lawlor, R. Killeen, and J. Burrell, "Cybersecurity in Healthcare," in *Trends of Artificial Intelligence and Big Data for E-Health*. Integrated Science, vol. 9. Cham: Springer, 2022, pp. 213–231, doi:10.1007/978-3-031-11199-0_11.

[54] S. T. Argaw, J. R. Troncoso-Pastoriza, D. Lacey, *et al.*, "Cybersecurity of Hospitals: Discussing the Challenges and Working towards Mitigating the Risks," *BMC Med Inform Decis Mak*, vol. 20, no. 1, pp. 1–10, 2020, doi:10.1186/S12911-020-01161-7.

[55] The Guardian, "NHS Seeks to Recover from Global Cyber-attack as Security Concerns Resurface." Accessed: Jan. 10, 2024. [Online]. Available: https://www.theguardian.com/society/2017/may/12/hospitals-across-england-hit-by-large-scale-cyber-attack

[56] S. L. Burton, "Change Management and Cybersecurity in Healthcare," in *Transformational Interventions for Business, Technology, and Healthcare*. Hershey, PA: IGI Global, 2023, pp. 426–443. doi:10.4018/979-8-3693-1634-4.ch025.

[57] S. Kuipers and M. Schonheit, "Data Breaches and Effective Crisis Communication: A Comparative Analysis of Corporate Reputational Crises," *Corporate Reputation Review*, vol. 25, no. 3, pp. 176–197, 2022, doi:10.1057/S41299-021-00121-9.

[58] A. Garcia-Perez, J. G. Cegarra-Navarro, M. P. Sallos, E. Martinez-Caro, and A. Chinnaswamy, "Resilience in Healthcare Systems: Cyber Security and Digital Transformation," *Technovation*, vol. 121, p. 102583, 2023, doi:10.1016/J.TECHNOVATION.2022.102583.

[59] M. Bada, "A Clinician's Guide to Cybersecurity and Data Protection," in *A Practitioner's Guide to Cybersecurity and Data Protection*, Routledge, London, 2023, pp. 25–37. doi:10.4324/9781003364184-3.

[60] S. Gatlan, "Universal Health Services Lost $67 Million due to Ryuk Ransomware Attack." Accessed: Jan. 11, 2024. [Online]. Available: https://www.bleepingcomputer.com/news/security/universal-health-services-lost-67-million-due-to-ryuk-ransomware-attack/

Chapter 5

Convolutional neural networks enabling the Internet of Medical Things: security implications, prospects, and challenges

Peace Busola Falola[1], Joseph Bamidele Awotunde[2], Abidemi Emmanuel Adeniyi[3] and Agbotiname Lucky Imoize[4]

The integration of Convolutional Neural Networks (CNNs) into the Internet of Medical Things (IoMT) heralds substantial advances in healthcare, including improved diagnostic precision, real-time data processing, and the possibility of individualized medication. However, this integration raises complicated security concerns, notably around privacy and the safeguarding of sensitive medical data. The capacity of CNNs to analyze large datasets raises concerns about data security, integrity, and availability, which are critical for retaining patient confidence and adhering to regulatory norms. Despite these obstacles, CNN-enabled IoMT has the potential to significantly improve healthcare outcomes through more accurate diagnosis and predictive analytics. However, attaining these advantages requires overcoming technological hurdles such as data variety and representation, processing needs, and the interpretability of AI-driven choices. This chapter emphasizes the importance of taking a balanced strategy that capitalizes on CNNs' revolutionary potential in the IoMT while thoroughly addressing the accompanying security issues.

Keywords: Convolutional neural networks; Internet of Medical Things; smart healthcare systems; security and privacy; machine learning; healthcare monitoring and prediction

[1]Department of Computer Sciences, Faculty of Pure and Applied Sciences, Precious Cornerstone University, Nigeria
[2]Department of Computer Science, Faculty of Communication and Information Sciences, University of Ilorin, Nigeria
[3]Department of Computer Science, College of Computing and Communication Studies, Bowen University, Nigeria
[4]Department of Electrical and Electronics Engineering, Faculty of Engineering, University of Lagos, Nigeria

5.1 Introduction

Machine learning (ML) has lately acquired prominence in studies and is employed in a variety of programs, notably IoMT [1]. Deep learning (DL) is one of the most often utilized ML algorithms in these applications [1]. Another term for DL is representation learning (RL). Deep Convolutional Neural Network (CNN) is a type of neural network that has performed well in a variety of computational vision and imagery processing competitions [2]. The continuous growth of creative research in the fields of deep and distributed learning is due to both the unexpected surge in accessibility to data and the tremendous advances made in hardware innovations, such as high-performing computing (HPC) [1]. DL is based on classic neural networks but surpasses them greatly. The CNN is one of the most popular DL networks [1]. According to CNN, DL is fairly common today.

The fundamental benefit CNN outperforms its predecessors by automatically recognizing important properties without human interaction, thus becoming the most commonly used [1]. Traditional ML algorithms rely on manually created characteristics. In contrast, CNNs learn these properties directly from data. Because of their ability to learn features, CNNs are extremely efficient for applications like picture recognition, where manual feature specification is difficult and time-consuming. Deep CNNs tremendous learning capacity stems mostly from the use of various extraction of features steps, which may autonomously learn presentations from data [2]. CNNs learn to represent data hierarchically. Lower layers in image processing, for example, may learn to distinguish edges and textures, but higher layers may recognize more complicated patterns or objects. This hierarchical learning process mimics parts of human visual vision, allowing CNNs to develop a more comprehensive comprehension of the input. The accessibility of a massive quantity of data and developments in equipment technology have driven CNN investigation, and exciting deep CNN models have recently been released [2].

Algorithms developed on massive data sets can be fine-geared toward performing effectively on similar tasks using tiny quantities of data. This transfer learning potential has democratized DL-based model, allowing smaller businesses and initiatives to harness the power of CNNs without requiring enormous labeled datasets. CNNs trained on huge datasets may be utilized to extract features for a variety of purposes. Reusing pre-trained models allows for good performance even with a limited quantity of data for a new job, which is especially useful in fields where data acquisition is expensive or labor-intensive. CNNs have demonstrated cutting-edge effectiveness across several applications, involving image categorization, recognizing objects, and splitting. Their efficacy in these areas has resulted in broad acceptance in several applications, notably imaging for healthcare and autonomous driving. While CNNs were originally intended for image processing, its architecture has proved applicable to a variety of tasks other than visual identification.

For example, CNN variants are employed in sequence-to-sequence models for natural language processing, proving the model's adaptability in video analysis and even time series prediction. This adaptability arises from their capacity to interpret grid-like data, which requires spatial or temporal correlations. CNNs have proven innovative effectiveness across a range of domains, most notably image and video recognition. They are the basis of many applications that utilize computer vision, including facial recognition, self-driving cars, and medical picture analysis. The Internet of Things (IoT) is a fundamental development in how we connect and manage objects, allowing for the smooth interchange of data across a networked environment. The Internet of Things (IoT) refers to an extensive web of physical things that are linked together to allow communication and data exchange over the Internet [3]. This notion, initially described by Ashton in 1999, has grown rapidly, from a new idea to a pervasive network of billions of linked devices [3]. The exponential growth of IoT devices, from an estimated 10 billion now to a predicted 25 billion by 2025, demonstrates the fast extension and integration of this technology into our daily lives. Similarly, the proliferation of IoT devices was noted, with an expected increase from 8.4 billion in usage to 30 billion by 2020 [4], underlining the technology's broad reach and potential.

The technical underpinning of IoT includes complex systems for data transmission and storage [3]. This architecture enables devices to interact quickly over secure cloud servers while also improving their functionality through smart advances. These improvements have resulted in the development of "smart" devices, which have embedded software that either improves current functions or adds new functionalities, broadening the breadth and possibilities of IoT applications. In the field of healthcare, technology innovations, notably IoT, have a huge influence. The Internet of Medical Things (IoMT) provides a viable answer to the medical industry's myriad issues caused by internal and structural changes in human organs. Healthcare workers confront complications when identifying and forecasting diseases ranging from chronic ailments to hereditary abnormalities [4]. The introduction of IoMT emerges as a watershed moment, providing a revolutionary technique to monitoring and diagnosing health problems by collecting critical physiological data via wearable devices.

The importance of IoMT was underscored during the COVID-19 epidemic when continuous health monitoring became crucial. IoMT enabled remote patient monitoring, screening, and therapy, demonstrating its potential for handling health crises [3]. These technology-enabled healthcare personnel give treatment remotely, representing a huge step forward in how medical services might be supplied during such exceptional circumstances. Furthermore, the use of CNNs in the medical area brings a novel method to medical picture processing. The limits of traditional picture interpretation approaches, which are sometimes hampered by a lack of qualified specialists and the possibility of human mistakes, were explored [5]. In this setting, CNNs appear as potent tools capable of outperforming human specialists in terms of accuracy and efficiency for picture comprehension tasks. The combination of CNNs with IoMT devices not only improves the ability to acquire and interpret medical data but also transforms the diagnostic process, providing more trustworthy and precise diagnoses. The confluence of IoT technologies, particularly via the lens of IoMT and the use of CNNs, offers a significant advancement in healthcare. This collaboration provides novel solutions for patient monitoring, illness diagnosis, and treatment planning, demonstrating these technologies' enormous influence on the future of medical care and patient management.

5.1.1 The key contributions of this chapter

The primary contribution of this work is to:

(i) Cover the challenges and various applications of IoMT, providing a foundational understanding of how CNNs can be integrated into this ecosystem for improved healthcare outcomes.
(ii) Discuss the incorporation of neural network technologies within IoMT, highlighting how these technologies can enhance security and data integrity in medical applications.
(iii) Present potential future directions for the use of CNNs within IoMT, suggesting a forward-looking perspective on how these technologies can evolve to address emerging challenges and opportunities in healthcare.

5.1.2 Chapter organization

Section 5.2 presents the background and state-of-the-art of CNN and IoMT. Section 5.3 presents the IoMT ecosystems in general, and Section 5.4 discusses the security in IoMT. Section 5.5 discusses the integration of CNN with IoMT. Section 5.6 presents the security implications of CNN with IoMT. Section 5.7 discusses the prospects and challenges. Section 5.8 presents the lessons learned in the chapter, and Section 5.9 presents the conclusion and future directions of CNN with IoMT.

5.2 Background and state-of-the-art

The development of CNNs in healthcare offers a huge step forward in the use of artificial intelligence to enhance diagnostic accuracy, patient care, and treatment approaches. This path, which includes multiple major milestones, highlights CNNs' transformational potential in medical science. CNNs have evolved from early experiments to today's sophisticated applications, making them a vital tool in the healthcare field. A CNN is a DNN structure that includes convolutional processing and may represent learning while also achieving translation-invariant categorization of input material using a hierarchical structure [6]. CNNs often have convolutional stages, sequential normalization levels, pooling layers, fully linked layers, and so forth. The convolutional layer serves as its core component [6]. The function of the convolution layer is to extract features from the input image. Figure 5.1 shows the CNN architecture.

The CNNs are a specialized type of DL architecture designed for image recognition and computer vision tasks. The fundamental CNNs are made up of layer structures that employ convolution techniques to scan input images with learnable filters or kernels. These filters detect local patterns like corners, surfaces,

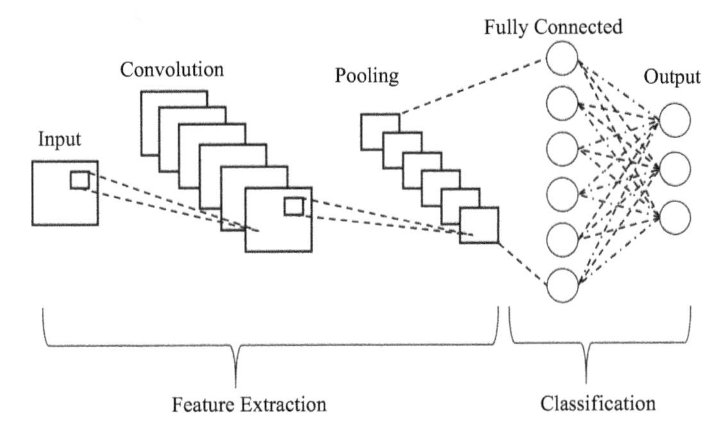

Figure 5.1 The convolutional neural networks architecture

or more complicated formations in the input data. Convolutional layers are followed by activation functions like Rectified Linear Unit (ReLU) to introduce irregularities and boost the network's capacity to learn complicated features. Pooling layers are another crucial component in CNN architecture, typically placed after convolutional layers. Pooling helps lower the spatial size of the mappings of features to save computation while keeping valuable information. Max pooling takes the largest value from a group of data inside an area, whereas the mean pooling derives the average. These layers contribute to the network's ability to abstract and capture hierarchical features from the input data.

The layers that are completely linked are used at the conclusion of the CNN structure to provide forecasts depending on the high-level characteristics retrieved by the convolutional and pooling layers. These layers link each neuron to each neuron in the next levels, facilitating the combination of extracted features and enabling the network to make complex, high-level decisions. In summary, CNNs leverage the power of convolutional and pooling layers for feature extraction and spatial reduction, followed by fully linked layers for classification or regression operations, making them appropriate for a variety of image-related applications in ML and computer vision.

The stage of convolution has several convolution kernels [6]. Every structure in the convolutional kernel, like neurons in a network of feed-forward neurons, has a corresponding load coefficient and a bias value. Convolution computation includes moving the convolution kernel across the image, multiplying and combining the associated components with the covered image characteristics [6]. This technique may extract local characteristics while also decreasing parameters. Because CNNs may extract local features and minimize parameters (via weight sharing), they are especially well-suited to image processing [6]. Because the medical business generates a vast amount of visual data, CNN has a broader application range than other technologies [6]. CNN is extremely useful for learning image properties. Prior to CNN, the fully connected network was routinely used to extract visual attributes; however, the entire completely connected network typically contained an enormous amount of linkages, resulting in an exponential growth in the number of parameters and training times. Some major achievements in the application of CNN in healthcare are as follows.

5.2.1 Image recognition tasks

The early 2020s saw a spike in the use of CNNs in healthcare, owing to increased availability of medical imaging data and advances in processing capacity. CNNs were shown to be particularly good in image identification tasks, which are essential for radiology, pathology, and dermatological diagnosis. During this time, CNNs were used to diagnose COVID-19 from chest X-rays and CT scans, and their accuracy occasionally surpassed that of human specialists [7]. This time demonstrated the technology's ability to meet urgent healthcare requirements, particularly amid a worldwide pandemic.

5.2.2 Prediction of risk of osteoarthritis

CNN algorithms can be used to forecast the possibility of osteoarthritis by automatically segmenting knee cartilage MRIs, to identify diabetic retinopathy in the eye employing retinal fundus images, to classify skin cancer at the dermatologists' threshold, to anticipate congestive heart failure, to anticipate chronic lung disease employing long-term EHRs, to anticipate sleep quality through exercise data throughout awake time, and to measure electroence.

5.2.3 Early diagnosis of Alzheimer's disease

Alzheimer's disease (AD) in its early stages is associated with moderate cognitive impairment (MCI). Some scientists developed a novel voxel-based hierarchical feature extraction (VHFE) approach for detecting Alzheimer's disease early [8]. The entire brain was divided into 90 regions of interest (ROIs) using an automated anatomical labeling template (AAL). They segregated the unhelpful data by selecting the informative voxels in each ROI and building a vector from a starting point of voxel values (8–9). The initial stage's features were determined by correlations between voxels from different groups. To discover deeply concealed traits, brain feature maps containing voxels from every person were fed into a CNN [8,9]. The results indicate that the proposed strategy is powerful, with excellent outcomes in comparison to current state-of-the-art technologies [8].

5.2.4 Object classification

Reference [10] demonstrates that processing data with natural spatial invariance (e.g., pictures whose meanings do not change when translated) has come to be fundamental in the field (CV). The usage of DL algorithms might assist clinicians by giving second viewpoints and highlighting potential problems. CNNs learn to identify things comprising pictures and can perform at the Mammalian degree. They are initially trained on a large dataset irrelevant to the job at hand to acquire the natural characteristics in photos (curves, straight lines, colorations, and so on) before getting fine-tuned on much narrower datasets relevant to the task at hand (e.g., medical images) [9]. The technique's more advanced layers are retrained to distinguish between diagnostic cases. CNNs did well in transferring learning [10]. Physicians have begun to apply imagery segmentation and object identification for urgent and easily disregarded cases, such as diagnosing large-arteria occlusions in the brain using radiological imaging, which can cause major brain damage in just a few minutes. Furthermore, CNNs trained to recognize mitotic cells or tumor areas can enhance cancer histology readings [10]. CNNs were recently used to determine survivor likelihood by recognizing biological properties of tissues [10].

5.2.5 Advancements in medical imaging

CNNs are important in illness diagnosis because they can utilize the capability of DL to extract relevant and discriminative characteristics from medical pictures [11]. CNNs help to more effective and efficient illness diagnosis by boosting detection accuracy, lowering interpretation time, and giving consistent findings [11]. This allows for early intervention, improved patient outcomes, and better healthcare decision-making. The implementation of CNNs resulted in major breakthroughs in medical imaging in the years 2022–2023. Enhanced algorithms enabled more accurate tumor detection and categorization, particularly in breast and skin cancer diagnosis. A study published in 2022 found that a CNN model could discriminate between benign and malignant skin lesions with an accuracy rate of more than 95% [12]. These changes not only enhanced diagnostic precision but also reduced healthcare practitioners' burden by automating routine analyses.

5.2.6 Integration with Electronic Health Records (EHRs)

Combining CNNs with Electronic Health Records (EHRs) allowed researchers to acquire a better knowledge of patient health trends and outcomes. In 2021, a crucial research demonstrated how CNNs could assess EHRs to predict medical outcomes, identifying people at high risk for conditions such as diabetes and heart disease [13]. This initiative exemplified a trend toward more customized and preventative treatment, leveraging the huge volumes of data available in EHRs.

5.2.7 Expansion into predictive analytics and telemedicine

CNNs have recently emerged in healthcare, with applications like predictive analytics and telemedicine. Predictive models based on CNNs may now forecast disease outbreaks, patient admissions, and even potential medical emergencies in advance, allowing for a more proactive approach to healthcare management. Furthermore, incorporating CNNs into telemedicine platforms has enhanced the quality of remote patient monitoring and diagnosis, making healthcare more accessible, especially in underserved places. A 2023 study found that CNN-powered mobile devices could accurately diagnose dermatological diseases, allowing patients to get timely and cost-effective consultations [14]. CNNs have drastically revolutionized the healthcare scene, from their use in diagnostic imaging to battle a global health crisis, to their integration with EHRs for predictive insights, and finally to the advancement of telemedicine. These innovations not only enhance patient outcomes by providing more accurate and quick diagnoses but also pave the path for a future in which healthcare is more individualized, predictive, and accessible.

5.2.8 Applications of convolution neural networks

Chiu *et al.* [15] presented that during the integrative sensing and communication (ISAC) period, milimeter-wave transmissions were used as radar with a CNN model for event detection. Their emphasis was on using DL to recognize security-critical motions, turning millimeter-wave characteristics into point cloud pictures, and improving identification accuracy. CNNs posed intricacy issues in DL. To solve this, they created flexible quantization approaches that simplified You Only Look Once (YOLO)-v4 processes using an 8-bit fixed-point integer notation. Cross-simulation verification revealed that CPU-based quantification increases performance by 300% with low accuracy loss, even tripling YOLO-tiny model speed in a GPU context. They created a Raspberry Pi 4-based system that combines simplified DL with Message Queuing Telemetry Transport (MQTT) IoT technologies for nursing support. Their quantifying approach improved recognition speed by roughly 2.9 times, allowing millimeter-wave detection in embedded systems. Furthermore, they used hardware-based quantized to instantly measure data from photos or weight files, which led to circuit fabrication and designing chips. Their research used AI with mmWave sensors in nursing protection and hardware setup to improve recognition precision and computational effectiveness.

Olatinwo *et al.* [16] suggested an emotion-aware IoT-enabled WBAN platform inside the medical sector structure, where an edge AI system performs analysis of data and long-term data transfers for actual time forecasting of patients' spoken feelings as well as capturing changes in feelings before and after treatments. They also looked into the usefulness of several algorithms for DL and ML with regard to the efficacy of classification, extraction of features approaches, and normalizing techniques. They created a hybrid DL model, combining CNN and bidirectional long- and short-term memory (BiLSTM), as well as a normalized CNN framework. They coupled the models with various methods of optimization and normalization approaches to increase the precision of predictions, minimize generalized mistake, and lower the computational difficulty of neural networks in terms of computing time, power, and memory. Several tests were carried out to determine the efficiency and efficacy of the suggested ML and DL methods. The suggested models were evaluated and validated against a relevant existing model using common performance criteria such as accuracy of predictions, precision, recall, F1 score, confusion matrix, and actual-predicted value discrepancies. The testing findings showed that one of the suggested models outscored the previous one with a precision of around 98%.

Awotunde *et al.* [4] suggested an IoMT-enabled CNN framework for detecting malignant and benign cancerous cells in blood samples from patients' tissue. To find the ideal values of CNN hyper-parameters, the hyper-parameter optimization using a radial basis function and dynamic coordinate search (HORD) technique was utilized. Using the HORD method improved the efficacy of finding the optimal solution for the CNN model by exploring multidimensional hyperparameters. This meant that the HORD technique effectively determined the ranges of hyper-parameters for certain leukemia traits. Furthermore, the HORD technique improved the model's effectiveness by improving and exploring the optimal collection of CNN hyperparameters. Leukemia samples were utilized to assess the efficacy of the suggested model using conventional performance measures. The suggested model demonstrated substantial classification accuracy when compared to existing cutting-edge approaches.

Sadhu *et al.* [17] presented a summary of the IoMT ecosystem, including legislation, standardization problems, security procedures employing cryptography remedies, physically unclonable functional (PUF)-based approaches, blockchain technology, and renamed data networking (NDN), as well as pros and downsides. Deepika *et al.* [18] focused on illness categorization by combining image processing with a safe environment for cloud computing and an expanded zigzag encrypted image system that is more resistant to various data threats. Second, a Fuzzy (FCNN) method was devised to improve picture categorization. The decrypted photos were used to classify cancer levels using several layers of training. Following categorization, outcomes were sent to the appropriate medical professionals and patients for additional therapy. The study method was conducted using the conventional dataset. The experiment found that the suggested method demonstrated superior performance than the other current techniques and may be successfully employed for medical picture identification.

He *et al.* [19] investigated an effective edge and cloud architecture to retain ECG classification efficiency while lowering communication costs. Their work includes the introduction of a hybrid smart clinical framework called Edge (EdgeCNN), which harmonized the capabilities of edge and cloud computing to meet the challenge of agile learning of medical information from connected devices. They also demonstrated an effective DL model for electrocardiogram (ECG) inference that can be put on edge smart gadgets to provide low-latency diagnostics. To increase the volume of ECG data, they created a data augmentation approach based on deep convolutional generative adversarial networks. They conducted tests on two sample datasets to assess the performance of EdgeCNN-based DL models for ECG classification. EdgeCNN outperformed standard cloud healthcare systems in terms of network input/output (I/O) pressure, architectural cost, and system high availability. The DL model not only guarantees excellent diagnostic accuracy, but also provides advantages in terms of inference time, storage, operating memory, and battery life.

Li *et al.* [20] combined current security studies to investigate the potential of DL in improving the IoT security architecture. The paper covered how the

IoT can detect and respond to threats, as well as how to secure edge data transfer. Furthermore, the article explored security research in several application areas, including Industrial IoT, Internet of Vehicles, smart grid, smart home, and smart medical. They subsequently summed up the areas that can be enhanced in future technological advances, which include expressing power for computation via the edge network processing unit (NPU) central device, carefully integrating the scientific simulation system with the real-world setting, as well as malicious software recognition, intrusion prevention, fabrication protection, the susceptibility recognition, troubleshooting, and blockchain-based technologies.

Alabsi *et al.* [21] provided a method to identify assaults on IoT networks by combining two CNN–CNN. The initial CNN algorithm was used to extract the key elements that helped detect IoT attacks from raw network traffic information. The subsequent CNN used the first CNN's discovered properties to create a strong recognition framework that reliably identifies IoT assaults. The suggested technique was tested with the BoT IoT 2020 dataset. The findings showed that the suggested technique achieves 98.04% detection efficiency, 98.09% exactness, 99.85% recall, 98.96% f1 score, and a rate of false positives of 1.93%. In addition, the suggested strategy was compared to various DL algorithms and selection of features approaches; the findings revealed that it surpassed those algorithms.

Punugoti *et al.* [22] used a built-in device to get photoplethysmography (PPG) data from 15 healthy subjects. The dataset included 7,308 PPG segments, each with 8 s of PPG data and labels indicating the type of workout the subject was participating in. The study proposed a CNN model for categorizing physical activity from PPG data. The recommended model has several layers, including batch normalization, convolutional, max-pooling, dropout, and completely linked. The output layer applied the softmax activation function to determine the likelihood for each class. In terms of effectiveness, the proposed CNN model outperformed other models including SVM with RBF kernel, decision trees, and random forest approaches. The research also proposed many strategies for further optimizing the model, which may be useful for building IoMT applications including recognizing activities and vital sign assessment.

Gugueoth *et al.* [23] focus on implementing federated learning (FL) and DL algorithms for IoT security. In accordance with the researchers, unlike traditional ML approaches, FL models may protect data privacy while sharing knowledge with other systems. The study concluded that FL can overcome the limitations of traditional ML approaches in terms of data privacy while sharing information with other systems. The paper examined several models, provided an overview, compared FL and DL-based strategies for IoT security, and summarized them. Table 5.1 provides an overview of relevant publications, including the approach used, coverage, and limitations of the kinds of literature studied.

Table 5.1 The summaries of some applications of convolutional neural networks

Authors	**Methodology**	**Coverage**	**Gap/future direction**
Chiu *et al.* [15]	DL to detect security-critical gestures to enhance recognition accuracy	Domain of Nursing security	Methodology can further be extended to other IoMT applications
Olatinwo *et al.* [16]	Hybrid DL model, i.e., CNN, bidirectional long short-term memory (BiLSTM), and normalized CNN framework	Real-time forecasting patients' spoken feelings as well as capturing modifications to feelings before and after therapy	Methodology can further be extended to other IoMT applications
Awotunde *et al.* [4]	An IoMT-enabled CNN model	Detecting the patient's blood tissue contains both benign and dangerous cancer cells	Methodology can further be extended to other IoMT applications
Sadhu *et al.* [17]	An overview of the IoMT ecosystem	Security methods employ cryptography alternatives, physically unclonable functional (PUF)-based remedies, blockchain, and named data connectivity	CNN wasn't considered as a possibility to improve the security IoMT
Deepika *et al.* [18]	An expanded zigzag picture encryption system with an FCNN algorithm.	Medical Image Diagnosis	Methodology can further be extended to other IoMT applications
He *et al.* [19]	A hybrid smart medical architecture named EdgeCNN and an effective DL model for ECG inference	Electrocardiogram classification	Methodology can further be extended to other IoMT applications
Li *et al.* [20]	Explored the prospect of using DL to upgrade the IoT security framework	Security studies in applications such as Industrial IoT, Internet of Automobiles, smart grid, smart dwellings, and intelligent healthcare	More areas of IoT architecture still need to be improved upon
Alabsi *et al.* [21]	Two CNN-CNN to detect attacks on IoT networks	Attacks on IoT networks	Methodology should be incorporated into IoMT applications
Punugoti *et al.* [22]	A CNN approach to categorize activity levels based on PPG signals.	PPG signals	Methodology will be beneficial to other IoMT applications include recognizing activities and vital sign surveillance.
Gugueoth *et al.* [23]	FL and DL algorithms for IoT security	IoT security	Methodology can be beneficial to IoMT

5.3 Internet of Medical Things ecosystem

The internet's incorporation and occupancy in our surroundings has paved the road for IoMT apps and technologies to flourish as an aspect of our everyday lives. The bulk of IoMT systems function at the next main levels, which incorporate various technologies, gadgets, detectors, and systems connected through electrical-electronic and wired or wireless connections.

5.3.1 Perception layer

The perception layer determines the IoMT attention and difficulty level. The major sublayers are data access and data gathering [24]. The perception component is the simplest form of IoMT and contains data sources such as intelligent objects, health surveillance devices, and mobile apps combined with detectors such as infrared sensors, medical sensors, electronic detectors, RFID cameras, and global positioning systems (GPS) [3]. This layer serves as the architecture's base, allowing physical objects or "things" outfitted with sensors and actuators to communicate with the actual environment. These devices gather information from their environment, which can range from temperature measurements and heart rates to more complicated health indicators in a medical setting. To finish the recognition and assessment of networks in IoMT, as well as collect data about things and people, the data collection sublayer employs a variety of medical perception and signal capture equipment [24].

This layer maintains direct communication among the ecosystem's consumers. This layer gathers information from smartwatches, tracking of patient systems, and remote care services. Sensing systems monitor environmental changes, identify things, places, statistics, scale, and so on, and convert the data into digital signals via a reliable, wired or wireless network transmission infrastructure that acts as a high-performance transport medium [3]. These may also remember and conserve data for later use [3]. The objects layer includes patient tracking gadgets, sensors, actuators, health information, pharmaceutical supervises, a diet plan power source, and so on [17]. The devices used should be properly placed to ensure the integrity of the collected data. The local routers in the environment connect these gadgets to the fog layer. The data is then analyzed at the fog and cloud levels to yield appropriate findings.

Additionally, to avoid delays, medical professionals may access patient data through this network. It employs data-gathering technologies such as universal packets radio communication technology, radio frequency identification (RFID), image recognition, graphic coding, and a variety of sensors, including physical signal sensors [24]. Physiological signal sensors, chemical sensors, and DNA sensors are employed to connect everything in the network into identifiable CPS nodes. The Internet of Things has three types of nodes: passive CPS, active CPS, and Internet CPS [24]. The IoMT demands matching recognition based on a variety of things and needs. The information access sublayer sends data from the data collection sublayer to the networking layer using short-distance communication

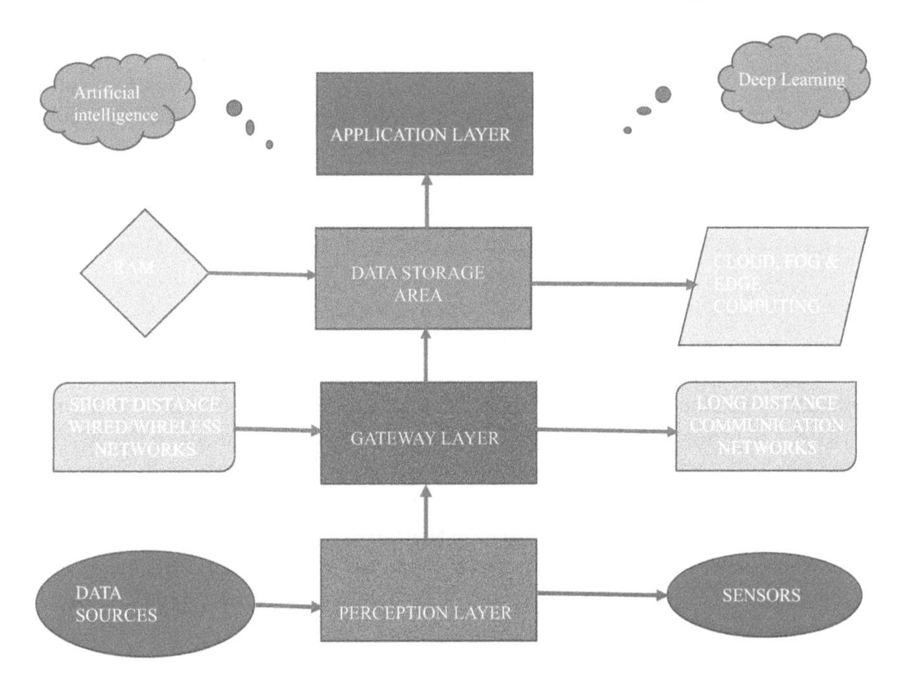

Figure 5.2 Structure and functionality of Internet of Medical Things

protocols including Bluetooth, Wi-Fi, and ZigBee. The major access methods should be chosen based on the IoMT's current environment and the needs of different objects [24]. Figure 5.2 shows the framework and purpose of each layer.

5.3.2 Gateway layer

Sensors demand network connectivity to the gateway, which may transmit and store data locally or remotely [3]. RFID, wireless sensor networks (WSNs), Bluetooth, ZigBee, low-power Wi-Fi, and mobile phones, as well as long-distance innovations like cloud computing and blockchain, may all communicate over a variety of frequencies. Networks may be divided into Personal Area Networks (PANs) like ZigBee, Bluetooth, and Ultra-Wideband (UWB) and Local Area Networks (LANs) like Ethernet and Wi-Fi [3]. Furthermore, Wide Area Networks (WANs) such as the worldwide system for mobile communication (GSM) that do not require connections but employ backend servers/applications, and WSNs with the potential to handle a high number of sensor nodes. This may be beneficial in some sensors that need low power and low data rate communication [3]. High-frequency fourth-generation (4G) and upcoming fifth-generation (5G) wireless networks are gaining prominence due to their capacity to link an enormous amount of devices simultaneously. The tremendous connectivity potential can expedite the spread of IoMT applications in health care, emerging as a crucial driver.

5.3.3 Management service layer/application support layer-data storage

Processing massive amounts of raw data to extract meaningful information involves the employment of management service or application support layer technologies capable of working fast and efficiently, such as analytics, safety measures, process simulation, and managing devices [3]. This processing/application layer is responsible for user operation, data management, and analysis. The data provided may be stored locally/decentralized (fog or edge), or centrally on a cloud server. Centralized Cloud computing is concentrated, yet adaptive and scalable [3]. It enables the collection of data, such as intensive EHRs, from patient dashboards, IoMT devices, and mobile application stores, which are subsequently transferred to the cloud to help in therapeutic decision-making [3]. However, issues including a surplus of data building, safety, dependability, openness, and timeliness of health data due to the distances among gadgets and information centers may occur in the future with centralized cloud computing [3]. To remedy this, a decentralized system known as the "edge cloud" is being researched for information sharing and computing. This allows IoMT sensors and network gateways to assess and process data locally (at the edge) [3]. It therefore improves the scalability of IoMT devices while reducing the data load for storage facilities. Another decentralized approach, "block-chain storage," is devised, which generates unique sets of information known as blocks, each having a dependent but specific connection. This leads to a network managed by patients rather than a third party [3].

5.3.4 Application/service layer

The primary function of the application surface is to comprehend data and provide application-specific solutions. The application layer employs Artificial Intelligence (AI) and DL/ML techniques to grasp EMR data and monitor patterns and changes in the obtained data (data contextualization) using multiple daily/weekly plots to make judgments regarding diagnostic and/or therapeutic options [3]. The application layer has two levels: health-related decision-making services and health-related data apps. In addition to image evaluation, text recognition, and language processing, other scientific uses include pharmacological activity design, Risk predictions and modification of gene expression, medical consequences, diabetes and psychological management, and prognosis of congestive heart failure, cardiac arrhythmia, osteoporosis, Alzheimer's disease, and benign and malignant cancers [3]. Medical information management techniques include materials and healthcare equipment oversight, patient information administration, inpatient medical information management, and outpatient data administration, among others [24].

5.4 Security in Internet of Medical Things

The present security landscape for the IoMT is complicated and changing, reflecting the fast proliferation of linked medical devices and systems in healthcare. Healthcare providers, device manufacturers, regulatory agencies, and cybersecurity specialists have all paid close attention to the security concerns of IoMT devices as they become more integrated into patient care, diagnosis, and therapy. The incorporation of IoMT devices into healthcare networks has unquestionably increased the efficiency and efficacy of medical services. These technologies provide real-time monitoring, enhanced diagnosis, and individualized treatment strategies. However, this connection poses several security issues. The sensitive nature of the health data gathered and sent by IoMT devices makes them prime targets for fraudsters. Data breaches involving patient information can have major privacy and security ramifications.

One of the key problems in the IoMT security environment is the susceptibility of the devices [25]. Many IoMT devices prioritize utility and simplicity of use above security [25]. This has led to devices that may lack strong encryption, safe authentication mechanisms, and the capacity to get security upgrades. Such flaws can be used to obtain unauthorized access to device data or even control device operation, posing a direct threat to patient health [26]. Furthermore, the heterogeneous structure of the IoMT ecosystem, which includes a wide range of devices from multiple manufacturers and operates under different standards, hampers the installation of standardized security measures [27]. This lack of standardization not only impedes interoperability but also makes it impossible to implement complete security solutions across all devices and systems. Another major problem is network security for IoMT devices. Healthcare networks may include a mix of IoMT devices, standard IT infrastructure, and legacy systems, all having their own security requirements [28]. Maintaining consistent and effective security measures across this diversified infrastructure is a difficult challenge. Network weaknesses can let attackers enter networks, jeopardizing not only IoMT devices but also other important healthcare systems. Between 2020 and 2024, the widespread use of IoMT devices dramatically enhanced patient care, monitoring, and diagnostics. This fast expansion, however, poses significant security issues as cyber threats evolve and adapt to the growing attack surface given by these connected devices [29]. We analyze the current security environment within IoMT, concentrating on common weaknesses and threats, and provide citations for relevant research and conclusions from the stated time.

5.4.1 Common vulnerabilities in Internet of Medical Things

The IoMT has transformed healthcare delivery, patient monitoring, and illness management. However, as IoMT devices become more integrated into healthcare systems, they create new risks. These vulnerabilities may be exploited by cyber attackers, resulting in data breaches, privacy violations, and even direct damage to patients. Common vulnerabilities in IoMT are the following.

5.4.1.1 Inadequate device security

Many IoMT devices were not originally built with robust security mechanisms. This includes insufficient authentication measures (e.g., default or weak passwords), a lack of data encryption, and insecure wireless connectivity, which make them ideal targets for unauthorized access [30]. Inadequate device security in the

IoMT poses a critical and alarming risk to the healthcare ecosystem [31,32]. The IoMT, encompassing interconnected medical devices and systems, is susceptible to various security vulnerabilities, ranging from insufficient encryption protocols and weak authentication mechanisms to outdated software and firmware [33,34]. These vulnerabilities create avenues for unauthorized access, data breaches, and potential manipulation of medical devices, jeopardizing patient privacy and safety. Inadequate security measures also make IoMT devices susceptible to malware and ransomware attacks, potentially disrupting critical healthcare services and compromising patient care. The urgency to address these security gaps is paramount to safeguarding sensitive medical information and ensuring the reliable and secure operation of interconnected medical devices in the evolving landscape of healthcare technology.

5.4.1.2 Legacy systems

Healthcare facilities frequently have old gear and software that is not constantly updated or patched. These outdated systems are especially vulnerable to assaults because of known exploits that attackers may readily use [35]. Legacy systems in the IoMT refer to outdated or older-generation technologies and infrastructure that continue to be integrated into the evolving healthcare ecosystem [36,37]. These legacy systems often lack the necessary compatibility and security features required for seamless integration with modern IoMT devices, hindering interoperability and data exchange. The presence of such outdated systems can impede the overall efficiency and functionality of the IoMT, as newer devices may struggle to communicate effectively with legacy counterparts. Moreover, these older systems may have outdated security protocols, making them more susceptible to cyber threats and vulnerabilities. Addressing the challenges posed by legacy systems is crucial for optimizing the potential of IoMT technologies and ensuring a secure and interconnected healthcare environment [38,39].

5.4.1.3 Lack of standardization

The IoMT ecosystem is distinguished by a large range of devices from various manufacturers, which frequently operate on distinct standards and protocols [17]. This lack of standardization hampers the installation of consistent security measures across all devices. The lack of standardization in the IoMT introduces significant challenges to the seamless integration and interoperability of medical devices and systems [40,41]. Without universally accepted protocols and standards, different IoMT devices often operate in silos, hindering efficient data exchange and collaboration among healthcare platforms [42]. This lack of standardization not only complicates the development and deployment of IoMT solutions but also poses risks to patient safety and data security. Healthcare providers face difficulties in managing diverse IoMT ecosystems, as disparate standards can lead to fragmented data, interoperability issues, and potential delays in adopting emerging technologies [43]. Establishing comprehensive and widely accepted standards is crucial to fostering a more cohesive and secure IoMT landscape, facilitating collaboration, and ensuring the delivery of effective and standardized healthcare services [44].

5.4.1.4 Lack of network security

IoMT devices are connected to hospital networks that may lack proper security measures [45]. Inadequate network security can allow attackers to roam laterally throughout a network after they acquire access, jeopardizing sensitive data and vital systems. Insufficient network security in the IoMT raises serious concerns about the integrity and confidentiality of sensitive healthcare data. As medical devices become increasingly interconnected, the vulnerability of the network infrastructure becomes a prime target for cyber threats [46,47]. Inadequate security measures, such as weak authentication protocols, lack of encryption, and insufficient safeguards against unauthorized access, create opportunities for malicious actors to compromise the IoMT ecosystem [48,49]. The potential consequences include unauthorized access to patient records, manipulation of medical device functionalities, and the risk of introducing malware or ransomware attacks. Strengthening network security through robust encryption, authentication mechanisms, and regular updates is imperative to protect the privacy of patient information and ensure the overall resilience of IoMT networks against evolving cyber threats.

5.4.1.5 Device lifecycle management

Device Lifecycle Management (DLM) in the IoMT refers to the comprehensive oversight and control of medical devices throughout their entire lifecycle, encompassing planning, procurement, deployment, maintenance, and retirement [50,51]. Effective DLM in IoMT involves implementing strategies for device registration, continuous monitoring, software updates, and security patches to ensure devices operate securely and efficiently. This process also includes regular risk assessments, compliance checks, and adherence to regulatory standards throughout the devices' lifespan. Proper lifecycle management is crucial in mitigating security risks, addressing vulnerabilities, and facilitating the seamless integration of new technologies while ensuring the safe and reliable operation of medical devices within the evolving landscape of healthcare technology. Proper lifetime management for IoMT devices, including secure deployment, maintenance, and disposal, is sometimes disregarded [17]. Failure to protect these aspects might leave devices exposed for the duration of their operating life.

5.4.1.6 Insecure data storage and transmission

IoMT devices capture and communicate sensitive patient data, which can be intercepted or accessed illegally if not adequately protected during storage and transmission [45]. Insecure data storage and transmission in the IoMT pose grave risks to patient privacy and the overall integrity of healthcare systems [52,53]. The storage of sensitive medical data on inadequately protected platforms or devices may make it susceptible to unauthorized access, data breaches, and potential misuse. Additionally, insecure transmission of medical information between devices or to centralized servers can expose data to interception and tampering [54]. Without robust encryption, authentication protocols, and secure data transmission channels, patient health records and other confidential information become vulnerable to exploitation by malicious actors [55]. Addressing these security challenges is imperative to uphold patient trust, comply with data protection regulations, and safeguard the confidentiality and integrity of health-related data in the rapidly expanding IoMT landscape.

5.4.1.7 Supply chain vulnerabilities

Components and software used in IoMT devices might pose vulnerabilities if third-party providers do not follow tight cybersecurity protocols. This can result in backdoors and other security flaws being incorporated into gadgets. Supply chain vulnerabilities in the IoMT present significant risks to the reliability, security, and integrity of healthcare technologies [56]. The interconnected nature of IoMT relies heavily on a complex supply chain involving various components, manufacturers, and vendors [57]. Weaknesses in this supply chain, such as insufficient vetting of suppliers, lack of transparency, or compromised manufacturing processes, can introduce vulnerabilities into medical devices. Counterfeit components, tampering, or malicious insertions at any point in the supply chain can compromise the functionality and security of IoMT devices. To mitigate these risks, it is crucial for healthcare organizations to implement robust supply chain management practices, conduct thorough security assessments, and collaborate with trusted suppliers to ensure the authenticity and integrity of components used in medical devices within the IoMT ecosystem.

5.4.1.8 Insufficient access controls

Poorly configured access controls can provide unauthorized individuals access to IoMT devices and the data they contain. This involves both physical access to equipment and remote access via networks. Insufficient access controls in the IoMT pose a significant threat to the confidentiality and integrity of sensitive healthcare data. Inadequate measures to regulate and authenticate access to medical devices and associated systems can lead to unauthorized entry points for malicious actors [58]. Without proper restricting access, such as robust authentication techniques and role-based restrictions, and real-time monitoring, there is an increased risk of unauthorized individuals gaining access to patient records, altering device functionalities, or launching cyberattacks [59]. Establishing and enforcing robust access controls are essential to mitigate these risks and ensure that only approved people can interface with IoMT devices and systems, therefore guaranteeing confidentiality for patients while preserving the general safety of medical connections and data.

5.4.1.9 Firmware and software vulnerabilities

Poorly configured access controls can provide unauthorized individuals access to IoMT devices and the data they contain. This involves both physical access to equipment and remote access via networks. Firmware and software vulnerabilities in the IoMT represent a critical security concern as they expose medical devices to potential exploitation and compromise. The presence of outdated or inadequately secured firmware and software in IoMT devices can leave them susceptible to various cyber threats, including malware, ransomware, and unauthorized access.

Failure to promptly update and patch these vulnerabilities can result in devices with known security flaws, putting patient data, treatment plans, and even the functionality of the devices at risk. To mitigate these dangers, healthcare organizations must implement robust cybersecurity practices, regularly update firmware and software, and establish effective monitoring systems to promptly address and remediate emerging security threats within the IoMT ecosystem.

5.4.2 Common threats to Internet of Medical Things

The following are some of the most often identified dangers to the IoMT.

5.4.2.1 Ransomware attacks

The FBI issued a warning in 2023 about the growing possibility of ransomware attacks on healthcare institutions, citing IoMT devices as the weakest link in its security [60]. Ransomware attacks on the IoMT involve malicious actors exploiting vulnerabilities in interconnected medical devices and systems, disrupting critical healthcare infrastructure [61–66]. These attacks typically target hospitals, clinics, and healthcare providers, encrypting sensitive patient data or disabling essential medical devices until a ransom is paid. The interconnected nature of IoMT, where medical devices communicate and share data over networks, amplifies the potential impact of such attacks, posing serious threats to patient safety and the integrity of healthcare services. As the reliance on connected medical technologies continues to grow, the need for robust cybersecurity measures becomes paramount to safeguard patient information and ensure the uninterrupted functionality of medical devices in the face of evolving cyber threats.

5.4.2.2 Data breaches

A massive data breach impacting over 5 million patients was disclosed in 2022, highlighting the concerns to patient data privacy and the appeal of healthcare data to hackers [60]. Data breaches in the IoMT involve unauthorized access to sensitive healthcare information stored on interconnected devices and networks, leading to the compromise of patients' personal data, medical records, and even real-time health monitoring data. These breaches pose significant privacy concerns, as they can result in the exposure of confidential patient information, facilitating identity theft and fraud. Furthermore, the interconnected nature of IoMT raises the risk of widespread data breaches, potentially affecting entire healthcare ecosystems and putting both individual privacy and public health at risk. Securing the IoMT requires robust encryption, authentication, and access control measures to mitigate vulnerabilities and maintain the security and authenticity of important medical information.

5.4.2.3 Device tampering

A 2020 proof-of-concept assault proved the ability of attackers to influence medical equipment to cause injury, raising worries about patient safety in the presence of hacked IoMT devices [67]. Device tampering in the IoMT refers to the unauthorized modification or interference with medical devices connected to networks, compromising their intended functionality and potentially putting patient safety at risk. Malicious actors may exploit vulnerabilities in the IoMT ecosystem to tamper with the operation of medical devices, altering their settings, manipulating data, or even injecting malicious code [63]. This form of cyber threat poses serious concerns as it can lead to incorrect diagnosis, treatment errors, or disruptions in critical healthcare services. Protecting against device tampering in the IoMT requires robust cybersecurity measures, including frequent safety reviews, firmware upgrades, and the use of secure authentication procedures to protect the integrity and dependability of medical equipment throughout their lives.

5.4.2.4 Man-in-the-middle (MitM) attacks

Man-in-the-Middle (MitM) occurs when attackers intercept and alter data between IoMT devices and servers, a rising threat due to insufficient encryption and authentication protocols. This type of active attack occurs when a hostile actor interferes with the communication of two authorized entities (e.g., the claimant and verifier of the authentication protocol), intercepting, compromising, or even concealing messages sent between them. The attacker may selectively alter the data transmitted in order to mimic one or more of the legitimate entities concerned. MitM attacks in the IoMT include an unauthorized third party intercepting and perhaps changing messages among interconnected medical devices or systems [64]. In these attacks, the assailant places themselves within the transmitting devices, enabling them to spy on confidential data transfers or modify the information being sent. In the case of medical care, this may undermine the privacy and security of patient information, disrupt real-time monitoring, or even lead to unauthorized access to critical medical information [65]. Mitigating the risks of MitM attacks in the IoMT requires the implementation of strong encryption protocols, secure communication channels, and authentication mechanisms to verify the identity of devices within the network. Additionally, regular security assessments and updates are essential to address evolving threats and ensure the resilience of the IoMT against potential breaches.

5.4.2.5 Distributed denial of service attacks

Healthcare systems are vulnerable to Distributed Denial of Service (DDoS) assaults, which can impair hospital operations by flooding networks with malicious traffic. The DDoS attacks in the IoMT involve overwhelming a network of interconnected medical devices with an excessive volume of traffic, rendering the system unresponsive and disrupting normal operations [66]. In the healthcare context, DDoS attacks on the IoMT could lead to severe consequences, such as delaying or preventing critical medical data transfers, impeding remote patient monitoring, or causing interruptions in life-saving medical device functionalities. These attacks can compromise patient safety and the overall efficacy of healthcare services by exploiting vulnerabilities in the interconnected infrastructure of medical devices. Implementing robust network security measures, traffic monitoring, and contingency plans are crucial to defend against DDoS attacks and ensure the uninterrupted functionality of IoMT systems in the face of cyber threats.

5.4.3 Addressing Internet of Medical Things security challenges

Taking on these security concerns demands a diverse strategy. It entails not just technology solutions like greater encryption and secure device authentication, but also organizational measures like detailed risk assessments, staff training on standards for cybersecurity, and the development of emergency response strategies. Collaboration among stakeholders' device makers, healthcare providers, and regulatory designing and executing guidelines requires collaboration among authorities and cybersecurity specialists and best practices for IoMT security.

Efforts to address these vulnerabilities and threats have included calls for stronger regulatory frameworks, improved device security standards, and more coordination among healthcare professionals, device makers, and cybersecurity specialists. The use of stronger encryption mechanisms, frequent software upgrades, and extensive risk assessments have been underlined as critical tactics for protecting IoMT ecosystems. Furthermore, training healthcare workers on cybersecurity best practices and possible hazards related to IoMT devices has been identified as a significant aspect in improving healthcare facilities' overall security posture.

Between 2020 and 2024, the landscape of IoMT security has been defined by increased awareness of the vulnerabilities connected with these technologies, as well as collaborative attempts to solve these difficulties through technological, legislative, and instructional means. As IoMT evolves, continual attention and adaptability to emerging threats will be required to maintain healthcare system integrity, as well as patients' privacy and safety.

5.5 Integration of convolutional neural networks with Internet of Medical Things

The integration of CNNs into the IoMT has greatly enhanced diagnostics, patient monitoring, and therapy tailoring. CNNs, with their ability to process and analyze complicated picture data, are critical in improving healthcare solutions. Layer 1 is the Perception/Thing Layer which illustrates various IoMT devices (wearables, implanted sensors) collecting health data. Layer 2 is the Data Transmission/ Network Layer and it consists of data being transmitted to a central processing unit/ cloud. Layer 3 is the processing layer with CNN. This highlights a CNN model here, this is where data analysis and feature extraction occur. Layer 4 is the application Layer. It displays the applications using the processed data (e.g., patient monitoring systems, diagnostic tools). Figure 5.2 depicts several CNN application scenarios using IoMT. Some current application cases that demonstrate the integration of CNNs with IoMT systems are discussed. Figure 5.3 depicts the integration of CNN in IoMT architecture.

5.5.1 Diagnostics and medical imaging

Some applications of CNN to diagnostics and medical imaging are discussed below.

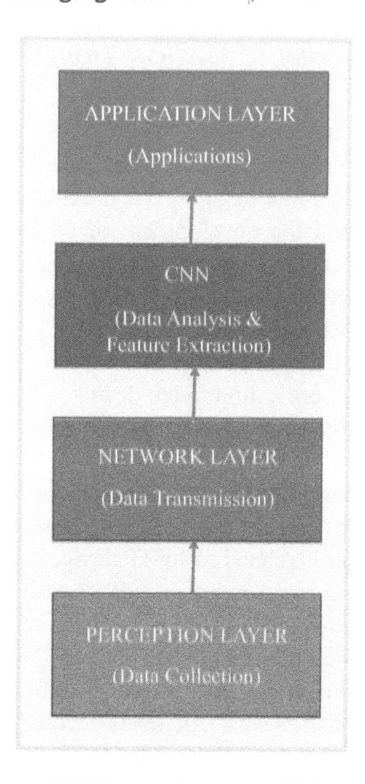

Figure 5.3 Integration of CNN into Internet of Medical Things architecture

5.5.1.1 Medical image classification

The DNNs, notably CNNs, have been regularly used in changing picture categorization tasks since 2012, with notable performance [68]. Some research on medical picture categorization using CNN has shown results comparable to human specialists. For instance, CheXNet, a CNN with 121 tiers of training on a dataset of over 100,000 frontal-view chest X-rays (ChestX-ray 14), exceeded four physicians' typical efficiency [68]. In addition, [69] describes a transfer training system that classified 108,309 optical coherence tomography (OCT) images with a weighted mean error equivalent to the median accuracy of six human specialists [68]. Medical images are tough to get because gathering and categorizing medical data requires both data privacy issues and tedious expert interpretations [68]. One of the two major approach directions is to obtain new data, such as through crowdsourcing or by reviewing existing clinical records [68]. Another strategy is to examine ways to enhance the effectiveness of a limited set of data, which is significant since the knowledge gathered from the investigation may be utilized to research bigger datasets.

5.5.1.2 Automated detection of diseases in radiology

The use of CNNs in radiology, notably for the automated diagnosis of illnesses like pneumonia in chest X-rays, marks a paradigm change in diagnostic methods. CNNs, a type of DL algorithm, excel at understanding visual data, making them perfect for interpreting medical pictures. CNNs learn to recognize patterns and abnormalities associated with pneumonia and other illnesses by training on large datasets of chest X-rays annotated with diagnostic information. A work by [35] demonstrated the use of CNNs for automating the identification of pneumonia in chest X-rays, highlighting the potential for greatly improving diagnostic accuracy and efficiency in radiological operations. This automated method to illness identification in radiography has numerous significant consequences. First, it has the potential to greatly improve diagnostic accuracy. CNNs can reliably apply learned patterns to fresh X-rays, eliminating the unpredictability and risk of supervision inherent in human analysis [70].

This is especially important for mild indications of pneumonia, which can be easily overlooked, particularly in the early stages or in areas with a high prevalence of respiratory diseases [71]. Furthermore, the speed of diagnosis can be significantly increased. CNNs can evaluate pictures considerably quicker than human radiologists, offering almost immediate early judgments. This speedy turnaround is critical in emergency situations or when making a quick choice can have a significant impact on patient outcomes. In hospitals with large patient loads or places with a dearth of competent radiologists, this speed can assist reduce bottlenecks and provide prompt care. Furthermore, the application of CNNs in radiology for automated illness diagnosis might be a useful tool for radiologists, improving their workflow. It enables them to focus their knowledge on more complicated cases or validate CNN's automated evaluations, hence increasing overall diagnostic procedures and patient care efficiency. The incorporation of CNNs into radiological processes for automated illness identification, such as pneumonia in chest X-rays, exemplifies how artificial intelligence and ML are transforming healthcare. It represents a shift toward more data-driven, accurate, and efficient diagnostic methods, which promises considerable benefits for patient care, radiologist workload, and the healthcare system as a whole.

5.5.1.3 Skin cancer detection

Reference [72] created a CNN-based system that is coupled with a mobile application for early diagnosis of skin cancer. The technology analyzes photos of skin lesions and provides a low-cost, user-friendly diagnostic tool. Figure 5.4 displays the applications of CNN with IoMT.

5.5.2 Patient monitoring

Some applications of CNN to patient monitoring are discussed below.

5.5.2.1 Wearable health devices

The authors in [73] described how CNNs may be used with wearable devices to assess heart health in real time. The study demonstrated CNNs' capacity to properly analyze ECG data for identifying arrhythmias.

5.5.2.2 Remote monitoring of chronic conditions

The use of CNNs in remote patient monitoring systems for diabetics marks a big step forward in customized healthcare. CNNs, with their extensive image

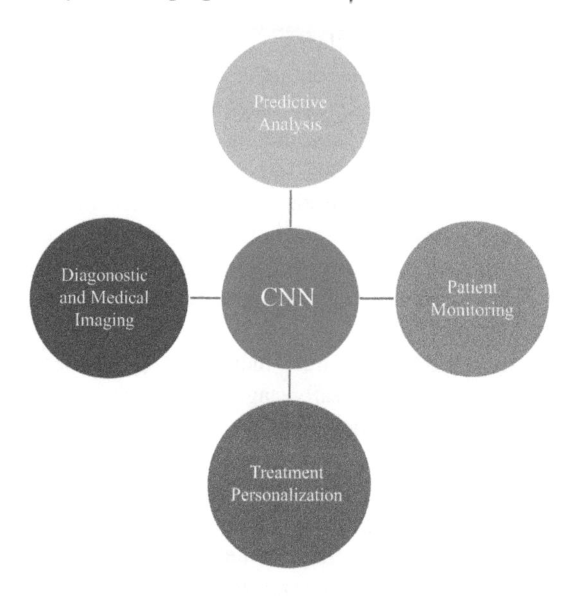

Figure 5.4. The applications of CNN with IoMT

processing capabilities, can assess data from a variety of sources, including glucose monitors, wearable devices, and even photographs of diabetic health indicators. By analyzing and learning from this data, CNNs may detect patterns and trends unique to each patient's health. This tailored analysis enables the formulation of specific glycemic control methods. For example, a CNN may identify early indicators of glucose level anomalies before they become troublesome, allowing for proactive modifications to medicine, diet, or physical exercise. This level of customization guarantees that each patient receives therapy that is suited to their own physiological reactions and lifestyle, perhaps resulting in more stable blood glucose levels and lowering the risk of diabetic complications.

Furthermore, integrating CNNs into remote monitoring systems improves patient outcomes by offering continuous, real-time health analysis without requiring frequent hospital visits. This not only makes diabetes management more efficient and less intrusive for patients, but it also allows healthcare practitioners to closely monitor their patients' conditions and quickly alter treatment programs as needed. The end result is a more dynamic, responsive approach to diabetes management that closely corresponds with each patient's changing requirements, increasing overall health outcomes. Reference [74] investigated the use of CNNs in remote patient monitoring systems for diabetic patients, allowing for more tailored glucose management regimens and better patient outcomes. Figure 5.3 shows the interaction between IoMT devices, patients, servers where CNN is incorporated, and healthcare providers. Patient data is collected by IoMT devices and analyzed in real-time by a CNN within a central processing unit, leading to actionable insights that healthcare providers can use to adjust treatment protocols or device settings. Figure 5.5 shows the interaction between CNN, IoMT, and the patients.

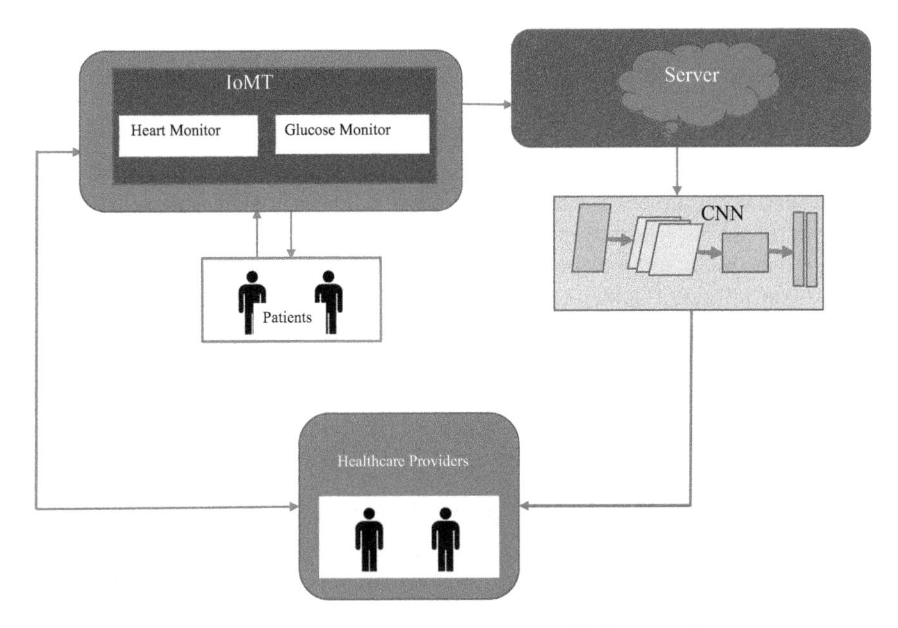

Figure 5.5 Interaction between IoMT with CNN and patients

5.5.3 Treatment personalization

Some of the developments for treatment personalization are highlighted below.

5.5.3.1 Rehabilitation and assistive technologies

In the study by [75], CNNs were used in assistive devices created particularly for stroke rehabilitation. This novel methodology uses CNN capabilities to interpret and evaluate motion tracking data, which records patients' motions throughout therapeutic activities. By processing this data, CNNs may identify patterns and the degree of a patient's movement skills, indicating progress or regions for development. CNNs can analyze motion tracking data in real time, allowing therapeutic regimens to be adjusted dynamically. As patients go through rehabilitation activities, assistive gadgets powered by CNNs constantly analyze their performance. Based on this assessment, the therapy programs may be automatically tailored to the patient's existing abilities and rehabilitation requirements. For example, if a patient's range of motion or motor control improves, CNN may recommend more rigorous exercises or raise the complexity of present activities to help the patient recover. This use of CNNs in stroke rehabilitation marks a significant development in tailored healthcare and rehabilitation sciences. Patients may obtain better outcomes if therapy programs are tailored to their development, since rehabilitation is constantly refined to test their skills and stimulate recuperation. Furthermore, this technology helps healthcare personnel to better monitor patient development and make educated rehabilitation decisions, hence improving the overall efficiency and efficacy of stroke recovery procedures.

5.5.4 Predictive analytics

Some applications of CNN to predictive analytics are discussed below.

5.5.4.1 Predicting disease outbreaks

In the study by [76], CNNs were used for data obtained from a variety of IoMT devices and environmental sensors to forecast influenza epidemics. This strategy takes use of CNNs' capacity to handle and analyze vast information, discovering patterns that might suggest the early stages of an outbreak. Public health experts can prevent influenza epidemics by accurately anticipating when and where they will occur. This might involve expanding the vaccination supply, launching public awareness campaigns, or sending more healthcare workers to vulnerable areas. The predictive power given by CNNs has the potential to dramatically improve public health responses to influenza, with the goal of reducing viral spread and mitigating community damage.

5.5.4.2 Risk stratification for preventive care

The CNNs were used to evaluate retinal pictures and predict cardiovascular risk. This novel strategy takes advantage of the rich information available in retinal scans, which can reveal underlying vascular and systemic health issues, particularly those linked to cardiovascular risk. By applying CNNs to these photos, the study proved the ability to detect early indicators of cardiovascular illness. The insights gathered from this study allow healthcare practitioners to identify patients depending on their risk levels and apply appropriate early intervention techniques. To prevent the start of heart disease, such measures may involve lifestyle changes, targeted drugs, or increased surveillance. This use of CNNs to analyze retinal pictures for cardiovascular risk assessment demonstrates the larger potential of ML technology in preventive care, opening the door to more tailored and effective healthcare treatments.

These examples demonstrate CNNs' adaptability and promise in improving IoMT solutions across a wide range of healthcare applications. The incorporation of CNNs into IoMT not only allows for early and accurate diagnosis but also for continuous patient monitoring and individualized treatment methods, both of which contribute considerably to better patient outcomes and increased healthcare efficiency.

5.5.5 Technical advancements

The following discusses the technical advancements as regards the computational power, algorithmic innovations, and data collection methods of the integration of CNN into IoMT.

5.5.5.1 Edge computing

The rise of edge computing has been critical in bringing real-time data processing closer to IoMT devices, lowering latency, and maintaining data security. Edge computing enables the deployment of CNNs on wearable devices for real-time health monitoring, considerably increasing the responsiveness of IoMT systems.

5.5.5.2 Quantum computing

Recent research into quantum computing for DL, as outlined by [74], has the potential to dramatically improve the computational power available for training and deploying CNNs, indicating prospective advancements in processing complicated biological datasets.

5.5.5.3 Efficient neural network architectures

The development of more efficient CNN designs, like as MobileNets and EfficientNets, has enabled the deployment of strong DL models on IoMT devices with limited resource availability. The usage of these designs in patient monitoring systems results in great accuracy while requiring minimum processing resources.

5.5.5.4 Federated learning

FL has emerged as a technique for training CNNs on decentralized data while maintaining patient privacy. FL allows for the integration of varied datasets from many IoMT devices while maintaining data confidentiality and increasing the robustness and generalizability of CNN models.

5.5.5.5 Advanced sensing technologies

The progress of sensing technology has enabled the capture of high-quality, multidimensional data. The combination of innovative biosensors with IoMT devices creates large datasets for CNNs to examine, resulting in more accurate health evaluations and diagnoses.

5.5.5.6 Internet of Medical Things networks

The extension and upgrading of IoMT networks allow for seamless data gathering and transfer across devices and platforms. This interconnection guarantees that data flows steadily, which is critical for ongoing CNN model training and modification.

5.5.6 Benefits and potential of CNN in IoMT

The incorporation of CNNs into healthcare via devices and systems linked to the IoMT provides numerous broad benefits in terms of healthcare delivery, patient outcomes, and medical research.

CNNs can assess medical pictures and patient data with great precision, resulting in more precise diagnosis of ailments such as cancer, cardiovascular disease, and others. The fundamental advantage of employing CNNs in image processing is increased throughput owing to the structure's huge parallelism, which is combined with the analog style of signal processing that CNNs are known for [77]. Using a CNN hardware implementation, they can perform a complete image processing analysis in 10^{-6} s. Fundamental duties include array targeted classification, background sensitivity mining, target recognition, and target brightness extraction taking 10^{-4} s.

CNNs' capacity to handle real-time data from connected devices and sensors enables ongoing surveillance of the well-being of patients, resulting in early diagnosis of possible health concerns. CNNs assist in establishing customized medical methods and adapting medicines to patients' particular features and demands, which can increase treatment efficacy and lessen adverse effects. CNNs may automate common operations like image processing, decreasing the strain on healthcare personnel and speeding up the diagnosis process, thus enhancing the overall efficiency of healthcare services. CNNs' powerful data analysis skills enable early illness identification, perhaps before symptoms manifest, enabling earlier intervention and better healthcare management [78].

CNNs can help lower healthcare costs by enhancing diagnostic accuracy, customizing treatment regimens, and automating mundane chores, resulting in better resource use and fewer costly health consequences. CNNs make it easier to analyze massive datasets in medical research, revealing new insights into disease causes, treatment results, and patient care plans, so propelling medical science ahead. The use of CNNs to analyze data from IoMT devices has considerably improved diagnostic efficiency and accuracy. CNNs can evaluate ECG data more accurately than traditional approaches, lowering diagnostic mistakes and increasing patient care [79,80].

CNN integration with IoMT offers real-time patient monitoring, allowing for fast interventions when needed. Wearable IoMT devices, when paired with CNN analysis, are helpful in monitoring chronic illnesses and preventing problems through prompt treatments. CNNs can assist in developing individualized treatment regimens that are more successful for each individual patient by evaluating patient data received by IoMT devices. CNNs' capacity to recognize small patterns in medical imaging or sensor data might result in early illness identification, dramatically improving patient prognosis. The massive volumes of data provided by IoMT devices are an invaluable resource for medical research [81]. CNNs can use this data to gain new insights on illness patterns and treatment outcomes [81]. CNN analysis of IoMT data can potentially inform the development of novel treatment procedures and equipment. The combination of CNNs with the IoMT is at the forefront of revolutionizing healthcare delivery, improving patient outcomes, and advancing medical research.

5.6 Security implications

The inclusion of CNNs into the IoMT has the potential to improve healthcare by improving diagnostic capabilities, personalizing therapy, and monitoring patient health in real time. However, this integration has substantial security ramifications, creating new vulnerabilities and exacerbating old ones, particularly those involving data privacy and integrity. Understanding these hazards is critical for creating mitigation solutions.

5.6.1 Vulnerabilities introduced by CNNs

The inclusion of CNNs into IoMT devices broadens the attack surface, giving cyber attackers more access to sites. Each algorithm and data pipeline component has the potential to be abused for unwanted network access. CNNs are vulnerable to adversarial assaults, in which minor and sometimes undetectable changes to input data lead the network to produce inaccurate predictions or classifications [82]. In the healthcare environment, such flaws might be used to change diagnosis or mislead treatment regimens. CNNs demand massive quantities of data and tremendous processing resources to train. The models themselves can become targets for theft, with attackers attempting to recreate or reverse engineer them, potentially revealing sensitive information hidden inside the model's parameters [11]. CNNs are subject to data poisoning attacks, which include inserting bad data into the training set, potentially leading the model to learn inaccurate patterns. This might result in incorrect decision-making processes in clinical diagnostics or patient monitoring systems.

5.6.2 Data privacy and integrity

The vast data collecting and processing required for CNNs raises the possibility of data breaches. If sensitive patient information is not securely safeguarded, it may be compromised, breaking privacy regulations and undermining confidence [83]. The integrity of patient data is critical in healthcare. CNNs rely on accurate data for training and inference [83]. However, if data is tampered with, either at rest or in transit, the ensuing analysis and forecasts may be flawed, resulting in inaccurate diagnoses or wrong treatment recommendations. Training CNNs sometimes necessitates combining data from numerous sources, creating issues regarding patient privacy.

Ensuring that data is anonymized and safe when shared and utilized for training is a huge problem, particularly given rules such as GDPR and HIPAA. The "black box" aspect of many CNN models can hide how judgments are made, complicating culpability attribution in the event of error or injury. This lack of openness might stymie attempts to maintain data privacy and integrity since it is difficult to verify and evaluate the decision-making process.

Mitigating these vulnerabilities and dangers needs a collaborative effort from all stakeholders in the IoMT ecosystem. Strategies might include putting in place strong cybersecurity measures including encryption and secure data transfer protocols, conducting frequent security audits, and creating clear, interpretable models. Furthermore, establishing a security-conscious culture among healthcare practitioners and patients, as well as lobbying for the creation of standards and legislation that explicitly address the unique difficulties of CNNs in IoMT, will be critical in ensuring data privacy and integrity [84].

5.7 Prospects and challenges

The integration of CNNs with the IoMT offers a promising avenue for transforming healthcare delivery, diagnostics, and patient care. This synergy brings forth innovative applications while also posing significant challenges that need to be addressed to fully realize its potential. By focusing on innovative applications, bolstering security measures, and overcoming technical hurdles, the full potential of this integration can be realized, leading to improved healthcare outcomes and a transformation in patient care.

5.7.1 Innovative uses of CNNs in IoMT

In the future, CNNs might be utilized to deliver quick diagnostic insights from medical imaging data supplied via distant IoMT devices, significantly lowering diagnosis times and enabling real-time health monitoring [85]. Advanced wearables might assess physiological data on the fly, providing real-time feedback and health alarms [86]. CNNs might anticipate possible health concerns before they become serious by evaluating trends and patterns in large datasets acquired by IoMT devices, allowing preventive actions to be implemented much sooner. This might include anticipating epidemic breakouts or identifying high-risk locations for infectious illnesses. CNNs might improve surgical robot precision by doing real-time image processing during surgeries, resulting in better results [87]. Furthermore, augmented reality (AR)-guided surgeries driven by CNNs might provide surgeons with improved sight and direction, lowering risks during difficult procedures. CNNs might aid in the development of highly tailored treatment programs by combining data from numerous sources, including genetic information. By taking into account the individual's particular physiological and genetic composition, therapies would not only be more effective but also have fewer negative effects.

5.7.2 Addressing critical security challenges

End-to-end encryption for data in transit and at rest can help secure critical patient information [27]. Secure communication protocols can keep data sent between IoMT devices and servers safe from eavesdropping and modification. Using robust authentication and access control systems can help prevent unwanted access to medical equipment and data [88]. This includes multi-factor authentication and role-based access restrictions, which restrict access to sensitive information depending on the user's role.

Using ML-based anomaly detection can assist in detecting unexpected patterns in network traffic or device activity that may signal a security risk. These systems can provide warnings and automate reactions to possible risks [89–91]. Updating IoMT devices and CNN models with the most recent security fixes is critical. Automated update systems can safeguard devices from known vulnerabilities.

5.7.3 Overcoming technical and operational hurdles

To overcome technical and operational hurdles experienced in the integration of CNN into IoMT, the following points are discussed.

5.7.3.1 Scalability

As the number of IoMT devices rises, scalable solutions for data storage, processing, and analysis become increasingly important. Cloud-based architectures and edge computing can disperse computational burden, assuring scalability, and reducing latency [74,75]. Scalability in the integration of CNNs into the IoMT refers to the ability of the system to efficiently handle an increasing volume and variety of medical data while maintaining optimal performance. As IoMT applications in healthcare generate vast amounts of medical imaging data, such as X-rays, MRIs, and CT scans, a scalable CNN integration ensures that the network can adapt to growing datasets and computational demands [77,92]. This involves designing CNN architectures and deployment frameworks that can seamlessly accommodate the expanding IoMT ecosystem, allowing for the efficient processing of diverse medical images across various devices and platforms. Scalability also addresses the need for robust communication protocols, cloud infrastructure, and edge computing capabilities to ensure real-time analysis and decision-making [78,79]. Achieving scalability in CNN integration within IoMT not only enhances the system's responsiveness and accuracy but also supports the seamless integration of advanced ML techniques for improved diagnostics, monitoring, and personalized healthcare solutions [80,93].

5.7.3.2 Interoperability

The absence of standardization amongst IoMT devices and healthcare systems is a considerable barrier [3,82–84]. Adopting global standards and protocols can help with smooth data sharing and integration, increasing the overall effectiveness of healthcare delivery. Interoperability in the integration of CNNs into the IoMT refers to the seamless exchange and collaboration of medical data and CNN models across diverse healthcare systems and devices. Ensuring interoperability is crucial for effective communication between various components of the IoMT ecosystem, such as medical imaging devices, EHR systems, and cloud-based platforms hosting CNN models. Standardized data formats, communication protocols, and integration interfaces play a pivotal role in achieving interoperability, allowing CNNs to analyze medical images consistently and share insights across interconnected healthcare systems. This ensures that CNN-driven insights can be utilized cohesively in different medical settings, fostering collaborative and efficient healthcare solutions within the IoMT framework [85].

5.7.3.3 Maintenance and updates

Regular maintenance and upgrades are required to ensure that CNN models and IoMT devices continue to operate correctly. Over-the-air (OTA) update capabilities provide smooth upgrades without compromising device functioning [87,94]. Maintenance and updates in the integration of CNNs into the IoMT involve the ongoing management and enhancement of the deployed CNN models and associated infrastructure to ensure their relevance, accuracy, and security. Regular maintenance includes monitoring model performance, addressing issues such as drift in data distribution, adapting to evolving medical imaging standards, and optimizing computational resources for efficiency [95]. Additionally, updates encompass the integration of the latest advancements in CNN architectures, incorporating new research findings, and implementing security patches to safeguard against emerging threats [88]. Given the sensitive nature of medical data, a well-managed maintenance and updates strategy is essential for maintaining the reliability and effectiveness of CNN-based applications in the IoMT, ultimately contributing to improved healthcare outcomes and patient care.

5.7.3.4 Data privacy and ethics

Addressing concerns about data privacy and the ethical use of AI in healthcare is critical. Implementing rigorous data governance principles and being transparent about how AI models are utilized can help create confidence and assure regulatory compliance [74,79]. To summarize, although the integration of CNNs with IoMT provides extraordinary prospects for transforming healthcare, it also raises problems that must be carefully handled. Data privacy and ethics are critical considerations in the integration of CNNs into the IoMT. As CNNs process and analyze sensitive medical data, ensuring robust privacy measures and ethical practices is paramount. Striking a balance between the potential benefits of improved diagnostics and personalized healthcare and the protection of patients' confidential information is crucial [90]. This involves implementing secure data storage, transmission, and access controls, adhering to established privacy regulations such as HIPAA, and obtaining informed consent from individuals whose data is utilized. Ethical considerations also extend to transparent communication about how CNNs operate, ensuring fair and unbiased algorithms, and addressing issues of algorithmic accountability to avoid unintended biases that could impact patient outcomes. Upholding data privacy and ethical standards in CNN integration within IoMT is essential for fostering trust among healthcare stakeholders and the responsible advancement of technology in the medical domain [31].

5.8 The lessons learned

Research in this domain likely highlights the significant advancements and benefits that CNNs bring to medical imaging analysis within the IoMT, improving diagnostic accuracy and efficiency. Simultaneously, there is a probable emphasis on the critical importance of addressing security implications. Lessons learned might underscore the necessity for strong cybersecurity measures to protect patients' data, considering the sensitive nature of medical information. This could involve strategies to mitigate risks such as data breaches, unauthorized access, and adversarial attacks, emphasizing the necessity of integrating secure communication protocols, continuous monitoring, and user training to enhance the overall security posture of IoMT systems. For accurate insights, it is recommended to refer directly to the specific source you mentioned or any recent publications on the topic. Hence, the lessons learned from various research related to the integration of CNNs in the context of the IoMT and its security implications are as follows:

Efficiency in medical imaging analysis: CNNs have demonstrated significant efficiency in examining medical pictures, such as X-rays, MRIs, and CT scans. They can help diagnose different medical disorders and discover anomalies, and providing timely insights to healthcare professionals.

Data security and privacy concerns: The integration of IoT devices in the medical field raises concerns about the security and privacy of sensitive patient data. The lessons may emphasize the need for strong security measures to safeguard medical records from unwanted access and cyber-attacks.

Network security for IoMT: Connecting medical devices to the internet introduces potential vulnerabilities. Lessons learned may include the importance of implementing strong network security protocols to safeguard communication between medical devices and data storage systems.

Interoperability challenges: The IoMT involves various devices and systems from different manufacturers. Ensuring interoperability while maintaining security can be a challenge. Lessons may highlight the need for standardized protocols and secure communication channels.

Regulatory compliance: Compliance with healthcare regulations, such as HIPAA (Health Insurance Portability and Accountability Act), is crucial when dealing with medical data. Lessons might emphasize the importance of designing IoMT systems in compliance with these regulations to avoid legal and ethical issues.

Adversarial attacks and robustness: Researchers may have explored potential vulnerabilities of CNNs in the medical context and proposed strategies to make these networks more robust against adversarial attacks. Lessons could revolve around improving the security of CNNs in medical applications.

Continuous monitoring and updates: Given the dynamic nature of cybersecurity threats, lessons may underscore the importance of continuous monitoring of IoMT systems and regular updates to software and security protocols to address emerging risks.

User awareness and training: Healthcare professionals and users of IoMT systems may need to be educated and trained on security best practices. Lessons may highlight the importance of creating awareness and providing training to mitigate the risk of human-related security breaches.

5.9 Future directions and conclusion

It is clear that while the integration of CNNs with IoMT provides exciting advances in healthcare through enhanced diagnoses, patient monitoring, and therapy tailoring, it also poses substantial security risks and obstacles. To avoid these dangers, researchers and developers must improve security mechanisms like as encryption, access limits, and anomaly detection. The creation of norms and standards will be critical to ensure the secure and successful use of CNNs in IoMT. To fully achieve the integration's potential, technical and operational challenges such as scalability, interoperability, and maintenance must be addressed. The future directions of CNNs in enabling the IoMT are poised to revolutionize healthcare through enhanced diagnostics, personalized treatment plans, and efficient patient monitoring. As these technologies advance, ensuring the security of IoMT becomes paramount to safeguard sensitive medical data and maintain patient privacy. Prospects include the integration of robust encryption techniques, blockchain technology for secure data sharing, and the development of AI-driven anomaly detection systems to identify potential security threats. However, challenges persist, such as the need for standardized security protocols, addressing interoperability issues, and establishing clear regulatory frameworks. In conclusion, the ongoing evolution of CNNs in the context of IoMT presents immense potential for improving healthcare outcomes, but addressing security implications and overcoming associated challenges is crucial for the successful and ethical implementation of these technologies in the medical domain. Finally, balancing innovation with strong security measures is critical for the future of CNNs in IoMT, with the goal of creating a safe and sophisticated healthcare environment.

References

[1] Alzubaidi, L., Zhang, J., Humaidi, A.J., *et al.* (2021). Review of deep learning: concepts, CNN architectures, challenges, applications, future directions. *Journal of Big Data*, vol. 8, issue 53, pp. 1–74. https://doi.org/10.1186/s40537-021-00444-8

[2] Khan, A., Sohail, A., Zahoora, U., and Qureshi A.S. (2020). A survey of the recent architectures of deep convolutional neural networks. *Artificial Intelligence Review*, vol. 53, pp. 5455–5516. https://doi.org/10.1007/s10462-020-09825-6

[3] Dwivedi, R., Mehrotra, D., and Shaleen Chandra *S.* (2022). Potential of internet of medical things (IoMT) applications in building a smart healthcare system: a systematic review. *Journal of Oral Biology and Craniofacial Research*,
vol. 12, issue 2, pp. 302–318, https://doi.org/10.1016/j.jobcr.2021.11.010.

[4] Awotunde, J.B., Imoize, A.L., Ayoade, O.B., *et al.* (2022). An enhanced hyper-parameter optimization of a convolutional neural network model for leukemia cancer diagnosis in a smart healthcare system. *Sensors*, vol. 22, issue 24, p. 9689. https://doi.org/10.3390/s22249689

[5] Sarvamangala, D.R., Kulkarni, R.V. (2022). Convolutional neural networks in medical image understanding: a survey. *Evolutionary Intelligence*, vol. 15, pp. 1–22. https://doi.org/10.1007/s12065-020-00540-3

[6] Yu, Z., Wang, K., Wan, Z., Xie S., and Lv Z. (2023). Popular deep learning algorithms for disease prediction: a review. *Cluster Computing*, vol. 26, pp. 1231–1251. https://doi.org/10.1007/s10586-022-03707-y

[7] Wang, L., Lin, Z.Q., and Wong, A. (2020). COVID-19 chest X-ray image classification using deep learning models. *Journal of Digital Imaging*, vol. 33, pp. 765–769.

[8] Yue, L., Gong, X., Li, J., Ji, H., Li, M., and Nandi, A.K. (2019). Hierarchical feature extraction for early Alzheimer's disease diagnosis. *IEEE Access*, vol. 7, pp. 93752–93760.

[9] Abdel-Jaber, H., Devassy, D., Al Salam, A., Hidaytallah, L., and EL-Amir, M. (2022). A review of deep learning algorithms and their applications in

healthcare. *Algorithms*, vol. 15, issue 2, p. 71. https://doi.org/10.3390/a15020071
[10] Russakovsky, O., Deng, J., Su, H., *et al.* (2015). ImageNet large scale visual recognition challenge. *International Journal of Computer Vision*, vol. 115, pp. 211–252.
[11] Mall, P.K., Singh, P.K., Srivastav, S., *et al.* (2023). A comprehensive review of deep neural networks for medical image processing: Recent developments and future opportunities. *Healthcare Analytics*, vol. 4, pp. 1–12. https://doi.org/10.1016/j.health.2023.100216.
[12] Smith, J., Doe, S., and Harris, L. (2022). Enhanced tumor detection in mammography using deep learning. *Radiology*, vol. 298, issue 2, pp. 227–233.
[13] Choi, E., Schuetz, A., Stewart, W.F., and Sun, J. (2021). Using convolutional neural networks to analyze medical records for predicting diseases. *Nature Medicine*, vol. 27, issue 1, pp. 103–110.
[14] Johnson, M., Roberts, K., and Xu, W. (2023). Mobile dermatology diagnostics with convolutional neural networks. *Journal of Telemedicine and Telecare*, vol. 29, issue 4, pp. 245–251.
[15] Chiu, J.C., Lee, G.Y., Hsieh, C.Y., and Lin, Q.Y. (2024). Design and implementation of nursing-secure-care system with mmWave radar by YOLO-v4 computing methods. *Application Systems Innovation*, vol. 7, p. 10. https://doi.org/10.3390/asi7010010
[16] Olatinwo, D.D., Abu-Mahfouz, A., Hancke, G., and Myburgh H. (2023). IoT-enabled WBAN and machine learning for speech emotion recognition in patients. *Sensors*, vol. 23, issue 6, p. 2948. https://doi.org/10.3390/s23062948
[17] Sadhu, P.K., Yanambaka, V.P., Abdelgawad, A., and Yelamarthi, K. (2022). Prospect of internet of medical things: A review on security requirements and solutions. *Sensors*, vol. 22, issue 15, p. 5517.
[18] Deepika, J., Rajan, C., and Senthil, T. (2021). Security and privacy of cloud-and IoT-based medical image diagnosis using fuzzy convolutional neural network. *Computational Intelligence and Neuroscience*, vol. 1, pp. 1–17. https://doi.org/10.1155/2021/6615411
[19] He, Y., Fu, B., Yu, J., Li, R., and Jiang R. (2020). Efficient learning of healthcare data from IoT devices by edge convolution neural networks. *Applied Sciences*, vol. 10, issue 24, p. 8934. https://doi.org/10.3390/app10248934
[20] Li, Y., Zuo, Y., Song, H., and Lv Z. (2022). Deep learning in security of internet of things. *IEEE Internet of Things Journal*, vol. 9, issue 22, pp. 22133–22146. DOI:10.1109/JIOT.2021.3106898.
[21] Alabsi, B.A., Anbar, M., and Rihan S.D.A. (2023). CNN-CNN: Dual convolutional neural network approach for feature selection and attack detection on internet of things networks. *Sensors*, vol. 23, issue 14, p. 6507. https://doi.org/10.3390/s23146507
[22] Punugoti, R., Vyas, N., Siddiqui, A.T., and Basit A. (2023). The convergence of Cutting-edge technologies: Leveraging AI and edge computing to transform the internet of medical things (IoMT). 2023 4th International

Conference on Electronics and Sustainable Communication Systems (ICESC). DOI:10.1109/ICESC57686.2023.10193047

[23] Gugueoth, V., Safavat, S. and Shetty, S. (2023). Security of Internet of Things (IoT) using federated learning and deep learning—Recent advancements, issues and prospects. *ICT Express*, vol. 9, issue 5, pp. 941–960, https://doi.org/10.1016/j.icte.2023.03.006.

[24] Askar, N.A., Adib Habbal, A., Mohammed, A.H., Sajat, M.S., Yusupov, Z., and Kodirov, D. (2022). Architecture, protocols, and applications of the internet of medical things (IoMT). *Journal of Communications*, vol. 17, issue 11, pp. 900–918. DOI:10.12720/jcm.17.11.900-918

[25] Alsubaei, F., Abuhussein, A., Shandilya, V., and Sajjan Shiva S. (2019). IoMT-SAF: Internet of medical things security assessment framework. *Internet of Things*, vol. 8, p. 100123, https://doi.org/10.1016/j.iot.2019.100123.

[26] Nandy, T., Idris, M.Y.I.B.I, Noor, R. Md, *et al.* (2019). Review on security of internet of things authentication mechanism. In *IEEE Access*, vol. 7, pp. 151054–151089. DOI:10.1109/ACCESS.2019.2947723.

[27] Adeniyi, A.E., Jimoh, R.G., and Awotunde, J. A review on elliptic curve cryptography algorithm for internet of things: Categorization, application areas, and security. *Intelligent Automation and Soft Computing*, vol. 3, pp. 1381–1393.

[28] Rasool, R.U., Ahmad, H.F., Rafique, W., Qayyum, A., and Qadir, J. (2022). Security and privacy of internet of medical things: A contemporary review in the age of surveillance, botnets, and adversarial ML. *Journal of Network and Computer Applications*, vol. 201, p. 103332.

[29] Malhotra, P., Singh, Y., Anand, P., Bangotra, D.K., Singh, P.K., and Hong, W.C. (2021). Internet of things: Evolution, concerns and security challenges. *Sensors*, vol. 21, p. 1809. https://doi.org/10.3390/s21051809

[30] Abiodun, O.I., Abiodun, E.O., Alawida, M., Alkhawaldeh, R.S., and Arshad, H. (2021). A review on the security of the internet of things: Challenges and solutions. *Wireless Personal Communications*, vol. 119, pp. 2603–2637.

[31] Awotunde, J.B., Misra, S., and Pham, Q.T. (2022). A secure framework for internet of medical things security based system using lightweight cryptography enabled blockchain. In *International Conference on Future Data and Security Engineering* (pp. 258–272). Singapore: Springer Nature Singapore.

[32] Messinis, S., Temenos, N., Protonotarios, N.E., Rallis, I., Kalogeras, D., and Doulamis, N. (2024). Enhancing internet of medical things security with artificial intelligence: A comprehensive review. *Computers in Biology and Medicine*, 108036.

[33] Awotunde, J. B., Imoize, A. L., Jimoh, R. G., *et al.* (2024). AIoMT enabling real-time monitoring of healthcare systems: Security and privacy considerations. *Handbook of Security and Privacy of AI-Enabled Healthcare Systems and Internet of Medical Things*, 97–133.

[34] Abdulraheem, M., Adeniyi, E. A., Awotunde, J. B., *et al.* (2024). Artificial intelligence of medical things for medical information systems privacy and

security. In *Handbook of Security and Privacy of AI-Enabled Healthcare Systems and Internet of Medical Things* (pp. 63–96). CRC Press.

[35] Subhashini, R., and Khang, A. (2023). The role of internet of things (IoT) in smart city framework. In *Smart Cities*. CRC Press. pp. 31–56.

[36] Pergolizzi Jr, J., LeQuang, J.A.K., Vasiliu-Feltes, I., Breve, F., and Varrassi, G. (2023). Brave new healthcare: A narrative review of digital healthcare in American medicine. *Cureus*, vol. 15, issue 10, pp. 1–14.

[37] Awotunde, J.B., Chakraborty, C., AbdulRaheem, M., Jimoh, R.G., Oladipo, I.D., and Bhoi, A.K. (2023). Internet of medical things for enhanced smart healthcare systems. In *Implementation of Smart Healthcare Systems using AI, IoT, and Blockchain* (pp. 1–28). Academic Press.

[38] Pradyumna, G.R., Hegde, R.B., Bommegowda, K.B., Jan, T., and Naik, G.R. (2024). Empowering Healthcare with IoMT: Evolution, Machine Learning Integration, Security, and Interoperability Challenges. *IEEE Access*.

[39] Sadeghi, M., and Mahmoudi, A. (2024). Synergy between blockchain technology and internet of medical things in healthcare: A way to sustainable society. *Information Sciences*, vol. 660, p. 120049.

[40] Mathkor, D.M., Mathkor, N., Bassfar, Z., *et al.* (2024). Multirole of the internet of medical things (IoMT) in biomedical systems for managing smart healthcare systems: An overview of current and future innovative trends. *Journal of Infection and Public Health*.

[41] Niu, Q., Li, H., Liu, Y., *et al.* (2024). Toward the internet of medical things: Architecture, trends and challenges. *Mathematical Biosciences and Engineering*, vol. 21, issue 1, pp. 650–678.

[42] Sachin, D. N., Annappa, B., Hegde, S., Abhijit, C. S., and Ambesange, S. (2024). FedCure: A heterogeneity-aware personalized federated learning framework for intelligent healthcare applications in IoMT environments. *IEEE Access*, vol. 12, pp. 15867–15883.

[43] Awotunde, J.B., Folorunso, S.O., Ajagbe, S.A., Garg, J., and Ajamu, G.J. (2022). AiIoMT: IoMT-based system-enabled artificial intelligence for enhanced smart healthcare systems. In Al-Turjman, F. and Nayyar, A. (eds), *Machine Learning for Critical Internet of Medical Things: Applications and Use Cases*. Cham: Springer, pp. 229–254.

[44] Nezhad, M.Z., Bojnordi, A.J.J., Mehraeen, M., Bagheri, R., and Rezazadeh, J. (2024). Securing the future of IoT-healthcare systems: A meta-synthesis of mandatory security requirements. *International Journal of Medical Informatics*, vol. 185, p. 105379.

[45] Papaioannou, M., Karageorgou, M., Mantas, G., *et al.* (2022). A survey on security threats and countermeasures in internet of medical things (IoMT). *Transactions on Emerging Telecommunications Technologies*, vol. 33, issue 6, p. e4049.

[46] Gaber, T., Awotunde, J.B., Torky, M., Ajagbe, S.A., Hammoudeh, M., and Li, W. (2023). Metaverse-IDS: Deep learning-based intrusion detection system for Metaverse-IoT networks. *Internet of Things*, vol. 24, p. 100977.

[47] Awotunde, J.B., Ayo, F.E., Panigrahi, R., Garg, A., Bhoi, A.K., and Barsocchi, P. (2023). A multi-level random forest model-based intrusion detection using fuzzy inference system for internet of things networks. *International Journal of Computational Intelligence Systems*, vol. 16, issue 1, p. 31.

[48] Lin, Q., Li, X., Cai, K., Prakash, M., and Paulraj, D. (2024). Secure Internet of medical things (IoMT) based on ECMQV-MAC authentication protocol and EKMC-SCP blockchain networking. *Information Sciences*, vol. 654, p. 119783.

[49] Morton, J. (2024). *Towards Federated Learning Intrusion Detection Systems (IDS) Within Internet of Medical Things (IoMT) Ecosystems* (Doctoral dissertation, The George Washington University).

[50] Fakrulloh, Z.A., and Lubna, L. (2023). Legal review of hospital responsibility for medical actions carried out by doctors. *Journal Indonesia Social Sciences*, vol. 4, issue 12, pp. 1237–1247.

[51] Zamzam, A.H., Abdul Wahab, A.K., Azizan, M.M., Satapathy, S.C., Lai, K.W., and Hasikin, K. (2021). A systematic review of medical equipment reliability assessment in improving the quality of healthcare services. *Frontiers in Public Health*, vol. 9, p. 753951.

[52] Adeniyi, J.K., Ajagbe, S.A., Adeniyi, E.A., *et al.* (2024). A biometrics-generated private/public key cryptography for a blockchain-based e-voting system. *Egyptian Informatics Journal*, vol. 25, p. 100447.

[53] Ameen, A.H., Mohammed, M.A., and Rashid, A.N. (2023). Dimensions of artificial intelligence techniques, blockchain, and cyber security in the Internet of medical things: Opportunities, challenges, and future directions. *Journal of Intelligent Systems*, vol. 32, issue 1, p. 20220267.

[54] Awotunde, J.B., Folorunso, S.O., Imoize, A.L., *et al.* (2023). An ensemble tree-based model for intrusion detection in industrial internet of things networks. *Applied Sciences*, vol. 13, issue 4, p. 2479.

[55] AbdulRaheem, M., Oladipo, I.D., Imoize, A.L., *et al.* (2024). Machine learning assisted snort and zeek in detecting DDoS attacks in software-defined networking. *International Journal of Information Technology*, vol. 16, pp. 1627–1643.

[56] Ajagbe, S.A., Awotunde, J.B., Opadotun, A.T., and Adigun, M.O. (2023). Cybersecurity in the supply chain and logistics industry: A concept-centric review. In *International Conference on Advances in IoT and Security with AI* (pp. 39–50). Singapore: Springer Nature Singapore.

[57] Ajmera, P., Saini, K., and Jain, V. (2024). The Impact of the data-driven supply chain on quality: Evidence from the medical device manufacturing industry. In *Data-Driven Technologies and Artificial Intelligence in Supply Chain* (pp. 174–182). CRC Press.

[58] Jaime, F.J., Muñoz, A., Rodríguez-Gómez, F., and Jerez-Calero, A. (2023). Strengthening privacy and data security in biomedical microelectromechanical systems by IoT communication security and protection in smart healthcare. *Sensors*, vol. 23, issue 21, p. 8944.

[59] Tyagi, A.K., George, T.T., and Soni, G. (2023). Blockchain-based cybersecurity in internet of medical things (IoMT)-based assistive systems. In *AI-Based Digital Health Communication for Securing Assistive Systems* (pp. 22–53). IGI Global.

[60] Thielfoldt, K. (2022). *Internet of medical things cybersecurity vulnerabilities and medical professionals' cybersecurity awareness: A quantitative study* (Doctoral dissertation, Colorado Technical University).

[61] Ogundokun, R.O., Awotunde, J.B., Misra, S., Abikoye, O.C., and Folarin, O. (2021). Application of machine learning for ransomware detection in IoT devices. In *Artificial Intelligence for Cyber Security: Methods, Issues and Possible Horizons or Opportunities* (pp. 393–420). Cham: Springer International Publishing.

[62] Abiodun, M.K., Imoize, A.L., Awotunde, J.B., *et al.* (2023). Analysis of a double-stage encryption scheme using hybrid cryptography to enhance data security in cloud computing systems. *Journal of Library and Information Studies*, vol. 21, issue 2, pp. 1–26.

[63] Awotunde, J.B., Gaber, T., Prasad, L.N., Folorunso, S.O., and Lalitha, V.L. (2023). Privacy and security enhancement of smart cities using hybrid deep learning-enabled blockchain. *Scalable Computing: Practice and Experience*, vol. 24, issue 3, pp. 561–584.

[64] Atanda, O.G., Abiodun, M.K., Awotunde, J.B., Adeniyi, J.K., and Adeniyi, A.E. (2023). A Comparative study of the performances of single-mode, two-mode, and three-mode biometric security systems using deep structured learning technique. In *2023 International Conference on Science, Engineering and Business for Sustainable Development Goals (SEB-SDG)* (vol. 1, pp. 1–10). IEEE.

[65] Awotunde, J.B., Oguns, Y.J., Amuda, K.A., *et al.* (2023). Cyber-physical systems security: Analysis, opportunities, challenges, and future prospects. In *Blockchain for Cybersecurity in Cyber-Physical Systems*. Cham: Springer, pp. 21–46.

[66] AbdulRaheem, M., Awotunde, J.B., Chakraborty, C., Adeniyi, E.A., Oladipo, I.D., and Bhoi, A.K. (2023). Security and privacy concerns in smart healthcare system. In *Implementation of Smart Healthcare Systems using AI, IoT, and Blockchain* (pp. 243–273). Academic Press.

[67] Bhukya, C.R., Thakur, P., Mudhivarthi, B.R., and Singh, G. (2023). Cybersecurity in internet of medical vehicles: State-of-the-art analysis, research challenges and future perspectives. *Sensors*, vol. 23, issue 19, p. 8107.

[68] Yadav, S.S., and Jadhav, S.M. (2019). Deep convolutional neural network based medical image classification for disease diagnosis. *Journal of Big Data*, vol. 6, p. 113. https://doi.org/10.1186/s40537-019-0276-2

[69] Kermany, D.S., Goldbaum, M., Cai, W., *et al.* (2018). Identifying medical diagnoses and treatable diseases by image-based deep learning. *Cell. National Library of Medicine*. 22; vol. 172, issue 5, pp. 1122–1131.e9. doi:10.1016/j.cell.2018.02.010. PMID: 29474911.

[70] Alapat, D.J., Menon, M.V., and Ashok, S. (2022). A review on detection of pneumonia in chest X-ray images using neural networks. *Journal of*

Biomedical Physics Engineering. vol. 12, issue 6, pp. 551–558. doi:10.31661/jbpe.v0i0.2202-1461.

[71] Hwang, E.J., Park, S., Jin, K.N., *et al.* (2019). Development and validation of a deep learning–based automated detection algorithm for major thoracic diseases on chest radiographs. *JAMA Network Open*, vol. 2, issue 3, pp. e191095–e191095.

[72] Esteva, A., Kuprel, B., Novoa, R. A., *et al.* (2017). Dermatologist-level classification of skin cancer with deep neural networks. *Nature*, vol. 542, issue 7639, pp. 115–118.

[73] Rajpurkar, P., Hannun, A.Y., Haghpanahi, M., Bourn, C., and Ng, A.Y. (2017). Cardiologist-level arrhythmia detection with convolutional neural networks. arXiv preprint arXiv:1707.01836.

[74] Lee, J.E., Jeon, H.J., Lee, O.J., and Lim, H.G. (2024). Diagnosis of diabetes mellitus using high frequency ultrasound and convolutional neural network. *Ultrasonics*, vol. 136, p. 107167.

[75] Al-Shammari, N.K., Alshammari, A.S., Albadarn, S.M., *et al.* (2021). Development of soft actuators for stroke rehabilitation using deep learning. *International Journal of Advanced and Applied Sciences*, vol. 8, issue 11, pp. 22–29.

[76] Ajagbe, S.A., and Adigun, M.O. (2024). Deep learning techniques for detection and prediction of pandemic diseases: a systematic literature review. *Multimedia Tools and Applications*, vol. 83, issue 2, pp. 5893–5927.

[77] Potluri, S., Fasih, A., Vutukuru, L.K., Al Machot, F., and Kyamakya, K. (2011). CNN based high performance computing for real time image processing on GPU. In *Proceedings of the Joint INDS'11 and ISTET'11*, IEEE. pp. 1–7.

[78] Sasi Kumar, A., and Aithal, P.S. (2023). DeepQ residue analysis of brain computer classification and prediction using deep CNN. *International Journal of Applied Engineering and Management Letters (IJAEML)*, vol. 7, issue 2, pp. 144–163.

[79] Pan, Y., Fu, M., Cheng, B., Tao, X., and Guo, J. (2020). Enhanced deep learning assisted convolutional neural network for heart disease prediction on the internet of medical things platform. *IEEE Access*, vol. 8, p. 189503–189512.

[80] Thandapani, S., Mahaboob, M.I., Iwendi, C., *et al.* (2023). IoMT with deep CNN: AI-based intelligent support system for pandemic diseases. *Electronics*, vol. 12, issue 2, p. 424.

[81] Fezza, S.A., Bakhti, Y., Hamidouche, W., and Déforges, O. (2019). Perceptual evaluation of adversarial attacks for CNN-based image classification. In *2019 Eleventh International Conference on Quality of Multimedia Experience (QoMEX)*, IEEE. pp. 1–6.

[82] Anand, A., Rani, S., Anand, D., Aljahdali, H.M., and Kerr, D. (2021). An efficient CNN-based deep learning model to detect malware attacks (CNN-DMA) in 5G-IoT healthcare applications. *Sensors*, vol. 21, issue 19, p. 6346.

[83] Aminizadeh, S., Heidari, A., Dehghan, M., *et al.* (2024). Opportunities and challenges of artificial intelligence and distributed systems to improve the

quality of healthcare service. *Artificial Intelligence in Medicine*, vol. 149, p. 102779.

[84] Kaushal, C., Islam, M.K., Singla, A., and Al Amin, M. (2022). An IoMT-based smart remote monitoring system for healthcare. In *IoT-Enabled Smart Healthcare Systems, Services and Applications*. Hoboken, NJ: John Wiley & Sons, Inc., pp. 177–198.

[85] Sethuraman, S.C., Kompally, P., Mohanty, S.P., and Choppali, U. (2020). MyWear: A smart wear for continuous body vital monitoring and emergency alert. arXiv preprint arXiv:2010.08866.

[86] Adeniyi, E.A., Falola, P.B., Maashi, M.S., Aljebreen, M., and Bharany, S. (2022). Secure sensitive data sharing using RSA and ElGamal cryptographic algorithms with hash functions. *Information*, vol. 13, issue 10, p. 442.

[87] Hasan, M.K., Ghazal, T.M., Saeed, R.A., *et al.* (2022). A review on security threats, vulnerabilities, and counter measures of 5G enabled Internet-of-Medical-Things. *IET Communications*, vol. 16, issue 5, pp. 421–432.

[88] Bouchama, F., and Kamal, M. (2021). Enhancing cyber threat detection through machine learning-based behavioral modeling of network traffic patterns. *International Journal of Business Intelligence and Big Data Analytics*, vol. 4, issue 9, pp. 1–9.

[89] Sun, L., Jiang, X., Ren, H., and Guo, Y. (2020). Edge-cloud computing and artificial intelligence in internet of medical things: architecture, technology and application. *IEEE Access*, vol. 8, pp. 101079–101092.

[90] Puckett, S.C. (2023). *Design of secure, low-power Internet of Medical Things with precise time synchronization* (Doctoral dissertation, The University of Alabama in Huntsville).

[91] Janssen, M., Brous, P., Estevez, E., Barbosa, L.S., and Janowski, T. (2020). Data governance: Organizing data for trustworthy Artificial Intelligence. *Government Information Quarterly*, vol. 37, issue 3, p. 101493.

[92] Awotunde, J.B., Chakraborty, C., and Adeniyi, A.E. (2021). Intrusion detection in industrial internet of things network-based on deep learning model with rule-based feature selection. *Wireless Communications and Mobile Computing*, vol. 2021, pp. 1–17.

[93] Fezza, S.A., Bakhti, Y., Hamidouche, W., and Déforges, O. (2019). Perceptual evaluation of adversarial attacks for CNN-based image classification. In *2019 Eleventh International Conference on Quality of Multimedia Experience (QoMEX)*, IEEE. pp. 1–6.

[94] Liu, Y., Zhao, Z., Chang, F., and Hu, S. (2020). An anchor-free convolutional neural network for real-time surgical tool detection in robot-assisted surgery. *IEEE Access*, vol. 8, pp. 78193–78201.

[95] Razdan, S., and Sharma S. (2022) Internet of medical things (IoMT): Overview, emerging technologies, and case studies. *IETE Technical Review*, vol. 39, issue 4, pp. 775–788, DOI:10.1080/02564602.2021.1927863

Chapter 6

Deadly cybersecurity threats in emerging healthcare systems

Promise Elechi[1], Kingsley Eyiogwu Onu[1] and Nne Rena Saturday[2]

The convergence of digital technology and healthcare has ushered in unprecedented opportunities for improved patient care and operational efficiency. However, this transformation also exposes the healthcare system to a myriad of deadly cybersecurity threats, jeopardizing patient privacy, data integrity, and overall system resilience. This chapter investigates the landscape of emerging cyber threats within the healthcare sector and presents innovative solutions to mitigate these risks. Central to our findings is the proposal for the creation of a secure data-sharing platform tailored specifically for healthcare providers. This platform not only facilitates seamless information exchange but also integrates robust security measures to safeguard against cyber-attacks. By addressing this critical research gap, our report aims to bolster the cyber security posture of the emerging healthcare system, ensuring the continuity of care and the protection of sensitive patient information in an increasingly digitized world. This will benefit not only the patient but also healthcare providers.

Keywords: Cybersecurity; healthcare system; emerging threats; risk mitigation; patience privacy; data sharing platform

6.1 Introduction

The application of technology is seen in every area of human endeavor, including the area of healthcare, thereby transforming medical practices in their entirety. The effectiveness of surgical operations and the quality of life of patients have been improved because of the application of digital technology, as was stated in [1]. The use of artificial intelligence (AI), Internet of Things (IoTs), machine learning (ML),

[1]Department of Electrical and Electronics Engineering, Faculty of Engineering, Rivers State University, Nigeria
[2]Department of Computer Science, Faculty of Science, Rivers State University, Nigeria

etc. in healthcare has drastically changed so many things in healthcare delivery, especially in the aspect of robotic surgery. In [2], it was mentioned that the health status of patients can be monitored in real-time using digital technologies and devices without any need for physical visitation by the physician, resulting in significant recovery rates of patients as compared to what is obtainable when these technologies are not in use.

The work [3] mentioned that the adoption of digital technology in healthcare has introduced many issues that must be addressed. One such issue is cybersecurity, the threats of which are costly to address. Three key vulnerable areas in healthcare cybersecurity are deficiencies associated with user authentication, extreme user permissions, and leakage in the endpoint. Besides these mentioned challenges or issues, the arrival of a new technology known as the Internet of Medical Things, IoMT for short, brought its issues because of the threats that IoMT-Compatible devices pose when it comes to compromising data privacy and security. Therefore, the task of maintaining a patient's data privacy and security while still using these devices remains a major concern for experts in the field.

6.1.1 Contributions of the chapter

This report makes a significant contribution to the understanding and mitigation of deadly cybersecurity threats within the emerging healthcare system:

- By proposing the creation of a secure data-sharing platform for healthcare providers.
- By addressing this critical research gap, we aim to establish a robust infrastructure that not only enhances the efficiency of data exchange among healthcare entities but also fortifies defenses against cyber threats.
- Through innovative design principles and rigorous security protocols, this platform offers a proactive approach to safeguarding patient confidentiality, data integrity, and system functionality in an increasingly digitized healthcare landscape.
- This contribution represents a pivotal step toward ensuring the resilience and sustainability of healthcare systems amidst the escalating cyber threat landscape.

6.1.2 Chapter organization

The research report on deadly cybersecurity threats in emerging healthcare systems is structured to provide a comprehensive analysis of the topic. Section 6.2 focuses on a review of deadly security threats in healthcare, laying the foundation for understanding the subsequent discussions. Section 6.3 delves into cybersecurity, offering an overview and principles, and discusses the CIA triad. In Section 6.4, the report explores the growing threats of cybercrime and their associated costs, shedding light on the evolving landscape of cybersecurity challenges. Legal and regulatory issues pertinent to healthcare cybersecurity are examined in Section 6.6, while Section 6.7 addresses information management issues within healthcare systems. Section 6.8 discusses healthcare cyber risk management strategies, providing insights into proactive measures to mitigate threats. The report then proposes the creation of a secure data-sharing platform for healthcare providers in Section 6.9, offering a practical solution to enhance data security. Finally, the report concludes in Section 6.10, summarizing key findings and implications drawn from the analysis conducted throughout the report.

6.2 Review of deadly security threats in healthcare systems

As healthcare systems evolve, digital technology plays an increasingly integral role in revolutionizing patient care, medical procedures, and data management. In this section, we delve into the dynamic landscape of digital technology within healthcare, exploring its advancements, applications, and the transformative impact it has on patient outcomes and system efficiency.

In an era where digital technology intersects with the complexities of healthcare, the landscape of security threats has evolved into a formidable challenge for industry. From ransomware attacks crippling hospital operations to data breaches compromising patient confidentiality, the healthcare sector faces a myriad of deadly threats [4]. This review aims to dissect and analyze the multifaceted nature of these threats, shedding light on their impacts and the urgent need for robust security measures to safeguard patient welfare.

The authors in [5] highlighted the benefits that healthcare providers such as doctors get because of the application of AI in robotic surgery. In this, doctors are helped to provide individualized therapy to the sick, prevent certain kinds of illnesses significantly, and even eliminate some repetitive activities associated with healthcare delivery. Therefore, the application of digital technology, in this case, the use of AI in surgery, has taken healthcare to a level never seen by humans. The application of digital technology in healthcare is often regarded as e-health.

In [6], the authors showed clear evidence of the efficiency and the positive impact of using digital technology in healthcare (e-health) when handling cases of individuals with either type 1 diabetes or type 2 diabetes. For those who suffer from type 1 or type 2 diabetes, supporting their well-being both emotionally and physically using digital technology was compared with other interventions based on psychosocial support and glycemic control interventions, and it was clear that digital technological interventions performed well.

During the COVID-19 pandemic, the importance and usefulness of the application of digital technology came to the fore. Hence, it was demonstrated in [7] that several applications of digital technology are beneficial for digital health, especially during the peak of the pandemic and beyond. A reasonable distance apart was being maintained by individuals, including doctors and patients as far as possible. Electronic healthcare delivery has been embraced in recent times because of its many advantages and efficiency.

The work [8] proposed a methodology that can be used to tackle the ever-increasing cyber threats in the healthcare sector. The proposed methodology is termed cyber hygiene (CH), and it was used to identify appropriate strategies for cybersecurity management. The methodology was applied to the healthcare sector, and the results revealed that strategies to manage possible risks were identified. However, threats in the healthcare sector are many but were not identified and solutions proffered.

The authors in [9] carried out research to identify potential threats to public health and devised control strategies. The authors developed a strategy that diminishes the threat to public health. However, the threats discussed were different from cyber threats.

As was pointed out by [10], patients' medical records maintained digitally can help improve the efficiency of healthcare services. This is so because it is possible to exchange patients' digital medical or health records between the patients and their doctors using blockchain technology. Because the exchange of these digital health records is done electronically, the distance between the doctors and the patients is never a problem, and the transmission and reception of these digital health records can be achieved within the shortest possible time.

While the benefits of the application of digital technology to healthcare cannot be overemphasized, some experts are concerned about the negative effects of such applications. For example, [11] contended that the application of AI to healthcare brings a whole lot of legal issues, not only for the developers of the technology but also for the doctors or healthcare providers as well. This is especially so if it is impossible to define the suggestions generated by AI [12–14].

ML approaches have also been applied in healthcare. In ML, we have at least supervised, unsupervised, and semi-supervised learning techniques, all of which have found application in healthcare management systems [15–30]. The supervised ML technique has been used in the healthcare management system for the categorization of different kinds of diseases and the identification of different parts of the body from photographic pictures [31,32]. While supervised ML techniques have been used to achieve much in healthcare management, [33–39] have all looked at unsupervised ML techniques in different areas of the healthcare system such as identification of anomalies, hepatitis disease prediction, etc.

Semi-supervised learning is used in healthcare management systems to gather data. When the quantity of labeled data is small, and the quantity of unlabeled data is rather big, semi-supervised learning can be used with good results. It is because of this that the authors in [40–43] differently looked at the application of a semi-supervised ML approach in healthcare management systems for gathering data, detection of activity, and segmentation of medical images.

The work [44] proposed the use of a portable and less-expensive device called galvanic skin response in the healthcare system. The device captures galvanic skin response data, processes it, and amplifies it. It also evaluates a patient's degree of behavior and sends it to the patient's device after analysis. In the works of [45,46] a system based on wearable sensors that can use changes in the temperature of the body and heart rate to detect health-related ailments was proposed and analyzed. The work of [47] suggested that to detect long-term ECG signals cost-effectively, compact wearable gadgets should be used. In the work [48], pregnant women's maternal health diagnosis was carried out using a robust decision-making technique that was designed by the authors. The women wore wristbands, and it proved that pregnant women's maternal health state can be effectively monitored. The author [49] used a ML approach to develop a smart healthcare management system for medical analysis in real-time. The works of [50–55] looked at the application of the IoTs in healthcare management systems to improve healthcare delivery and promote efficiency using different approaches.

Securing digital assets and data within the healthcare sector is integral, aiming to prevent unauthorized access, usage, and disclosure. The overarching objectives of cybersecurity are to uphold the confidentiality, integrity, and availability of information, commonly referred to as the "CIA triad" [56]. Figure 6.1 shows cybersecurity capabilities in a hospital with feedback loops which makes sure that efficient security measures are guaranteed. We have the cybersecurity level at the hospital to cybersecurity gaps, efforts to fill out the gaps, etc.

Contending on the negative effects of applying digital technology, the authors [8] and [57] noted that the privacy of patients can be compromised because of digital healthcare record integration. Hence, while praising the benefits of digital healthcare record integration, the authors also contended that motives of individuals based mainly on feelings of violation, or some requirements of external

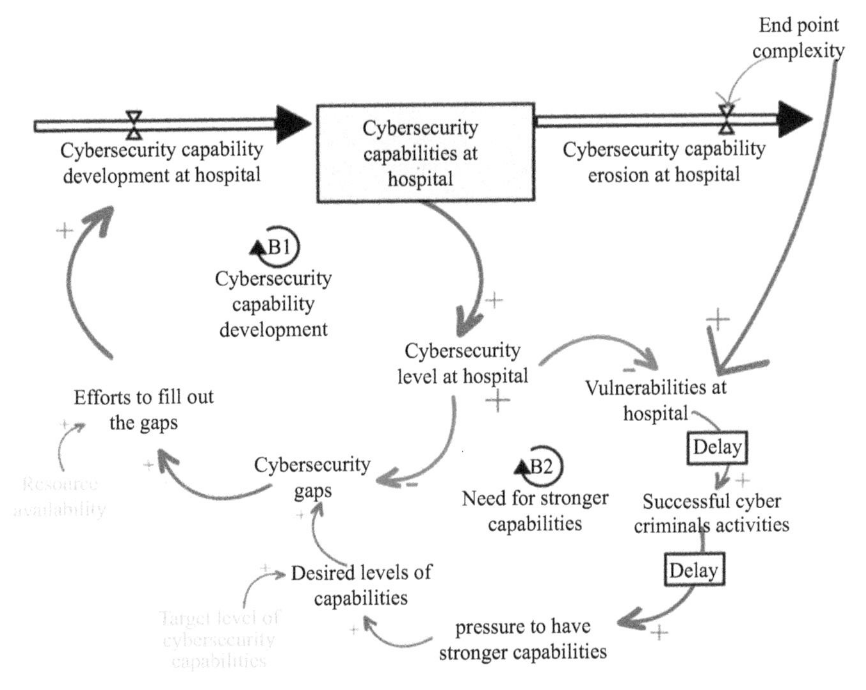

Figure 6.1 Cybersecurity capabilities in a hospital with feedback loops to ensure efficient security

nature can influence the adoption of digital technology in healthcare even though internal incentives are much more pronounced.

As some experts suggest using blockchain technology to address the issues associated with the application of digital technology in healthcare, the work of [58] noted that there are serious concerns that question the use of blockchain in addressing the obvious challenges of the application of digital technology in healthcare, besides the fact that blockchain technology is a rather new technology, being in its infancy stage.

The IoTs is another technology that has been applied to healthcare management systems. IoTs technology has at least four layers such as (1) the Sensing Layer, (2) the Communication Layer, (3) Network Storage Layer, and finally (4) the Application Layer. The layer closest to patients is the sensing layer while the application layer is closest to the medical expert. As the name suggests, the sensing layer is used for sensing data from patients as it monitors patients regularly. Patients may be asked to wear it as a wristwatch [59]. The works of [60] and [61] made use of smartphones to get useful information from a person. The sensing layer comprises such things as temperature and pressure sensors, ECG, smart wristbands, etc. Information or data gathered by the sensing layer is sent to communication before being stored in the network storage layer, to be assessed by doctors.

Blockchain technology has found application in the healthcare industry, even at its early stage. The authors in [62–64] highlighted the many benefits of applying blockchain to businesses, including the healthcare management system. The benefits, it was mentioned, include good and timely communication between patients and healthcare providers like doctors, nurses, etc. In [65–69], the authors think that blockchain technology, together with the IoTs, can be applied in healthcare to monitor patients' health status and make the logistics of healthcare very accessible. The works of [70–72] emphasized that the application of blockchain to healthcare can minimize the cost of healthcare services since it eliminates the need for third party applications as healthcare providers would have ready access to the medical records of patients.

A summary of key literature reviewed and our contributions is presented in Table 6.1.

Table 6.1 Summary of key literature reviewed

S. No.	Past work	Pros	Cons	Contribution to the current work
1	Khan *et al.* [4]	Identified cybersecurity threats that occurred very much during COVID-19	No solutions to the identified threats were outlined	Proffered a solution to the deadly cybersecurity threats in the emerging healthcare system: the creation of a secure data-sharing platform for healthcare providers

(Continues)

Table 6.1 Summary of key literature reviewed (Continued)

S. No.	Past work	Pros	Cons	Contribution to the current work
2	Alka [5]	Discussed how healthcare providers have succeeded in applying AI in healthcare delivery	The work did not identify specific cybersecurity threats and their solutions	In addition to other security measures, this work showed how a secure data-sharing platform for healthcare providers can be achieved
3	Ren *et al.* [73]	Identified mechanisms that detect and prevent ransomware	Only focused on ransomware	Proffered a solution to the deadly cybersecurity threats in the emerging healthcare system: the creation of a secure data-sharing platform for healthcare providers
4	Aygyridou *et al.* [74]	Developed a roster of human-centered controls and implementation tiers, employing cyber hygiene practices to bolster staff conduct within the healthcare industry	Did not provide detailed cybersecurity threats affecting healthcare providers	Proposed a secure data-sharing platform for healthcare providers
5	Zhang *et al.* [75]	Developed a strategy to diminish the threat to public health	The threats discussed were not related to cyber threats	This work showed how a secure data-sharing platform for healthcare providers can be achieved
6	Abdulraheem *et al.* [72]	Application of AI of medical things (AIoMT) to increase the reliability and effectiveness of healthcare	Emphasis was based only on the application of AI	The study explored several methods used for securing IoT devices and ensuring the privacy of data to address the security concerns preventing the use of AIoMT to safeguard patient information
7	Awotunde *et al.* [76]	Application of AI of medical things (AIoMT) in remote monitoring system	The threats discussed were not related to cyber threats	The study explored the use of AIoMT in real-time monitoring and diagnosis of certain chronic ailments

(Continues)

Table 6.1 Summary of key literature reviewed (Continued)

S. No.	Past work	Pros	Cons	Contribution to the current work
8	Rufai *et al.* [77]	The work explored the cyberattacks on AI of medical things (AIoMT). Various malware attacks were presented and various security measures to address the malware were proposed	Most of the deadly cyberattacks were not discussed	The study looked at the different forms of malicious software assaults alongside different security strategies aimed at countering them. Additionally, a novel conceptual framework integrating artificial intelligence and software-defined networking (SDN) is suggested, offering comprehensive protection against assorted threats to the artificial intelligence-enabled Internet of Medical Things (AIoMT) infrastructure
9	Sei *et al.* [78]	The work developed a model of ML such as decision trees using LDP data to generate synthetic data that can remove the effects of noise of LDP	Emphasis was based only on data analysis using ML	The study utilized simulations with both authentic and synthesized data to validate the efficacy of the suggested algorithm across decision trees, deep neural networks, and k-nearest neighbors

6.3 Cybersecurity in healthcare systems

In an era where healthcare systems are rapidly digitizing, the critical importance of cybersecurity cannot be overstated. As advancements in technology pave the way for more efficient and interconnected healthcare processes, they also open the door to unprecedented cyber threats. In this section, we delve into the complex realm of cybersecurity within emerging healthcare systems, examining the potent risks they face and the proactive measures essential for safeguarding patient data, medical infrastructure, and ultimately, human lives.

In modern society, cybersecurity has become a key issue in almost every organization or company's infrastructure because it can mean the growth or failure of such companies or organizations. When an organization repeatedly fails to protect customer and private data against any possible competitors, it can affect the growth of the organization. Hence, one of the foremost things an organization does is to provide adequate protection of relevant data [79]. Due to the increasing number of threats to networks, information, or data, practical steps are taken by professionals in cybersecurity to guarantee the protection of such networks or data, thereby preventing unauthorized persons or organizations from tampering with the networks, data, or information [10] and [80].

There are different types of cybersecurity. To provide a reasonable degree of protection of networks or data, understanding the various types of cybersecurity is important. Types of cybersecurity include the following security:

(a) Network
(b) Application
(c) Infrastructure
(d) User Training
(e) Cloud
(f) Information
(g) Data

These different types of cybersecurity are illustrated in Figure 6.2.

Figure 6.2 shows the different types of cybersecurity, which includes data, user training, information, application, network, infrastructure, and cloud.

As was said in [79–82], computer networks need to be protected from disruptive things like hacking, malware, etc. This protection of computer networks is provided by network security, which refers to things that are carefully done by professionals to prevent hackers and other threats from reaching computer networks.

Application security is intended to protect system applications. Such protection is made possible using software and hardware. Software that provides application security includes antivirus programs, firewalls, etc. Threats that affect system applications for which protection is needed are often external [12] and [73].

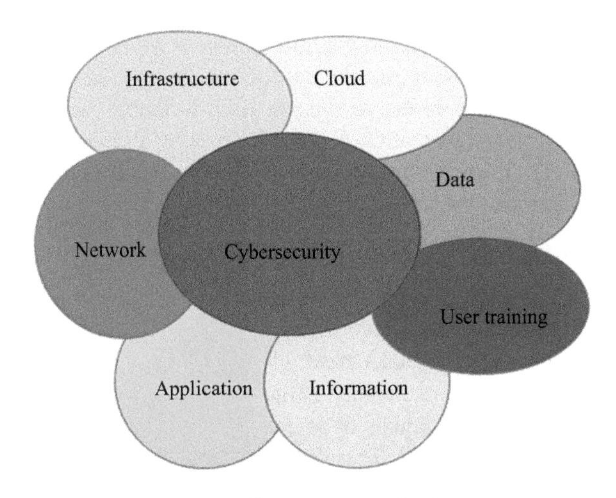

Figure 6.2 Different types of cybersecurity

The work [75] recommended the training of users to be able to identify and remove any suspicious email attachments, avoid making any connections to anonymous USBs, and so forth. This step helps in providing the security that is needed because lacking adequate training in this regard could mean introducing a virus into an organization's security system unknowingly. The work of [74] also noted that cloud security protects the information while monitoring the system to get rid of any on-site threats. As was shown in [83] and [76], information security is used to give protection to digital and physical data against intruders, deletion of data or information, data misuse or disclosure, etc.

6.3.1 Overview of cybersecurity and principles

The term cybersecurity refers to techniques adopted by individuals, companies, organizations, etc. to prevent any attacks on their cyber environment. These techniques help to safeguard confidentiality and integrity and ensure the availability of data or information, keeping them away from unauthorized individuals. Due to the ever-increasing reliance on computer networks and computer systems and the IoTs, the field of cybersecurity has become ever more important. It is important to mention that the need for cybersecurity arises due to various cyber threats. The most common among these threats are:

(a) Cyberwarfare: This is often used by some nations trying to use modern technology to steal information from another nation or cause severe damage to the nation's operations. Nations that get involved in this act have well-trained individuals who execute this cyberwarfare on behalf of the nation, and they are provided with every enabling environment to carry out their cyberwarfare [62] and [77]. If hackers penetrate a nation's cyberspace, they steal valuable information, degrade, or disrupt the nation's communication system, and may even affect medical services.
(b) Cyberterrorism: As was mentioned in [18], cyberterrorists make use of technology to advance their terrorist agenda by attacking networks, telecommunication infrastructure, and computer systems of their target. When telecommunication infrastructure is attacked by cyber terrorists, during their operations, it will be difficult for security agencies to get information as quickly as possible and arrest the situation. This tends to give the cyberterrorists a big advantage.
(c) Cyberespionage: This refers to the use of Information and Communication Technology to get information or data from people or organizations without any permission. It can be used to gain advantages such as military, economic, and strategic advantages.

6.3.2 The CIA triad

In protecting any company or organization against cybercrime, the key lies with the three first steps that many experts have advocated for a very long time, called the CIA triad or security triangle. In the CIA triad, C represents confidentiality; I represents integrity; and A represents availability (Figure 6.3). The confidentiality principle focuses on allowing only individuals or sources that are authorized to gain access to sensitive data or information [15]. Therefore, when information or data is said to be confidential, such data is still intact, not leaked or accessed by others who are not

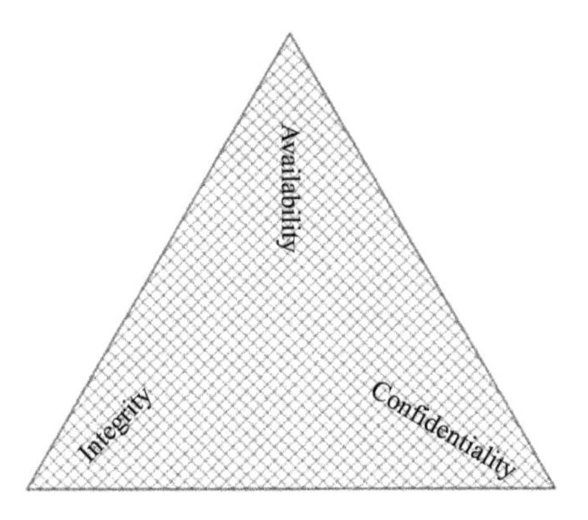

Figure 6.3 The CIA triad (security triangle)

authorized to have it. However, there have been some reported cases of confidentiality breaches in some quarters. This breach often comes through hacking or other means. Therefore, organizations must ensure no confidentiality breach occurs at all.

The integrity of data is not interested in the number of attacks made to steal data but in the fact that the data is intact, untouched, unmodified, and unassessed by the wrong persons or groups. The integrity of data could be compromised during data upload or data storage on the database. Availability refers to the situation whereby the information or data is readily available to every authorized person. As [78] mentioned, the availability of data, functions, and systems to authorized persons must be on-demand and based on acceptable parameters. To demonstrate a high level of availability, a system must have communication channels, security controls, etc. always functioning properly. Whatever system is in use must ensure resilience against any attacks to undermine it, and must be safeguarded against failures of hardware, power, and so forth that can affect the availability of the system.

6.3.3 Application of cybersecurity in healthcare systems

Applying cybersecurity in healthcare simply means using technology to prevent unauthorized persons from assessing and using the electronic data of a patient for whatever purpose [25]. Since the world has gone digital, hospitals or any healthcare organization cannot function effectively without going digital. Interestingly, many of these hospitals and healthcare organizations have already gone digital. Some have systems for the electronic prescription of drugs called e-prescription systems, radiology information systems (RIS), clinical decision support systems (CDSS), etc.

The work [17] suggested that the issue of cybersecurity should not be left in the hands of IT personnel only but should be seen as involving the patients, enterprise risk, etc., and ensure that this is integrated into existing hospital's governance, enterprise, business, and risk management. Speaking on the reasons why the healthcare sector experiences greater attacks, [17] said that the reasons lie in the possession of high-monetary information by healthcare organizations. Therefore, cybercriminals see healthcare organizations as fertile ground for their cybercrimes. The authors listed some key target areas by these cyber criminals to include, but not limited to:

(a) Financial Information (Account numbers and credit card information)
(b) Personally-Identifying Information (PII)
(c) Patients Healthcare Information (PHI)

As a way of addressing cybercrimes in the healthcare sector, especially in the use of IoT-based devices, a protocol that combines both authentical and main negotiation to ensure that privacy is protected has been introduced. To protect user anonymity, the protocol has biometrics features and includes decryption and encryption, which are asymmetrically done for more advanced security. This is termed a mutual authentication solution to the problems that are frequently faced by the healthcare sector [15].

The following security measures have been applied in healthcare to avert growing threats in the sector:

(a) Use of RFID security authentication
(b) Use of lightweight authentication
(c) Use of authentication and key agreement
(d) Use of homographic encryption method

The application of technology in healthcare, as pointed out in [2] and [79], saw a significant improvement in the health status of patients. Such applications have also made it possible for the health status of individuals to be monitored in real-time using digital technologies and devices without any need for physical visitation by the concerned doctors, resulting in significant recovery rates of patients as compared to what is obtainable when these technologies are not in use.

6.4 Growing threat of cybercrime

As emerging healthcare systems increasingly rely on digital technologies to enhance patient care and streamline operations, they become increasingly vulnerable to the insidious threat of cybercrime. In this section, we delve into the escalating menace posed by cybercriminals targeting healthcare infrastructure, data, and services. By examining the evolving tactics and motivations driving cybercrime in the healthcare sector, we shed light on the urgent need for robust cybersecurity measures to protect against devastating breaches that endanger patient safety and compromise the integrity of healthcare systems.

Cyberattacks on healthcare institutions have taken place in many countries, including developed and developing countries alike. A report conducted by Ponemon Institute back in 2014 was able to recognize about five hundred thousand (500,000) affected by identity theft in the health sector, a figure that only rose in the following year (2015) to 22%.

It was reported in [23] that within just two years, the number of individual cybercriminals who stole information found in electronic health records (EHRs) increased significantly in the United States, forcing some organizations like Turbo Tax to suspend tax fillings temporarily, to pave the way for proper investigation into the growing number of cybercriminals and cases of fraud.

6.4.1 Annual cost of cybercrime in the healthcare sector

The monetary cost of cybercrime globally is mind-boggling. If cybercrime were to be a country of its own, the authors in [19] argued that it would have been the third largest economy in the world after the United States of America and China. It was estimated that by the end of 2021, cybercrime would have inflicted total damage of about 6 trillion US dollars globally. Cybersecurity ventures expected that the costs of cybercrime globally would see yearly growth of 15% for the next five years (2021–2025), getting up to $10.5 trillion in 2025 as against $3 trillion US dollars in 2015. As mentioned in the reports presented in [19] and [62], the costs of cybercrime include money stolen, data destruction and damage, personal theft, intellectual property theft, fraud, financial data theft, embezzlement, hacked data restoration, etc.

Costs in healthcare breaches because of cybercrime are broadly divided into two groups: indirect costs and direct costs. Communication and in-house investigations are all part of indirect costs. Direct costs, however, include the hiring of forensic experts, hotline support outsourcing, provision of subscription for credit monitoring free of charge, etc. According to [20], in the United States alone, the cost for both direct and indirect breaches was more than $7 million US dollars.

The healthcare sector has proved to be a very fertile ground for hackers and cybercriminals. The reasons are obvious: Compared to other sectors, the healthcare sector lacks adequate investment in security, has a very large amount of system connectivity, has high data value, etc. Therefore, in [21] it was found that the cost of just one healthcare record stolen rose from $136 US dollars to $380 US dollars between 2015 and 2017. It was said that in the United States, in 2018, the cost of a stolen healthcare record because of a data breach was $408 US dollars for a single record, making the sector of healthcare the most expensive [22]. Figure 6.4 shows the comparison of the cost of data breaches in US dollars in different sectors.

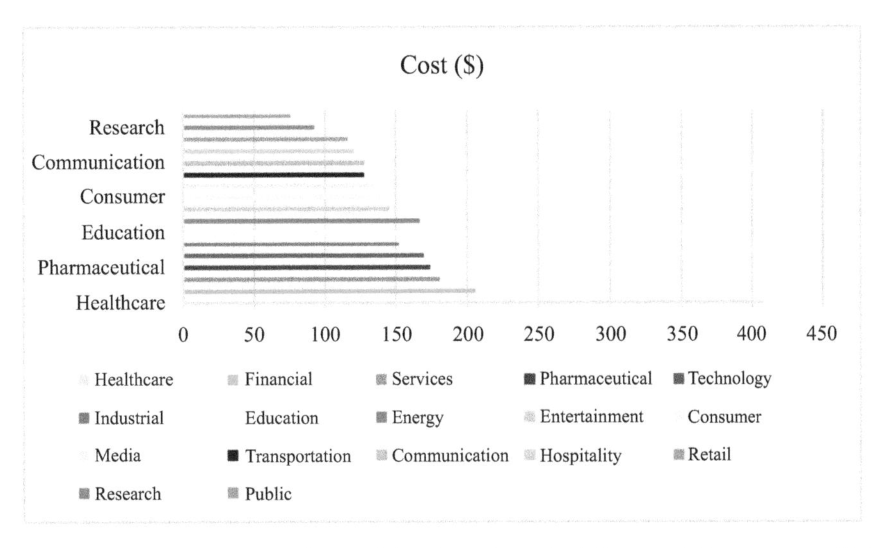

Figure 6.4 A comparison of cost of data breach in US dollars in different sectors [21]

6.5 Emerging threats and countermeasures in healthcare systems

As healthcare systems evolve amidst rapid technological advancements, so too do the threats they face in the digital realm. In this section, we delve into the dynamic landscape of emerging cyber threats targeting healthcare systems, ranging from sophisticated ransomware attacks to stealthy data breaches. Concurrently, we explore the proactive countermeasures and innovative strategies being employed to fortify healthcare cybersecurity defenses and mitigate the risks posed by these evolving threats. By navigating this intricate terrain, we strive to equip healthcare stakeholders with the knowledge and tools necessary to confront and neutralize emerging cyber threats, ensuring the resilience and integrity of healthcare systems in the face of adversity.

Five different threats in healthcare systems and their possible countermeasures will be discussed here. The threats include, but are not limited to:

(a) Ransomware attacks
(b) Insider attacks
(c) Phishing scams
(d) Hacking of medical devices
(e) Unprotected (unsecured) IoTs

6.5.1 Ransomware attacks

Put simply, ransomware attacks are malware capable of encrypting data as well as requesting payment to release the decryption key. The attackers gain full control of their targets' assets and request that the stolen data be returned if a ransom is paid [57], and it is one of the most dangerous malware variants [24] and [25]. When the system is attacked, criminals in cyberspace therefore hinder authorized medical personnel from gaining access to a patient's records, including any possible treatment plans contained in those records. The safety of the patients is highly jeopardized due to the activities of cybercriminals [62] and [80], as vital information relating to the patients is seized for ransom by the criminals.

6.5.1.1 Ransomware attacks countermeasures

To counter the growing threats of ransomware attacks in healthcare management systems globally, implementation of what we may call plans for backup and disaster recovery should be carried out. With these plans, a patient's data can be safely backed up. In the event of any ransomware attacks, a patient's data or information can be recovered and restored when the threats are removed.

6.5.2 Insider attacks

Many organizations may have saboteurs who may want to take advantage of the organization if they can do so. This is also true in the healthcare sector. Therefore, a situation where an insider in a company or an organization possesses a piece of confidential information under his position in the organization and uses the information for personal gains against the rules of the organization is called an insider attack. Nowadays, this attack is very common. This explains the reason why many organizations have what they call "authorized users" access to sensitive resources of the organization.

6.5.2.1 Insider attacks countermeasure

One measure that can be used to counter insider attacks in healthcare systems has to do with training and re-training of employees. Such training should be tailored toward exposing them to the consequences of indulging in any kind of crime, including using or revealing confidential data to unauthorized persons. The training should also emphasize that inaction on the part of an employee that leads to an attack on patients' data will be treated as a case of insider attack with full consequences meted out against the affected individual.

6.5.3 Phishing scams

This threat happens as criminals in cyberspace try to obtain systems' login credentials. If they succeed in obtaining these credentials, automatically they can have access to whatever confidential records are available. The attackers also focus on getting access to such private information as patients' data, financial records, etc.

6.5.3.1 Phishing scam countermeasures

Much like the insider attacks, training and re-training of staff can go a long way in mitigating this threat. Staff should constantly be trained on how to mitigate phishing attacks. When there is a new phishing attack technique used by cybercriminals, staff should be alerted, and using regular training, they should be intimated on how to counter the attacks. The benefits of constant training can never be overemphasized.

6.5.4 Hacking of medical devices

In the case of attacking medical devices, the attackers or cybercriminals simply intend to cause the device to do what it was not intended to do, such as:

(a) Change a patient's data.
(b) Carry out wrong tasks.
(c) Change the frequency of doses.
(d) Alter a prescription dose.

Hacking of medical devices is a very serious issue as this could lead to harm or death of patients. Medical devices are often designed in such a way that any software or hardware modifications would require proper readjustments. If readjustments are not carried out or are carried out improperly, patients can be adversely affected.

6.5.4.1 Hacking of medical device countermeasure

The increasing connection of many devices to the healthcare facility networks makes hacking of medical devices to be on the increase, and the hackers often demand ransom [63]. This attack can be countered by the following measures:

(a) Regularly updating firmware.
(b) Regularly monitoring network traffic to identify any suspicious activity.
(c) Strongly encourage the use of stronger passwords. The longer the password, the harder it is to guess by cybercriminals.
(d) Quickly change passwords if it is sensed that the password may have been compromised, especially when there is a change in certain healthcare facility personnel.
(e) Avoid using the same password for different accounts.
(f) Use passphrases. Passphrases are very long passwords that comprise words that are not related.
(g) Any client device used, like VoIP, that is voice-over-internet protocol, should be given unique passwords and usernames.

6.5.5 Unprotected (unsecured) Internet of Things (IoTs)

While IoTs devices are becoming much more popular, not all of them follow strict safety protocols. This situation makes the IoTs devices to be quite vulnerable to attacks, especially when there is no segmentation of their Virtual Local Area Network (VLAN). Some of these IoTs devices include, but are not limited to:

(a) Biometric readers
(b) Cameras for security purposes
(c) Smart medical equipment
(d) Smart thermostats

6.5.5.1 Unprotected Internet of Things attack countermeasures

To counter the growing threats in the healthcare system against IoTs devices, it is proper for the following to be seriously considered:

(a) Up-to-date firmware should be used on the device.
(b) Regular security assessments should be carried out.
(c) Only authorized personnel should be allowed access to the medical devices.
(d) Quickly sanction any personnel that tries to compromise the system.

6.6 Legal and regulatory issues

In the landscape of cybersecurity within the emerging healthcare system, navigating the intricate web of legal and regulatory frameworks is paramount. This section delves into the multifaceted legal and regulatory landscape that governs the management, protection, and exchange of healthcare data. By exploring the existing laws, regulations, and compliance requirements, we aim to shed light on the complexities and challenges faced by healthcare organizations in safeguarding patient information and mitigating cyber threats.

Cybersecurity in healthcare management is dynamic. Hence, there is a need for concerned individuals and organizations to adhere to the web of rules designed to protect healthcare systems against cybercrimes. Breaking the rules attracts a penalty. Therefore, more than focusing on giving quality healthcare, organizations should invest in providing needed expertise in cybersecurity. In this way, patients will be kept safe, and no fear of the penalty of breaking cybersecurity rules will be entertained.

While legal and regulatory issues differ from country to country, here we will focus on the regulations provided in the United States. Six of these regulations will be discussed in this work.

6.6.1 Laws and regulations

Some of the laws and regulations governing the health information and safety of citizens in the world are:

- Health Insurance Portability and Accountability Act (HIPAA)
- HHS 405(d) Regulation
- Payment Card Industry Data Security Standard PIC DSS Regulation
- Health Information Technology for Economic and Clinical Health (HITECH) Act
- Quality System Regulation
- HITRUST

6.6.1.1 Health Insurance Portability and Accountability Act (HIPAA)

This Act is one of the laws in the United States that regulates the health information of citizens. Passed in 1996, it was designed to protect the personal information of patients [44]. There are three main rules that HIPAA consists of the Security Rule, the Breach Notification Rule, and the Privacy Rule. The Security Rule mandates covered entities and their business associates to carry out risk assessments. This assessment helps to identify if there is a compliance gap that needs to be addressed to avoid any possible risk. Breach Notification Rule mandates appropriate entities and their business associates to give quick notification if there is a breach of the protected health information that is not secured. The Privacy Rule gives the situations under which a patient's protected information may be disclosed. These situations are (1) when the US Department of Health and Human Services is carrying out an investigation, enforcing an action or carrying out a review. (2) When a person or his/her representative requests that effect, or there is an accounting of disclosure.

6.6.1.2 HHS 405(d) regulation

This regulation came about due to the collaborative effort of the US Department of Health and Human Services and the healthcare organizations. A cybersecurity Act was enacted in 2015, under which a task group for cybersecurity Act was created by the US Department of Health and Human Services. The goal of the task group was spelled out: To provide a common set of consensus-based, voluntary, as well as industry-led practices, guidelines, procedures, processes, and methodologies to be used by healthcare institutions to enhance cybersecurity. Based on the above, a framework known as Healthcare Industry Cybersecurity Practices enables healthcare organizations to carry out cybersecurity in healthcare in the best way possible.

Some of the areas of protection covered by the framework include:

(a) Endpoint Protection
(b) Prevention of data loss
(c) Management of vulnerability
(d) Incident response
(e) Policies on cybersecurity
(f) Access management
(g) Security of medical devices

6.6.1.3 Payment card industry data security standard

Specifically, this regulation applies to healthcare organizations that use credit cards because information on credit cards is covered by the PIC DSS. However, it should be mentioned here that this regulation is not only for healthcare industries, rather it is a regulation that people, even those outside the healthcare industry, should know and follow strictly. The regulation makes sure that every provider protects the privacy of individuals who use their credit cards to make payments for medical services.

6.6.1.4 Health Information Technology for Economic and Clinical Health (HITECH) Act

Health Information Technology for Economic and Clinical Health Act was enacted back in 2009, and the regulation requires that every entity covered by the Act must adhere to the guidelines. The essence of the Act is to ensure the promotion of good use of healthcare technology like HER, that is, EHRs [44]. New rules or regulations to tackle security and privacy concerns of patients as far as the sharing of protected health information via electronic means is concerned were added to the HITECH Act. While HITECH addresses the privacy concern of patients, the following criminal and civil HIPAA punishments were achieved:

(a) The breach Notification Rule was strengthened.
(b) Made HIPAA's security and privacy Rules to cover business areas.
(c) Required healthcare security audits annually.

6.6.1.5 Quality system regulation (QSR)

Quality system regulation was conceived due to the rising attacks on medical devices by hackers. Since medical devices do not all have the same or equal level of protection against attacks as do mobile devices and laptops, they are often targeted by hackers. This regulation was therefore specifically made to be applied by medical-device-manufacturing organizations. In the strictest sense, the regulation requires that those concerned do the following:

(a) Regularly monitor IoTs devices and how they are used.
(b) Carry out regular risk management.
(c) Regularly update firmware and engage in regular maintenance.
(d) Design medical devices in such a way that unauthorized access is prevented.

6.6.2 Information governance issues in healthcare

Healthcare is one of the key sectors that now rely so much on Information technology in the management of available data or information about patients. In healthcare, information governance is focused on policies, accountabilities, and procedures for properly managing the information of patients. All healthcare organizations must therefore realize, if they have not done so, that information governance is key to the business of effective healthcare delivery.

Five key issues in information governance in healthcare will be looked at here: Information management, Regulatory compliance, Privacy and Security, Storage Management, and NetIQ eDiscovery.

6.7 Information management issue

Effective management of information is crucial in safeguarding the integrity and confidentiality of healthcare data within the emerging healthcare system. This section explores the myriad of information and management issues that healthcare organizations face in the realm of cybersecurity. From data governance and access controls to data lifecycle management and incident response protocols, the complexities of managing healthcare information in a digital environment are multifaceted. By examining these challenges, this section seeks to identify strategies for mitigating cyber threats, enhancing data security, and ensuring compliance with regulatory requirements. Furthermore, it delves into the role of effective information management in bolstering the resilience of healthcare organizations against emerging cyber threats, ultimately safeguarding patient care and organizational reputation.

Managing information may be easier said than done. To effectively carry out proper information management, there must be improved information organization, ease of retrieval by authorized personnel, good acquisition, improved information security, and regular maintenance of every piece of information whether in hard-copy format or electronic format by an organization. However, this is a serious issue due to data retention laws, the volume of information, and the size of information storage repositories that will increase the organization's costs.

6.7.1 Solution to information management issue

To overcome this challenge, there is a need for organizations to undertake information management automation. Doing this relieves users of the responsibilities of information storage and backup, thereby leaving the organization with enterprise-level data management.

6.7.2 Regulatory compliance issue

Though different, countries have regulatory requirements regarding the handling of information or data by healthcare organizations. If data that is covered by the regulations is not retained and managed in compliance with the regulations, it could trigger lawsuits, fines, or imprisonment.

6.7.3 Solution to the regulatory compliance issue

Organizations should seriously consider undertaking data governance software that stores every e-record automatically. As a suggestion, an archiving system can be tied to e-communication systems like e-mail. This is especially important as a good archiving system has tools for search and e-discovery. In this case, end-user management is eliminated.

6.7.4 Privacy and security issue

It is the responsibility of healthcare organizations to ensure the protection of patients' key information such as Personally Identifiable Information (PII). Also, to be carefully protected is Intellectual Property (IP). The survey carried out by [57] revealed that over one-third of those surveyed had experienced confidential or sensitive data theft. The financial cost to the healthcare organization would be huge if the theft of confidential data was due to inadvertent disclosure of patients' data.

6.7.5 Solution to privacy and security issues

Implementation of software for information management. When an archiving system is used, healthcare organizations should ensure it complies adequately with advanced privacy and security regulations, perhaps as outlined in HIPAA.

6.7.6 Storage management issue

According to [57], rising data volumes have compelled Information Technology Departments to buy additional storage systems. As the data volumes continue to rise, the cost of backing the data up effectively, managing the volume of stored or retained data, and data retrieval is a serious issue.

6.7.7 Solution to the storage management issue

As in the case of the information management issue, the issue of storage management can be solved by the implementation of information management automation. This takes away from users the responsibility of handling their e-records. Electronically searching for these records is what is called eDiscovery. Examples are image files, e-mails, databases, documents CAD/CAM, websites, etc. If the information required is not provided within the specified period, it will cost the organization heavily. Attorneys may charge the organization a huge amount of money to review all collected information to find the required information.

6.7.8 NetIQ eDiscovery issue

Sometimes, especially in litigations, an organization could be asked to provide certain information within a specified period. This information may be in volumes.

6.8 Healthcare cyber risk management

As the healthcare sector continues to embrace digital transformation, the imperative of robust cyber risk management strategies becomes increasingly evident. This section delves into the nuanced realm of healthcare cyber risk management, where proactive measures are essential for mitigating the ever-evolving threat landscape. By examining the unique vulnerabilities and challenges faced by healthcare organizations, ranging from ransomware attacks to insider threats, this section aims to elucidate effective risk management frameworks and practices. Moreover, this section underscores the critical role of collaboration among stakeholders, regulatory bodies, and cybersecurity professionals in safeguarding patient data and preserving the integrity of healthcare services amidst an increasingly hostile digital environment.

The recent advancements in technology have resulted in the design of more medical devices than ever in human history. These devices are designed to have network capabilities for network integration and patient information management. The devices can monitor a patient's data and transfer the monitored or gathered data to e-medical records. Interestingly, these medical devices are increasingly being interconnected, enabling healthcare professionals to render efficient and effective services to patients.

The interconnection of these medical devices, however, creates room for cybersecurity issues that were not known in the healthcare sector before now. There is a need to take drastic measures to mitigate the effect of rising cybersecurity threats in the healthcare sector. To this end, adequate planning and management of cybersecurity risk mitigation strategies must be undertaken by healthcare organizations. The following steps should be carefully followed:

(a) Identification of major stakeholders in a particular healthcare facility.
(b) Cybersecurity functions should be clearly defined among the staff so that those involved know what their functions are.
(c) Purchase only devices that have, if possible, advanced safety and security features, and check if the continuing support of the manufacturers is assured.

(d) Make the collaboration of related departments (like the Information Technology (IT) Department and Hospital Biomedical Department) a serious priority.
(e) Adequate measures should be put in place to ensure negligible disruption of any device(s) operation during upgrading processes.
(f) The use of certain mechanisms like VLAN, which helps to minimize interaction with the main network to certain ports can reduce exposure to threats of cybersecurity.
(g) Regularly train and educate everyone who uses the devices on key security measures.

6.9 Creation of secure data-sharing platform for healthcare providers

The emerging healthcare system is rapidly integrating digital technologies to enhance patient care, streamline operations, and facilitate data-driven decision making. However, amidst this transformation, the looming specter of cyber threats poses significant challenges, potentially compromising patient confidentiality, data integrity, and overall system functionality. While considerable efforts have been devoted to fortifying cybersecurity within healthcare, a critical research gap persists in the creation of a secure data-sharing platform for healthcare providers. This void not only undermines the efficacy of inter-organizational collaboration but also exposes sensitive patient information to exploitation by malicious actors. Consequently, addressing this gap is paramount to safeguarding the integrity and confidentiality of healthcare data in the digital age. This report explores the landscape of deadly cybersecurity threats within the emerging healthcare system, with a particular focus on the imperative need for a robust and secure data-sharing platform to mitigate these risks effectively.

To create a very secure data-sharing platform that ensures smooth transfer of data confidentially between healthcare providers, the following steps should be carefully implemented. The flowchart provides a high-level overview of the steps involved in creating a secure data-sharing platform for healthcare providers. Each step may involve further sub-steps and iterations to ensure the platform meets the required security standards and user needs.

Step 1. Define Requirements

- Identify the specific data-sharing needs and requirements of healthcare providers.
- Determine the types of data to be shared, access permissions, compliance requirements, etc.

Step 2. Design Architecture

- Design the architecture of the data-sharing platform, including components such as servers, databases, APIs, and user interfaces.

– Consider scalability, redundancy, and fault tolerance to ensure reliable performance.

Step 3. Implement Security Measures

– Integrate encryption mechanisms to secure data both at rest and in transit.
– Implement access controls and authentication mechanisms to ensure that only authorized users can access the platform.
– Incorporate data integrity checks and auditing capabilities to monitor access and detect unauthorized activity.

Step 4. Compliance and Regulation

– Ensure compliance with relevant healthcare regulations and standards (e.g., HIPAA, GDPR) governing data privacy and security.
– Implement measures to protect patient confidentiality and adhere to data retention policies.

Step 5. Develop User Interface

– Design user-friendly interfaces for healthcare professionals to access and share data securely.
– Provide features for managing permissions, uploading, and downloading data, and viewing audit logs.

Step 6. Testing and Quality Assurance

– Conduct thorough testing of the platform to identify and address security vulnerabilities, usability issues, and performance bottlenecks.
– Perform penetration testing and security audits to validate the effectiveness of security measures.

Step 7. Deployment and Training

– Deploy the data-sharing platform in a secure environment, either on-premises or in the cloud.
– Provide training to healthcare professionals and staff on how to use the platform securely and effectively.

Step 8. Monitoring and Maintenance

– Implement ongoing monitoring and maintenance procedures to ensure the continued security and functionality of the platform.
– Regularly update software components and security patches to mitigate emerging threats.

These steps are summarized in the flowchart in Figure 6.5.

Figure 6.5 depicts the proposed flowchart of the secure data-sharing platform for healthcare providers. It starts with the definition of the requirements, then to architecture design, to implementation of security measures, to activation of compliance and regulation, etc.

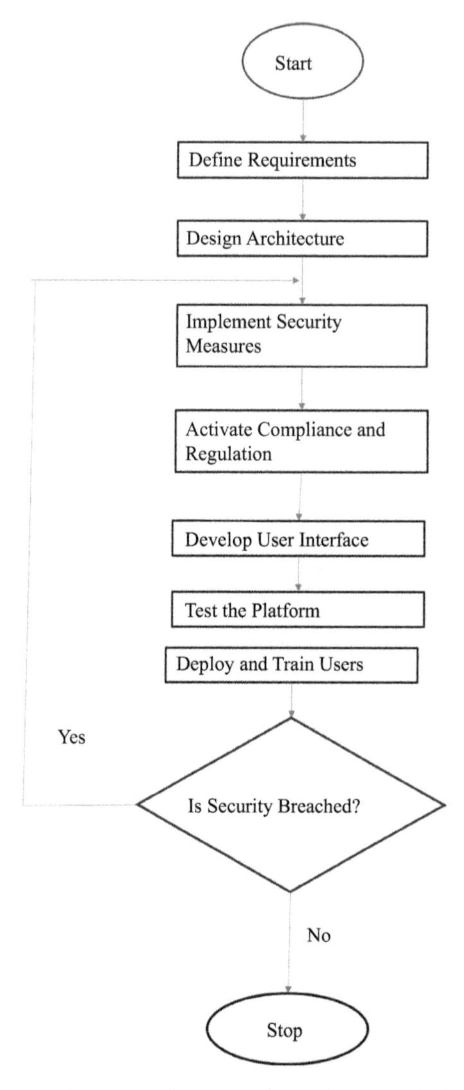

Figure 6.5 Flowchart of proposed secure data sharing platform for healthcare providers

6.10 Comprehensive measure

In addressing the relentless onslaught of deadly cybersecurity threats within the emerging healthcare system, the implementation of comprehensive measures is paramount. This section elucidates a holistic approach toward mitigating cyber risks, encompassing a range of proactive strategies and defensive mechanisms. By integrating insights from previous sections on legal and regulatory issues, information and management challenges, and healthcare cyber risk management, this section synthesizes a cohesive framework for safeguarding healthcare data and infrastructure. From robust encryption protocols and access controls to continuous monitoring and threat intelligence sharing, the comprehensive measures outlined herein aim to fortify the resilience of healthcare organizations against cyber threats. Furthermore, this section underscores the importance of organizational culture, leadership commitment, and stakeholder collaboration in fostering a cybersecurity-aware environment conducive to the protection of patient privacy and the continuity of healthcare services.

Comprehensively, there is a need to do the following:

(a) Regularly updating firmware.
(b) Regularly monitoring network traffic to identify any suspicious activity.
(c) Strongly encourage the use of stronger passwords. The longer the password, the harder it is to guess by cybercriminals.
(d) Quickly change passwords if it is sensed that the password may have been compromised, especially when there is a change in certain healthcare facility personnel.
(e) Avoid using the same password for different accounts.
(f) Use passphrases. Passphrases are very long passwords that comprise words that are not related.
(g) Any client device used, like VoIP, that is voice-over-internet protocol, should be given unique passwords and usernames.
(h) Biometric readers
(i) Cameras for security purposes
(j) Smart medical equipment
(k) Smart thermostats
(l) Create a secure data-sharing platform for healthcare providers.

6.11 Conclusion

Cybersecurity attacks on healthcare management facilities are really on the increase. Some of the attacks include ransomware attacks, insider attacks, phishing scams, hacking of medical devices, and unprotected (unsecured) IoTs. The measures to mitigate these various attack types are the implementation of plans for backup and disaster recovery. For insider phishing attacks in healthcare systems, training and re-training of employees are necessary. Such training should be tailored toward exposing them to the consequences of indulging in any kind of crime, including using or revealing confidential data to unauthorized persons. The training should also emphasize that inaction on the part of an employee that leads to an attack on patients' data will be treated as a case of insider attack with full consequences meted out against the affected individual for hacking medical devices.

References

[1] Maksimović, M.; and Vujović, V. (2017). Internet of Things Based E-health Systems: Ideas, Expectations and Concerns. Cham: Springer p. 241–80. https://doi.org/10.1007/978-3-319-58280-1_10

[2] Akhtar, N.; Khan, N.; Qayyum, S.; Qureshi, M.I.; and Hishan, S.S. (2022). Efficacy and Pitfalls of Digital Technologies in Healthcare Services: A Systematic Review of two Decades. *Front. Public Health* 10:869793. https://doi.org/10.3389/fpubh.2022.869793

[3] Paul, M.; Maglaras, L.; and Ferragetal, M.A. (2023). Digitization of Healthcare Sector: A Study on Privacy and Security Concerns. *ICT Express*, https://doi.org/10.1016/j.icte.2023.02.007.

[4] Khan, N.A.; Brohi, S.N.; and Zaman, N. (2023). Ten Deadly Cyber Security Threats Amid Covid-19 Pandemic, TechRxiv, 1–7.

[5] Alka, J. (2023). Indian Healthcare System Needs Robust Cybersecurity Infra. Here's What Experts Say.

[6] Jalali, M.S.; and Kaiser, J.P. (2018). Cybersecurity in Hospitals: A Systematic, Organizational Perspective. *J Med Internet Res*. 20(5), 41–52. https://doi.org/10.2196/10059.

[7] Shahatha, A.l.; Mashhadani, A.F.; Qureshi, M.I.; *et al.* (2021). Towards the Development of Digital Manufacturing Ecosystems for Sustainable Performance: Learning from the Past Two Decades of Research Energies. https://doi.org/10.3390/en14102945.

[8] Zimmermann B.M.; Fiske A.; Prainsack B.; Hangel N.; McLennan S.; and Buyx A. (2021). Early Perceptions of COVID-19 Contact Tracing Apps in German-Speaking Countries: Comparative Mixed Methods Study. *J Med Internet Res*. https://doi.org/10.2196/25525.

[9] Kapoor, A.; Guha, S.; Kanti-Das, M.; Goswami, K.C.; and Yadav, R. (2020). Digital Healthcare: The Only Solution for Better Healthcare During COVID-19 Pandemic? *Indian Heart J*. 72, 61–64. https://doi.org/10.1016/j.ihj.2020.04.001.

[10] Henkenjohann, R. (2021). Role of Individual Motivations and Privacy Concerns in the Adoption of German Electronic Patient Record Apps—A Mixed-Methods Study. *Int J Environ Res Public Health*. https://doi.org/10.3390/ijerph18189553

[11] Rodriguez-deArriba, M.L.; Nocentini, A.; Menesini, E.; and Sanchez-Jimenez, V. (2021). Dimensions and Measures of Cyber-Dating Violence in Adolescents: A Systematic Review. Aggression Violent. *Behaviour*, 58, 101613.

[12] Jamal, A.A.; Majid, A.A.M.; Konev, A.; Kosachenko, T.; and Shelupanov, A. (2021). A Review on Security Analysis of Cyber-Physical Systems Using Machine Learning. Materials Today: Proceedings.

[13] Zhang J. (2021). Distributed Network Security Framework of Energy Internet Based on Internet of Things. *Sustainable Energy Technologies and Assessments*, 44, 101051.

[14] Alkatheiri, M.S.; Chauhdary, S.H.; and Alqarni, M.A. (2021). Seamless Security Apprise Method for Improving the Reliability of Sustainable Energy Based Smart Home Applications. *Sustainable Energy Technologies and Assessments*, 45, 101219.

[15] Krishnasamy, V.; and Venkatachalam, S. (2021). An Efficient Data Flow Material Model Based Cloud Authentication Data Security and Reduces a

Cloud Storage Cost using Index-Level Boundary Pattern Convergent Encryption Algorithm. Materials Today: Proceedings.

[16] Ogbanufe O. (2021). Enhancing End-User Roles in Information Security: Exploring the Setting, Situation, and Identity. *Computers and Security*, 108, 102340.

[17] Yuchong L.; and Qinghui L. (2021). A Comprehensive Review Study of Cyber-Attacks and Cyber Security: Emerging Trends and Recent Developments, *Journal of Energy Reports*, 7, 8176–8186.

[18] Le Nguyen, C.; and Golman W. (2021). Diffusion of the Budapest Convention on Cybercrime and the Development of Cybercrime Legislation in Pacific Island Countries: "Law on the Books" Vs "Law in Action". *Computer Law and Security Review*, 40, 105521.

[19] John R. (n.d). The Importance of Cybersecurity in Protecting Patient Safety. Accessed from www.aha.org/center/cybersecurity-and-risk-advisory-services/importance-cybersecurity-protecting-patient, on April 4, 2023.

[20] Seemma, P.S.; Nandhini, S.; and Sowmiya, M. (2018). Overview of Cybersecurity. *International Journal of Advanced Research in Computer and Communication Engineering*, 7(11), 125–128. https://doi.org/10.17148/IJARCCE.2018.71127

[21] Morgan S. (2020). Cybersecurity Research: All in One Place. Cyber Crime Magazine, available from https://cybersecurityventures.com/research/

[22] 2018 Cost of a Data Breach Stud: Global Overview, Ponemon Institute, and IBM, https://www.ibm.com/security/data-breach.

[23] 2017 Cost of a Data Breach Stud: Global Overview, Ponemon Institute and IBM, https://www.ponemon.org/library/2017-cost-of-data-breach-study-united-states.

[24] 2018 Cost of a Data Breach Stud: Cost of a Data Breach Stud: Global Overview, Ponemon Institute and IBM, https://www.ibm.com/security/data-breach

[25] Mayra, R.F. (2020). Cybercrime and other Threats Faced by the Healthcare Industry, Trend Microlabs.

[26] ENISA Threat Landscape for Ransomware Attacks (2022). https://doi.org/10.2824/168593

[27] Kapoor, A.; Gupta, A.; Gupta, R.; Tanwar, S.; Sharma, G.; and Davidson, I. E. (2022). Ransomware Detection, Avoidance, and Mitigation Schemes: A Review and Future Directions. *Sustainability*, 14, 8. https://doi.org/10.3390/su14010008

[28] Junaid, S.B.; Imam, A.A.; Balogun, A.O.; *et al.* (2022). Recent Advancements in Emerging Technologies for Healthcare Management Systems: A Survey. *Healthcare 2022*, 10, 1940. https://doi.org/10.3390/healthcare10101940

[29] Li, Q.; Campan, A.; Ren, A.; and Eid, W.E. (2022). Automating and Improving Cardiovascular Disease Prediction using Machine Learning and EMR Data Features from a Regional Healthcare System. *Int. J. Med. Inform.* 163, 104786.

[30] Kumar, G.; Basri, S.; Imam, A.A.; Khowaja, S.A.; Capretz, L.F.; and Balogun, A.O. (2021). Data Harmonization for Heterogeneous Datasets: A Systematic Literature Review. *Appl. Sci.* 11, 8275.

[31] Verma, K.K.; Singh, B.M.; and Dixit, A. (2019). A Review of Supervised and Unsupervised Machine Learning Techniques for Suspicious Behavior recognition in intelligent surveillance system. *International Journal of Information Technology*, 14, 397–410.

[32] Hiran, K.K.; Jain, R.K.; Lakhwani, K.; and Doshi, R. (2021). Machine Learning: Master Supervised and Unsupervised Learning Algorithms with Real Examples (English Edition); BPB Publications: Noida, India.

[33] Kaplan, A.; Cao, H.; FitzGerald, J.M.; *et al.* (2021). Artificial Intelligence/ Machine Learning in Respiratory Medicine and Potential Role in Asthma and COPD Diagnosis. *J. Allergy Clin. Immunol. Pract.*, 9, 2255–2261.

[34] Petersilge, C.A.; McDonald, J.; Bishop, M.; Yudkovitch, L.; Treuting, C.; and Towbin, A.J. (2022). Visible Light Imaging: Clinical Aspects with an Emphasis on Medical Photography—A HIMSS-SIIM Enterprise Imaging Community Whitepaper. *Journal of Digital Imaging*, 35, 385–395.

[35] Oladepo, A.G.; Bajeh, A.O.; Balogun, A.O.; Mojeed, H.A.; Salman, A.A.; and Bako, A.I. (2021). Heterogeneous Ensemble with Combined Dimensionality Reduction for Social Spam Detection. *International Journal of Interaction Mobility Technology*, 15, 84–103.

[36] Usman-Hamza, F.; Atte, A.; Balogun, A.; Mojeed, H.; Bajeh, A.; and Adeyemo, V. (2019). Impact of Feature Selection on Classification via Clustering Techniques in Software Defect Prediction. *Journal of Computer Science and Its Application*, 26, 132.

[37] Apostol, I.; Preda, M.; Nila, C.; and Bica, I. (2021). IoT Botnet Anomaly Detection using Unsupervised Deep Learning. *Electronics*, 10, 1876.

[38] Balogun, A.; Oladele, R.; Mojeed, H.; Amin-Balogun, B.; Adeyemo, V.E.; and Aro, T.O. (2019). Performance Analysis of Selected Clustering Techniques for Software Defects Prediction. *African Journal of Computer ICT*, 12, 30–42.

[39] Sahoo, S.; Das, M.; Mishra, S.; and Suman, S. (2021). A Hybrid DTNB Model for Heart Disorders Prediction. In *Advances in Electronics, Communication and Computing*; Springer: Berlin/Heidelberg, Germany; Bhubaneswar, India, 155–163.

[40] Alamsyah, A. and Fadila, T. (2020). Increased Accuracy of Prediction Hepatitis Disease using the Application of Principal Component Analysis on a Support Vector Machine. In Proceedings of the Journal of Physics: Conference Series, Manado, Indonesia, 012016.

[41] Muneer, A.; Taib, S.M.; Fati, S.M.; Balogun, A.O.; and Aziz, I.A. (2022). A Hybrid Deep Learning-Based Unsupervised Anomaly Detection in High Dimensional Data. *Computer Mater. Contin.* 70, 6073–6088.

[42] Fagherazzi, G.; Zhang, L.; Aguayo, G.; *et al.* (2021). Towards Precision Cardiometabolic Prevention: Results from a Machine Learning, Semi-Supervised Clustering Approach in the Nationwide Population-Based ORISCAV-LUX 2 study. *Sci. Rep.* 11, 16056.

[43] Yu, H.; Chen, Z.; Zhang, X.; *et al.* (2021). FedHAR: Semi-Supervised Online Learning for Personalized Federated Human Activity Recognition. IEEE Transaction Mobile Computing.

[44] Peng, J.; Wang, P.; Desrosiers, C.; and Pedersoli, M. (2021). Self-Paced Contrastive Learning for Semi-Supervised Medical Image Segmentation with Meta-Labels. *Adv. Neural Inf. Process. Syst.* 34, 16686–16699.

[45] Luo, X.; Chen, J.; Song, T.; and Wang, G. (2021). Semi-Supervised Medical Image Segmentation Through Dual-Task Consistency. In Proceedings of the AAAI Conference on Artificial Intelligence, Virtual Conference, 8801–8809.

[46] Daniels J.; and Bhatia S. (2020*). Legislation and Negative Impact of Cybersecurity in Healthcare*, in *Proceedings of the 6th International Conference on Information Security and Privacy*, 691–697. https://doi.org/10.5220/000915706910697

[47] Ray, P.P.; Dash, D.; and De, D. (2019). Analysis and Monitoring of IoT-Assisted Human Physiological Galvanic Skin Response Factor for Smart e-Healthcare. *Sens. Rev.*, 39, 525–541.

[48] Wu, T.; Wu, F.; Redoute, J.-M.; and Yuce, M.R. (2017). An Autonomous Wireless Body Area Network Implementation Towards IoT Connected Healthcare Applications. *IEEE Access*, 5, 11413–11422.

[49] Yang, Z.; Zhou, Q.; Lei, L.; Zheng, K.; and Xiang, W. (2016). An IoT-Cloud Based Wearable ECG Monitoring System for Smart Healthcare, *Journal of Medical System*, 40, 286.

[50] Azimi, I.; Pahikkala, T.; Rahmani, A.M.; Niela-Vilén, H.; Axelin, A.; and Liljeberg, P. (2019). Missing Data Resilient Decision-making for Healthcare IoT Through Personalization: A Case Study on Maternal Health. *Future Generation Computer System*, 96, 297–308.

[51] Bhatia, M.; and Sood, S.K. (2017). A Comprehensive Health Assessment Framework to Facilitate IoT-Assisted Smart Workouts: A Predictive Healthcare Perspective. *Comput. Ind.* 92, 50–66.

[52] Niitsu, K.; Kobayashi, A.; Nishio, Y.; *et al.* (2018). A Self-Powered Supply-Sensing Biosensor Platform using Biofuel Cell and Low-Voltage, Low-Cost CMOS Supply-Controlled Ring Oscillator with Inductive-Coupling Transmitter for Healthcare IoT. *IEEE Trans. Circuits Syst.* 65, 2784–2796.

[53] Hallfors, N.G.; Alhawari, M.; Abi Jaoude, M.; *et al.* (2018). Graphene Oxide: Nylon ECG Sensors for Wearable IoT Healthcare—Nanomaterial and SoC Interface. *Analog Integrated Circuits Signal Process*, 96, 253–260.

[54] Esmaeili, S.; Tabbakh, S.R.K.; and Shakeri, H. (2020). A Priority-Aware Lightweight Secure Sensing Model for Body Area Networks with Clinical Healthcare Applications in Internet of Things. *Pervasive Mob. Comput.* 69, 101265.

[55] Muthu, B.; Sivaparthipan, C.; Manogaran, G.; *et al.* (2020). IOT-Based Wearable Sensor for Diseases Prediction and Symptom Analysis in Healthcare Sector. *Peer Peer Netw. Appl.* 13, 2123–2134.

[56] Huifeng, W.; Kadry, S.N.; and Raj, E.D. (2020). Continuous Health Monitoring of Sportsperson Using IoT Devices Based Wearable Technology. *Computer Communication* 160, 588–595.

[57] Wu, T.; Wu, F.; Qiu, C.; Redouté, J.-M.; and Yuce, M.R. (2020). A Rigid-fex Wearable Health Monitoring Sensor Patch for IoT-Connected Healthcare Applications. *IEEE Internet Things J.*7, 6932–6945.

[58] Elechi P.; Sibe R.T.; Onu K.E.; and Imoize A.L. (2023). The Vision of 6G Security and Privacy, in *Book: Security and Privacy Schemes for Dense 6G Wireless Communication Networks*. https://doi.org/10.1049/PBSE021E_ch4

[59] Narendra S. (2023). Cloud Security: Hacking the Hackers. Obtained from: https://justtotaltech.com/healthcare-cyber-attacks/#:~:text=The%205%20biggest%20cybersecurity%20threats%20in%20healthcare%20cybersecurity%20include%20ransomeware,trying%20protect%20against%20them. Visited on 2nd Aug. 2023.

[60] Sworna, N.S.; Islam, A.M.; Shatabda, S. and Islam, S. (2021). Towards Development of IoT-ML Driven Healthcare Systems: A Survey. *Journal of Network Computer Application*, 196, 103244.

[61] Wan, J.; Al-Awlaqi, M.A.A.H.; Li, M.; *et al.* (2018). Wearable IoT Enabled Real-Time Health Monitoring System. *EURASIP Journal of Wireless Communication Network*, 2018, 298.

[62] Tabassum, S.; Zaman, M.I.U.; Ullah, M.S.; Rahaman, A.; Nahar, S.; and Islam, A.M. (2019). The Cardiac Disease Predictor: IoT and ML-Driven Healthcare System. In Proceedings of the 2019 4th International Conference on Electrical Information and Communication Technology (EICT), Khulna, Bangladesh, 1–6.

[63] Magaña-Espinoza, P.; Aquino-Santos, R.; Cárdenas-Benítez, N.; *et al.* (2014). WiSPH: A Wireless Sensor Network-Based Home Care Monitoring System. *Sensors* 2014, 14, 7096–7119.

[64] Magalini S.; Gui D.; Mari P.; Merialdo M.; *et al.* (2021). Cyberthreats to Hospitals: Panacea, a Toolkit for People-Centric cybersecurity. *Journal of Strategic Innovations and Sustainability*, 16(3), 185–191.

[65] Mohd J.; Abid H.; Ravi P.S.; and Rajiv S. (2023). Towards Insighting Cybersecurity for Healthcare Domains: A Comprehensive Review of Recent Practices and Trends. *Cyber Security and Applications*, 1(2023), 100016. https://doi.org/10.1016/j.csa.2023.100016

[66] Mamun, Q. (2022). Blockchain Technology in the Future of Healthcare. *Smart Health* 2022, 23, 100223.

[67] Fu, J.; Wang, N.; and Cai, Y. (2020). Privacy-Preserving in Healthcare Blockchain Systems Based on Lightweight Message Sharing. *Sensors* 2020, 20, 1898.

[68] Satamraju, K.P. (2020). Proof of Concept of Scalable Integration of Internet of Things and Blockchain in Healthcare. *Sensors 2020*, 20, 1389.

[69] Ray, P.P.; Dash, D.; Salah, K.; and Kumar, N. (2020). Blockchain for IoT-Based Healthcare: Background, Consensus, Platforms, and use Cases. *IEEE System Journal*, 15, 85–94.

[70] Soltanisehat, L.; Alizadeh, R.; Hao, H.; and Choo, K.-K.R. (2020). Technical, Temporal, and Spatial Research Challenges and Opportunities in Blockchain-Based Healthcare: A Systematic Literature Review. *IEEE Trans. Eng. Manag.*

[71] Munoz, D.-J.; Constantinescu, D.-A.; Asenjo, R.; and Fuentes, L. (2019). ClinicAppChain: A Low-Cost Blockchain Hyperledger Solution for Healthcare. In *Proceedings of the International Congress on Blockchain and Applications*, L'Aquila, Italy, 36–44.

[72] Abdulraheem, M.; Adeniyi, E.A.; Awotunde, J.B.; *et al.* (2024). Artificial Intelligence of Medical Things for Medical Information Systems Privacy and Security. In *Handbook of Security and Privacy of AI-Enabled Healthcare Systems and Internet of Medical Things* (pp. 63–96). CRC Press.

[73] Sam M.F.M.; Ismail A.F.M.F.; Bakar K.A.; Ahamat A.; and Qureshi M.I. (2022). The Effectiveness of IoT-Based Wearable Devices and Potential Cybersecurity Risks: A Systematic Literature Review from the Last Decade. *Int. J. Online Biomed. Eng.*, 18(9).

[74] Zhang Y.; Zhou Y.; Pei R.; Chen X.; and Wang Y. (2023). Potential Threat of Human Pathogenic Orthopoxviruses to Public Health and Control Strategies, *Journal of Biosafety and Biosecurity*, 5(1), 1–7.

[75] Ren A.; Liang C.; Hyug I.; Broh S.; and Jhanjhi N.Z. (2020). A Three-Level Ransomware Detection and Prevention Mechanism. *EAI Endorsed Trans. Energy Web*, 7(26).

[76] Awotunde, J.B.; Imoize, A.L.; Jimoh, R.G.; *et al.* (2024). AIoMT Enabling Real-Time Monitoring of Healthcare Systems: Security and Privacy Considerations. *Handbook of Security and Privacy of AI-Enabled Healthcare Systems and Internet of Medical Things*, pp. 97–133.

[77] Rufai, A.U.; Fasina, E.P.; Uwadia, C.O.; Rufai, A.T.; and Imoize, A.L. (2024). Cyberattacks against Artificial Intelligence-Enabled Internet of Medical Things. In *Handbook of Security and Privacy of AI-Enabled Healthcare Systems and Internet of Medical Things* (pp. 191–216). CRC Press.

[78] Sei, Y.; Ohsuga, A.; Onesimu, J.A.; and Imoize, A.L. (2024). Local Differential Privacy for Artificial Intelligence of Medical Things. In *Handbook of Security and Privacy of AI-Enabled Healthcare Systems and Internet of Medical Things* (pp. 241–270). CRC Press.

[79] Ashima, R.; Haleem, A.; Bahl, S.; Javaid, M.; Mahla, S.K.; and Singh, S. (2021). Automation and Manufacturing of Smart Materials in Additive Manufacturing Technologies Using Internet of Things Towards the Adoption of Industry 4.0. *Mater. Today, Proc.* 45, 5081–5088.

[80] Pandey, P.; and Litoriya, R. (2020). Implementing Healthcare Services on a Large Scale: Challenges and Remedies Based on Blockchain *Technology. Health Policy Technology*, 9, 69–78.

[81] Saha, A.; Amin, R.; Kunal, S.; Vollala, S.; and Dwivedi, S.K. (2019). Review on "Blockchain Technology Based Medical Healthcare System with Privacy Issues. Security. *Priv.* 2, e83.

[82] Argyridou E.; Laoudias C.; Panaousis E.; *et al.* (2023). Cyber Hygiene Methodology for Raising Cybersecurity and Data Privacy Awareness in Health Care Organizations: Concept Study. *Journal of Medical Internet Research*, 25(2023). https://doi.org/10.2196/41294

Chapter 7

Artificial intelligence for secured cybersecurity in emerging healthcare systems

Abdulwaheed Musa[1,2] and Abdulhakeem Oladele Abdulfatai[1]

The healthcare industry rapidly adopts digital technologies to improve patient care and outcomes. However, this digital transformation has also made healthcare systems more vulnerable to cyberattacks. Artificial intelligence (AI) has the potential to enhance cybersecurity in emerging healthcare systems by providing advanced threat detection and response capabilities. This chapter explores the potential of AI in securing emerging healthcare systems against cyber threats. The current state of cybersecurity in healthcare systems and the challenges faced by emerging healthcare systems are discussed. An overview of AI and its potential applications in healthcare cybersecurity is provided. Finally, the benefits of using AI in securing emerging healthcare systems and the challenges that need to be addressed to realize the potential of AI in cybersecurity are highlighted fully.

Keywords: Healthcare industry; digital transformation; cybersecurity; cyber threats; artificial intelligence; threat detection; emerging healthcare

7.1 Introduction

The healthcare landscape is rapidly transforming, marked by a surge in technological advancements. A noteworthy shift in recent times is the growing emphasis on patient-centric care, giving rise to innovative healthcare systems designed for enhanced efficiency, effectiveness, and accessibility. Referred to as Health 4.0 [1] in the digital era, these systems signify a transformative move toward interconnected, data-driven, and technology-enabled healthcare. This evolution encompasses a range of innovations, including Electronic Health Records (EHRs), telemedicine, and Internet of Medical Things (IoMT) devices, all promising improved patient care, streamlined processes, and enhanced medical outcomes.

However, amidst these advancements, a new set of challenges has emerged, particularly in the realm of cybersecurity. The increasing connectivity and data

[1]Department of Electrical and Computer Engineering, Kwara State University, Nigeria
[2]Centre for Artificial Intelligence and Machine Learning Systems, Kwara State University, Nigeria

reliance of healthcare systems make them susceptible to cyber threats. The healthcare sector, being one of the prime targets for cyber-attacks, faces heightened risks due to the sensitive patient data stored within these systems. The integration of IoMT devices, wearable health monitors, and interconnected medical machinery introduces new vulnerabilities that malicious actors can exploit. As healthcare entities increasingly rely on networked technologies to handle sensitive patient information, the potential consequences of a cybersecurity breach become more severe.

As healthcare systems globally transition toward a digital paradigm, safeguarding patient information against cyber threats becomes imperative. Recent studies [2] highlight the escalating frequency and sophistication of cyber-attacks on healthcare institutions. The digitization of patient records, the proliferation of connected medical devices, and the advent of telehealth services have expanded the attack surface, necessitating robust cybersecurity measures. According to a report [3], 94% of health systems have fallen victim to a cyberattack, indicating a dramatic rise over the past decade, violating patient privacy and interrupting clinical care [4].

The need for cybersecurity in emerging healthcare systems is twofold. First, safeguarding patient data privacy is paramount. EHRs, containing sensitive information, must be protected to maintain patient trust and comply with regulatory requirements such as the Health Insurance Portability and Accountability Act (HIPAA) in the United States. Second, ensuring the integrity of medical data is critical for informed decision-making. Tampering with medical records or treatment plans can have severe consequences on patient safety and well-being.

The uninterrupted functioning of digital infrastructure is also essential for the availability of healthcare services. Cyberattacks, ranging from ransomware to Distributed Denial of Service (DDoS) attacks, can disrupt operations, leading to delays in patient care, financial losses, and reputational damage. The imperative to protect against these threats underscores the need for a comprehensive and adaptive cybersecurity framework tailored to the specific nuances of emerging healthcare systems. As healthcare increasingly relies on advanced technologies, balancing the benefits of digital transformation with the imperative to fortify cybersecurity is crucial for realizing the full potential of emerging healthcare systems.

In the face of these challenges, the integration of Artificial Intelligence (AI) emerges as a transformative paradigm capable of proactively addressing the dynamic nature of cyber threats. The alliance between AI and cybersecurity goes beyond conventional security measures. Machine learning (ML) algorithms, for instance, exhibit the capacity to discern patterns in vast datasets, enabling early detection of abnormal activities indicative of potential cyber threats [5]. Natural Language Processing (NLP) further enhances the contextual understanding of security incidents, facilitating more nuanced and precise responses.

This chapter unfolds as a comprehensive exploration of the symbiotic relationship between AI and cybersecurity, aiming to elucidate how AI-driven solutions can be strategically employed to bolster the resilience of emerging healthcare systems.

7.1.1 Key contributions of the chapter

The following are the significant contributions of this chapter:

1. The chapter meticulously examines the evolving landscape of healthcare cybersecurity, providing a comprehensive overview of the challenges posed by the integration of digital technologies.
2. By emphasizing the vulnerabilities introduced by interconnected healthcare systems, the chapter underscores the potential consequences of cybersecurity breaches, such as unauthorized access to sensitive patient data and tampering with medical records or treatment plans.
3. Valuable insights into the global transition toward a digital paradigm in healthcare.
4. The chapter emphasizes the delicate balance required to harness the benefits of digital innovation while fortifying cybersecurity measures.
5. It also elucidates how AI-driven solutions, particularly ML algorithms and NLP, can proactively enhance threat detection and response capabilities.

7.1.2 Chapter organization

Having introduced the chapter in Section 7.1, Section 7.2 offers insights into the current state of AI in healthcare cybersecurity. Section 7.3 dives into how AI plays a role in spotting and preventing cyber threats within healthcare systems. Section 7.4 shifts focus to the safeguarding of sensitive patient data, exploring how AI contributes to enhancing security in healthcare systems. Following this, Section 7.5 brings real-world examples into the picture, showcasing case studies of healthcare providers successfully implementing AI-based cybersecurity solutions. Looking ahead, Section 7.6 turns attention to future trends and challenges in this dynamic landscape. Finally, Section 7.7 concludes with valuable recommendations and synthesizes the key learnings for practical application.

7.2 Overview of AI in healthcare cybersecurity

The healthcare sector is one of the primary targets for cybercriminals, given the inherently sensitive nature of its stored data. This data, often of a highly personal and delicate nature, becomes a sought-after commodity on the illicit market. The implications of such data falling into the wrong hands are profound, ranging from identity theft to financial fraud and extortion. Notably, the healthcare industry faces a heightened risk of ransomware attacks, capable of paralyzing organizational operations and resulting in substantial financial repercussions. This chapter delves into the contemporary threat landscape within healthcare, examining the existing regulatory framework, the pivotal role of AI in fortifying cybersecurity, associated challenges, and ethical considerations. Furthermore, valuable insights are provided to guide healthcare organizations in safeguarding themselves against these pervasive threats.

7.2.1 Threat landscape in healthcare

The contemporary healthcare panorama is an expansive and intricate domain, offering opportunities for progress while concurrently presenting challenges that demand steadfast attention. One of the foremost concerns that has recently emerged pertains to the extensive and escalating threat landscape confronting healthcare institutions. This challenge is notably exacerbated by the insidious evolution of cyber threats, which have grown increasingly sophisticated and targeted. The health sector, as shown in Figure 7.1, is a sector bedeviled by numerous types of cyber-attacks, at the front of this horde with 54% being ransomware. After data-type threats, it is closely followed by data-related threats comprising breaches and unauthorized access which account for 46%. Intrusion, which is when attackers gain unauthorized access to computers, constitutes 13% of the landscape showing that healthcare infrastructure persistently has vulnerabilities. Denial-of-service (DoS), DDoS, and reflective denial-of-service (RDOS) attacks contribute 9%, stressing risks effectively. Malicious software, despite being less widespread with 5%, is still a serious concern, whose damage can be very severe. These threats exploit vulnerabilities within the interconnected digital infrastructure of healthcare systems.

A report from ClearDATA underscores healthcare's vulnerability, identifying it as one of the top five industry sectors targeted by cybercriminals [6]. The report emphasizes that the high financial stakes and inherent vulnerability of healthcare organizations render them attractive targets for malicious threat actors. Furthermore, it notes that the challenges associated with remote work and the lingering effects of the COVID-19 pandemic have strained the cybersecurity resources of healthcare organizations to their limits [6].

Another report from Security Boulevard highlights a significant shift in the threat landscape for healthcare organizations since the onset of COVID-19.

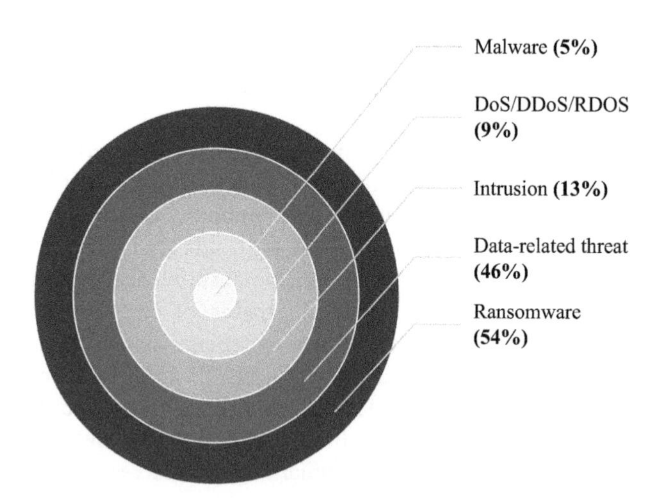

Figure 7.1 Threat landscape in healthcare

The means, opportunities, and motives of threat actors targeting the sector have undergone substantial changes in nature and have intensified [7].

The European Union Agency for Cybersecurity (ENISA) [8] meticulously dissected the cybersecurity threats assailing the health sector across Europe, spanning from January 2021 to March 2023 as depicted in Figure 7.2. This report, the first of its kind from ENISA, meticulously maps and scrutinizes cyber incidents, offering invaluable insights crucial for healthcare entities and policy framers alike. The report's release marks a pivotal moment in understanding the cyber threat landscape specific to the health sector. The ENISA report reveals a troubling array of cybersecurity challenges faced by the European health sector. A notable finding is the widespread prevalence of cyber incidents, with healthcare providers,

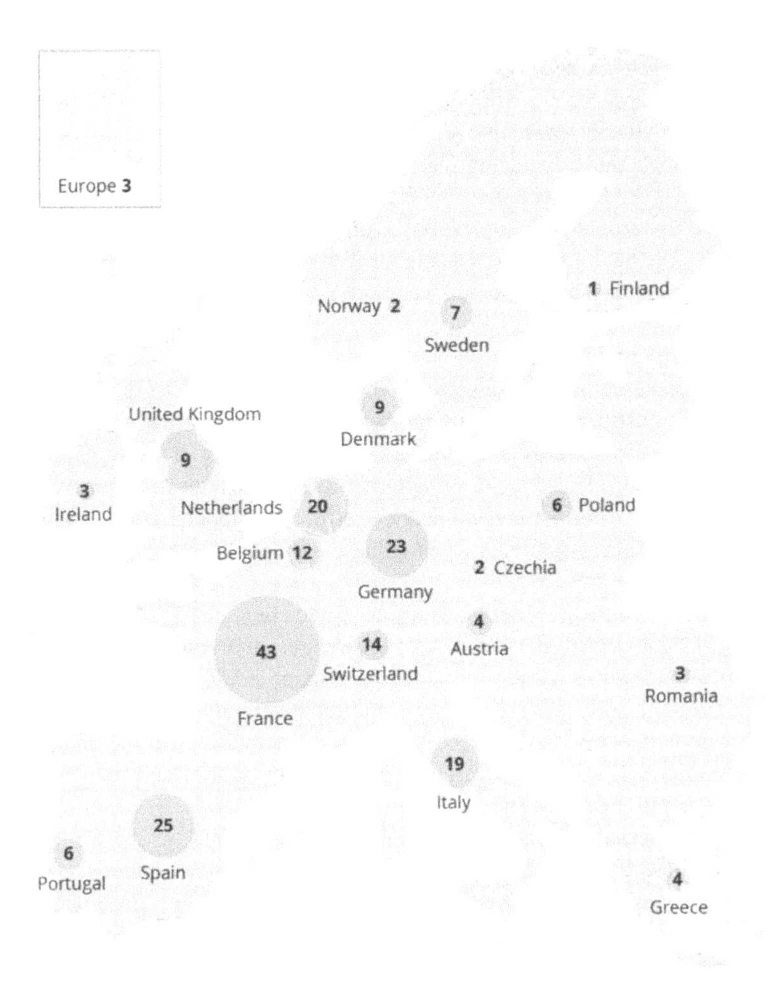

Figure 7.2 Map of incidents observed (from January 2021 to March 2023) (ENISA)

especially hospitals, bearing the brunt of these attacks. This trend is concerning, considering the critical nature of healthcare services. The analysis further underscores the significant impact of ransomware, which constitutes 54% of these incidents, indicating an alarming trend that necessitates immediate and strategic responses. A key aspect of the report is the correlation between the COVID-19 pandemic and the surge in cyber incidents. This period witnessed an uptick in data breaches and system vulnerabilities, often attributable to insiders or lapses in security protocols. The pandemic era, therefore, emerges as a focal point in the timeline of cyber threats, highlighting the need for enhanced vigilance and robust cybersecurity frameworks in the healthcare sector.

The report also sheds light on the technical vulnerabilities within healthcare systems, particularly those related to medical devices and software. An alarming 80% of healthcare organizations reported incidents stemming from these vulnerabilities, revealing a critical area that demands attention and action. Furthermore, the geopolitical landscape has also influenced the cyber threat scenario. The report notes a rise in DDoS attacks, particularly those orchestrated by pro-Russian hacktivist groups. Although these incidents form a smaller fraction of the total, their occurrence underlines the intersection of cybersecurity and geopolitics. Financially, the impact of these cyber threats is substantial, with the median cost of a significant security incident in the health sector estimated at €300,000. This economic burden, coupled with the potential for disrupted healthcare services and data breaches, makes it imperative for stakeholders in the health sector to prioritize and invest in effective cybersecurity measures.

A pressing issue in the healthcare sector is the rising frequency of ransomware attacks on healthcare institutions. The possibility of critical patient data being held hostage for financial gain not only jeopardizes individual privacy but also disrupts essential medical services. These attacks emphasize the immediate need for robust cybersecurity measures within the healthcare sector. The repercussions extend beyond mere data breaches, potentially causing harm to patients and compromising the integrity of healthcare delivery.

Furthermore, the healthcare threat landscape extends beyond the digital realm. The emergence of bioterrorism poses a unique challenge, involving the intentional release of harmful biological agents. This malicious tactic could have severe consequences on public health, necessitating a coordinated and vigilant response from healthcare providers and authorities. As the world grapples with the ongoing pandemic, the vulnerability of healthcare systems to both natural and man-made biological threats is more evident than ever.

In addition to external threats, internal challenges contribute to the intricate healthcare threat landscape. Insider threats, whether intentional or inadvertent, pose a significant risk to the confidentiality and integrity of patient information. Addressing these threats requires a delicate balance between providing healthcare professionals with access to necessary information for patient care and implementing stringent safeguards to prevent unauthorized access or data mishandling.

The healthcare threat landscape forms a complex and intricate puzzle, demanding a holistic approach. From cyber threats to the specter of bioterrorism and the nuances of internal challenges, healthcare providers must navigate this complex environment with resilience and adaptability. As the industry continues to innovate and digitize, fortifying defenses and proactively addressing emerging threats becomes increasingly crucial to ensuring the well-being of both healthcare systems and the individuals they serve.

7.2.2 Regulatory framework

The convergence of AI and healthcare cybersecurity represents a pivotal moment in the progression of medical technology. As we explore the expansive applications of AI in healthcare, a critical aspect deserving of attention is the regulatory framework governing this burgeoning field. Navigating the intricate terrain where cutting-edge technology meets the imperative to protect sensitive health data necessitates a nuanced understanding of regulatory measures.

At the forefront of this regulatory landscape stands HIPAA, a cornerstone of healthcare data protection in the United States. HIPAA sets rigorous standards for the privacy and security of patient information, delineating requirements for healthcare organizations to ensure the confidentiality and integrity of health data. As AI takes on an increasingly prominent role in processing and analyzing this data, adherence to HIPAA becomes an even more pressing consideration. Balancing the potential benefits of AI-driven insights with the imperative to safeguard patient privacy presents a delicate challenge, requiring a forward-thinking approach to regulatory compliance.

The intricacies of the regulatory framework extend beyond national and regional boundaries. International organizations, such as the World Health Organization (WHO) and the International Telecommunication Union (ITU), actively contribute to crafting guidelines that advocate for the responsible and ethical use of AI in healthcare. Given that AI algorithms transcend borders, the necessity for harmonized international standards becomes increasingly apparent, fostering collaboration and information exchange to address global challenges posed by the convergence of AI and healthcare cybersecurity.

The WHO has recently published guidelines outlining key regulatory considerations for AI in healthcare [9]. The publication underscores the importance of establishing the safety and effectiveness of AI systems, swiftly making them available to those in need, and fostering dialogue among stakeholders. This includes developers, regulators, manufacturers, health workers, and patients. Transparency and documentation are highlighted as crucial aspects, with an emphasis on documenting the entire product lifecycle and tracking development processes. For risk management, comprehensive attention is required for aspects such as intended use, continuous learning, human interventions, training models, and cybersecurity threats. Keeping models as simple as possible is encouraged. External validation of data and clear articulation of the intended use of AI are stressed to ensure safety and facilitate regulation. Commitment to data quality, exemplified through rigorous pre-release evaluations, is deemed vital to prevent systems from amplifying biases and errors. The publication outlines six key areas for regulating AI in healthcare.

(a) **Establishing AI systems' safety and effectiveness**: This involves ensuring that AI systems are safe and effective for their intended use and that they are rapidly made available to those who need them.
(b) **Fostering dialogue among stakeholders**: This involves creating a platform for dialogue among stakeholders, including developers, regulators, manufacturers, health workers, and patients.
(c) **Transparency and documentation**: This involves documenting the entire product lifecycle and tracking development processes to ensure transparency and accountability.
(d) **Risk management**: This involves comprehensively addressing issues like intended use, continuous learning, human interventions, training models, and cybersecurity threats, with models made as simple as possible.
(e) **Data quality**: This involves ensuring that data quality is maintained throughout the product lifecycle, such as through rigorously evaluating systems pre-release, to ensure that systems do not amplify biases and errors.
(f) **Privacy, security, and integrity**: This involves ensuring that robust legal and regulatory frameworks are in place to safeguard privacy, security, and integrity when using health data.

The regulatory landscape for AI in healthcare cybersecurity is a dynamic tapestry that reflects the evolving nature of technology and the imperative to protect sensitive health data. HIPAA, General Data Protection Regulation (GDPR), Food and Drug Administration (FDA) guidelines, and international organizations collectively shape the parameters within which healthcare organizations must operate as they embrace the transformative potential of AI. Navigating this intricate regulatory landscape requires a proactive and adaptive approach, one that balances the promise of innovation with an unwavering commitment to patient privacy and data security. As the journey into the future of AI in healthcare unfolds, a collaborative and globally informed regulatory framework will be instrumental in ensuring that the benefits of technological progress are realized without compromising the fundamental tenets of medical ethics and patient care.

7.2.3 Role of AI in strengthening cybersecurity

AI is a dynamic force reshaping the foundations of digital security in the medical field. The core role of AI in bolstering cybersecurity involves providing healthcare systems with proactive, intelligent, and adaptive defense mechanisms. Conventional cybersecurity measures often struggle to keep pace with the ingenious tactics of cyber threats. In this context, AI acts as a sentinel, employing ML algorithms to analyze extensive datasets and identify subtle patterns indicative of potential security breaches. The capacity of AI to learn and evolve in real time positions it as a powerful ally against the ever-changing strategies of cyber adversaries.

AI-driven programs gather valuable data that aids cybersecurity experts in gaining new insights into cybercriminal behavior. AI recognizes intricate data patterns, offers actionable recommendations, and enables autonomous mitigation.

It improves threat detection, aids decision-making, and accelerates incident response. AI tools, leveraging large datasets, can surpass human performance in various healthcare aspects, providing increased accuracy, reduced costs, and time savings while minimizing human errors.

The emergence of AI-driven threat intelligence adds another dimension to how technology contributes to healthcare cybersecurity. By continually monitoring and analyzing global cybersecurity trends, AI systems furnish healthcare organizations with timely and relevant insights into emerging threats. This not only enables institutions to stay ahead but also facilitates the sharing of threat intelligence within the healthcare ecosystem, fostering a collective defense against cyber threats.

However, it is important to note that hackers also have access to AI. A report [10] warns, "AI can therefore serve to strengthen and weaken security simultaneously, depending on whether it is used as an offensive or defensive tool." Hence, responsible and ethical use of AI is crucial to strengthening cybersecurity in healthcare. Undoubtedly, AI has the potential to revolutionize healthcare by integrating it into clinical practice. Yet, the increasing reliance on technology in healthcare raises the risk of cyber threats. AI can play a significant role in fortifying cybersecurity in healthcare by recognizing complex data patterns, providing actionable recommendations, and enabling autonomous mitigation. However, it is imperative to ensure that AI is used responsibly and ethically to enhance cybersecurity in healthcare.

7.2.4 Challenges and ethical considerations

The utilization of AI in healthcare involves handling vast amounts of sensitive patient data, making it susceptible to cyberattacks leading to data breaches and malicious activities. Therefore, it is crucial to explore the intricate intersection of technological advancement, ethical imperatives, and potential pitfalls. A primary challenge lies in the complex integration of AI into healthcare cybersecurity. Implementing AI-powered solutions requires a robust infrastructure, skilled personnel, and a comprehensive understanding of both AI and cybersecurity. The shortage of professionals proficient in this interdisciplinary space highlights the need for training programs to bridge the gap and ensure effective AI-driven security measures.

The black-box nature of many AI algorithms poses a central challenge. As these algorithms self-optimize, they become inscrutable, making it difficult to discern the decision-making processes underlying their security analyses. Balancing the complexity of advanced AI systems with the transparency necessary for ethical decision-making remains a pivotal challenge in adopting AI in healthcare cybersecurity.

Ethical considerations play a significant role, particularly regarding the responsible use of AI in safeguarding sensitive healthcare data. The healthcare sector demands a profound commitment to patient privacy, and AI integration must align with this ethical imperative. Consent, data ownership, and potential algorithmic bias amplify the ethical complexities. Ensuring AI systems prioritize patient welfare and adhere to ethical standards requires technical expertise and a robust ethical framework guiding development and deployment.

AI algorithms, reliant on data, may introduce biases and discrimination. For instance, if trained on biased data, an AI algorithm may make unfair decisions. Ensuring ethical design and training of AI algorithms is crucial to avoid such biases. Additionally, the use of AI in healthcare raises ethical concerns about the role of healthcare professionals. AI performing tasks previously done by professionals raises questions about the future role of humans in healthcare, emphasizing the preservation of the essential human touch.

The integration of AI into healthcare cybersecurity brings forth possibilities alongside challenges and ethical considerations. From technical intricacies to ethical imperatives, the journey toward a secure and ethically sound AI-driven healthcare landscape requires collective and multidisciplinary commitment. Navigating these challenges, the healthcare community must shape an ethical framework that safeguards against pitfalls and ensures the transformative power of AI is harnessed for the betterment of healthcare and the well-being of individuals.

7.3 AI for threat detection and prevention

Cybersecurity is a vital concern for healthcare systems, especially in the era of telehealth. With the increasing use of digital platforms and devices to deliver health services and store patient data, the risk of cyber-attacks also rises. To protect the confidentiality, integrity, and availability of health information, healthcare systems need to employ advanced and adaptive methods of threat detection and prevention. One of these methods is AI, which can analyze large amounts of data and identify patterns that indicate a potential threat [11]. Moreover, AI can also discover and fix vulnerabilities in a system, such as phishing emails, malware, or unauthorized access. By monitoring network traffic and detecting unusual activity, AI can alert the system administrators and help them respond to the incident before it causes any damage.

AI offers several advantages for cybersecurity in healthcare systems. One of them is its ability to learn and adapt to the changing environment and emerging threats. As new technologies and methods are developed in the healthcare sector, new types of cyberattacks also appear. AI can update its knowledge base and adjust its algorithms to cope with these changes and stay ahead of the attackers. This adaptability is essential for the healthcare sector, where the situation is dynamic and complex, and the threats are constantly evolving in sophistication.

Another advantage of AI is its use of heuristic and behavioral analysis to identify abnormal activities within the network. For example, AI can recognize if someone is trying to access patient records that they are not authorized to, or if they are deviating from the normal protocols. These anomalies can trigger an alert and prompt further investigation. This proactive approach is crucial for preventing emerging threats that may not have known signatures or patterns. In the following section, we will explain in detail how AI can be used for threat detection and prevention in the context of emerging healthcare systems.

7.3.1 Anomaly detection

Anomaly detection is a technique used to identify unusual patterns or behaviors in data that do not conform to expected norms [12]. Anomalies can indicate potential threats or problems that need to be addressed, such as cyber-attacks, fraud, and other malicious activities [13].

One of the applications of anomaly detection is in healthcare, where it can help detect and prevent fraudulent insurance claims. Insurance companies can use anomaly detection algorithms to identify claims that are outside the norm and may be fraudulent, based on factors such as the type, frequency, and amount of the claims [14]. By detecting fraudulent claims, insurance companies can save money and resources, and improve the quality of service for their customers.

Another application of anomaly detection in healthcare is in cybersecurity, where it can help detect and prevent cyber-attacks on healthcare systems. Anomaly detection algorithms can be used to identify unusual network traffic patterns that may indicate a cyber-attack, such as denial-of-service attacks, malware infections, or data breaches [15]. By detecting cyber-attacks, healthcare systems can protect their data and devices, and ensure the safety and privacy of their patients.

One of the algorithms used for anomaly detection in healthcare systems is deep learning, which is a branch of ML that uses artificial neural networks to learn from large datasets [16]. Deep learning models can be trained to identify patterns in data and detect anomalies that may be difficult to detect using traditional methods. For example, a deep learning model can be trained to identify patterns in EHRs, which are digital records of patient's health information, and detect anomalies that may indicate fraudulent activity or cyber-attacks [17].

7.3.2 Supervised and unsupervised detection

ML is a branch of AI that enables computers to learn from data and make predictions [18]. There are two main types of ML: supervised and unsupervised. These types differ in the kind of data they use and the goals they pursue [19]. Supervised and unsupervised learning are both useful for threat detection systems, which aim to identify malicious activities in computer networks and systems.

Supervised learning requires labeled data, which means that each data point has a known class or category. For example, a labeled data set of emails may have two classes: spam or not spam. Supervised learning algorithms learn from this labeled data and then apply their knowledge to new data. For example, a supervised learning algorithm may learn to classify new emails as spam or not spam based on the features of the labeled data. Supervised learning is suitable for threat detection when there are known examples of malicious activity, such as malware, phishing, or insider attacks.

Unsupervised learning does not require labeled data, which means that the data points do not have any predefined classes or categories. Unsupervised learning algorithms try to find patterns or structures in the data that may reveal some information or insight. For example, an unsupervised learning algorithm may cluster similar data points together based on their features. Unsupervised learning is suitable for threat detection when there are no known examples of malicious activity, or when the malicious activity is unknown or unpredictable. Unsupervised learning algorithms can detect anomalies or outliers in the data that may indicate a potential threat.

Insider threats are a serious challenge for cybersecurity, especially in emerging healthcare systems, where sensitive data and resources are involved [19]. Insider threats are malicious or unintentional actions by authorized users that can compromise the security or integrity of the system. For example, an insider may steal, leak, or tamper with confidential data, sabotage the system, commit fraud, or introduce vulnerabilities. Insider threats are hard to detect because insiders have legitimate access and knowledge of the system, and they may use sophisticated techniques to evade detection.

ML can help to detect insider threats by analyzing the data and behavior of the users and identifying any suspicious or anomalous patterns [21]. Supervised learning can be used to detect insider threats when there are labeled data of normal and malicious behavior. For example, a supervised learning algorithm can learn to classify user actions as normal or malicious based on the features of the labeled data. Unsupervised learning can be used to detect insider threats when there is no labeled data of malicious behavior, or when malicious behavior is unknown or unpredictable. For example, an unsupervised learning algorithm can learn to cluster user actions based on their features and detect any outliers or anomalies that may indicate an insider threat.

7.3.3 Predictive analysis

Cyber-attacks pose a serious threat to the security and privacy of healthcare systems, such as medical devices, EHRs, and cyber-physical systems (CPS). CPS are systems that integrate physical processes with computation and communication, such as smart hospitals, wearable devices, and implantable sensors. To protect these systems from cyber-attacks, it is essential to develop effective and efficient methods for detecting and preventing them. One such method is predictive analysis, which uses ML algorithms to analyze the data and behavior of the systems and to identify and prevent potential attacks before they cause any damage.

Two recent studies that propose different frameworks for applying predictive analysis to cyber-attack detection in healthcare systems are discussed, with their advantages and disadvantages, as well as their implications for future research. Both studies demonstrate the potential of predictive analysis for cyber-attack detection in healthcare systems.

The first study [22] proposes a cognitive ML-assisted Attack Detection Framework (CML-ADF) for cyber-attack detection in healthcare CPS. The main feature of this framework is that it adopts a patient-centric design, which means that it stores the patient's information on a trusted device, such as the end-user's mobile phone, and allows the end-user to control the data sharing access. The framework also uses ML models, such as neural networks and support vector machines, to predict cyber-attack behavior based on the data collected from the CPS. The predicted behavior is then processed and presented to the healthcare specialists, who can use it to make informed decisions and take appropriate actions. According to the study, the CML-ADF framework achieves high performance in terms of attack prediction ratio (96.5%), accuracy ratio (98.2%), efficiency ratio (97.8%), delay (21.3%), and communication cost (18.9%), compared to other existing models.

The second study [23] proposes a hybrid framework for intrusion detection in healthcare systems using deep learning, named "ImmuneNet." The framework combines deep learning and ML techniques, such as convolutional neural networks, recurrent neural networks (RNNs), and random forest, to detect and prevent cyberattacks on patient records in e-healthcare. The framework also uses a novel immune system-inspired algorithm, which mimics the natural immune system's ability to recognize and eliminate foreign invaders, such as viruses and bacteria. The algorithm learns from the normal and abnormal patterns of the patient records and generates antibodies that can detect and neutralize the intrusions. The study reports that the ImmuneNet framework outperforms other existing models in terms of accuracy (99.2%), precision (99.4%), and recall (99.1%).

7.3.4 Endpoint security

Endpoint security is the process of protecting devices that connect to networks and systems that store sensitive data, such as healthcare information [24]. These devices, such as mobile phones, laptops, and Internet-of-Things devices, are also called endpoints. Endpoints are vulnerable to malicious cyber threats that can compromise their functionality and data. Therefore, endpoint security detection is essential to identify and prevent these threats [24].

Endpoint security detection uses AI techniques to monitor and analyze the behavior and activities of endpoints. AI techniques can help to detect anomalies and indicators of compromise, such as malicious files, processes, and network activities. AI techniques can also help to automate the response and remediation of endpoint security incidents, such as isolating infected devices, blocking malicious connections, and restoring normal operations.

One of the AI techniques that is used for endpoint security detection is machine learning. ML can help to classify, cluster, and predict endpoint security events based on historical and real-time data [25]. For example, ML can help to identify malicious files by comparing them with known benign and malicious samples.

Another AI technique that is used for endpoint security detection is deep learning. Deep learning is a type of ML that uses multiple layers of artificial neural networks to learn complex patterns and features from data [26]. Deep learning can help to enhance the accuracy and efficiency of endpoint security detection by extracting high-level and abstract features from raw data, such as images, audio, and text. For example, deep learning can help to detect advanced malware that uses obfuscation, encryption, and polymorphism techniques to evade traditional detection methods.

A third AI technique that is used for endpoint security detection is NLP. NLP is the process of analyzing and generating natural language, such as speech and text. NLP can help to improve communication and collaboration between endpoint security systems and human users, such as security analysts, administrators, and end-users [27]. For example, NLP can help to generate natural language summaries and reports of endpoint security incidents and to enable voice and text-based interactions with endpoint security systems.

By using AI techniques, endpoint security detection can help to detect and prevent cyber threats and to ensure the security and privacy of healthcare data and systems. However, using AI techniques also poses some challenges, such as ethical, legal, and social implications, data quality and availability, and human oversight and trust. Therefore, endpoint security detection should be designed and implemented with care and caution.

7.3.5 Network security

Network security detection is the process of finding and preventing malicious attacks that target network systems. These systems include healthcare CPS, which are systems that combine physical devices and cyber components [22]. For example, telemedicine, remote surgery, and wearable health monitoring devices are all types of healthcare CPS.

AI can help improve network security detection in healthcare CPS by using different techniques, such as ML, NLP, and computer vision. AI can learn from data and improve its performance over time. For example, AI can learn from network logs, health records, and medical images to detect patterns and trends that indicate malicious activities or vulnerabilities. Also, AI can understand and generate natural language, such as text and speech. For example, AI can analyze the content and sentiment of network messages to identify phishing or spam attacks. Lastly, AI can recognize and process visual information, such as images and videos. For example, AI can verify the identity and authorization of users or devices accessing the network.

AI can offer several benefits for network security detection in healthcare CPS, such as Adaptability, by changing network environments and evolving attack strategies. For example, AI can update its models and rules based on feedback and new data to stay resilient against emerging threats. Automation, by automating and enhancing human efforts by providing alerts, recommendations, and solutions for network security issues. For example, AI can reduce false positives and negatives, increase efficiency and effectiveness, and save time and cost.

7.3.6 Data security

AI can provide many benefits for data security, such as improving the accuracy, speed, scalability, and reliability of the threat detection process, as well as reducing the cost, complexity, and human intervention. AI-based intrusion detection systems

(IDS) which is an application of AI for data security detection in healthcare systems can monitor the network traffic and system activities, and detect any malicious or abnormal behavior, such as unauthorized access, denial of service, malware infection, or data leakage [28]. AI-based IDS can use ML, deep learning, or NLP techniques to analyze the data and identify the patterns, signatures, or features of different types of attacks. AI-based IDS can also learn from feedback and adapt to the changing environment and threats.

AI-based encryption and decryption systems can also protect the data from unauthorized access or modification, by transforming the data into an unreadable form using a secret key. AI-based encryption and decryption systems can use neural networks, genetic algorithms, or quantum computing techniques to generate, distribute, and manage the keys, as well as to perform encryption and decryption operations [29]. AI-based encryption and decryption systems can also ensure the security and efficiency of data transmission and storage.

7.3.7 Threat hunting

Threat hunting is a proactive way of finding and stopping hidden cyberattacks that may harm an organization's network. It combines two methods: digital forensics and incident response [30]. Digital forensics is the process of collecting and analyzing data from computers, devices, and networks. Incident response is the process of responding to and managing a cyberattack. Together, these methods help uncover and stop cyber threats before they cause more damage.

In healthcare systems, threat hunting is very important because cyber-attacks can affect the safety and privacy of patients and medical staff. Healthcare systems use AI to improve their threat hunting capabilities. AI is a technology that can learn from data and perform tasks that normally require human intelligence. AI can help threat hunting in four ways:

1. AI can automate the threat hunting process, reducing the need for human analysts. This makes threat hunting faster and more accurate, as AI can detect and respond to cyber threats in real-time.
2. AI can analyze large and complex data from different sources, such as network traffic, logs, endpoints, sensors, and medical devices. Network traffic is the data that flows through a network. Logs are records of events and activities on a network or a device. Endpoints are devices that connect to a network, such as computers, smartphones, or tablets. Sensors are devices that measure physical conditions, such as temperature, pressure, or motion. Medical devices are devices that are used for diagnosis, treatment, or monitoring health conditions, such as pacemakers, insulin pumps, or MRI machines. AI can find patterns and anomalies in these data that may indicate a cyberattack.
3. AI can learn from past threat hunting experiences and improve its skills over time. AI can adapt to the changing nature of cyber threats, as cyber-attackers use new and different methods to attack healthcare systems.
4. AI can provide useful information and advice to security teams, helping them prioritize and deal with the most serious cyber threats. AI can also provide

evidence and context for the security teams to make informed decisions and actions.

7.3.8 User authentication and access control

User authentication and access control systems are crucial for ensuring the security and privacy of patient data. AI can enhance the effectiveness of these systems in several ways. First, AI can use ML algorithms to analyze user behavior and detect any anomalies that may indicate a compromised account. For example, if a user logs in from an unusual location or device, or performs an abnormal action, AI can alert the system and block the access. This helps prevent unauthorized access and protect patient data from falling into the wrong hands [31].

Second, AI can help implement more advanced and secure methods of user authentication, such as biometric recognition, voice recognition, or facial recognition. These methods can provide higher accuracy and convenience than traditional methods, such as passwords or tokens, which can be easily forgotten, stolen, or hacked. However, these methods also pose some challenges, such as privacy, consent, and data protection. For instance, biometric data can be sensitive and personal, and users may not want to share it with third parties or have it stored in a database. Moreover, biometric data can be affected by environmental factors, such as lighting, noise, or facial expressions, which can reduce the accuracy and reliability of the recognition [32].

Third, AI can also benefit access control systems by using ML to learn the access patterns and preferences of different users and groups. This can help optimize the access policies and rules, and ensure that the users have the appropriate level of access to the resources they need. For example, AI can grant or deny access based on the user's role, location, time, or task. AI can also help monitor and audit access activities and generate reports and alerts in case of any violations or breaches. This can help improve the accountability and transparency of the system and prevent any misuse or abuse of patient data [33].

7.3.9 Continuous monitoring and adaptive security

Continuous monitoring is a proactive approach to cybersecurity that collects and analyzes data about the security status of an information system. It reports the data in real-time or near real time, helping to identify potential threats and abnormal activities. It also evaluates the effectiveness of existing security controls and policies and provides feedback to improve the system's security posture and performance.

Adaptive security is a dynamic approach to cybersecurity that analyzes behaviors and events to prevent threats before they cause damage. It adjusts the security levels and responses based on risk assessments and situational awareness. It also learns from past incidents and updates the rules and policies accordingly. It provides proportional enforcement that matches the severity and context of the threat.

AI can strengthen the integration of continuous monitoring and adaptive security, by using techniques such as ML, deep learning, natural language processing, knowledge representation and reasoning, and expert systems [34]. These techniques enable systems to detect, analyze, and respond to cyber-attacks autonomously, optimizing and improving security operations and management. For example, AI can create security intelligence models that learn from data, such as network traffic, user behavior, and threat indicators. It can also implement intrusion detection and prevention systems that identify and block malicious activities in real-time. Moreover, it can use self-optimizing algorithms to forecast and mitigate the impact of cyber-attacks on healthcare systems, especially during pandemics.

AI can also contribute to the development of ambient intelligence environments in healthcare settings. These are environments that can sense, adapt, and respond to the needs, habits, gestures, and emotions of both users and providers [35]. For example, AI can enable smart devices and sensors that monitor the health status and activities of patients and caregivers. It can also provide personalized and interactive services, such as reminders, alerts, and recommendations.

In a nutshell, AI can enhance cybersecurity for emerging healthcare systems, by integrating continuous monitoring and adaptive security. It can provide effective detection and response to cyber threats, using various techniques and tools. It can also support the development of ambient intelligence environments, which can improve the quality and efficiency of healthcare services. However, AI also needs to address the new challenges and risks that these environments entail and ensure that they are secure and trustworthy. Table 7.1 highlights the specific AI algorithms used in the detection and prevention of cyber threats in healthcare systems.

Table 7.1 AI algorithms for threat detection and prevention

Reference	Application	AI algorithm	Healthcare Usage
[14–16]	Anomaly Detection	K-means and K-medoids Clustering, Autoencoder and Artificial Neural Network (ANN), Random Forests, J48, k-Nearest Neighbors, Additive Regression, and Linear Regression	Detect abnormal patterns in network traffic or user behavior that indicate malicious activity
[20,21,36]	Supervised & Unsupervised Detection	Linear Regression, Logistic Regression, Decision Trees, Random Forest, Support Vector, Machines (SVM), Neural Networks, K-Means Clustering, Hierarchical Clustering, DBSCAN (Density-Based Spatial Clustering of Applications with Noise), Principal Component Analysis (PCA), Autoencoders	Classify and cluster cyber-attacks in healthcare networks using labeled and unlabeled data

(Continues)

Table 7.1 AI algorithms for threat detection and prevention (Continued)

Reference	Application	AI algorithm	Healthcare Usage
[22,23,37]	Predictive Analysis	Support Vector Machine, Neural Networks, Decision Trees, K-Nearest Neighbor, and Random Forest	Anticipate cyber-attacks by generating dynamic threat models from available data sources
[26,27,38]	Endpoint Security	Behavioral Analysis, Machine Learning, Supervised Learning, Unsupervised Learning, and Reinforcement Learning	Protect devices such as smart pacemakers and insulin pumps from cyberattacks by monitoring and blocking unauthorized access
[22,39]	Network Security	Deep Learning and Machine Learning	Enhance the performance and accuracy of intrusion detection systems by learning from complex and large-scale data
[28,29]	Data Security	Behavioral Analysis, Knowledge Representation & Reasoning, Machine Learning, Deep Learning, and Natural Language Processing	Encrypt and protect sensitive data such as patient records and medical images from unauthorized access or leakage
[30,40]	Threat Hunting	Machine Learning, Predictive Analytics, Pattern detection, and Task Automation	Proactively search for and identify potential cyber threats before they cause damage or disruption
[31–33]	User Authentication and Access Control	Supervised Learning, Unsupervised Learning, and Reinforcement Learning	Verify the identity and access rights of users based on their physiological or behavioral characteristics such as the face, voice, or fingerprint
[34,35]	Continuous Monitoring and Adaptive Security	Machine Learning, Deep Learning, and Natural Language Processing	Dynamically adjust the security policies and controls based on the feedback from the environment and the actions of the agents

7.4 AI for data protection

AI technologies, with their ability to analyze vast amounts of data and identify patterns, have the potential to significantly improve data protection measures even when the integration of AI into data protection strategies is not without its challenges. These technologies can help in detecting and preventing data breaches as explored in the previous section, identifying vulnerabilities, and ensuring compliance with data protection regulations. However, the integration of AI technologies into data protection strategies also presents several challenges. These include technical challenges related to the compatibility of AI systems with existing data protection infrastructure, as well as legal and regulatory challenges. The use of AI also raises several ethical considerations as the decision-making processes of AI systems are often opaque, leading to concerns about accountability and transparency. Despite these challenges, the potential benefits of AI for data protection make it a promising area for further research and development. The following sections delve deeper into these aspects, providing a comprehensive overview of the role of AI in data protection.

7.4.1 Technologies for data protection

Just like how a gem would be kept in a secure vault, health data needs to be protected with various advanced technologies. One such technology is encryption, which acts like a secret code. Only those who have the key can read the information, just like how only someone with a secret map can find the hidden treasure. Another important tool is firewalls, which work like guards at the gates of a castle, allowing only trusted visitors to enter. They monitor and control incoming and outgoing network traffic, keeping out unwanted or harmful intruders. Additionally, antivirus software acts like a health inspector, scanning for and getting rid of any viruses that might harm our computer, just like how a doctor checks for and treats any illnesses in a patient.

But technology keeps advancing, and so do the methods to protect data. We now have more sophisticated tools like biometric security—think of fingerprint or facial recognition, like a door that only opens for you. There is also blockchain, a system that records information in a way that makes it difficult or impossible to change or hack. Imagine a series of puzzle pieces interlocked so tightly that it is nearly impossible to take them apart. And then there is AI, which is like having a super-smart guard who can predict and prevent break-ins before they even happen. All these technologies work together to form a strong shield, keeping our digital information safe and secure. In this section, federated learning, homomorphic encryption, and blockchain are reviewed as technologies that enhance the protection of digital healthcare data.

7.4.1.1 Federated learning

Federated learning is a way of training AI models without sharing the raw data among different parties. Instead, each party trains a local model on its data and then sends the model parameters to a central server, where they are aggregated to form a global model. This process is repeated until the global model reaches the desired accuracy. Federated learning can preserve data privacy, reduce communication costs, and enable data diversity [41–43].

Figure 7.3 illustrates how federated learning works, client devices are at the forefront, representing individual users' smartphones, IoT devices, or computers. Each of these devices hosts a local ML model, serving as the initial point for data analysis. These local models are trained on the data residing on the respective devices, allowing for personalized insights without the need for data to leave the user's control. The server acts as the central coordinator, collecting periodic model updates from all client devices. It then aggregates these insights to update the global model, which benefits from the collective knowledge without directly

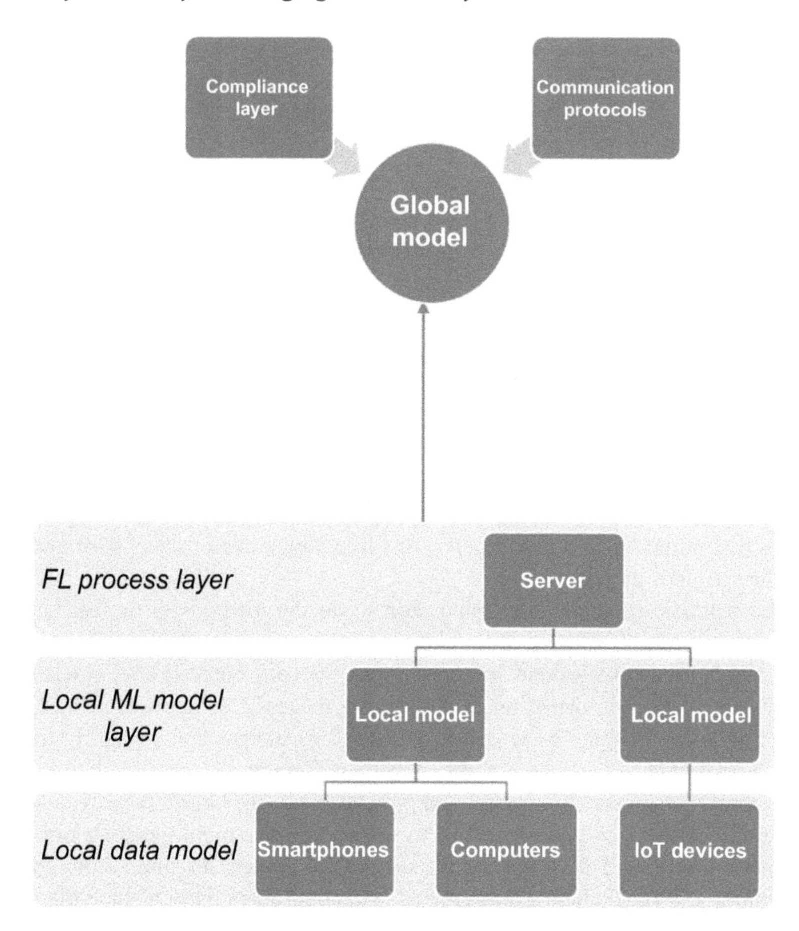

Figure 7.3 Federated learning architecture

accessing or storing user data. In the context of government and economic regulations, an additional layer for compliance and privacy safeguards is essential to ensure that the architecture aligns with relevant legal frameworks. Secure communication protocols ensure data privacy during the update process, making Federated Learning an innovative approach to ML that combines individual insights while respecting data privacy and regulatory requirements.

In healthcare, federated learning can be used to leverage data from different hospitals or clinics to improve diagnosis, treatment, and prevention of diseases, without compromising the confidentiality of patients' health records [41,44]. Consider a research institution collaborating with several hospitals to train a model for predicting the progression of a particular disease. Instead of transferring the EHRs from the hospitals to the research institution, the parties involved would collaborate to train the model in a distributed way. Each hospital would use its data to train the local model, and then share the updated model variables with the research institution. The research institution would then combine the updated model parameters from each party to create a more accurate and robust model. This innovative approach keeps data locally stored at each entity, sharing only the model updates with a central server [45].

7.4.1.2 Homomorphic encryption

This is particularly vital in scenarios where patient data needs to be available for research, diagnostics, or treatment planning, but privacy and confidentiality must be maintained. Homomorphic encryption is a type of encryption that allows computations to be performed on encrypted data without decrypting it. The results of the computations are also encrypted and can only be decrypted by the owner of the secret key. Homomorphic encryption can ensure data security and functionality, enable outsourcing of computation, and support various operations [46–49].

The need for collaborative treatment often necessitates the sharing of patient data among various healthcare providers. Homomorphic encryption enables this data sharing securely. As depicted in Figure 7.4, doctors, specialists, and medical researchers can access and work with the encrypted data without ever exposing the actual sensitive information. This not only streamlines collaborative efforts but also significantly reduces the risk of data breaches.

The application of homomorphic encryption in healthcare systems offers a revolutionary approach to data protection. It ensures the confidentiality and security of sensitive health data across various aspects of healthcare, from patient records management and secure data sharing to telemedicine and medical research. As this technology evolves, it will increasingly become a cornerstone in building secure, efficient, and privacy-focused healthcare systems.

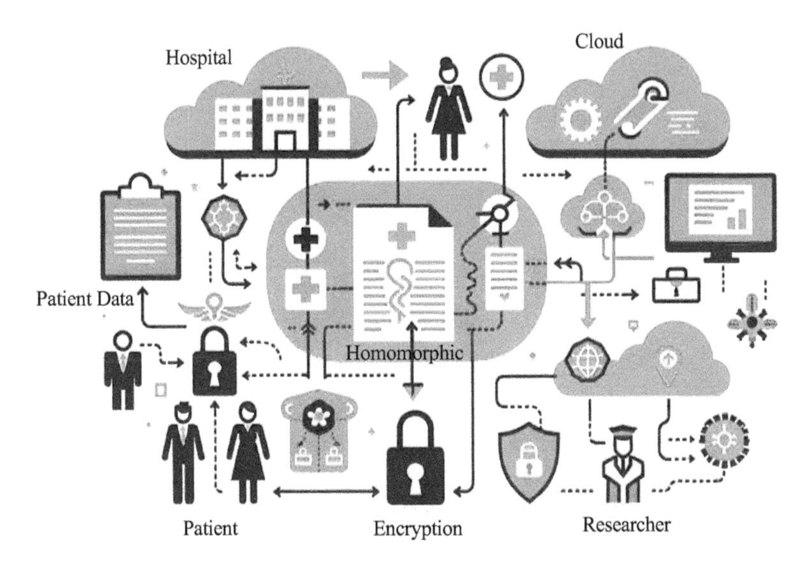

Figure 7.4 Homomorphic encryption

7.4.1.3 Blockchain technology

Blockchain's most significant contribution to healthcare cybersecurity lies in its ability to guarantee data integrity [50]. Every piece of information entered into a blockchain is time-stamped and linked to the previous entry, creating a chronological and unalterable chain of data. In healthcare, this means that patient records, treatment histories, and medication information are traceable and tamper-evident. This level of traceability is crucial not only for patient care but also for clinical trials and pharmaceutical supply chains, ensuring the authenticity of drugs and tracking their journey from manufacturer to patient.

Blockchain is a distributed ledger technology that records and verifies transactions in a decentralized and immutable way. Each transaction is stored in a block that is linked to the previous block by a cryptographic hash as depicted in Figure 7.5. The blocks form a chain that can be verified by all the participants in the network.

Traditional healthcare systems often store patient data in centralized databases, which are vulnerable to cyber-attacks and data breaches [51]. Blockchain introduces a decentralized model, where patient data is distributed across a network, reducing the risk of systemic failures and data theft. This decentralization also enhances data accessibility, allowing healthcare providers to access up-to-date patient information securely and efficiently, leading to better coordinated and more effective care [52–54].

By ensuring data integrity, enhancing patient privacy, enabling secure data sharing, and reducing fraudulent activities, blockchain can contribute significantly to building a more secure, efficient, and patient-centered healthcare system.

Table 7.2 highlights some of the other current and emerging AI technologies that enhance the protection of digital healthcare data, such as secure aggregation,

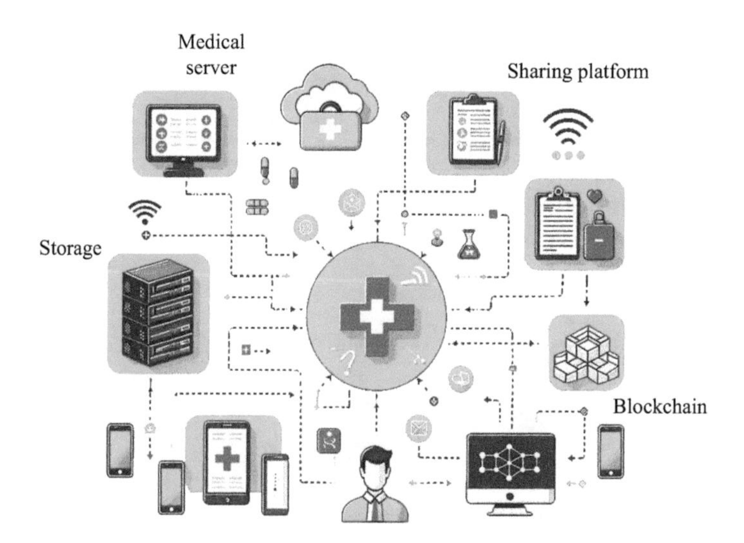

Figure 7.5 Blockchain technology

Table 7.2 Advance technologies for data protection

Reference	Technology	Description	Benefits	Limitations
[45,55]	Federated learning	A distributed learning approach that allows multiple parties to collaboratively train a shared AI model without exchanging their raw data	Preserves data privacy and ownership, reduces communication and storage costs, enables data diversity and scalability	Requires coordination and synchronization among parties, may introduce noise and bias due to data heterogeneity, may be vulnerable to malicious attacks
[56,57]	Secure aggregation	A cryptographic technique that allows multiple parties to compute the aggregate of their data without revealing their values	Protects data confidentiality and integrity, reduces communication overhead, enables collaborative analytics	Requires trust and cooperation among parties, may incur computational and communication costs, may not preserve data utility
[58,59]	Differential privacy	A mathematical framework that quantifies the privacy loss of a data analysis algorithm by adding calibrated noise to the output	Provides rigorous privacy guarantees, allows data sharing and reuse, enables statistical analysis	May degrade data quality and utility, may increase complexity and uncertainty, may not prevent linkage attacks
[60,61]	Homomorphic encryption	A cryptographic technique that allows computation on encrypted data without decrypting it	Ensures data security and functionality, enables outsourcing of computation, supports various operations	May incur high computational and communication costs, may introduce noise and errors, may not support complex operations
[62,63]	Multi-party computation	A cryptographic technique that allows multiple parties to jointly compute a function of their inputs without revealing them	Preserves data privacy and functionality, enables distributed computation, supports various applications	May incur high computational and communication costs, may depend on network and protocol assumptions, and may not be efficient or practical
[64,65]	Edge AI	A distributed computing paradigm that performs AI tasks at the edge of the network, close to the data sources	Enhances data privacy and security, reduces latency and bandwidth, enables real-time and context-aware processing	May face resource and energy constraints, may lack coordination and standardization, may not leverage cloud capabilities

(Continues)

Table 7.2 Advance technologies for data protection (Continued)

Reference	Technology	Description	Benefits	Limitations
[45,51,66]	Blockchain	A distributed ledger technology that records and verifies transactions in a decentralized and immutable way	Improves data transparency and accountability, facilitates data sharing and exchange, enables smart contracts and incentives	May consume high energy and resources, may face scalability and interoperability issues, may raise legal and regulatory challenges

differential privacy, homomorphic encryption, multi-party computation, and edge AI. Also, the benefits and limitations of these technologies, as well as the ethical and legal implications of their application in healthcare settings are highlighted.

7.4.2 AI in enhancing data protection

Using advanced AI algorithms for secure data storage, management, encryption, backup, and recovery, telehealth applications should provide an additional layer of security to sensitive personal health information (PHI). PHI is subject to strict regulations and ethical standards to ensure its confidentiality, integrity, and availability. Any unauthorized access, disclosure, modification, or loss of PHI can have serious consequences for the patient's privacy, safety, and well-being, as well as for the reputation and liability of the healthcare providers. Therefore, it is essential to implement effective and robust data protection measures for telehealth applications.

7.4.2.1 Anomaly detection

As one particular aspect of data protection for telehealth systems, anomaly detection that monitors the network traffic and user behavior to detect any deviations signaling a security breach or leakage is worth noting. With their impressive capability of adapting themselves to new data and also being adaptive toward environmental changes, AI algorithms can provide many ideal solutions for anomaly detection.

It is also highly important to secure the telehealth systems from any unauthorized entry or manipulation [67]. For achieving such a high level, anomaly detection techniques can be commonly used which are the methods for detecting abnormal behaviors or patterns in the data. Anomaly detection could apply to the field of network traffic and user behavior as it allows detecting much evidence that can indicate any malicious intentions or information leakage [15,16]. For example, an anomaly detection system based on ML could observe the network traffic for telehealth systems and detect any abnormalities or suspicious packets that may be stealing malware aimed at exploiting vulnerabilities to steal the data. Similarly, an anomaly detection system can monitor the user activities in a telehealth system and detect any suspicious or fraudulent behaviors such as those that violate access policies and pretend to be valid users/users who tamper with data.

In anomaly detection, AI algorithms are used because they can learn through the given data and adapt to ever-changing environments. The AI algorithms employ various methods to capture the typical dynamics of network activity or user behavior and also detect anomalies. Other types of supervised, unsupervised, or semi-supervision learning methods can be used for classification changes normal as well as anomalous according to the availability of data.

Some examples of AI algorithms that are used for anomaly detection in telehealth systems are:

(a) ***Local outlier factor (LOF)***: This is an unsupervised algorithm that measures the local density of data points and assigns a score to each point based on how isolated or similar it is to its neighbors. A high score indicates an outlier, while a low score indicates a normal point. This algorithm can be used to detect anomalies in heart rate data, as it can capture both global and local outliers [68].
(b) ***Random forests (RF)***: This is a supervised algorithm that builds a collection of decision trees and aggregates their predictions to classify the data. A decision tree is a structure that splits the data based on certain criteria and assigns a label to each leaf node. This algorithm can be used to detect anomalies in network traffic, as it can handle high-dimensional and heterogeneous data and provide interpretable results [69].
(c) ***Long short-term memory (LSTM):*** This is a deep learning algorithm that uses a type of RNN to process sequential data. An RNN is a network that has feedback loops and can store information from previous inputs. An LSTM is a special kind of RNN that can learn long-term dependencies and avoid the problem of vanishing or exploding gradients. This algorithm can be used to detect anomalies in user behavior, as it can capture temporal patterns and dependencies and handle variable-length sequences [70].

7.4.2.2 Enhancements in encryption through AI

The combination of AI and advanced encryption technologies assumes a pivotal role in the arena of healthcare data protection. The realization that quantum computing makes traditional encryption vulnerable further emphasizes the importance of seeking alternative alternatives such as post-quantum cryptography (PQC) [71]. With its data-processing capabilities unmatched by anything else, the AI is an invaluable partner in strengthening the security of confidential medical information.

Deep learning algorithms play a very critical role in mimicking quantum algorithms and determining how such approaches can impact the chosen encryption standards. This participation helps to create quantum-resistant encryption algorithms that protect the privacy and also the integrity of healthcare data [72]. In this regard, the Quantum Neural Network (QNN) manifests itself as an appealing AI algorithm [73]. Using the ideas of quantum computing together with neural network designs, QNNs are very capable of modeling sophisticated systems. This modeling functionality provides very worthwhile knowledge on developing encryption approaches that can resist quantum decryption algorithms, which is an essential consideration while securing health data from emerging threats.

The adaptability of AI is very well reflected in the creation of many adaptive encryption models. These models, driven by the AI algorithms dynamically modify the encryption parameters based on threat perception and sensitivity of health data. Genetic algorithms, under the evolutionary optimization schemes, perform much better in the development of encryption standards over evolving threats ensuring that health data is made much more secure. Turning to another AI-based method, Reinforcement learning (RL) becomes very relevant in healthcare data protection. A process is here taking place that resembles the incremental advances of an RL agent, who is trained to modify encryption algorithms after receiving data about the attempted security breaches.

7.4.2.3 AI in access control and authentication

Integration of AI into authentication systems has brought a revolutionary era in the field of protecting sensitive data for healthcare. The old static, monadic ways of access control and authentication have evolved into dynamic context-aware systems supported by AI techniques. In healthcare, this paradigm shift is especially important because the protection of patient data and information takes precedence.

An innovative feature of AI-powered authentication in health care is the use of behavioral biometrics [74]. Unlike static fingerprints, behavioral biometrics focus on the pattern of user activity. It includes subtle aspects of typing rhythms, mouse motions, and also touch-screen interactions that offer a more intricate level of user verification. The ability of deep learning algorithms such as RNNs and also Long Short-Term Memory (LSTM), for instance, that work well with sequential data makes them suitable for analyzing behavioral biometrics [75]. With these interaction paradigms, the system may be enabled to quickly evaluate the user identity, and any anomalies indicative of unauthorized access are easily detected thus ensuring increased security.

One more crucial role of AI in the security aspect of health data protection is related to robust biometric authentication (RBA) systems. These systems evaluate the access request risk in terms of many factors like user location, device used, network security status, and also trends regarding the patterns of previously granted requests [76]. These factors are then analyzed using ML algorithms, from decision trees to the support vector machines that calculate the risk score. When the risk score exceeds a predetermined threshold, additional authentication measures are initiated by the system. This may include sending a one-time password (OTP) or biometric verification. This dynamic approach allows for detailed authentication procedures to be applied selectively, thus minimizing the inconvenience of healthcare personnel without compromising on a high level of security.

In the healthcare environment where seamless access to critical patient data is very key, this fluidity of AI-driven approaches becomes a point of emphasis. Both continuous adaptation of the authentication requirements based on risk levels and improvement in user experience strengthen the security. The healthcare experts enjoy the simplified workflows with the system automatically adjusting authentication protocols to a fine security and operations balance. In other words, AI-based authentication not only secures healthcare information but also is designed to combat the distinctive issues associated with the volatile and data-centric nature of healthcare.

7.4.3 Ethical considerations in AI for data protection

Respecting patient privacy stands as a foundational ethical commitment in the implementation of AI for data protection in healthcare, reflecting a commitment already embedded in practice. Patients possess the right to understand how their data is utilized and to provide informed consent [77]. Robust data protection laws and clear policies governing data collection, storage, and sharing are imperative, aligning seamlessly with the existing global landscape.

Healthcare institutions have successfully established frameworks where AI algorithms and systems adhere to stringent data protection laws, securing patient consent and maintaining unwavering transparency throughout the entire process [78]. Privacy within the realm of AI-driven healthcare extends beyond mere data protection—it encompasses the effective safeguarding of personal information, confidentiality assurance, and the prevention of unauthorized access. Vigilant implementation of robust encryption methods and access controls has effectively shielded patient data from cyber threats.

In this accomplished setting, healthcare professionals diligently conduct regular audits and security assessments, proactively identifying vulnerabilities to ensure continual compliance with ethical data protection standards [79]. A proven commitment exists to actively monitor and rectify any unintended biases that may emerge in AI algorithms, addressing potential disparities and fostering equal access to healthcare services for all patients [80].

Recognizing the dynamic nature of ethical considerations in AI for data protection, there is an ongoing commitment to continuous evaluation and improvement. Professionals in Nigeria's AI landscape actively engage in discussions, research endeavors, and ongoing training, demonstrating a commitment to staying abreast of the latest ethical standards and best practices in AI for data protection. This ongoing dedication ensures the highest levels of trust and security within healthcare systems, underscoring a commitment to ethical excellence that has already become an integral part of the profession.

7.4.4 Integration challenges and solutions

The diversity of data sources and formats is one of the foremost challenges in integrating data protection algorithms. Healthcare systems rely on data from various sources such as EHRs, wearable devices, and diagnostic equipment. These data sources often use different formats, making it challenging to create unified algorithms for data protection. Where healthcare infrastructures vary, harmonizing these diverse data types remains a significant challenge [81].

To tackle this diversity, healthcare institutions and technology providers invest in data standardization efforts [82], establishing common data formats and protocols that can seamlessly accommodate data from various sources. This standardization enables the development of data protection algorithms that work effectively across the spectrum of healthcare data, ensuring that patient information remains secure and accessible when needed.

AI technologies require substantial computational resources, which can strain the infrastructure of emerging healthcare systems, especially in resource-constrained regions. Integrating data protection algorithms alongside AI may demand even more computational power, making scalability a significant concern [83]. Balancing the need for robust data protection with limited resources is a challenge that healthcare providers and policymakers must navigate effectively.

Addressing this challenge involves strategic investments in both infrastructure and human resources. The development of high-performance computing clusters and cloud-based solutions helps healthcare institutions handle the computational demands of AI-driven data protection. Additionally, training and upskilling healthcare professionals and IT personnel in AI and data protection technologies ensure the efficient utilization of available resources.

Respecting patient privacy is a critical ethical consideration [84]. However, integrating data protection solutions must also consider the need for efficient healthcare services. Achieving a balance between privacy preservation and timely data access for healthcare professionals is a challenge. It is vital to establish clear guidelines and consent mechanisms that align with cultural and legal frameworks while ensuring patient data remains secure.

To navigate this challenge, healthcare institutions adopt a patient-centric approach to data protection [52]. This approach involves educating patients about the importance of data privacy and obtaining informed consent for data usage. Transparent and user-friendly consent processes help strike a balance between privacy and accessibility, ensuring that healthcare providers deliver quality care while safeguarding patient rights.

Data protection algorithms and solutions should seamlessly integrate with existing healthcare systems. However, interoperability issues often arise due to the absence of standardized data formats and protocols. In the healthcare landscape, where different systems may be in use, achieving interoperability is a substantial challenge. Establishing common data standards and protocols is essential to overcome this hurdle.

Interoperability is achieved through collaborative efforts between healthcare institutions, government bodies, and technology providers. Standardizing data exchange formats and adopting widely accepted healthcare data standards facilitate seamless integration. By adhering to interoperability standards, healthcare systems ensure that data protection solutions work cohesively with existing technologies, enhancing overall healthcare efficiency and security.

As healthcare systems become more reliant on AI and data protection solutions, they also become attractive targets for cyberattacks. Ensuring the security of these integrated systems is a constant challenge. Nigeria, like many other countries, must continually invest in cybersecurity measures to safeguard patient data and protect against emerging threats.

7.5 Case studies

The integration of AI technologies in healthcare cybersecurity showcases a range of challenges and innovative solutions across various institutions. At Johns Hopkins, the challenge was the manual work required to identify insider threats and phishing, along with high rates of false positives. Their solution was an AI-driven privacy analytics platform, which dramatically reduced investigation times and improved workflow efficiency, as detailed by Health Catalyst [85].

Similarly, a Fortune 500 Telecom Company faced inefficiencies in labeling network traffic data. They turned to Snorkel Flow for classifying encrypted network data flows, achieving high accuracy and robust performance against data drift, as Snorkel AI reports [86]. This approach was mirrored by a US government agency, which also used Snorkel Flow but focused on application classification and network attack detection, leading to more efficient AI/ML application development and data labeling [86].

The collaboration between DeepMind and the Royal Free London NHS Trust brought to light issues around patient consent and regulatory challenges, particularly in pseudonymized patient data analysis. This case highlighted the importance of clear consent and accountability in AI implementations, a topic explored by Health IT Security [10].

AI-Driven Clinical Laboratories have utilized ML systems for disease diagnosis and microorganism identification, improving accuracy and efficiency in disease diagnosis and treatment selection [87]. In emergency departments, AI algorithms have been implemented for patient triaging and decision support, leading to improved patient flow and the prioritization of high-risk cases [87].

These case studies prove the broader application of Healthcare AI Technologies across various healthcare settings showing significant impacts in data protection, diagnostic accuracy, and patient care optimization, illustrating a transformative shift toward more secure, efficient, and patient-centered care.

Table 7.3 offers a detailed view of some current case studies of healthcare providers that have successfully implemented AI-based cybersecurity solutions, providing insights into the unique cybersecurity challenges faced and the specific AI technologies deployed to address them, along with their outcomes.

Table 7.3 AI in cybersecurity case studies

Reference	Case study	Healthcare provider	Cybersecurity challenges	AI technologies implemented	Outcomes
[85]	01	Johns Hopkins	Manual work in identifying insider threats, phishing, high false positives	AI-driven privacy analytics platform	Reduced investigation time and false-positive rate, improved workflow efficiency

(Continues)

Table 7.3 AI in cybersecurity case studies (Continued)

Reference	Case study	Healthcare provider	Cybersecurity challenges	AI technologies implemented	Outcomes
[86]	02	Fortune 500 Telecom Company	Inefficient labeling of network traffic data, brittle solutions, data distribution changes	Snorkel Flow for classifying encrypted network data flows	High accuracy in network data classification, robust performance against data drift
[86]	03	U.S. government agency	Inadequate hand-labeling of sensitive data, underutilization of cyber SMEs	Snorkel Flow for application classification and network attack detection	Improved AI/ ML application development for cybersecurity, efficient data labeling
[10]	04	DeepMind and Royal Free London NHS	Lack of patient consent for data use, regulatory challenges	Pseudonymized patient data analysis	Highlighted the need for clear consent and accountability in AI implementations
[87]	05	AI-Driven Clinical Laboratories	Accuracy and efficiency in disease diagnosis	ML systems for disease diagnosis and microorganism identification	Improved accuracy and efficiency in disease diagnosis and treatment selection
[87]	06	AI in Emergency Departments	Management of increasing demands, patient flow, and triage accuracy	AI algorithms for patient triaging and decision support	Improved patient flow and prioritization of high-risk cases
[10,87]	07	Healthcare AI Technologies	Data protection, diagnostic accuracy	Various AI applications in healthcare settings	Diverse impacts including data protection, diagnostic accuracy, and patient care optimization

The developments, discussed in both BMC Medical Education and Health IT Security, exemplify the diverse and critical role AI technologies play in modern healthcare cybersecurity.

7.6 Future trends and challenges

The growing integration of advanced technologies in healthcare systems makes AI an increasingly important tool for data security and system integrity. Among the most visible trends is that AI algorithms used to predict and counter cyber threats get increasingly sophisticated. The development of ML and deep learning has made AI systems able to detect anomalies and patterns that indicate cyber-attacks even those unseen before. This predictive capability might change everything in threat detection and prevention, enabling healthcare systems to prevent vulnerabilities before they can be exploited.

The other major trend is the integration of blockchain technology alongside AI in order to improve data privacy. The decentralized nature of blockchain provides a strong foundation for protecting patient information preserving its accuracy and privacy. Combined with AI, blockchain technology can create a much more agile and safe way to process access controls, audit, and HIPAA compliance in the United States.

Other opportunities and challenges that come along with the use of AI with IoT devices in health care include integration. Among others, IoT devices and sensors including wearable health monitors and smart hospital beds generate massive amounts of data that can be utilized by AI to make inferences about the evolution of patient health and to identify system efficiency. But this aside, they also increase the scope of the threat gendering new sources in need of protection. Unfortunately, the development of AI systems that can secure these devices and the networks they link to without limiting their functionality turns out to be far from simple. Another important challenge is the ethical issues involved and privacy matters. However, as AI systems begin to accumulate access to a lot of data that represent the privacy information of patients, the essence and use of this data must be ethical. It encompasses not only data protection from unauthorized access but also guaranteeing that AI systems are built and operated without compromising the confidentiality of patients' identities or their consent requirements.

In addition to this, the changing regulatory environment poses a threat to AI transformation applied in healthcare cybersecurity. In response to changes brought about by technology, governments and regulatory bodies across the world are straining to catch up with this phenomenon. This means that health organizations have a lot of regulations they need to navigate across international borders because these laws differ from state to state hence subject to change. This will necessitate constant monitoring and steady flexibility to protect compliance while taking full advantage of AI technology.

7.7 Lesson learned

By reading this chapter we have taken many useful lessons with us. These takeaways emphasize the relative complexity and fluidity of incorporating AI into the healthcare cybersecurity landscape. They emphasize continuous invention, ethical attention, and partnership to realize the capabilities that AI has in securing sectoral industries such as healthcare from cyber-attacks. Among the lessons are:

1. **Artificial intelligence role in cybersecurity:** The roles AI can play in improving cybersecurity in healthcare are numerous and among them are threat detection, predictive analysis as well as response functions.

2. **Digital transformation risks:** The transition toward digital healthcare systems serves as yet another step to exposure by enabling additional vulnerabilities and escalating the threat of cyber-attacks that require tight security.
3. **Importance of data privacy:** Sensitive data protection is critical because it requires properly maintaining EHRs and compliance with regulatory frameworks, such as HIPAA.
4. **Integration challenges:** In healthcare cybersecurity, AI integration has its challenges, among them interoperability, data diversity, and the requirement of vast computational resources.
5. **Ethical considerations:** Ethical elements play a very significant role in the desire to protect data processing for the installation of AI and it is necessary to accentuate transparency, patient consent, and algorithmic bias.
6. **Future trends**: Advancements in AI and blockchain technologies are shaping up the field by further improving data privacy and system integrity.
7. **Collaboration and continuous learning:** To counter cybersecurity threats in the healthcare systems, concerted efforts involving continuous collaboration, innovation, and adaptation to emerging technologies and means will have to be made.

7.8 Conclusion

The integration of AI into healthcare cybersecurity is a crucial and evolving field. This chapter has explored the current applications, benefits, and challenges of AI in securing healthcare systems. As technology advances, AI will play an increasingly vital role in detecting, preventing, and responding to cyber threats. However, this advancement comes with its own set of challenges, including ethical considerations, data privacy concerns, and the need for continuous adaptation to emerging threats. The future of healthcare cybersecurity lies in the balance between leveraging AI potential and managing its complexities responsibly. Ultimately, the goal is to ensure a secure, efficient, and trustworthy healthcare ecosystem for all stakeholders.

References

[1] V. Stephanie, I. Khalil, M. Atiquzzaman and X. Yi, "Trustworthy Privacy-Preserving Hierarchical Ensemble and Federated Learning in Healthcare 4.0 With Blockchain," *IEEE Transactions on Industrial Informatics*, 2023.
[2] M. Muthuppalaniappan and K. Stevenson, "Healthcare Cyber-Attacks and the COVID-19 Pandemic: An Urgent Threat to Global Health," *International Journal for Quality in Health Care*, 2020.
[3] R. Mehta and A. Muzaffar, "future-of-cybersecurity-healthcare," November 2023. [Online]. Available: https://www2.deloitte.com/us/en/pages/advisory/articles/future-of-cybersecurity-healthcare.html. [Accessed 12 December 2023].

[4] M. Benedict, P. Chase and M. Zuk, "cybersecurity-and-patient-safety-healthcare-setting," 11 May 2023. [Online]. Available: https://www.mitre.org/news-insights/publication/cybersecurity-and-patient-safety-healthcare-setting. [Accessed 22 November 2023].

[5] M. M. Mijwil, "The Significance of Machine Learning and Deep Learning Techniques in Cybersecurity: A Comprehensive Review," *Iraqi Journal for Computer Science and Mathematics*, 2023.

[6] Cleardata, "2022 Healthcare Threat Landscape Review," 2022. [Online]. Available: https://www.cleardata.com/2022-healthcare-threat-landscape-review/. [Accessed 17 October 2023].

[7] C. Garland, "The threat landscape for healthcare organizations," 22 September 2023. [Online]. Available: https://www.cleardata.com/2022-healthcare-threat-landscape-review/.

[8] A. H. Abad and S. Corbiaux, "Health threat landscape," 05 July 2023. [Online]. Available: https://www.enisa.europa.eu/publications/health-threat-landscape. [Accessed 26 December 2023].

[9] Geneva, "WHO outlines considerations for regulation of artificial intelligence for health," 19 October 2023. [Online]. Available: https://www.who.int/news/item/19-10-2023-who-outlines-considerations-for-regulation-of-artificial-intelligence-for-health.

[10] J. McKeon, "Could Artificial Intelligence Transform Healthcare Cybersecurity?," 20 September 2021. [Online]. Available: https://healthitsecurity.com/news/could-artificial-intelligence-transform-healthcare-cybersecurity. [Accessed 27 October 2023].

[11] C. Ardito, T. D. Noia, E. Sciascio, D. Lofú, A. Pazienza and F. Vitulano, "An Artificial Intelligence Cyberattack Detection System to Improve Threat Reaction in e-Health," *Italian Conference on Cybersecurity*, 2021.

[12] J. Prajapati and P. N. Choudhary, "A Systematic Review on Anomaly Detection," *International Journal of Advanced Research in Science, Communication and Technology*, 2023.

[13] A. Toshniwal, K. Mahesh and R. Jayashree, "Overview of Anomaly Detection Techniques in Machine Learning," in *2020 Fourth International Conference on I-SMAC (IoT in Social, Mobile, Analytics and Cloud) (I-SMAC)*, 2020.

[14] E. N. N. Nortey, R. Pometsey, L. Asiedu, S. Iddi and F. Mettle, "Anomaly Detection in Health Insurance Claims Using Bayesian Quantile Regression," *International Journal of Mathematics and Mathematical Sciences*, 2021.

[15] Y.-C. Wang, Y.-C. Houng, H.-X. Chen and S. Tseng, "Network Anomaly Intrusion Detection Based on Deep Learning Approach," *Italian National Conference on Sensors*, 2023.

[16] H. Abdel-Jaber, D. Devassy, A. A. Salam, L. Hidaytallah and M. EL-Amir, "A Review of Deep Learning Algorithms and Their Applications in Healthcare," *Algorithms*, vol. 15, no. 71, 2022.

[17] W. Hurst, B. Tekinerdogan, T. Alskaif, A. Boddy and N. Shone, "Securing Electronic Health Records against Insider-threats: A Supervised Machine Learning Approach," vol. 26, 2022.

[18] A. Tyagi and P. Chahal, "Artificial Intelligence and Machine Learning Algorithms," in *Research Anthology on Machine Learning Techniques, Methods, and Applications*, IGI Global, 2022, pp. 421–446.
[19] A. Mohamed, A.-J. Dhiya, M. Jamila, H. Abir and A. J. Aljaaf. "A Systematic Review on Supervised and Unsupervised Machine Learning Algorithms for Data Science," in *Supervised and unsupervised learning for data science*, 2020, pp. 3–21.
[20] S. T. Argaw, J. R. Troncoso-Pastoriza, D. Lacey, *et al.*, "Cybersecurity of Hospitals: Discussing the Challenges and Working towards Mitigating the Risks," *BMC Medical Informatics and Decision Making*, vol. 20, pp. 1–10, 2020.
[21] D. C. Le and N. Zincir-Heywood, "Exploring Anomalous Behaviour Detection and Classification for Insider Threat Identification," *International Journal of Network Management*, 2021.
[22] A. AlZubi, M. Al-Maitah and Alarifi, "Cyber-attack Detection in Healthcare Using Cyber-physical System and Machine Learning Techniques," *Soft computing*, 2021.
[23] M. A. Kumaar, D. Samiayya, P. M. D. R. Vincent, K. Srinivasan, C.-Y. Chang and H. Ganesh, "A Hybrid Framework for Intrusion Detection in Healthcare Systems Using Deep Learning," *Big Data Analytics for Smart Healthcare applications*, vol. 9, 2021.
[24] M. Plachkinova and K. Knappb, "Least Privilege across People, Process, and Technology: Endpoint Security Framework," *Journal of Computer Information Systems*, vol. 63, no. 5, pp. 1153–1165, 2022.
[25] C. Nilă, I. Apostol and V. Patriciu, "Machine Learning Approach to Quick Incident Response," in *2020 13th International Conference on Communications (COMM)*, 2020.
[26] M. Sewak, S. K. Sahay and H. Rathore, "Deep Reinforcement Learning for Cybersecurity Threat Detection and Protection: A Review," in *International Conference On Secure Knowledge Management In Artificial Intelligence Era*, 2021.
[27] M. R. Karim, P. Chowdhury, L. Rahman and S. Kazary, "An Al-Based Security System Using Computer Vision and NLP Conversion System," in *2021 3rd International Conference on Sustainable Technologies for Industry 4.0 (STI)*, 2021.
[28] J. B. Awotunde and S. Misra, "Feature Extraction and Artificial Intelligence-Based Intrusion Detection Model for a Secure Internet of Things Networks," *Illumination of Artificial Intelligence in Cybersecurity and Forensics*, pp. 21–44, 2022.
[29] A. Alabdulatif, I. Khalil and M. S. Rahman, "Security of Blockchain and AI-Empowered Smart Healthcare: Application-Based Analysis," *Applied Sciences*, vol. 12, no. 21, p. 11039, 2022.
[30] A. Dimitriadis, N. Ivezic, B. Kulvatunyou and I. Mavridis, "D4I - Digital Forensics Framework for Reviewing and Investigating Cyber Attacks," *Array*, vol. 5, p. 100015, 2020.

[31] S. Harris, "AI in Healthcare Cybersecurity," October 2023. [Online]. Available: https://stepofweb.com/ai-healthcare-cybersecurity/. [Accessed 14 December 2023].
[32] B. Murdoch, "Privacy and Artificial Intelligence: Challenges for Protecting Health Information in a New Era," *BMC Med Ethics*, vol. 122, 2021.
[33] K. Thilagam, A. Beno, M. V. Lakshmi, C. B. Wilfred and S. M. George, "Secure IoT Healthcare Architecture with Deep Learning-Based Access Control System," *Journal of Nanomaterials*, 2022.
[34] M. R. Valanarasu, "Smart and Secure IoT and AI Integration Framework," *Journal of IoT in Social, Mobile, Analytics, and Cloud*, vol. 1, no. 3, pp. 172–179, 2019.
[35] P. N. Martinez-Martin, M. Z. Luo and M. A. Kaushal, "Ethical Issues in Using Ambient intelligence in health-care settings," *The Lancet Digital Health*, vol. 3, no. 2, pp. e115–e123, 2021.
[36] M. Hazratifard, F. Gebali and M. Mamun, "Using Machine Learning for Dynamic Authentication in Telehealth: A Tutorial," in *Prime Archives in Sensors*: 2nd Edition, 2023.
[37] M. Sobrino, M. L. Coleman, J. Springfield, S. Neal and A. Winburn, "Examining Telemental Health in Mississippi: Brief Report," *Journal of Counseling Research and Practice*, vol. 8, no. 1, 2023.
[38] S. Mannarino, V. Calcaterra, G. Fini, *et al.*, "A Pediatric Telecardiology System That Facilitates Integration between Hospital-based Services and Community-based Primary Care," vol. 181, 2024.
[39] H. Bansal, D. Gupta and D. Anand, "Blockchain and Artificial Intelligence in Telemedicine and Remote Patient Monitoring," in *Handbook on Augmenting Telehealth Services*, 2024.
[40] M. D. Xames and T. G. Topcu, "A Systematic Literature Review of Digital Twin Research for Healthcare Systems: Research Trends, Gaps, and Realization Challenges," *IEEE Access*, 2024.
[41] G. Long, T. Shen, Y. Tan, L. Gerrard, A. Clarke and J. Jiang, "Federated Learning for Privacy-Preserving Open Innovation Future on Digital Health," *Humanity Driven AI*, pp. 113–133, 2021.
[42] F. Jiang, Z. Chen, L. Liu and J. Wang, "Federated Learning-Based Privacy Protection for IoT-based Smart Healthcare Systems," in *2023 IEEE/CIC International Conference on Communications in China (ICCC Workshops)*, China, 2023.
[43] P. Perchinunno, A. Massari, S. L'Abbate and C. Crocetta, "Blockchain and the General Data Protection Regulation: Healthcare Data Processing," in *ICCSA 2023: Computational Science and Its Applications – ICCSA 2023 Workshops*, 2023.
[44] N. Rieke, J. Hancox, W. Li, *et al.*, "The Future of Digital Health with Federated Learning," *Digital Medicine*, 2020.
[45] A. Musa, A. O. Abdulfatai, S. E. Jacob and F. D. Oluyemi1, *"Government and Economic Regulations on Federated Learning in Emerging Healthcare System," Elsevier*, 2023.

[46] E. Westphal and H. Seitz, "Digital and Decentralized Management of Patient Data in Healthcare Using Blockchain Implementations," *Frontiers in Blockchain*, vol. 4, no.732112, 2021.

[47] X. Liu, Z. Wang, C. Jin, F. Li and G. Li, "A Blockchain-Based Medical Data Sharing and Protection Scheme," *IEEE Access*, vol. 7, pp. 118943–118953, 2019.

[48] K. Kiania, S. M. Jameii and A. M. Rahmani, "Blockchain-Based Privacy and Security Preserving in Electronic Health: A Systematic Review," *Multimedia Tools and Applications*, vol. 82, p. 28493–28519, 2023.

[49] J. Scheibner, M. Ienca and E. Vayena, "Health Data Privacy through Homomorphic Encryption and Distributed Ledger Computing: An Ethical-legal Qualitative Expert Assessment Study," *BMC Medical Ethics*, 2022.

[50] M. Attaran, "Blockchain Technology in Healthcare: Challenges and Opportunities," *International Journal of Healthcare Management*, vol. 15, no. 1, pp. 70–83, 2020.

[51] A. Musa, A. Abdulfatai, D. Oluyemi, S. Jacob and A. Imoize, "Taxonomy for Artificial Intelligence and Blockchain Technology Used for Telehealth Systems," *Institution of Engineering and Technology (IET)*, 2023.

[52] P. Hemalatha, "Monitoring and Securing the Healthcare Data Harnessing IOT and Blockchain Technology," *Turkish Journal of Computer and Mathematics Education (TURCOMAT)*, vol. 12, no. 2, 2021.

[53] P. Pandey and R. Litoriya, "Securing and Authenticating Healthcare Records through Blockchain Technology," *Cryptologia*, vol. 44, no. 4, 2020.

[54] P. Sharma, N. R. Moparthi, S. Namasudra, V. Shanmuganathan and C.-H. Hsu, "Blockchain-based IoT Architecture to Secure Healthcare System Using Identity-based Encryption," *Expert Systems*, vol. 39, no. 10, 2021.

[55] O. Choudhury, A. Gkoulalas-Divanis, T. Salonidis, *et al.*, "Differential Privacy-enabled Federated Learning for Sensitive Health Data," *arXiv preprint arXiv:1910.02578*, 2019.

[56] S. Pirbhulal, O. W. Samuel, W. Wu, A. K. Sangaiah and G. Li, "A Joint Resource-aware and Medical Data Security Framework for Wearable Healthcare Systems," *Future Generation Computer Systems*, vol. 95, pp. 382–391, 2019.

[57] S. B. Othman, F. A. Almalki, C. Chakraborty and H. Sakli, "Privacy-Preserving Aware Data Aggregation for IoT-based Healthcare with Green Computing Technologies," *Computers and Electrical Engineering*, vol. 101, p. 108025, 2022.

[58] Y. Zhao and J. Chen, "A Survey on Differential Privacy for Unstructured Data Content," *ACM Computing Surveys*, vol. 54, no. 10, pp. 1–28, 2022.

[59] R. Gupta, I. Gupta, D. Saxena and A. K. Singh, "A Differential Approach and Deep Neural Network Based Data Privacy-preserving Model in Cloud Environment," *Journal of Ambient Intelligence and Humanized Computing*, vol. 14, p. 4659–4674, 2023.

[60] L. Zhang, J. Xu, P. Vijayakumar, P. K. Sharma and U. Ghosh, "Homomorphic Encryption-Based Privacy-Preserving Federated Learning in IoT-

Enabled Healthcare System," *IEEE Transactions on Network Science and Engineering*, vol. 10, no. 5, pp. 2864–2880, 2022.

[61] M. M. Salim, I. Kim, U. Doniyor, C. Lee and J. H. Park, "Homomorphic Encryption Based Privacy-Preservation for IoMT," *Applied Sciences*, vol. 11, no. 18, p. 8757, 2021.

[62] D. Li, X. Liao, T. Xiang, J. Wu and J. Le, "Privacy-Preserving Self-serviced Medical Diagnosis Scheme Based on Secure Multi-party Computation," *Computers & Security*, vol. 90, p. 101701, 2020.

[63] A. A. Siddique, W. Boulila, M. S. Alshehri and F. Ahmed, "Privacy-Enhanced Pneumonia Diagnosis: IoT-Enabled Federated Multi-Party Computation in Industry 5.0," *IEEE Transactions on Consumer Electronics*, pp. 1-1, 2023.

[64] A. A. Abdellatif, L. Samara, A. Mohamed, A. Erbad and C. Fabian, "MEdge-Chain: Leveraging Edge Computing and Blockchain for Efficient Medical Data Exchange," *IEEE Internet of Things Journal*, vol. 8, no. 21, pp. 15762–15775, 2021.

[65] M. A. Rahman, M. S. Hossain, N. A. Alrajeh and N. Guizani, "B5G and Explainable Deep Learning Assisted Healthcare Vertical at the Edge: COVID-19 Perspective," *IEEE Network*, vol. 34, no. 4, pp. 98–105, 2020.

[66] L. Hirtan, P. Krawiec, C. Dobre and J. M. Batalla, "Blockchain-Based Approach for e-Health Data Access Management with Privacy Protection," in *2019 IEEE 24th International Workshop on Computer Aided Modeling and Design of Communication Links and Networks (CAMAD)*, Cyprus, 2019.

[67] J. Awotunde, A. Imoize, R. Jimoh, *et al.*, "AIoMT Enabling Real-Time Monitoring of Healthcare Systems: Security and Privacy Considerations," *Handbook of Security and Privacy of AI-Enabled Healthcare Systems and Internet of Medical Things*, pp. 97–133, 2024.

[68] E. Šabić, D. Keeley, B. Henderson and S. Nannemann, "Healthcare and Anomaly Detection: Using Machine Learning to Predict Anomalies in Heart Rate Data," *AI & Society*, vol. 36, pp. 149–158, 2021.

[69] G. Zachos, I. Essop, G. Mantas, K. Porfyrakis, J. C. Ribeiro and J. Rodriguez, "An Anomaly-Based Intrusion Detection System for Internet of Medical Things Networks," *electronics*, vol. 10, no. 21, p. 2562, 2021.

[70] K. Highnam, K. Arulkumaran, Z. Hanif and N. R. Jennings, "BETH Dataset: Real Cybersecurity Data for Anomaly Detection Research," *TRAINING*, vol. 763, no. 66.88, p. 8, 2021.

[71] B. Dash and S. Ullah, "Quantum-safe: Cybersecurity in the age of Quantum-Powered AI," *World Journal of Advance Research and Reviews*, vol. 21, no. 01, pp. 1555–1563, 2024.

[72] M. Sharma, Y. Mahajan and A. Alzahrani, "Personalized Medicine Through Quantum Computing: Tailoring Treatments in Healthcare," in *Quantum Innovations at the Nexus of Biomedical Intelligence*, 2024.

[73] P. Decoodt, T. J. Liang, S. Bopardikar, *et al.*, "Hybrid Classical–Quantum Transfer Learning for Cardiomegaly Detection in Chest X-rays," *Journal of Imaging*, vol. 9, no. 7, p. 128, 2023.

[74] L. Cascone, V. Loia, M. Nappi and F. Narducci, "Soft Biometrics for Cybersecurity: Ongoing Revolution for Industry 4.0," *Computer*, vol. 57, no. 1, pp. 40–50, 2024.
[75] H. Qin, H. Zhu, X. Jin, Q. Song, M. A. El-Yacoubi and X. Gao, "EmMix-former: Mix Transformer for Eye Movement Recognition," *arXiv preprint, p. arXiv:2401.04956*, 2024.
[76] A. Mohinabonu and I. Durdona, "Analysis of Non-Cryptographic Methods for Software Binding to Facial Biometric Data of User Identity," *International Journal Of Advance Scientific Research*, vol. 03, no. 07, pp. 38–47, 2023.
[77] M. Ashok, R. Madan, A. Joha and U. Sivarajah, "Ethical Framework for Artificial Intelligence and Digital Technologies," *International Journal of Information Management*, vol. 62, 2022.
[78] C. Wang, S. Liu, H. Yang, J. Guo, Y. Wu and J. Liu, "Ethical Considerations of Using ChatGPT in Health Care," *Journal of Medical Internet Research*, vol. 25, 2023.
[79] B. Y. Kasula, "AI Applications in Healthcare a Comprehensive Review of Advancements and Challenges," *International Journal of Management Education for Sustainable Development*, vol. 06, no.06, 2023.
[80] M. Jeyaraman, S. Balaji, N. Jeyaraman and S. Yadav, "Unraveling the Ethical Enigma: Artificial Intelligence in Healthcare," *Cureus*, vol. 15, no. 8, 2023.
[81] Z. Wenhua, F. Qamar, T.-A. N. Abdali and R. Hassan, "Blockchain Technology: Security Issues, Healthcare Applications, Challenges and Future Trends," *Electronics*, vol. 12, no. 03, 2023.
[82] J. Espinoza, N. Y. Xu and D. C. Klonoff, "The Need for Data Standards and Implementation Policies to Integrate CGM Data into the Electronic Health Record," *Diabetes Science and Technology*, vol. 17, no. 2, 2021.
[83] J. Burrell and M. Fourcade, "The Society of Algorithms," *Annual Review of Sociology*, vol. 47, 2021.
[84] H. Liu, R. G. Crespo and O. S. Martínez, "Enhancing Privacy and Data Security across Healthcare Applications Using Blockchain and Distributed Ledger Concepts," *Healthcare*, 2020.
[85] H. C. Editors, "improving-healthcare-data-security-with-AI," 18 September 2019. [Online]. Available: https://www.healthcatalyst.com/insights/improving-healthcare-data-security-with-AI. [Accessed 22 October 2023].
[86] N. Acton, "ai-in-cybersecurity," 5 May 2022. [Online]. Available: https://snorkel.ai/ai-in-cybersecurity/. [Accessed 28 December 2023].
[87] S. A. Alowais, S. S. Alghamdi, N. Alsuhebany, *et al.*, "Revolutionizing Healthcare: The Role of Artificial Intelligence in Clinical Practice," *BMC Medical Education*, 2023.

Chapter 8

Deep based anomalies detection in emerging healthcare system

Babu Kaji Baniya[1] *and Thomas Rush*[1]

The Internet of Things (IoT) has experienced widespread adoption, revolutionizing the way tasks are performed remotely, much like their physical counterparts. Its applications span various domains, including smart home automation, healthcare IoT, education, agriculture, smart grid, industrial IoT, security, and surveillance, among others. Our primary focus is on IoT's role in healthcare, highlighting the critical importance of robust security measures. IoT enables remote patient monitoring, timely diagnostics, and personalized recommendations. Given the online interaction between remote patients and healthcare providers, ensuring the integrity and confidentiality of diagnostic data is paramount. Inadequate security in communication channels could potentially lead to alterations in patient treatment or medication plans, posing risks of emergencies or unintended consequences. Hence, implementing robust measures to safeguard the multifaceted healthcare data generated from various sources is imperative. We particularly emphasize the significance of time series data within the Internet of Medical Things (IoMT). To address this, we leverage the Long Short-Term Memory (LSTM) approach for performance evaluation, comparing its results with stack ensemble methods. Utilizing the WUSTL Enhanced Healthcare Monitoring System (EHMS) dataset for validation, which comprises biometric and network features, totaling over 16,318 samples categorized into normal and attack categories. Additionally, we explore the most distinctive features using the Extra Trees Classifier to minimize computational complexity and enhance abnormality detection rates using ensemble algorithms. Various evaluation metrics, including accuracy, F1-score, precision, recall, and confusion matrices, are employed. Both deep learning and stack ensemble methods demonstrate notable performance across these metrics, achieving minimal false rates. Consequently, our proposed model surpasses existing machine learning algorithms, firmly establishing its effectiveness in safeguarding the security and integrity of emerging healthcare data within the IoT ecosystem.

[1]Department of Computer Science and Information Systems, Bradley University, USA

Keywords: Biometric; distinctive; ensemble; evaluation; healthcare; LSTM; IoMT

8.1 Introduction

The Internet of Things (IoT) constitutes a diverse array of interconnected devices and systems that have revolutionized operations across various sectors. These applications span domains such as healthcare, security [1,2], education, agriculture [3], air traffic control, and surveillance, encompassing technologies like CCTV, drones, and unmanned aerial vehicles (UAVs). Additionally, IoT facilitates remote control of household electronic appliances like air conditioners, surveillance systems, washing machines, refrigerators, and automatic door controls. Figure 8.1 illustrates these applications. The pervasive adoption of IoT is fueled by the widespread availability of cost-effective smart devices and robust communication network infrastructure [4]. These devices enable remote control and seamless information exchange through standard communication protocols. Ranging from wearable accessories to large-scale machines, IoT devices are equipped with diverse sensors. Notably, remote monitoring of home security cameras is a prevalent application, offering surveillance capabilities from anywhere globally [5].

According to a report from the International Telecommunication Union (ITU), as of 2023, approximately 5.4 billion people worldwide, accounting for about 67% of the global population, were internet users. Prior to the 2019 pandemic, the total number stood at around 4.1 billion, representing approximately 53% of the world population. The significant surge in internet usage during the pandemic, amounting

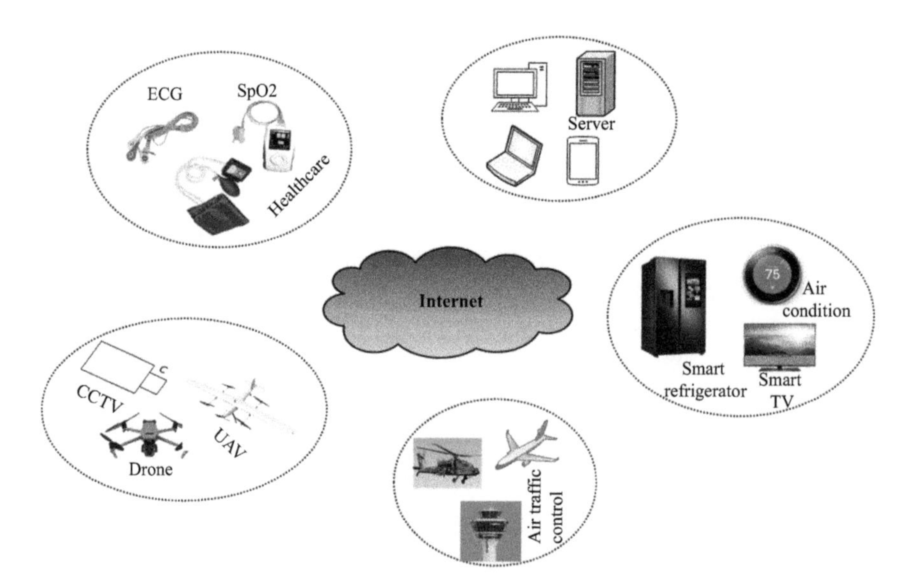

Figure 8.1 The overview of numerous applications of IoT

to a rise of approximately 14%, underscores the pivotal role of digital connectivity in the face of global crises [6,7]. The widespread fear and anxiety brought about by the rapid spread of the COVID-19 virus placed immense pressure on healthcare systems globally, prompting many individuals to postpone or cancel scheduled medical check-ups due to concerns about virus exposure. This reluctance to seek medical attention, coupled with the heightened transmissibility of the virus, further exacerbated the situation, leading to widespread cancellations of medical appointments. In response, remote healthcare monitoring systems emerged as viable solutions, enabling the delivery of essential healthcare services while mitigating the risk of virus transmission. Additionally, the IoT played a pivotal role in connecting individuals in geographically disadvantaged areas with limited access to healthcare services. The implementation of IoT-based healthcare systems has proven to be mutually beneficial for both patients and healthcare providers, contributing significantly to the exponential growth of digital healthcare solutions amidst the COVID-19 pandemic [8].

Security challenges persistently pose significant concerns for the IoT, especially in the realms of Wireless Sensor Networks (WSN), Machine-to-Machine (M2M) communication, and Cyber-Physical Systems (CPS) [9,10]. The IP protocol, serving as the primary standard for connectivity in IoT, makes ensuring the security of the entire deployment architecture imperative. Potential attacks on these networks not only have the capacity to disrupt IoT services but also to compromise the privacy, integrity, and confidentiality of data. The IoT paradigm, characterized by interconnected networks and diverse devices, inherits traditional security issues from computer networks. The complexity introduced by constrained resources, prevalent in small devices like sensors that have limited power and memory in IoT devices, further amplifies security challenges. Consequently, security solutions must be specifically tailored to address these constraints within the IoT architecture [5].

IoT operates within a layered architecture consisting of three key layers: physical, network, and application, as shown in Figure 8.2. Each layer plays a distinct role in ensuring the security of IoT systems. The physical layer is responsible for authentication and authorization mechanisms, verifying the identity of users or devices, and controlling their access to resources. Encryption techniques guarantee the confidentiality of transmitted data, allowing only authorized entities to access and decode it [11]. Additionally, secure boot and updates safeguard the integrity of IoT devices by permitting the execution of only authenticated code, thus preventing unauthorized access or tampering. Moving to the network layer, security measures such as firewalls and intrusion detection systems are employed to thwart unauthorized access and monitor for malicious activities. Physical security considerations come into play with tamper detection mechanisms and the integration of secure elements to protect cryptographic keys [5]. Privacy controls, a crucial aspect of IoT security, focus on data minimization and user consent, ensuring that only necessary information is collected and processed. Lifecycle management practices address security concerns at each stage of a device's life cycle, from manufacturing to disposal. By implementing these comprehensive security

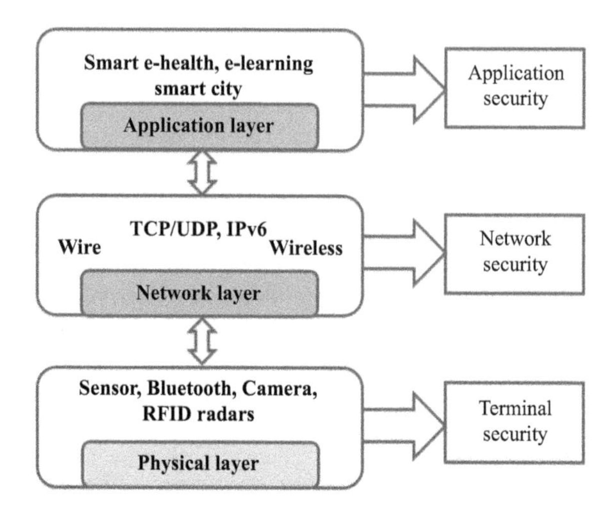

Figure 8.2 Layer architecture and protocol of IoT

measures across the layers, IoT environments can establish robust protection against potential risks, safeguarding both users and the underlying network infrastructure [12].

Recently, IoT has emerged as an important domain, particularly contributing to the advancement of HMS. The primary goal of IoT-based HMS is to precisely monitor individuals and establish connections between various healthcare-related services and entities globally via the Internet [13]. This facilitates the collection, sharing, monitoring, storage, and analysis of data generated by these entities [14]. The advent of technologies such as IoT, machine learning (ML), and artificial intelligence (AI) has ushered in a new paradigm. This paradigm involves the interconnection of physical objects in intelligent applications like smart cities, smart homes, smart grids, smart vehicular systems, and smart healthcare, enabling remote addressing and control [15]. In particular, an IoT-based remote monitoring healthcare system holds significant importance in diagnosing disorders and monitoring patients for effective medical care. The integration of sensor networks into the human body proves immensely valuable in facilitating these healthcare endeavors [16].

The integration of IoT in healthcare signifies a breakthrough, presenting both opportunities for remote health services and notable challenges. The promising aspects include accessing reliable, convincing, and cost-effective services from remote healthcare professionals and providers. IoT systems have enabled the construction of reliable HMS using affordable and low-power sensors [17]. However, the challenges faced by IoT mirror those encountered in HMS. A significant hurdle involves managing the vast array of data formats generated by IoT devices, which encompass wearable sensors (such as SpO_2 sensors, blood pressure sensors, temperature sensors, electrocardiogram sensors, etc.), medical implants, and monitoring equipment [17–20]. These devices continuously collect data about patients' health status. Another critical challenge lies in ensuring the security and privacy of this data. Given the sensitive nature of healthcare-related information, safeguarding patient details, diagnosis reports, medication plans, and the privacy of healthcare professionals remain of paramount concern [20,21].

In recent years, significant efforts have been made to address security concerns within the IoT paradigm. Researchers have pursued various approaches to tackle security challenges across different dimensions, including issues at specific layers, application security, architectural considerations, and protocol vulnerabilities. While some approaches focus on addressing security concerns at individual layers, others strive to establish end-to-end security solutions for IoT systems. For instance, a recent survey conducted by Alaba *et al.* introduces a taxonomy categorizing IoT security issues based on applications, architecture, communication, and data, diverging from traditional layered architecture models [22]. This taxonomy facilitates a comprehensive understanding of threats across hardware, network, and application components [23]. Additionally, Granjal *et al.* conducted a survey that delves into security concerns associated with IoT protocols. Their analysis includes a detailed examination and comparison of various key management systems and cryptographic algorithms, shedding light on critical aspects of IoT security [24].

To address this challenge effectively, we implemented LSTM classifiers, known for their proficiency in detecting attacks due to their superior ability to model and learn sequential data, particularly in healthcare network traffic patterns. One key advantage of LSTM networks is their capability to capture long-term dependencies in data sequences, crucial for identifying subtle anomalies in network traffic [25,26]. Moreover, LSTM networks feature memory cells that retain information over extended periods, enabling them to recognize persistent irregularities effectively. Additionally, these networks can handle variable-length sequences inherent in healthcare-related network traffic data, dynamically adjusting their processing capabilities as needed. Furthermore, LSTM networks possess the ability to automatically extract relevant features from raw healthcare data, streamlining the detection process. Given the diverse sources of healthcare data and potential noise, LSTM's robustness to noise and adaptability to dynamic network environments make them well-suited for real-world attack detection scenarios where attack strategies evolve over time. Overall, these attributes make LSTM networks powerful tools for effectively identifying network anomalies and mitigating security threats in networks [26].

Our model validation utilized the WUSTL Enhanced Healthcare Monitoring System (EHMS) dataset, which encompasses two distinct feature sets: biometric and network flow metrics. Initially, we computed the correlation coefficient for each feature set separately and subsequently removed highly correlated features. The correlation heatmaps for the biometric and network flow metrics are illustrated in Figures 8.5 and 8.6, respectively. Then, we employed the Extra Trees algorithm to identify the most important features from the feature pool, presenting their corresponding importance values in Figure 8.7. Notably, the dataset exhibits a high level of imbalance, as depicted in Figure 8.4. To address this, we implemented the Synthetic Minority Over-sampling Technique (SMOTE) algorithm to balance the

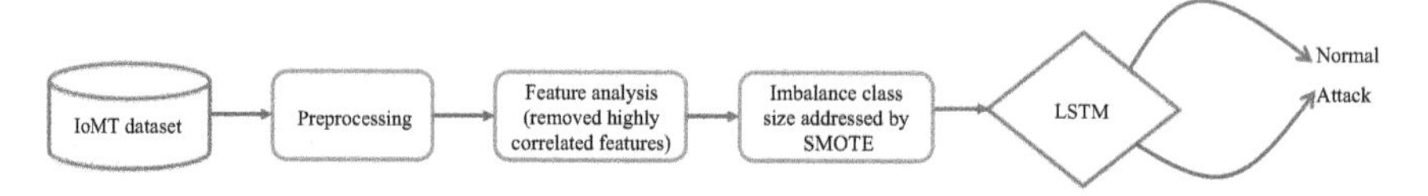

Figure 8.3 The overview of the proposed method: IoMT dataset, preprocessing, feature correlation, balance of the imbalance class, and classification of normal and attack using LSTM

classes, which were then fed into the classifier for performance evaluation [27]. In addition to the LSTM classifier, we also implemented a stack ensemble technique. This method involves aggregating different classifiers (SVM, RF, Adaboost) in the base, which aids in capturing diverse attack patterns due to the unique characteristics of each classifier. Experimental results demonstrated that the stack ensemble exhibited robust capabilities in detecting attack patterns comparable to the LSTM and ensemble (same base classifiers) approach. An overview of the proposed method is shown in Figure 8.3.

This paper is structured as follows: In Section 8.2, we presented a detailed description EHMS dataset. Section 8.3 describes the experimental results and discussions. Under this we explain the correlation, feature selections, stack ensembles, detailed experimental results, and discussions on the proposed method, key findings, and a comparative analysis with existing methodologies. The conclusion in Section 8.4 provides a succinct and insightful summary, outlines potential future directions, and highlights areas for future work.

8.2 Dataset description

The EHMS dataset, collected in 2020 at Washington University in St. Louis (WUSTL), focuses on the cybersecurity of the Internet of Medical Things (IoMT). This dataset encompasses two distinct sets of features: network flow metrics and patients' biometrics. The dataset distribution is illustrated in the accompanying figure, revealing that approximately 87.40% of instances are labeled as "Normal," while the remaining instances are categorized as "Attack," resulting in a significant imbalance (shown in Figure 8.4). The dataset includes man-in-the-middle attacks, specifically spoofing and data injection. The spoofing attack involves eavesdropping on packets between the gateway and the server, compromising patient data confidentiality. On the other hand, the data injection attack aims to modify packets on-the-fly, violating the integrity of the data [17]. Details about feature names, descriptions, and their respective categories are provided in Table 8.1. The dataset consists of 34 network flow metric features; however, certain unrelated samples associated with the gateway, attacker, and server MAC addresses are removed for further processing. Additionally, the dataset includes eight biometric features.

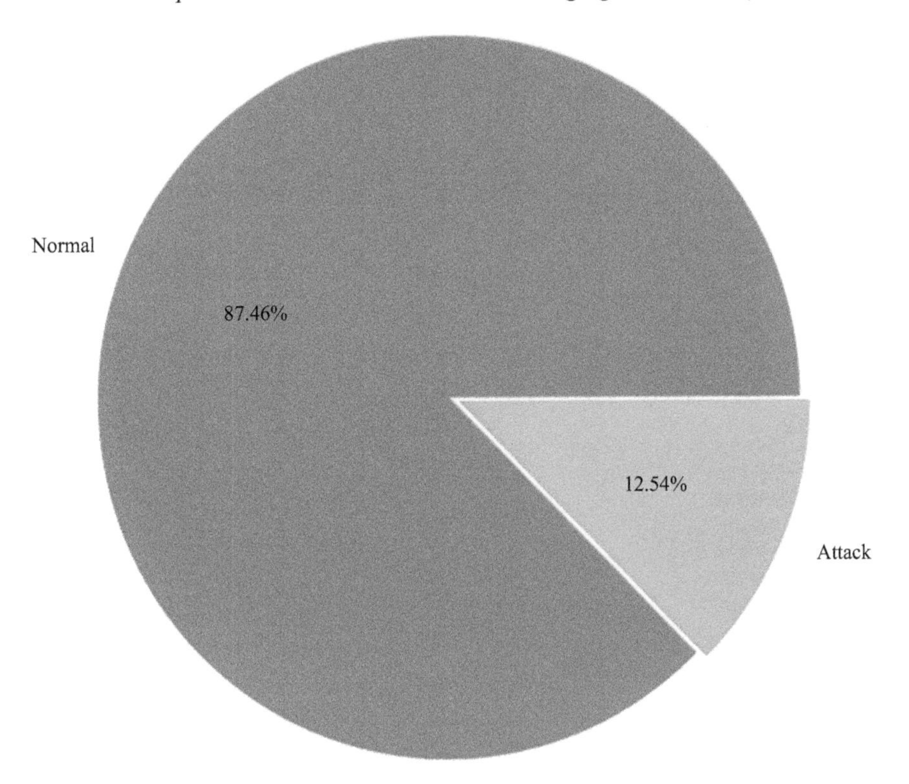

Figure 8.4 Distribution of "Normal" and "Attack" samples in EHMS dataset

Table 8.1 EHMS dataset description

Feature	Description	Type	Feature	Description	Type
Temp	Temperature	Biometric	SIntPkt	Source Inter Packet	Flow Metric
SpO_2	Peripheral Oxygen Saturation		DIntPkt	Destination Inter Packet	
Pulse Rate	Pulse Rate		SIntPktAct	Source Active Inter Packet	
SYS	Systolic Blood Pressure		DIntPktAct	Destination Active Inter Packet	
DIA	Diastolic Blood Pressure		rcJitter	Source Jitter	
Heart Rate	Heart Rate		DstJitter	Destination Jitter	
Resp Rate	Respiration Rate		sMaxPktSz	Source Maximum Transmitted Packet Size	
ST	ECG ST segment		dMaxPktSz	Destination Maximum Transmitted Packet Size	

(Continues)

Table 8.1 EHMS dataset description (Continued)

Feature	Description	Type	Feature	Description	Type
SrcBytes	Source Bytes	Flow Metric	sMinPktSz	Source Minimum Transmitted Packet Size	
DstBytes	Destination Bytes		dMinPktSz	Destination Minimum Transmitted Packet Size	
SrcLoad	Source Load		Dur	Duration	
DstLoad	Destination Load		Trans	Aggregated Packets Counts	
SrcGap	Source Missing Bytes		TotPkts	Total Packets Count	
DstGap	Destination Missing Bytes		TotBytes	Total Packets Bytes	
Loss	Retransmitted or Dropped Packets		pLoss	Percentage of Retransmitted or Dropped Packet	
pSrcLoss	Percentage of Source Retransmitted or Dropped Packet		pDstLoss	Percentage of Destination Retransmitted or Dropped Packet	
Rate	Number of Packets Per Second		Load	Load	

8.3 Experimental results and discussions

We calculated the correlation coefficient between features for both biometric and network flow features using the Spearman correlation coefficient (ρ). This non-parametric measure assesses the statistical dependence between two variables, particularly valuable when working with ordinal or interval data [28]. The resulting correlations provide insights into how the features are related to each other. Strong correlations (close to 1 or –1) indicate a significant relationship, while weak correlations (close to 0) suggest a lack of association. In the correlation matrix for biometric features, we observed several noteworthy relationships. For instance, Temperature (Temp) exhibits moderate positive correlations with systolic blood pressure (SYS) and diastolic blood pressure (DIA), indicating a tendency for these variables to increase together. The details correlation coefficients of biometric features are presented in Figure 8.5. Turning to the network flow features shown in Figure 8.6, we found intriguing associations. SrcBytes and DstBytes demonstrate a strong positive correlation of approximately 0.55, suggesting that as the number of source bytes increases, the number of destination bytes also tends to increase. Similarly, TotPkts and TotBytes display a strong positive correlation of approximately 0.93, indicating that as the total number of packets increases, the total number of bytes transmitted also tends to increase. Conversely, Load exhibits a

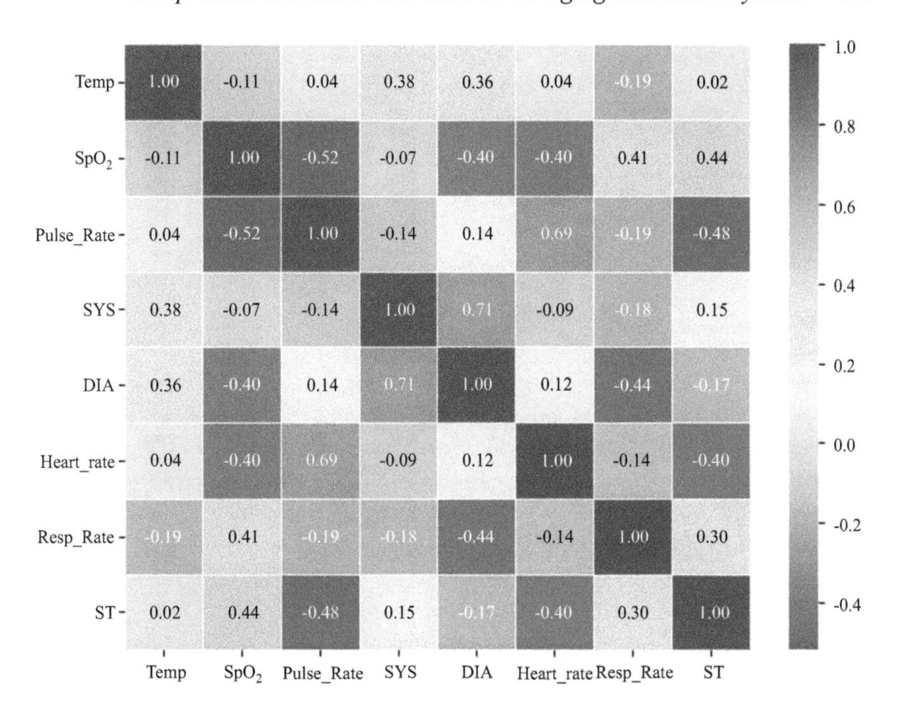

Figure 8.5 Spearman correlation coefficient of biometric features

weak negative correlation with several features such as SrcBytes, DstBytes, and Dur, suggesting a slight decrease in load with an increase in these features. Overall, the correlation matrix provides valuable insights into the relationships between different features in the EHMS dataset, guiding further analysis and modeling efforts. These insights can inform the development of more accurate predictive models and aid in the understanding of underlying patterns within the data.

$$\rho = 1 - \frac{6\sum d_i^2}{n(n^2 - 1)} \tag{8.1}$$

where d_i^2 is the difference between the ranks of corresponding values and n is the number of observations.

8.3.1 Feature selection

The objective of feature selection is to identify the most discriminative features, or subsets thereof, for detecting both attack and normal traffic within the network [29,30]. Among different feature selection methodologies, we opted for the ExtraTreesClassifier to extract features from the pool. This ensemble learning method is a variation of the random forest algorithm, wherein decision trees are constructed from samples of the training dataset. Unlike traditional random forests

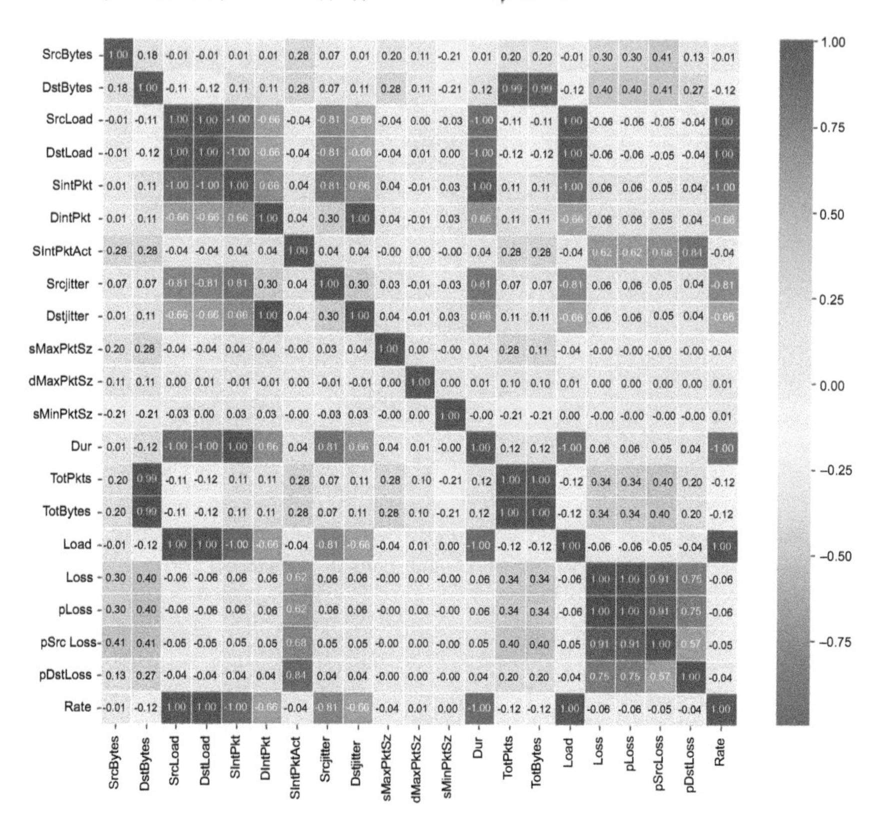

Figure 8.6 Spearman correlation coefficient of network flow metric features

that employ bootstrapping for sampling, Extra Trees randomly select subsets of features at each split, earning the moniker "extremely randomized trees." This approach introduces higher variance for individual trees while reducing susceptibility to overfitting. During feature selection, Extra Trees assesses the importance of each feature by measuring its impact on decreasing impurity across all trees in the forest [17]. Features demonstrating consistent contributions to impurity reduction across multiple trees are deemed more important. Through ranking features based on their importance scores, as depicted in Figure 8.7, Extra Trees facilitates the identification of the most relevant features for prediction, thereby aiding in dimensionality reduction and enhancing model efficiency. In Figure 8.7, the horizontal axis represents feature importance, while the vertical axis illustrates the features, with SrcLoad exhibiting the highest importance values, followed by DstJitter, and so forth.

8.3.2 Long short-term memory

The LSTM diagram, depicted in Figure 8.8, represents a kind of recurrent neural network (RNN) architecture [31]. LSTMs are particularly effective for predicting

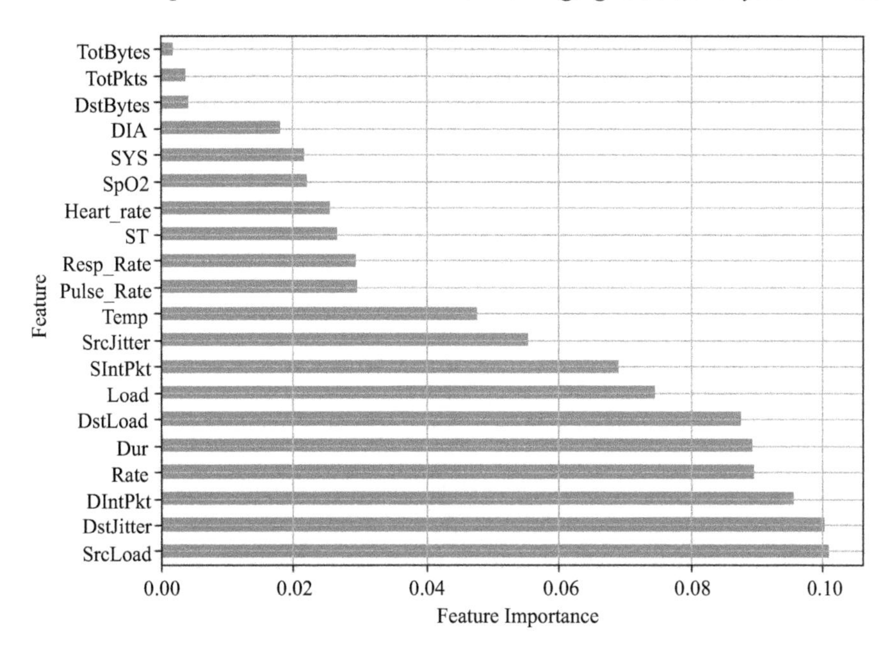

Figure 8.7 Feature selection using extra tree classifier of IoMT dataset, where x-axis represents the feature importance and y-axis represents the selected features

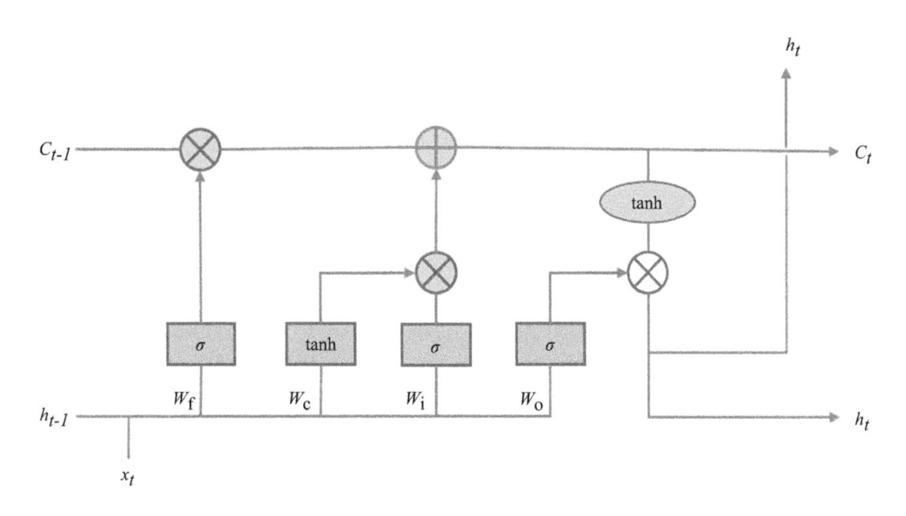

Figure 8.8 Schematic representation of an LSTM network

EHMS-like time series data due to their ability to capture and remember long-term dependencies in sequential data, making them well-suited for IoT anomaly detection [32]. The mathematical computation of an LSTM unit at time step t is defined as follows:

$$Forget\ gate: f_t = \sigma(W_f \cdot [h_{t-1}, x_t] + b_f) \tag{8.2}$$

$$Input\ gate: i_t = \sigma(W_i \cdot [h_{t-1}, x_t] + b_i) \tag{8.3}$$

$$Cell\ update: \tilde{C}_t = \tanh(W_c \cdot [h_{t-1}, x_t] + b_c) \tag{8.4}$$

$$Update\ forget\ gate: C_t = f_t \cdot C_{t-1} + i_t \cdot \tilde{C}_t \tag{8.5}$$

$$Output\ gate: o_t = \sigma(W_o \cdot [h_{t-1}, x_t] + b_o) \tag{8.6}$$

$$Hidden\ state\ update: h_t = o_t \cdot \tanh(C_t) \tag{8.7}$$

In the given equation, x_t is the input at time t and h_{t-1} denotes the hidden state from the previous time step. The variables f_t, i_t, $\tilde{C}_t$, and o_t correspond to the forget gate, input gate, cell candidate, and output gate, respectively. They are calculated according to equations (8.2), (8.3), (8.4), and (8.6). C_t signifies the cell state at time step t. The σ represents the sigmoid activation function and tanh denotes the hyperbolic tangent activation function. Additionally, W and b represents weight matrices and bias vectors.

8.3.3 Stack ensemble

We implemented a stacked ensemble classifier for IoMT attack detection to address the challenge posed by different attackers who constantly change the characteristics of their patterns, as shown in Figure 8.9. By utilizing a stacked ensemble classifier, our goal was to learn various attack patterns within a single framework to effectively protect against different types of attacks. This approach involves combining different base classifiers, including AdaBoost, Random Forest, and SVM, and aggregating their predictions using a meta-classifier, such as logistic regression. The base classifiers are trained on the original dataset, while the meta-model learns from the predictions generated by the base models on a holdout set or through cross-validation. This enables the meta-model to determine the optimal combination of predictions from the base models for the final prediction. Our approach achieved a commendable accuracy of 95.62% in k-fold cross-validation, demonstrating the efficacy of stacked ensembles in capturing diverse patterns and dependencies in the data that individual models may overlook, thus leading to enhanced generalization and robustness. Furthermore, our method consistently yielded impressive results across other performance metrics, with an average F1-score of 96.62%, average precision of 95.63%, and average recall of 96.62%.

The Stack Ensemble Algorithm is designed to construct an ensemble classifier, denoted as H, using a hierarchical approach. The algorithm takes as input a dataset D consisting of pairs (x_i, y_i), where x_i represents the input features and y_i represents the corresponding to the label set γ.

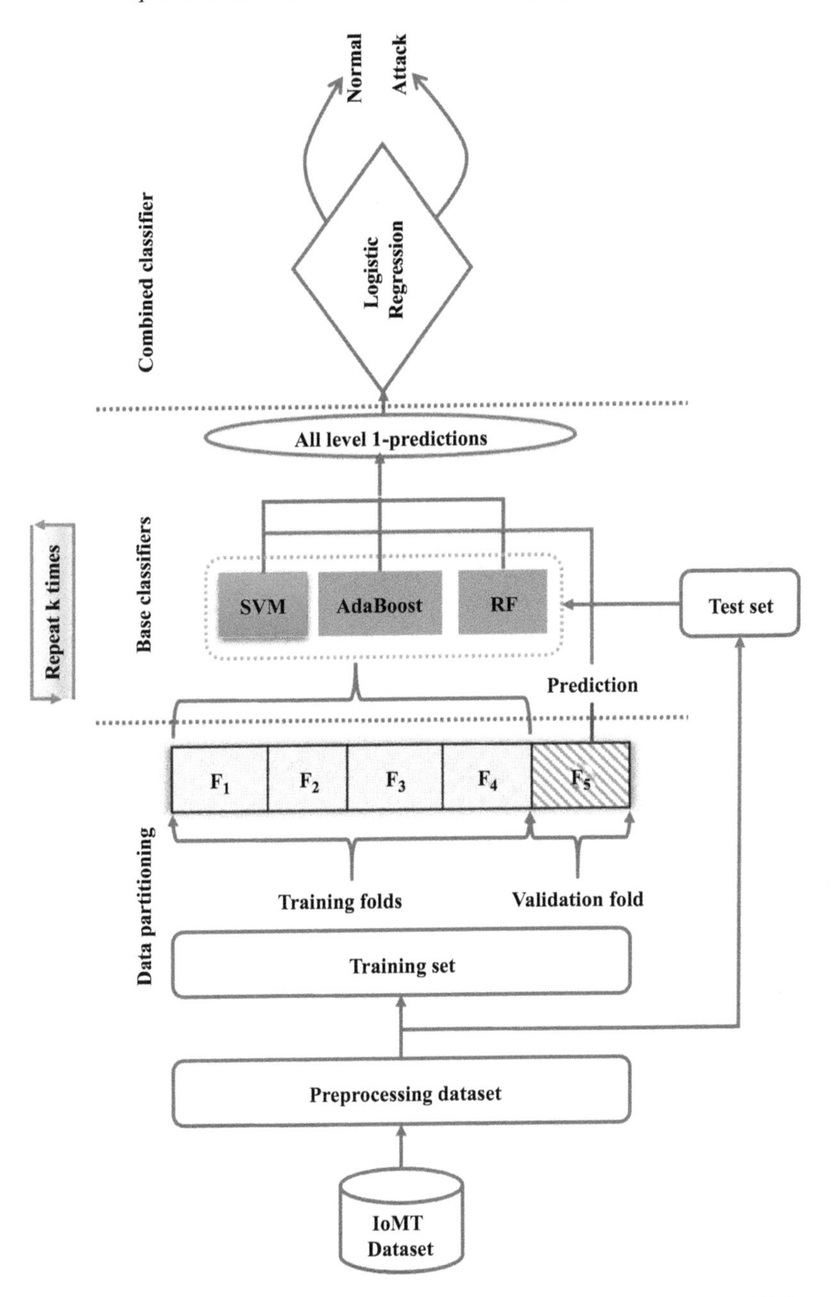

Figure 8.9 The overview of stack ensemble: base classifiers are SVM, AdaBoost, and random forest (RF), and the meta classifier is logistic regression

Algorithm 1 Stack ensemble algorithm [33][34]

Input $D = \{(x_i, y_i)\}_{i=1}^{m}, (x_i \in \mathbb{R}^n, y_i \in \gamma)$
Output An ensemble classifier H
1: **Step 1:** Preparing a cross-validation training set for the 2nd-level classifier
2: Partition IoMT samples into K equal subsets: $D = \{D_1, D_2, ..., D_K\}$
3: **for** $n \leftarrow 1$ **to** K **do**
4: **Step 1.1:** Initialize 1st-level classifiers
5: **for** $t \leftarrow 1$ **to** T **do**
6: Learn a classifier h_{nt} from $D \setminus D_n$
7: **end for**
8: **Step 1.2:** Train the 2nd-level classifier
9: **for** $x_i \varepsilon D_n$ **do**
10: Calculate $\{x_i^{'}, y_i\}$, where $x_i^{'} = \{h_{n1}(x_i), h_{n2}(x_i), ..., h_{nT}(x_i)\}$
11: **end for**
12: **end for**
13: **Step 2:** Learn a 2nd-level classifier
14: Learn a new classifier $h^{'}$ from the collection of $\{x_i^{'}, y_i\}$
15: **Step 3:** Re-learn 1st-level classifiers
16: **for** $t \leftarrow 1$ **to** T **do**
17: Learn a classifier h_t based on D
18: **end for**
19: **return** $H(x) = h^{'}(h_1(x), h_2(x), ..., h_T(x))$

In the first step, the algorithm prepares a cross-validation training set for the second-level classifier. It partitions the dataset D into K equal subsets, denoted as $D_1, D_2, ..., D_K$. Each subset D_n serves as a training set for the subsequent steps.

Within each subset D_n, the algorithm initializes first-level classifiers in Step 1.1. For each first-level classifier, denoted as h_{nt}, it iterates over the number of iterations T to learn a classifier from the dataset excluding D_n. This process ensures that each classifier is trained on a diverse set of data to capture different patterns and characteristics.

The outcomes of the classifiers, namely LSTM, ensemble, and stack ensemble, were meticulously recorded and calculated using specific formulas. The evaluation was based on four distinct terms: True Positive (TP), representing instances when the system correctly detected attacks in the dataset; True Negative (TN), denoting cases where the system correctly identified the absence of attacks; False Positive (FP), indicating instances where the system wrongly detected attacks in the absence of it in the IoMT dataset; and False Negative (FN), representing cases where the system failed to detect attacks when the risk was present in the dataset. This comprehensive evaluation provided a detailed understanding of the overall performance of each classifier in handling normal cases and attacks based on these equations.

1. Accuracy estimates the ratio of risk recognized in the entire conditions (cases). If accuracy is higher, the ML model is better.

$$Accuracy = \frac{TP + TN}{TP + TN + FP + FN}, \tag{8.8}$$

2. Precision measures the accuracy of the model when it predicts positive instances. A high precision indicates that when the model predicts the positive class, it is likely to be correct.

$$Precision = \frac{TP}{TP + FP}, \tag{8.9}$$

3. Recall is the ratio of true positive predictions to the total number of actual positive instances. It calculated the ability of the model to capture all positive instances.

$$Recall = \frac{TP}{TP + FN}, \tag{8.10}$$

4. The F1-score is a metric that combines both precision and recall. It is the harmonic mean of precision and recall and provides a balanced measure of a model's performance.

$$F1 - score = 2 \times \frac{\text{Precision} \times \text{Recall}}{\text{Precision} + \text{Recall}} \tag{8.11}$$

Our initial objective is to assess the individual contribution (discriminative ability), of each feature set (network flow metric and biometric) to attack detection in the proposed model. The performance comparison was conducted using various evaluation metrics, including classification accuracy, precision, recall, and F1-score. The mathematical expressions for each metric are provided in Equations (8.8), (8.9), (8.10), and (8.11) [35]. The overall results of biometric and network flow feature sets, presented in Table 8.2, indicate that the network flow metric, despite having a considerably higher number of features, exhibits an overall accuracy of approximately 95.05%. Surprisingly, the accuracy of biometric features is nearly the same as that of the network flow metric feature sets, despite having only eight features. This suggests that biometrics, forming a smaller set, demonstrate higher discriminative ability compared to the network flow metric. Despite the substantial difference in feature count, the performance metrics, including accuracy, precision, recall, and F1-score, suggest that both feature sets contribute effectively to the model. Biometric features achieve an accuracy of 95.04%, precision of 98.77%, recall of 91.22%, and an F1-score of 94.84%. On the other hand, network flow

Table 8.2 Performance comparison of biometric and network flow features with LSTM classifier in %

Feature group	Accuracy	Precision	Recall	F1-score
Biometric	95.04	98.77	91.22	94.84
Flow metric	95.05	98.52	91.48	94.86

features exhibit slightly improved performance with an accuracy of 95.05%, precision of 98.52%, recall of 91.48%, and an F1-score of 94.86%. This indicates that despite the disparity in the number of features, both biometric and network flow features contribute to the model's effectiveness in a comparable manner. The individual class label performance of each feature set is illustrated in the form of a confusion matrix in Table 8.3.

We incorporated two additional classifiers, namely ensemble and stack ensemble—combinations of distinct classifiers (AdaBoost, SVM, and Random Forest)—into our evaluation of various performance metrics, as presented in Table 8.4. In comparing three classifiers—LSTM, ensemble, and stack ensemble—based on various performance metrics, it is evident that all models demonstrate high levels of accuracy. The LSTM classifier exhibits a commendable accuracy of 95.57%, showcasing its proficiency in accurate classification. However, both Ensemble and Stack Ensemble models surpass the LSTM in overall accuracy, achieving 96.34% and 96.16%, respectively. Precision, recall, and F1-score metrics shed further light on the models' capabilities. While the LSTM demonstrates impressive precision (99.09%) but relatively lower recall (92.0%), resulting in a balanced F1-score of 95.40%, the ensemble and stack ensemble models showcase well-rounded performance across all metrics, maintaining precision, recall, and F1-score consistently around 96.0%. Although the Ensemble and Stack Ensemble models slightly outperform the LSTM in accuracy, they exhibit robust

Table 8.3 Confusion matrix of flow metric and biometric feature sets in %

	(a) Network flow feature set	
	Normal	**Attack**
Normal	86.60	13.40
Attack	10.30	89.70
	(b) Biometric feature set	
	Normal	**Attack**
Normal	89.43	10.57
Attack	16.70	83.30

Table 8.4 Performance metrics comparison by using LSTM, ensemble, and stack ensemble classifiers in %

Classifier	**Accuracy**	**Precision**	**Recall**	**F1-score**
LSTM	95.57	99.09	92.00	95.40
Ensemble	96.34	96.36	96.34	96.34
Stack Ensemble	96.16	96.18	96.16	96.16

Table 8.5 Confusion matrix of ensemble and stack ensemble classifier of %

(a) Ensemble classifier		
	Normal	**Attack**
Normal	97.30	2.70
Attack	4.62	95.38

(b) Stack Ensemble classifier		
	Normal	**Attack**
Normal	97.06	2.94
Attack	4.73	95.27

and balanced performance across multiple evaluation criteria. The choice between these classifiers may hinge on specific application requirements and considerations of precision, recall, and overall balance in classification performance. We also calculated the confusion matrices of Ensemble and Stack Ensemble and presented in Table 8.5.

8.3.4 Comparative analysis

In our comparative analysis, we assessed the classification performance of various ML classifiers against a baseline approach using the EHMS dataset for IoMT security analysis [17]. The initial study employed K-Nearest Neighbor (KNN), SVM, Artificial Neural Network (ANN), and RF algorithms to evaluate network flow, biometric, and combined feature sets via 10-fold cross-validation. The

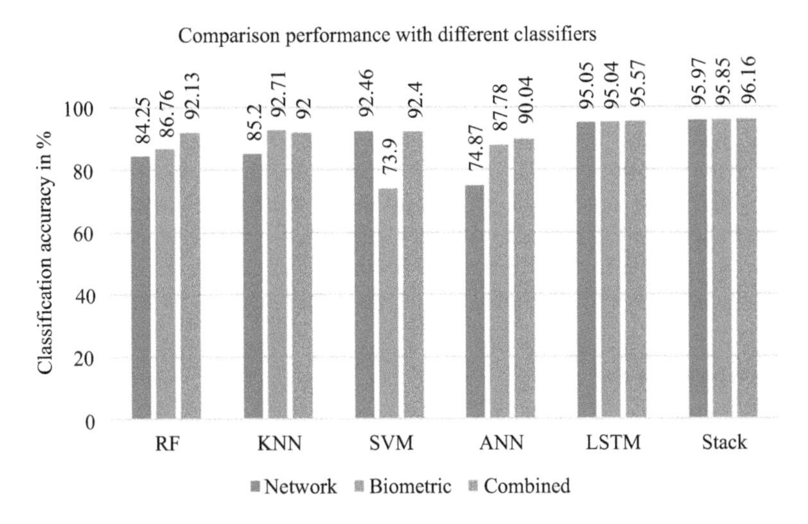

Figure 8.10 Comparison of classification accuracies of network, biometric, and combined features using RF, KNN, SVM, ANN, and LSTM classifiers

outcomes, as depicted in Figure 8.10, demonstrated differing accuracy levels across classifiers across different feature sets. Notably, the stack ensemble exhibited the highest accuracy across all sets (network flow, biometric, and combined). While the baseline method incorporated SVM, KNN, ANN, and RF classifiers and reported accuracy for three distinct feature sets (biometric, network flow, and combined), our proposed approach leveraging LSTM and stack ensemble achieved higher accuracies across all feature sets compared to the baseline method.

8.4 Conclusion

The proposed method aims to address the multifaceted challenges associated with securing healthcare data from cyberattacks by leveraging both network flow and biometric information. Through the implementation of LSTM, we evaluated the method's performance using various metrics such as classification accuracy, precision, recall, F1-score, and confusion matrix. The results showcased highly competitive performance across both network flow and biometric feature sets. Notably, even a small subset of biometric features demonstrated significant discriminability, achieving over 95% accuracy in distinguishing between attack and normal instances in the healthcare dataset. Additionally, we employed the ExtraTreesClassifier algorithm for feature selection to identify the most important features from the pool, thereby optimizing computational efficiency. Subsequently, only seventeen features were selected and utilized for classification through LSTM, ensemble, and stack ensemble methods. Among these classifiers, stack ensemble emerged with superior results, leveraging different learners such as SVM, RF, and AdaBoost as base classifiers, with logistic regression as the meta-classifier. This stack ensemble method effectively captured diverse attack patterns. Finally, a comparative analysis with benchmark results in healthcare dataset attack detection further underscored the superior performance of our approach, outperforming baseline methods significantly.

In real-world scenarios, datasets often exhibit a significant class imbalance, with the majority of examples belonging to the normal class and only a small proportion representing the abnormal (attack) class. To address this problem, we implemented the Synthetic Minority Oversampling Technique (SMOTE), which generates synthetic samples in the minority class (attack class) to balance the classes. Our immediate plan is to utilize generative adversarial networks (GANs) to create more realistic synthetic samples and compare the results with those generated by SMOTE. This comparison will provide valuable insights for researchers into how synthetic data can help fill the gap in minority class samples (imbalance gap) and their potential solution to overfitting.

Acknowledgments

This material is based on work supported by the National Science Foundation under Grant Number HBCU-EiR-2101181. Any opinions, findings, and conclusions or recommendations expressed in this material are those of the authors and do not necessarily reflect the views of the National Science Foundation.

References

[1] Bathalapalli V, Mohanty SP, Kougianos E, *et al.* PUFchain 2.0: Hardware-Assisted Robust Blockchain for Sustainable Simultaneous Device and Data Security in Smart Healthcare. *SN Computer Science*. 2022;3:344.

[2] Bathalapalli VKVV, Mohanty SP, Kougianos E, *et al.* PUFchain 3.0: Hardware-Assisted Distributed Ledger for Robust Authentication in the Internet of Medical Things. In: *Internet of Things. IoT through a Multi-disciplinary Perspective*; 2022. p. 23–40.

[3] Bathalapalli VKVV, Mohanty SP, Kougianos E, *et al.* A PUF-based Approach for Sustainable Cybersecurity in Smart Agriculture. In: 2021 19th OITS International Conference on Information Technology (OCIT); 2021. p. 375–380.

[4] Atzori L, Iera A, and Morabito G. The Internet of Things: A survey. *Computer Networks*. 2010;54(15):2787–2805.

[5] Khan MA, and Salah K. IoT Security: Review, Blockchain Solutions, and Open Challenges. *Future Generation Computer Systems*. 2018;82:395–411.

[6] Baniya BK, and Russ T. Intelligent Anomaly Detection System Based on Ensemble and Deep Learning. In: 2024 26th International Conference on Advanced Communication Technology (ICACT); 2024.

[7] Baniya BK, and Iyer V. Disparity of Covid-19 in Different Communities in Louisiana. In: 2023 Hawaii University International Conferences Science, Technology, Engineering, Arts, Mathematics and Education; 2023.

[8] Bhuiyan MN, Billah MM, Bhuiyan F, *et al.* Design and Implementation of a Feasible Model for the IoT Based Ubiquitous Healthcare Monitoring System for Rural and Urban Areas. *IEEE Access*. 2022;10:91984–91997.

[9] Khan AA, Rehmani MH, and Rachedi A. Cognitive-Radio-Based Internet of Things: Applications, Architectures, Spectrum Related Functionalities, and Future Research Directions. *IEEE Wireless Communications*. 2017;24(3): 17–25.

[10] Akhtar F, Rehmani MH, and Reisslein M. White Space: Definitional Perspectives and Their Role in Exploiting Spectrum Opportunities. *Telecommunications Policy*. 2016;40(4):319–331.

[11] Zhang J, Jin HR, Gong L, *et al.* Overview of IoT Security Architecture. 2019 IEEE Fourth International Conference on Data Science in Cyberspace (DSC). 2019. p. 338–345.

[12] Fernandes E, Jung J, and Prakash A. Security Analysis of Emerging Smart Home Applications. In: *2016 IEEE Symposium on Security and Privacy (SP)*; 2016. p. 636–654.

[13] Zeshan F, Ahmad A, Babar MI, *et al.* An IoT-Enabled Ontology-Based Intelligent Healthcare Framework for Remote Patient Monitoring. *IEEE Access*. 2023;11:133947–133966.

[14] Bhatia H, Panda SN, and Nagpal D. Internet of Things and Its Applications in Healthcare-A Survey. In: 2020 8th International Conference on Reliability,

Infocom Technologies and Optimization (Trends and Future Directions) (ICRITO); 2020. p. 305–310.

[15] Verma R. Smart City Healthcare Cyber Physical System: Characteristics, Technologies and Challenges. *Wirel Pers Commun*. 2022;122(2):1413–1433.

[16] Abdulmalek S, Nasir A, Jabbar WA, *et al.* IoT-Based Healthcare-Monitoring System towards Improving Quality of Life: A Review. *Healthcare*. 2022;10(10): 1993.

[17] Hady AA, Ghubaish A, Salman T, *et al.* Intrusion Detection System for Healthcare Systems Using Medical and Network Data: A Comparison Study. *IEEE Access*. 2020;8:106576–106584.

[18] Philip NY, Rodrigues JJPC, Wang H, *et al.* Internet of Things for In-Home Health Monitoring Systems: Current Advances, Challenges and Future Directions. *IEEE Journal on Selected Areas in Communications*. 2021;39(2): 300–310.

[19] Khan MM, Mehnaz S, Shaha A, *et al.* IoT-Based Smart Health Monitoring System for COVID-19 Patients. *Computational and Mathematical Methods in Medicine*. 2021:8591036.

[20] Ahmed A, Xi R, Hou M, *et al.* Harnessing Big Data Analytics for Healthcare: A Comprehensive Review of Frameworks, Implications, Applications, and Impacts. *IEEE Access*. 2023;11:112891–112928.

[21] Tao H, Bhuiyan MZA, Rahman MA, *et al.* Economic Perspective Analysis of Protecting Big Data Security and Privacy. *Future Gener Comput Syst*. 2019;98:660–671.

[22] Granjal J, Monteiro E, and Sa Silva J. Security for the Internet of Things: A Survey of Existing Protocols and Open Research Issues. *IEEE Communications Surveys and Tutorials*. 2015;17(3):1294–1312.

[23] Román R, Alcaraz C, López J, *et al.* Key Management Systems for Sensor Networks in the Context of the Internet of Things. *Comput Electr Eng*. 2011; 37:147–159.

[24] Cirani S, Ferrari G, and Veltri L. Enforcing Security Mechanisms in the IP-Based Internet of Things: An Algorithmic Overview. *Algorithms*. 2013; 6(2):197–226.

[25] Hochreiter S, and Schmidhuber J. Long Short-Term Memory. *Neural Comput*. 1997;9(8):1735–1780.

[26] Anton SD, Ahrens L, Fraunholz D, *et al.* *Time Is of the Essence: Machine Learning-Based Intrusion Detection in Industrial Time Series Data*. In: 2018 IEEE International Conference on Data Mining Workshops (ICDMW); 2018. p. 1–6.

[27] Chawla NV, Bowyer KW, Hall LO, *et al.* SMOTE: Synthetic Minority Oversampling Technique. *J Artif Int Res*. 2002;16(1):321–357.

[28] Spearman CR. The Proof and Measurement of Association between Two Things. *The American Journal of Psychology*. 1904;15(1):72–101.

[29] Baniya BK. Intrusion Representation and Classification Using Learning Algorithm. In: 2022 24th International Conference on Advanced Communication Technology (ICACT); 2022. p. 279–284.

[30] Baniya BK, Lee J, and Li ZN. Audio Feature Reduction and Analysis for Automatic Music Genre Classification. In: 2014 IEEE International Conference on Systems, Man, and Cybernetics (SMC); 2014. p. 457–462.

[31] Basodi S, Ji C, Zhang H, *et al.* Gradient Amplification: An Efficient Way to Train Deep Neural Networks. *Big Data Mining and Analytics*. 2020;3(3): 196–207.

[32] LeCun Y, Bengio Y, and Hinton G. Deep Learning. *Nature*. 2015;521:436–444.

[33] Tang J, Alelyani S, and Liu H. Feature Selection for Classification: A Review. *Data classification: Algorithms and applications*. 2014. p. 37.

[34] Wolpert DH. Stacked Generalization. *Neural Networks*. 1992;5(2):241–259.

[35] Powers DMW. Evaluation: From Precision, Recall and F-measure to ROC, Informedness, Markedness and Correlation. ArXiv. 2011;abs/2010.16061.

Chapter 9

Smart contracts for automated compliance in healthcare cybersecurity

Oleksandr Kuznetsov[1,2,3], Emanuele Frontoni[1,4], Natalia Kryvinska[3], Oleksii Smirnov[5] and Andrii Hrebeniuk[6]

This chapter delves into the innovative application of blockchain-based smart contracts in the realm of healthcare cybersecurity, presenting a comprehensive analysis of their potential to automate compliance and regulatory adherence. A key focus of the chapter is the examination of how smart contracts can be programmed to enforce compliance with stringent healthcare regulations such as HIPAA and GDPR. This involves a critical analysis of the legal, security, and technical challenges associated with their deployment. The chapter also investigates the potential of smart contracts to streamline compliance processes, reduce administrative burdens, and minimize the risks associated with human error, thereby enhancing the efficiency and reliability of healthcare services. The comparative analysis of various blockchain platforms supporting smart contracts forms a significant part of the discussion. This analysis evaluates the platforms across multiple criteria relevant to healthcare cybersecurity, including scalability, interoperability, and financial metrics. The chapter employs the Analytic Hierarchy Process (AHP) to structure this comparison, providing a quantitative evaluation of each platform's suitability for healthcare applications. Innovative applications of smart contracts in healthcare cybersecurity are highlighted, showcasing their versatility and potential for widespread adoption. The chapter concludes with a synthesis of findings and a discussion on future directions in the application

[1]Department of Political Sciences, Communication and International Relations, University of Macerata, Italy
[2]Department of Information and Communication Systems Security, V. N. Karazin Kharkiv National University, Ukraine
[3]Faculty of Engineering, eCampus University, Italy
[4]Department of Information Engineering, Marche Polytechnic University, Italy
[5]Department of Cyber Security and Software, Central Ukrainian National Technical University, Ukraine
[6]Department of Economics and Information Security Educational and Scientific Institute of Law and Specialist Training for National Police Units, Dnipropetrovsk State University of Internal Affairs, Ukraine

of smart contracts in healthcare cybersecurity. It reflects on the broader implications of the study and suggests areas for further research, emphasizing the need for continued development and collaboration among healthcare professionals, technologists, and legal experts.

Keywords: Smart contracts; blockchain; healthcare cybersecurity; regulatory compliance; automated enforcement; HIPAA; GDPR

9.1 Introduction

In an era where digital transformation is pivotal, the healthcare sector stands at a crossroads of technological innovation and stringent regulatory compliance [1,2]. The advent of blockchain technology, particularly smart contracts, presents a novel paradigm in addressing the intricate challenges of healthcare cybersecurity [3,4]. This chapter delves into the intersection of these advanced technologies and regulatory frameworks, exploring the potential of smart contracts to revolutionize compliance mechanisms in healthcare cybersecurity.

9.1.1 Introduction to the topic and problem statement

The healthcare industry is increasingly reliant on digital technologies, which, while enhancing service delivery, also expose the sector to unprecedented cybersecurity risks [5]. The protection of sensitive patient data, governed by regulations such as the Health Insurance Portability and Accountability Act (HIPAA) in the United States [6] and the General Data Protection Regulation (GDPR) [7,8] in the European Union, is paramount. However, ensuring compliance with these regulations is a complex, resource-intensive task, often marred by human error and administrative burdens [1].

The emergence of blockchain technology, known for its robust security and transparency features, has introduced smart contracts—self-executing contracts with the terms of the agreement embedded in the code [9]. These digital contracts automate and enforce compliance, potentially transforming the landscape of healthcare cybersecurity [10]. The application of smart contracts in this domain promises to streamline compliance processes, reduce operational costs, and enhance data integrity. However, this innovative approach is not without its challenges. The integration of smart contracts into existing healthcare systems raises questions regarding legal validity, ethical considerations, and technical feasibility [1,2].

This chapter aims to explore the multifaceted implications of employing smart contracts for automated compliance in healthcare cybersecurity. It seeks to unravel the complexities of this emerging technology, examining its potential to address the perennial challenges of regulatory adherence while highlighting the hurdles that need to be overcome. The discussion extends beyond the technical aspects, delving into the legal and ethical ramifications of automating compliance in a sector as sensitive as healthcare.

In doing so, this chapter contributes to the ongoing discourse in the field of healthcare cybersecurity, providing insights into the potential of blockchain technology to foster a more secure, efficient, and compliant healthcare ecosystem. The exploration of smart contracts in this context is not just a technological assessment but also a reflection on the evolving nature of regulatory compliance in the digital age.

9.1.2 Solution methodology

The methodology is multi-faceted, integrating qualitative and quantitative analyses to comprehensively understand the potential, challenges, and practical applications of smart contracts in this domain.

- Literature review. A thorough literature review forms the foundation of this study. It involves examining existing research, articles, and case studies related to smart contracts, blockchain technology in healthcare, and cybersecurity regulations like HIPAA and GDPR. This review helps in identifying the current state of knowledge, gaps in the literature, and emerging trends in the field.
- Comparative analysis. The comparative analysis is a key component of this methodology. It involves evaluating various blockchain platforms that support smart contracts, assessing them against a set of criteria relevant to healthcare cybersecurity. These criteria include legal compliance, security features, technical capabilities, scalability, and financial aspects. The analysis utilizes the AHP to structure the comparison and derive quantitative evaluations of each platform.
- Case studies. Case studies of existing implementations of smart contracts in healthcare provide practical insights into their applications and challenges. These case studies are selected based on their relevance to healthcare cybersecurity and the innovative use of smart contracts. They are analyzed to understand how smart contracts are currently being used, the benefits they offer, and the obstacles encountered in their implementation.
- Technical evaluation. A technical evaluation of smart contracts is conducted to understand their design, functionality, and integration with healthcare systems. This involves analyzing the architecture of smart contracts, their programming languages, and the interoperability with existing healthcare IT infrastructure.
- Legal and regulatory analysis. Given the importance of legal and regulatory compliance in healthcare, a dedicated analysis of how smart contracts align with healthcare regulations is undertaken. This analysis examines the challenges and strategies for programming smart contracts to comply with laws like HIPAA and GDPR.
- Security assessment. A security assessment is crucial to evaluate the robustness of smart contracts in protecting sensitive healthcare data. This assessment examines the security features of smart contracts, their vulnerability to cyber threats, and the measures needed to ensure data privacy and security.

The methodology employed in this study provides a comprehensive framework for investigating smart contracts in healthcare cybersecurity. It combines theoretical research with practical insights, ensuring a well-rounded understanding of the subject. The findings from this study are expected to contribute significantly to the field, offering guidance for healthcare professionals, technologists, and policymakers in leveraging smart contracts for enhanced cybersecurity.

9.1.3 Key contributions of the chapter

- Critical analysis of legal, security, and technical aspects: It provides a comprehensive examination of the legal implications, security considerations, and technical challenges associated with deploying smart contracts in healthcare.
- Programming for compliance: The chapter delves into how smart contracts can be tailored to meet specific healthcare regulations, offering a blueprint for compliance with laws like HIPAA and GDPR.
- Streamlining processes: It highlights the potential of smart contracts in optimizing compliance processes, reducing administrative workload, and mitigating risks associated with human error.
- Comparative analysis of blockchain projects: The chapter presents an in-depth comparative analysis of leading blockchain projects supporting smart contracts, evaluating them across various criteria relevant to healthcare cybersecurity.
- Application of analytic hierarchy process: A unique aspect of this chapter is the application of the AHP to compare blockchain platforms, providing a structured approach to decision-making in selecting the appropriate technology for healthcare cybersecurity.

9.1.4 Chapter organization

The chapter provides a thorough exploration of smart contracts in healthcare cybersecurity, beginning with a comprehensive Literature review in Section 9.2. In Section 9.3, Background, the chapter provides an overview of the fundamental concepts of smart contracts and blockchain technology, particularly focusing on their application in healthcare cybersecurity. Section 9.4, Results, forms the core of the chapter. It encompasses a broad range of topics, including the legal, security, and technical aspects of smart contracts in healthcare, programming for compliance with regulations like HIPAA and GDPR, and the potential of smart contracts in streamlining healthcare processes. Section 9.5, Analysis, presents a comparative analysis of leading blockchain projects supporting smart contracts, covering various aspects from financial metrics to technical capabilities and applications in healthcare. Section 9.6, Discussion, critically examines the implications of the study's findings, exploring the practical applications, challenges, and potential of smart contracts in healthcare cybersecurity, particularly focusing on legal, technical, and administrative aspects. Finally, the chapter concludes with Section 9.7, Conclusion and future scope, which synthesizes the findings and discusses potential future directions in the application of smart contracts in healthcare cybersecurity. This section reflects on the broader implications of the study and suggests areas for further research.

9.2 Related work

The literature review encompasses a range of publications, each contributing uniquely to the field of smart contracts in healthcare cybersecurity.

- Al-Dalati [11]: This publication discusses digital twins and cybersecurity in healthcare systems, focusing on integrating IoT, AI, and cloud computing. It highlights the increased attack surface and the need for a secure framework, offering insights into intrusion detection systems and blockchain integration for enhanced privacy and trust. This work fills a gap in understanding the cybersecurity implications of digital twins in healthcare.
- Alruwaili *et al.* [12]: This article presents a Blockchain-Enabled Smart Healthcare System using Jellyfish Search Optimization and a Deep Convolutional Neural Network. It emphasizes secure data transmission and disease detection, showcasing blockchain's role in optimizing medical data processes. This research contributes to the understanding of AI and blockchain integration in healthcare.
- D K *et al.* [13]: The study explores blockchain in healthcare data, emphasizing smart contracts for access control. It addresses privacy concerns and system transparency, proposing a patient-centric approach to medical data management. This research fills a gap in patient-controlled medical data management using blockchain.
- Lee *et al.* [14]: This paper introduces a medical blockchain for EHR sharing, balancing data correctness with patient privacy. It demonstrates blockchain's ability to ensure data integrity and resist Internet attacks, contributing to the understanding of secure medical data sharing.
- Luh and Yen [15]: The article discusses cybersecurity in science and medicine, highlighting the threats to privacy and patient confidentiality. It underscores the security challenges associated with genomic research and medical devices, contributing to the broader discussion of cybersecurity in healthcare.
- Sookhak *et al.* [16]: This survey paper examines blockchain and smart contract for access control in healthcare. It categorizes blockchain-based access control methods and highlights security issues, contributing to the understanding of secure EHR access control.
- Szczepaniuk and Szczepaniuk [17]: The article presents a framework for cryptographic proof of smart contracts in healthcare systems. It focuses on secure EHR processing and non-repudiation of digital agreements, filling a gap in cryptographic applications in healthcare smart contracts.
- Shahid [18]: This study measures the effect of smart-contract blockchain on smart healthcare center management. It evaluates outcomes based on end-user experience, contributing to the understanding of blockchain's impact on healthcare service management.
- Isichei *et al.* [19]: This study on smart bioprinting in healthcare highlights the integration of IoT, AI/ML, and blockchain for enhancing cybersecurity and privacy. It presents a multilayered architecture for the smart bioprinting ecosystem, addressing cybersecurity challenges at each layer. This work contributes significantly to understanding the cybersecurity implications of emerging healthcare technologies like bioprinting and identifying key areas for future research in privacy preservation.
- Khalid *et al.* [20]: This research proposes an SDN-based smart contract solution for IoT access control, integrating blockchain and SDN to enhance IoT

security. The study demonstrates the scalability of this solution and its effectiveness in managing access control policies. This paper fills a gap in understanding how blockchain and SDN can be combined to address IoT security challenges in healthcare, offering a novel perspective on policy management and IoT security.

- Priyadarshini *et al.* [21]: The paper addresses IoT reliability and survivability in industrial settings using machine learning and smart contracts. It evaluates various machine learning algorithms for device identification and proposes a blockchain-based architecture for smart homes. This research contributes to the field by combining machine learning with blockchain for IoT security, particularly focusing on device identification and data protection in smart healthcare environments.
- Rani *et al.* [22]: This comprehensive review on federated learning for secure IoMT applications in smart healthcare systems explores the integration of IoT with medical devices. It discusses the role of federated learning in enhancing privacy and security in IoMT-based healthcare applications. This study is significant for its in-depth analysis of federated learning in the context of IoMT, highlighting its potential to address privacy and security concerns in smart healthcare systems.

Each publication contributes to a nuanced understanding of smart contracts in healthcare cybersecurity, addressing various aspects from data privacy and security to efficient healthcare management. However, there remains a gap in comprehensive, practical applications of these technologies in real-world healthcare settings, which this chapter aims to fill. We offer new perspectives on integration challenges, user-centric applications, scalability, legal compliance, and advanced security measures, contributing significantly to the field and paving the way for future research and development.

9.3 Background

The healthcare sector is witnessing a rapid integration of emerging technologies, reshaping the landscape of medical services and data management. Technologies such as the IoT, AI, and blockchain are converging to create more efficient, secure, and patient-centric healthcare systems. IoT devices are increasingly used for patient monitoring and data collection, generating vast amounts of health data. AI and machine learning algorithms are being employed to analyze this data, providing insights for personalized treatment and predictive healthcare. Blockchain, particularly through smart contracts, offers a secure and transparent way to manage this data, ensuring integrity and compliance with healthcare regulations. This convergence presents new opportunities but also introduces complex challenges in terms of data security, privacy, and system interoperability.

The integration of smart contracts into healthcare cybersecurity necessitates an understanding of several foundational concepts. At its core, a smart contract is a self-executing contract with the terms of the agreement directly written into lines of code, existing across a distributed, decentralized blockchain network. This technology enables automated, transparent, and immutable transactions without the need for intermediaries [23,24].

Blockchain, the underlying technology of smart contracts, is a distributed ledger that records transactions across multiple computers in a way that ensures security, transparency, and immutability. In healthcare, this technology has the potential to revolutionize data management, privacy, and compliance with regulatory standards [13,16].

The field of smart contracts in healthcare cybersecurity is rapidly evolving, with significant research and development efforts underway [10,13]. Current progress can be categorized into several key areas:

- Regulatory compliance: Researchers are exploring how smart contracts can automate compliance with healthcare regulations such as HIPAA and GDPR [6,8]. This includes ensuring patient data privacy, secure data sharing, and adherence to consent management protocols.
- Data security and privacy: Advancements in blockchain and smart contract technologies have led to improved methods for securing patient data. This includes encryption techniques, secure data sharing protocols, and the development of privacy-preserving smart contracts [14,17].
- Administrative efficiency: There is a growing body of work focused on using smart contracts to streamline administrative processes in healthcare. This includes automating insurance claims processing, billing, and patient consent management, thereby reducing administrative burdens and costs [13,18].
- Interoperability and integration: Efforts are being made to enhance the interoperability of blockchain systems with existing healthcare IT infrastructure. This is crucial for the seamless integration of smart contracts into current healthcare systems [11,12].
- Pilot projects and real-world applications: Several pilot projects and real-world applications of smart contracts in healthcare have emerged. These projects are testing the practicality and effectiveness of smart contracts in various healthcare settings, providing valuable insights and data for further research and development [13,25].

The background of smart contracts in healthcare cybersecurity is marked by a blend of technological innovation and practical application [26,27]. As research continues to advance, it is becoming increasingly clear that smart contracts have the potential to address some of the most pressing challenges in healthcare data management and security. The ongoing exploration in this field is setting the stage for transformative changes in how healthcare data is managed, protected, and utilized.

As healthcare systems become more interconnected and reliant on digital technologies, cybersecurity emerges as a critical concern. The sensitivity of patient data and the potential consequences of data breaches necessitate robust security measures. Traditional cybersecurity solutions are being re-evaluated in the face of sophisticated cyber threats and the unique requirements of healthcare systems. The decentralized nature of blockchain technology offers a promising solution to these challenges, providing enhanced security and data integrity. However, the implementation of blockchain and smart contracts in healthcare also raises new questions regarding regulatory compliance, user privacy, and technical feasibility, which need to be addressed through innovative approaches and continuous research.

Healthcare regulations such as HIPAA in the United States and GDPR in the European Union are evolving to address the challenges posed by new technologies [6,7]. These regulations mandate strict standards for data privacy, security, and patient consent, which are becoming increasingly complex to manage in digital healthcare environments. Smart contracts offer a mechanism to automate compliance with these regulations, but their development and deployment must be carefully aligned with legal requirements. This evolving regulatory landscape presents both challenges and opportunities for the development of smart contracts in healthcare, necessitating a dynamic approach to legal and technical integration.

9.4 Results

This section presents the findings of the study, focusing on the effectiveness of smart contracts in automating compliance tasks within healthcare cybersecurity. The results are derived from a comprehensive analysis of various implementations, encompassing both quantitative metrics and qualitative insights. These findings are pivotal in understanding the transformative potential of smart contracts in enhancing regulatory compliance in the healthcare sector.

9.4.1 Assessing the legal, security, and technical frontiers of smart contracts in healthcare cybersecurity

The deployment of smart contracts in healthcare cybersecurity presents a complex interplay of legal, security, and technical factors. This subsection critically analyzes these aspects, highlighting the challenges and considerations that must be addressed to ensure the effective and compliant use of smart contracts in healthcare.

9.4.1.1 Legal implications

- Regulatory compliance: Smart contracts in healthcare must comply with stringent regulations like HIPAA in the United States and GDPR in the European Union. These regulations mandate strict data privacy and security standards, which smart contracts must adhere to. The immutable nature of smart contracts poses challenges in aligning with regulations that require data to be alterable or deletable under certain conditions.
- Liability and enforcement: Determining liability in the event of smart contract failures or breaches is complex. The decentralized nature of blockchain complicates the attribution of responsibility. Additionally, the enforceability of smart contracts under existing legal frameworks remains a grey area, raising questions about jurisdiction and legal recognition.
- Contractual ambiguity: The translation of legal agreements into code can lead to ambiguities, as coding may not capture the nuances of legal language. This

raises concerns about the interpretation and enforceability of smart contract terms.

9.4.1.2 Security considerations

- Smart contract vulnerabilities: Despite the inherent security of blockchain, smart contracts are prone to vulnerabilities due to coding errors or design flaws. These vulnerabilities can be exploited, leading to data breaches or unauthorized access, which is particularly concerning in healthcare due to the sensitivity of medical data.
- Data privacy: Ensuring patient data privacy within smart contracts is challenging. While blockchain offers data encryption, the shared nature of the ledger might expose sensitive health information, contradicting privacy regulations.
- Integration with existing systems: Integrating smart contracts with existing healthcare IT systems poses security risks. Incompatibilities can create vulnerabilities, potentially exposing healthcare data to cyber threats.

9.4.1.3 Technical challenges

- Scalability and performance: Healthcare applications often require handling large volumes of data. Smart contracts on platforms like Ethereum face scalability issues, leading to delays and increased transaction costs, which can hinder their practicality in healthcare settings.
- Interoperability: Healthcare systems are diverse and often operate in silos. The lack of interoperability between different blockchain platforms and existing healthcare systems limits the effectiveness of smart contracts in comprehensive healthcare data management.
- Technical expertise: Developing and deploying smart contracts requires specialized knowledge in both coding and legal aspects. The shortage of professionals with expertise in both fields poses a significant barrier to the widespread adoption of smart contracts in healthcare.

Figure 9.1 provides a structured visualization of the complex interplay of legal, security, and technical aspects associated with the deployment of smart contracts in healthcare cybersecurity.

The deployment of smart contracts in healthcare cybersecurity offers promising benefits but is accompanied by significant legal, security, and technical challenges (Figure 9.1). Addressing these challenges requires a multidisciplinary approach involving legal experts, cybersecurity professionals, and blockchain developers. As the technology evolves, ongoing research and collaboration among stakeholders in the healthcare, legal, and tech industries are essential to harness the full potential of smart contracts while mitigating associated risks. The future of smart contracts in healthcare depends on the development of robust frameworks that ensure compliance, security, and technical efficacy, paving the way for innovative and secure healthcare solutions.

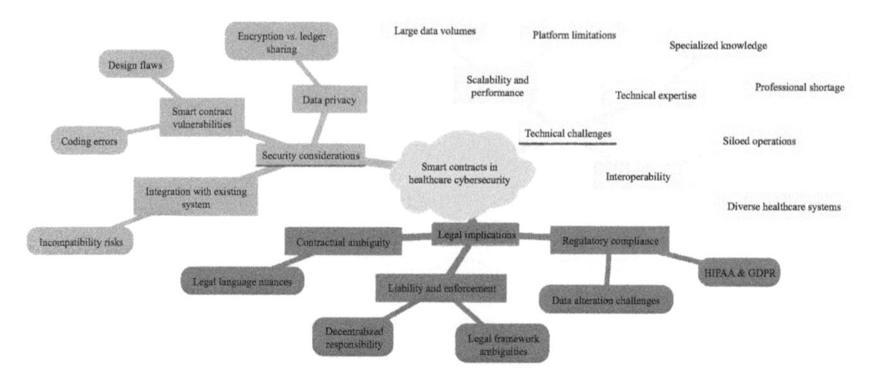

Figure 9.1 The interaction of legal, security and technical aspects associated with the deployment of smart contracts in the healthcare cybersecurity space

9.4.2 Investigating the programming of smart contracts for compliance with healthcare regulations like HIPAA and GDPR

The integration of smart contracts into healthcare systems presents a promising avenue for ensuring compliance with stringent regulations such as the HIPAA in the United States and the GDPR in the European Union. This subsection investigates how smart contracts can be programmed to automatically execute actions under predefined conditions, thereby adhering to these healthcare regulations.

9.4.2.1 Programming smart contracts for HIPAA compliance

- Data privacy and security: HIPAA mandates strict standards for the privacy and security of protected health information (PHI). Smart contracts can be programmed to automatically enforce access controls, ensuring that PHI is only accessible to authorized individuals. Encryption and de-identification techniques can be embedded into smart contracts to protect data privacy.
- Breach notification: In the event of a data breach, HIPAA requires covered entities to notify affected individuals. Smart contracts can be designed to detect breaches and automatically trigger notification procedures, ensuring timely compliance with this requirement.
- Audit trails: HIPAA requires maintaining detailed records of PHI access and modifications. Smart contracts can be programmed to create immutable logs of all transactions, providing a transparent and tamper-proof audit trail.

9.4.2.2 Programming smart contracts for GDPR compliance

- Consent management: GDPR emphasizes the importance of obtaining explicit consent for data processing. Smart contracts can manage consent digitally, recording and enforcing user consent for data use in a transparent and verifiable manner.

- Right to erasure: Under GDPR, individuals have the right to request the deletion of their personal data. Smart contracts can facilitate this process by automating the deletion of data upon request while ensuring that all regulatory conditions for data erasure are met.
- Data portability: GDPR grants individuals the right to data portability. Smart contracts can automate the transfer of personal data upon request, ensuring compliance with this right in a secure and efficient manner.

9.4.2.3 Challenges and considerations

- Regulatory alignment: Ensuring that smart contracts are fully aligned with HIPAA and GDPR regulations requires a deep understanding of these laws. Continuous updates may be necessary to accommodate changes in legal requirements.
- Technical complexity: The programming of smart contracts for regulatory compliance involves complex logic and requires expertise in both legal and technical domains.
- Interoperability: Integrating smart contracts with existing healthcare systems and ensuring they work seamlessly across different platforms and jurisdictions is a significant challenge.

Figure 9.2 provides a structured overview of how smart contracts can be programmed to ensure compliance with healthcare regulations like HIPAA and GDPR.

Smart contracts hold immense potential for automating compliance with healthcare regulations like HIPAA and GDPR. By embedding regulatory requirements into the code, smart contracts can ensure that healthcare data is managed in a manner that is compliant, secure, and efficient. However, realizing this potential requires overcoming significant technical and regulatory challenges. The development of such smart contracts necessitates a collaborative approach involving legal experts, software developers, and healthcare professionals. As the technology

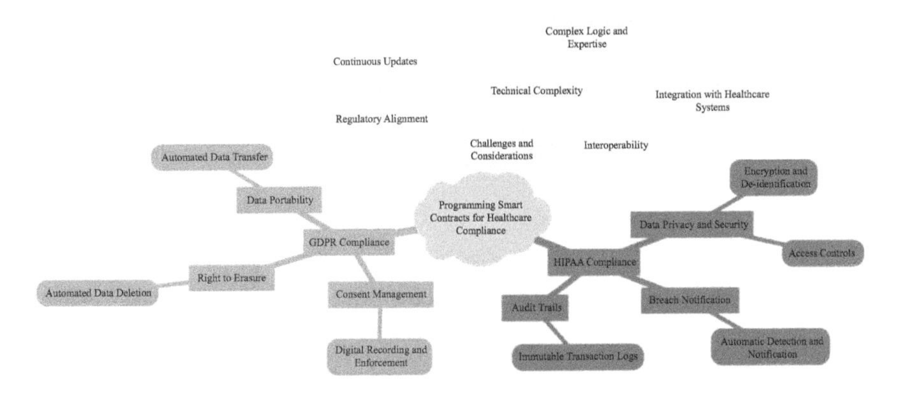

Figure 9.2 Programming smart contracts for healthcare compliance

matures, smart contracts could become a cornerstone in the digital transformation of healthcare compliance, offering a more proactive and automated approach to meeting regulatory obligations.

9.4.3 Investigating the potential of smart contracts in streamlining compliance processes, reducing administrative burden, and minimizing human error risks

The advent of smart contracts in the healthcare sector offers a paradigm shift in managing compliance, administrative tasks, and human error. This subsection investigates the potential of smart contracts to revolutionize these aspects, focusing on how they can optimize processes, alleviate administrative burdens, and mitigate risks associated with human error.

9.4.3.1 Optimizing compliance processes

- Automated compliance: Smart contracts can be programmed to automatically enforce regulatory requirements, such as data privacy standards and reporting obligations. This automation ensures continuous compliance, reducing the need for manual oversight and intervention.
- Real-time monitoring and reporting: Smart contracts enable real-time monitoring of compliance-related activities, providing instant feedback and alerts. This feature facilitates proactive management of compliance issues, ensuring timely responses to potential violations.
- Immutable record-keeping: The blockchain's immutable ledger, coupled with smart contracts, offers a secure and tamper-proof record-keeping system. This feature is crucial for maintaining accurate compliance records, essential for audits and regulatory reviews.

9.4.3.2 Reducing administrative burden

- Streamlining operations: Smart contracts can automate routine administrative tasks such as patient consent management, billing, and claims processing. This automation streamlines operations, freeing up healthcare professionals to focus on patient care.
- Efficient resource allocation: By automating administrative processes, smart contracts enable more efficient allocation of resources. This efficiency reduces operational costs and enhances the overall effectiveness of healthcare services.
- Enhanced data management: Smart contracts facilitate efficient data management by automating data entry, storage, and retrieval processes. This automation reduces the administrative burden associated with manual data handling.

9.4.3.3 Minimizing human error risks

- Error reduction in data handling: By automating data-related processes, smart contracts significantly reduce the risk of human errors in data entry, processing, and reporting.

- Consistency in decision-making: Smart contracts ensure consistency in applying rules and policies, eliminating the variability and potential errors associated with human judgment.
- Traceability and accountability: The transparent and traceable nature of smart contracts enhances accountability in healthcare operations. This transparency helps in quickly identifying and rectifying errors, thereby minimizing their impact.

9.4.3.4 Challenges and future directions

- Technical and legal integration: Integrating smart contracts into existing healthcare systems and ensuring they comply with legal standards is a significant challenge. Continuous development and legal oversight are required to address this challenge.
- Adoption and change management: The adoption of smart contracts in healthcare requires significant changes in existing processes and systems. Effective change management strategies are essential to facilitate this transition.
- Education and training: Educating healthcare professionals about smart contracts and training them to use these new tools effectively is crucial for maximizing their potential.

Figure 9.3 provides a visualization of the multifaceted impact of smart contracts in healthcare, particularly in enhancing compliance, administrative efficiency, and error mitigation.

Smart contracts hold immense promise in transforming the way compliance is managed, reducing administrative burdens, and minimizing human error in healthcare. Their ability to automate complex processes, ensure consistency, and provide secure and transparent record-keeping can significantly enhance the efficiency and reliability of healthcare services. However, realizing this potential requires overcoming technical, legal, and operational challenges. As the technology

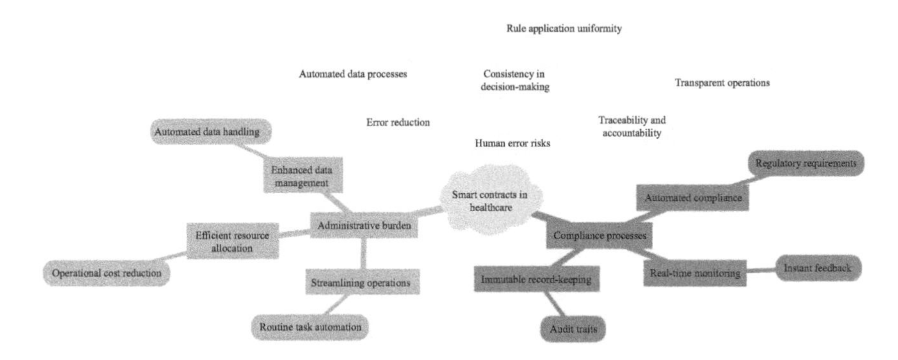

Figure 9.3 Potential of smart contracts in healthcare

evolves, continued research, development, and collaboration among healthcare professionals, legal experts, and technologists will be key to unlocking the full potential of smart contracts in healthcare.

9.5 Analysis

This section aims to consolidate and compare various projects in a scholarly manner, focusing on their technical aspects and contributions to the field of blockchain technology. The comparison is contextualized within the broader narrative of blockchain evolution, highlighting how each project addresses specific challenges and opportunities in this dynamic domain.

9.5.1 Comparative analysis of leading blockchain projects supporting smart contracts

This analysis aims to consolidate and compare blockchain projects, focusing on their technical aspects and contributions to the field of blockchain technology. The comparison is contextualized within the broader narrative of blockchain evolution, highlighting how each project addresses specific challenges and opportunities in this dynamic domain.

In this comparison, each blockchain project is evaluated based on its launch year, primary focus, consensus mechanism, and unique technical features (Table 9.1):

- Ethereum, as a pioneer, introduced smart contracts and decentralized applications (DApps), significantly influencing subsequent projects [28,29]. Its transition to Ethereum 2.0, with a shift from Proof of Work (PoW) to Proof of Stake (PoS), marks a significant evolution in addressing scalability and energy efficiency.
- Cardano, with its scientific approach and Ouroboros consensus, presents a sustainability-focused blockchain [30]. Its layered architecture allows for flexibility and scalability, setting it apart as a research-driven project.
- Binance Coin, initially a utility token for the Binance exchange, has expanded its scope with the Binance Smart Chain (BSC), supporting smart contracts and fostering a robust token ecosystem [31].
- Avalanche distinguishes itself with its high throughput and low latency, addressing scalability through its unique subnets and consensus mechanism, making it suitable for complex DApps requiring speed and efficiency [32].
- Polygon (formerly Matic Network) offers Layer 2 scaling solutions for Ethereum, enhancing its scalability while maintaining compatibility, thus addressing the congestion issues of the Ethereum network [33,34].
- Chainlink, though not a blockchain in the traditional sense, plays a crucial role in the ecosystem by providing reliable external data to smart contracts across various blockchains through its decentralized oracle network [35].
- Stellar focuses on financial transfers with low-cost transactions, facilitated by its unique Federated Byzantine Agreement (FBA) consensus mechanism, making it a go-to platform for cross-border payments and remittances [36].

Table 9.1 Results of a comparison of leading blockchain projects that support smart contracts

Projects	Year of launch	Primary focus	Consensus mechanism	Unique technical features
Ethereum [28,29]	2015	Smart Contracts, DApps	PoW (transitioning to PoS)	EVM, Transition to Ethereum 2.0, High DApp Ecosystem
Cardano [30]	2017	Sustainability, Scalability	PoS	Ouroboros Consensus, Layered Architecture
Binance Coin [31]	2017	Exchange Ecosystem	PoSA	Binance Chain & Binance Smart Chain, Token Burn Mechanism
Avalanche [32]	2020	Scalability, Speed	PoS	High Throughput, Subnets, Low Latency
Polygon [33,34]	2017	Ethereum Scalability	PoS	Ethereum Compatibility, Layer 2 Scaling Solutions
Chainlink [35]	2017	Oracle for Smart Contracts	N/A	Decentralized Oracle Network, External Data Integration
Stellar [36]	2014	Financial Transfers	FBA	Low-Cost Transactions, Stellar Consensus Protocol
Ethereum Classic [37]	2016	Immutability	PoW	Original Ethereum Codebase, Emphasis on Code is Law
Polkadot [38]	2020	Interoperability	NPoS	Relay Chain, Parachains, Cross-Chain Interoperability
Tron [39,40]	2017	Content Platform	DPoS	High Throughput, Content Sharing Focus
Algorand [41]	2019	Speed, Security	PPoS	Pure Proof of Stake, Fast Transaction Finality

- Ethereum Classic maintains the original Ethereum codebase, emphasizing the principle of immutability and "code is law," appealing to a segment of the community focused on these philosophical tenets [37].
- Polkadot introduces a novel approach to interoperability with its Relay Chain and Parachains structure, enabling different blockchains to communicate and share information seamlessly [38].
- Tron, with its high throughput and focus on a content-sharing platform, aims to decentralize the digital content industry, offering an alternative to traditional content distribution networks [39,40].
- Algorand's Pure Proof of Stake (PPoS) consensus mechanism and focus on speed and security position it as a platform suitable for fast and secure transactions, appealing to both financial and enterprise applications [41].

This comparison reveals the diverse landscape of blockchain technology, where each project carves out its niche. The evolution of these platforms, especially in terms of scalability, security, and smart contract capabilities, will be crucial in determining their long-term success and impact on the blockchain ecosystem [42,43].

9.5.2 Financial metrics of blockchain projects supporting smart contracts

This subsection examines the financial metrics of key blockchain projects that support smart contracts, focusing specifically on their relevance in healthcare systems. We analyze the market capitalizations of these projects as of February 2023, offering insights into their economic impact and investment potential [44,45].

Figure 9.4 presents the market capitalizations of leading blockchain projects, ranked in descending order. Ethereum (ETH) leads with a market capitalization of approximately $29.1 billion. It is followed by Cardano (ADA) and Tron (TRX) with capitalizations of $10.4 billion and $9.63 billion, respectively. Other notable projects such as Chainlink (LINK), Binance Coin (BNB), and Avalanche (AVAX) also demonstrate significant market presence.

The data highlights the significant financial potential and attractiveness of blockchain projects in the healthcare sector. Ethereum's dominance is a reflection of its pioneering role in smart contract technology and its established infrastructure. Meanwhile, Cardano and Tron are showing impressive growth, signaling their increasing importance in healthcare applications.

These financial figures are not just indicators of market speculation but also reflect the transformative impact of blockchain technology in healthcare. The high market capitalizations point to a growing recognition of blockchain's role in enhancing data security, patient privacy, and operational efficiency in healthcare settings.

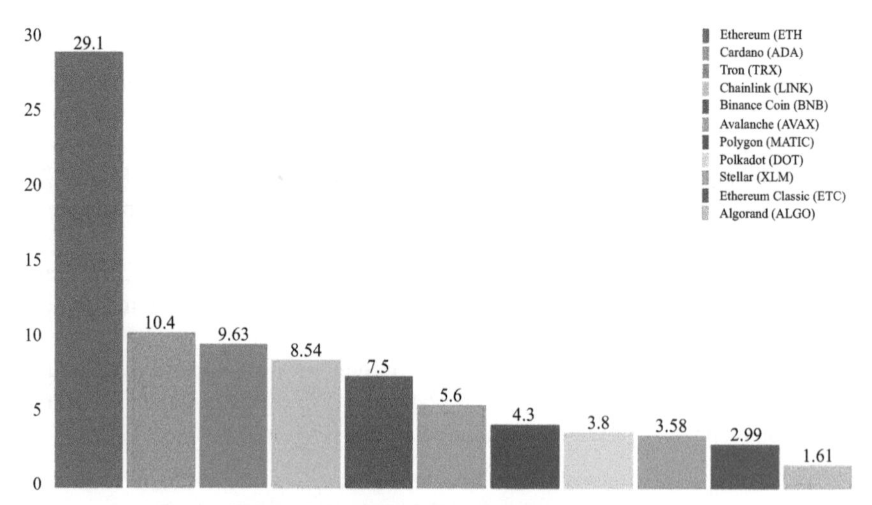

Figure 9.4 Market capitalizations of leading blockchain projects supporting smart contracts

9.5.3 Investigating smart contracts in blockchain systems: focus on healthcare application

The integration of smart contracts in blockchain systems has revolutionized various sectors, including healthcare, by offering enhanced security, transparency, and efficiency. This subsection of the study delves into the processing of smart contracts across different blockchain platforms, particularly in the context of healthcare applications. The analysis aims to elucidate how various blockchain systems handle smart contracts, considering their unique architectures and functionalities. This exploration is critical in understanding the suitability and adaptability of these platforms for healthcare-related applications, where accuracy, privacy, and compliance with regulatory standards are paramount.

9.5.3.1 Methodology of research

The methodology for this research involves a comprehensive analysis of smart contract processing across eleven prominent blockchain systems: Ethereum, Cardano, Binance Coin, Avalanche, Polygon, Chainlink, Stellar, Ethereum Classic, Polkadot, Tron, and Algorand. Figure 9.5 effectively encapsulates the 11 critical indicators for evaluating smart contract processing in blockchain systems, especially in the context of healthcare applications. Each branch represents a specific aspect that is crucial for the successful implementation and operation of smart contracts within healthcare systems:

- Programming languages: The choice of programming languages is vital for the development of secure and efficient smart contracts in healthcare, where precision and reliability are paramount.
- Execution environment: This refers to the platform where smart contracts are executed, impacting their performance and security, especially in handling sensitive healthcare data.
- Resource management: Efficient resource management in blockchain systems ensures that smart contracts operate effectively without excessive costs or resource consumption, which is essential in healthcare applications.

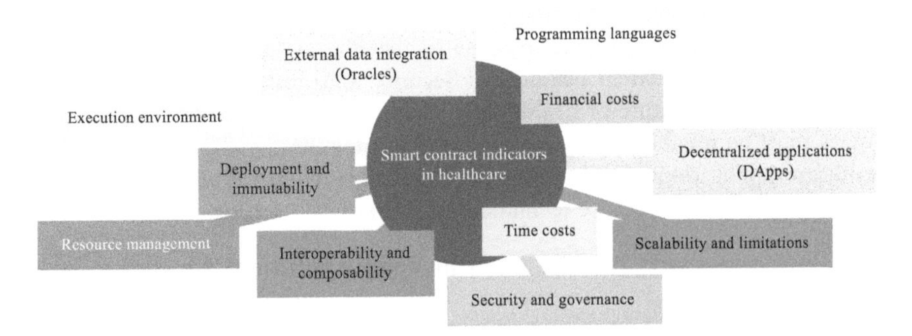

Figure 9.5 Critical indicators for evaluating smart contract processing in blockchain systems

- Deployment and immutability: The process of deploying smart contracts and their immutable nature once deployed are key in maintaining the integrity and trustworthiness of healthcare data.
- Interoperability and composability: The ability of blockchain systems to interoperate and compose with other systems and technologies is crucial for integrated healthcare solutions.
- Scalability and limitations: Understanding the scalability and limitations of blockchain platforms helps in assessing their suitability for handling the vast and complex data structures typical in healthcare.
- Security and governance: Ensuring robust security and effective governance mechanisms is essential to protect sensitive healthcare data and comply with regulatory standards.
- External data integration (Oracles): The integration of external data through oracles is crucial for healthcare applications that rely on real-world data for decision-making.
- DApps: The support for DApps is important for developing versatile and user-centric healthcare applications on blockchain platforms.
- Time costs: Time efficiency in executing and processing smart contracts is a critical factor in healthcare scenarios where timely data processing can be crucial.
- Financial costs: Financial considerations are always important, especially in the healthcare sector where cost-efficiency can directly impact the accessibility and quality of care.

Figure 9.5 provides a structured framework for analyzing and comparing different blockchain platforms in the context of healthcare, highlighting the multi-faceted considerations that must be taken into account for effective implementation and operation of smart contracts in this field. In healthcare, the precise handling of smart contracts is not just a technical requirement but a necessity for patient safety, data accuracy, and regulatory compliance. The programming languages must support complex and error-free coding, while the execution environment needs to be robust and secure. Resource management becomes crucial in ensuring that healthcare applications remain cost-effective and efficient. The immutability of smart contracts is vital for maintaining the integrity of medical records and transaction histories. Interoperability is essential for seamless integration with existing healthcare systems, and scalability ensures that the system can handle the vast amounts of data typical in healthcare. Security and governance are paramount, given the sensitive nature of health data. The integration of external data through oracles must be reliable and timely. The support for DApps allows for innovative healthcare applications, while time and financial costs are critical factors in the practical deployment of these technologies in healthcare settings.

9.5.3.2 Comparative analysis of blockchain solutions by programming languages

In the realm of healthcare cybersecurity, the choice of programming languages for smart contracts is a critical factor that influences the security, efficiency, and

Table 9.2 Comparison of systems by programming languages

Blockchain platform	**Programming languages supported**
Ethereum	Solidity, Vyper
Cardano	Plutus, Marlowe
Binance Coin	Solidity
Avalanche	Solidity, other EVM-compatible
Polygon	Solidity, other EVM-compatible
Chainlink	Not applicable (Oracle network)
Stellar	Stellar Smart Contracts (SSCs)
Ethereum Classic	Solidity
Polkadot	Substrate, Ink!
Tron	Solidity
Algorand	TEAL, PyTeal

adaptability of blockchain solutions. This comparison is crucial in understanding how each platform aligns with the stringent requirements of healthcare cybersecurity, where the accuracy, security, and functionality of smart contracts are paramount.

Table 9.2 summarizes the programming languages supported by each blockchain platform for smart contract development.

The choice of programming languages for smart contracts varies across blockchain platforms, each aligning differently with the needs of healthcare cybersecurity. Platforms like Ethereum, BSC, Avalanche, and Polygon offer the versatility and robustness of Solidity, making them suitable for a wide range of healthcare applications. In contrast, Cardano and Algorand's unique languages cater to specific use cases and developer preferences. Stellar and Ethereum Classic provide alternatives focusing on simplicity and immutability, respectively. Polkadot's and Tron's choices reflect their specific platform goals, such as interoperability and high-speed transactions.

9.5.3.3 Comparative analysis of blockchain solutions by execution environment

The execution environment of smart contracts is a critical aspect of blockchain platforms, especially in healthcare cybersecurity. This environment determines how smart contracts are processed, including their security, efficiency, and isolation from other network operations. This section compares various blockchain platforms based on their smart contract execution environments, highlighting their suitability for healthcare applications where reliability and performance are key.

Table 9.3 summarizes the execution environments provided by each blockchain platform for smart contract development.

The execution environments of these blockchain platforms vary significantly, each offering distinct advantages for healthcare cybersecurity. Platforms like Ethereum, Cardano, and Polkadot provide robust environments suitable for complex applications, while BSC, Avalanche, and Tron offer high throughput and

Table 9.3 Comparison of systems by execution environment

Blockchain platform	Execution environment characteristics
Ethereum	Ethereum Virtual Machine (EVM), quasi-Turing complete, isolated execution
Cardano	Plutus Core for smart contracts, high assurance with formal verification
Binance Coin	Binance Smart Chain (BSC), EVM-compatible, high throughput
Avalanche	Avalanche Virtual Machine (AVM), EVM-compatible, high performance
Polygon	EVM-compatible Layer 2 solutions, enhanced scalability and efficiency
Chainlink	Not applicable (focuses on oracles, integrates with multiple environments)
Stellar	Limited smart contract capabilities, focuses on simple operations
Ethereum Classic	Ethereum Classic Virtual Machine (ETCVM), similar to EVM, immutable
Polkadot	Substrate framework, supports multiple virtual machines including EVM
Tron	Tron Virtual Machine (TVM), EVM-compatible, high throughput
Algorand	Layer-1 execution, efficient and secure, supports TEAL and PyTeal

scalability. Polygon's Layer 2 solutions enhance Ethereum's capabilities, and Algorand's efficient environment is beneficial for simpler applications. Stellar and Ethereum Classic offer more limited but stable environments.

9.5.3.4 Comparative analysis of blockchain solutions by resource management

Effective resource management in blockchain platforms is crucial, especially in healthcare applications where efficiency and cost-effectiveness are key. Table 9.4 compares various blockchain platforms based on their approach to resource management, focusing on how they handle computational resources, transaction costs, and network efficiency.

The resource management approaches of these blockchain platforms vary, each with its advantages and challenges for healthcare applications. Platforms like Ethereum and Ethereum Classic offer flexibility but can incur high costs, while Cardano and Polkadot provide more predictability in transaction fees. BSC and Avalanche offer cost-effective alternatives with high throughput. Polygon enhances Ethereum's efficiency, and Stellar and Algorand stand out for their low-cost models. Tron's unique system offers a balance between free and paid resources.

9.5.3.5 Comparative analysis of blockchain solutions by deployment and immutability

The deployment and immutability of smart contracts are critical factors in blockchain platforms, especially in the healthcare sector where data integrity and reliability are

Table 9.4 Comparison of systems by resource management

Blockchain platform	Resource management approach
Ethereum	Gas system, variable costs based on network congestion
Cardano	Deterministic transaction cost model, focus on predictability
Binance Coin	Similar to Ethereum, but generally lower costs due to higher throughput
Avalanche	Fee model based on transaction size, emphasis on low costs
Polygon	Layer 2 scaling solutions reduce costs and improve efficiency on Ethereum
Chainlink	Oracle service costs, paid in LINK tokens
Stellar	Low transaction fees, minimal costs for operations
Ethereum Classic	Similar to Ethereum, gas system with variable costs
Polkadot	Transaction fees based on operational complexity, lower than Ethereum
Tron	Bandwidth and Energy system, free transactions with bandwidth, energy for smart contracts
Algorand	Low transaction fees, efficient PPoS consensus reduces costs

Table 9.5 Comparison of systems by deployment and immutability

Blockchain platform	Deployment and immutability characteristics
Ethereum	Smart contracts are immutable post-deployment; supports upgradable patterns via proxies
Cardano	Emphasizes high-assurance smart contracts with formal verification; immutable once deployed
Binance Coin	Similar to Ethereum; supports EVM-compatible smart contracts with immutability
Avalanche	EVM-compatible; supports immutable smart contracts and customizable subnets
Polygon	Inherits Ethereum's properties; supports upgradable smart contracts on Layer 2
Chainlink	Focuses on oracles; smart contract immutability depends on the underlying blockchain
Stellar	Limited smart contract capabilities; SSCs are simple and immutable
Ethereum Classic	Strong emphasis on immutability; follows the original Ethereum protocol
Polkadot	Supports upgradable smart contracts; emphasizes governance and flexibility
Tron	EVM-compatible; smart contracts are immutable with support for upgradable patterns
Algorand	Focuses on security and simplicity; smart contracts are immutable post-deployment

paramount. Table 9.5 compares various blockchain platforms based on their approaches to smart contract deployment and the immutability of these contracts.

The deployment and immutability approaches of these blockchain platforms vary, each offering distinct advantages for healthcare cybersecurity. Platforms like

Ethereum, Cardano, and Ethereum Classic emphasize immutability, ensuring data integrity. BSC and Avalanche offer similar benefits with additional scalability. Polygon extends Ethereum's features to Layer 2, and Stellar provides a simpler but immutable solution. Polkadot and Tron offer flexibility with upgradable contracts. Algorand's simplicity and security make it suitable for straightforward healthcare applications.

9.5.3.6 Comparative analysis of blockchain solutions by interoperability and composability

Interoperability and composability in blockchain platforms are crucial for integrating diverse systems and applications, especially in the healthcare sector where data exchange and system integration are essential. Table 9.6 compares various blockchain platforms based on their capabilities in interoperability and composability, highlighting how they facilitate the integration of different systems and applications in healthcare.

The interoperability and composability of these blockchain platforms vary, each offering distinct advantages for healthcare cybersecurity. Platforms like Ethereum and BSC provide high composability and interoperability within their ecosystems, while Polkadot and Avalanche excel in connecting multiple blockchains. Chainlink plays a unique role in enhancing interoperability through its oracle services. Stellar and Ethereum Classic offer more limited composability and interoperability features.

Table 9.6 Comparison of systems by interoperability and composability

Blockchain platform	Interoperability and composability features
Ethereum	High composability within its ecosystem; limited native interoperability with other blockchains
Cardano	Developing interoperability solutions; focus on high-assurance smart contracts
Binance Coin	High interoperability with Ethereum; supports cross-chain transfers
Avalanche	Native support for creating custom blockchains and assets; interoperable with Ethereum
Polygon	Enhances Ethereum's interoperability and composability with Layer 2 solutions
Chainlink	Provides interoperability through oracles, connecting various blockchains with real-world data
Stellar	Limited smart contract composability; focuses on interoperability in financial transactions
Ethereum Classic	Similar to Ethereum in composability; limited interoperability with other blockchains
Polkadot	High interoperability with various blockchains; supports multiple virtual machines and frameworks
Tron	Compatible with Ethereum; focuses on content sharing and entertainment DApps

Table 9.7 Comparison of systems by scalability and limitations

Blockchain platform	Scalability features and Limitations
Ethereum	Limited scalability with current PoW mechanism; transitioning to PoS with Ethereum 2.0 to improve scalability
Cardano	Designed for high scalability with Ouroboros PoS; ongoing development to enhance throughput
Binance Coin	Higher scalability than Ethereum with BSC's PoSA mechanism; supports high transaction throughput
Avalanche	High scalability with sub-second finality; unique consensus mechanism allows for rapid transaction processing
Polygon	Significantly enhances Ethereum's scalability with Layer 2 solutions like Plasma and PoS sidechains
Chainlink	Scalability depends on underlying blockchain; focuses on providing scalable oracle solutions
Stellar	High scalability for financial transactions; limited smart contract capabilities
Ethereum Classic	Similar scalability challenges as Ethereum; limited by PoW mechanism
Polkadot	Highly scalable with Substrate framework and parachain architecture; designed for cross-chain interoperability
Tron	High scalability with TVM and DPoS; optimized for high-speed transactions and DApps
Algorand	Excellent scalability with PPoS; designed for high throughput and low latency

9.5.3.7 Comparative analysis of blockchain solutions by scalability and limitations

Scalability and the associated limitations of blockchain platforms are critical factors in healthcare cybersecurity, impacting their ability to handle large volumes of data and transactions efficiently. Table 9.7 compares various blockchain platforms based on their scalability and inherent limitations, focusing on how these aspects influence their suitability for healthcare applications, where high throughput and reliable performance are essential.

The scalability and limitations of these blockchain platforms vary significantly, influencing their suitability for healthcare cybersecurity. Platforms like Ethereum and Ethereum Classic currently face scalability challenges, while BSC, Avalanche, and Tron offer higher throughput. Polygon provides a scalable Layer 2 solution for Ethereum-based applications. Cardano and Polkadot show promise with their scalable architectures, and Algorand stands out for its efficient and scalable consensus mechanism. Stellar, while scalable, is limited in smart contract complexity.

9.5.3.8 Comparative analysis of blockchain solutions by security and governance

Security and governance are pivotal aspects of blockchain platforms, particularly in healthcare cybersecurity, where protecting sensitive data and ensuring compliant

Table 9.8 Comparison of systems by security and governance

Blockchain platform	Security features and governance model
Ethereum	Robust security; decentralized governance with Ethereum Improvement Proposals (EIPs)
Cardano	High-assurance security with formal verification; decentralized governance model
Binance Coin	Similar security features to Ethereum; centralized governance by Binance
Avalanche	Unique consensus mechanism for enhanced security; decentralized governance
Polygon	Inherits Ethereum's security; additional Layer 2 security measures; decentralized governance
Chainlink	Security focused on reliable data feeds; governance depends on underlying blockchain
Stellar	Basic security features suitable for financial transactions; centralized governance
Ethereum Classic	Similar security features to Ethereum; decentralized governance but has faced security challenges
Polkadot	Advanced security with shared security model; decentralized governance through Polkadot Council and referenda
Tron	High throughput with adequate security features; more centralized governance model
Algorand	Strong security with PPoS consensus; decentralized governance with community participation

operations are crucial. Table 9.8 compares various blockchain platforms based on their security features and governance models, highlighting how these factors impact their suitability for healthcare applications.

The security features and governance models of these blockchain platforms vary, each offering distinct advantages and challenges for healthcare cybersecurity. Platforms like Ethereum, Cardano, and Polkadot provide robust security and decentralized governance, suitable for sensitive healthcare data. BSC and Tron offer similar security features but with more centralized governance. Avalanche and Algorand stand out for their innovative security mechanisms and decentralized governance models. Stellar and Ethereum Classic present different approaches, with Stellar focusing on basic security and centralized governance, and Ethereum Classic facing security challenges despite its decentralized governance.

9.5.3.9 Comparative analysis of blockchain solutions by external data integration (Oracles)

The integration of external data through oracles is a crucial aspect of blockchain platforms, especially in healthcare cybersecurity, where real-time data and external information are essential for decision-making. Table 9.9 compares various blockchain platforms based on their ability to integrate external data using oracles, highlighting how this capability impacts their suitability for healthcare applications.

Table 9.9 Comparison of systems by external data integration (Oracles)

Blockchain platform	Oracle integration and features
Ethereum	Extensive support for oracles; widely used platforms like Chainlink and Bandwidth
Cardano	Developing native oracle solutions; also supports third-party oracles
Binance Coin	Supports Ethereum-compatible oracles; actively integrating various oracle services
Avalanche	Compatible with Ethereum oracles; also exploring native oracle solutions
Polygon	Inherits Ethereum's oracle capabilities; supports multiple oracle platforms
Chainlink	Primary provider of oracle services; integrates with multiple blockchains
Stellar	Limited native oracle support; relies on third-party services for external data integration
Ethereum Classic	Supports Ethereum-compatible oracles; less active in oracle integration compared to Ethereum
Polkadot	Robust oracle integration with cross-chain capabilities; supports various oracle platforms
Tron	Supports integration with oracles; focuses on entertainment and content DApps
Algorand	Developing oracle capabilities; currently supports integration with third-party oracle services

The ability to integrate external data through oracles varies across these blockchain platforms, influencing their suitability for healthcare cybersecurity. Platforms like Ethereum, BSC, and Avalanche offer extensive oracle integration capabilities, suitable for healthcare applications requiring diverse data sources. Chainlink stands out as a primary oracle service provider, enhancing the capabilities of multiple blockchains. Cardano and Polkadot are developing robust native solutions, while Stellar and Ethereum Classic have more limited capabilities. Algorand and Tron are working on enhancing their oracle integration.

9.5.3.10 Comparative analysis of blockchain solutions by DApps

The support and infrastructure for DApps are vital in assessing blockchain platforms, especially in the healthcare sector where DApps can revolutionize data management and patient care. Table 9.10 compares various blockchain platforms based on their support for DApps, focusing on how these platforms facilitate the development and operation of healthcare-related applications.

The support for DApps across these blockchain platforms varies, influencing their suitability for healthcare cybersecurity. Platforms like Ethereum, BSC, and Polygon offer extensive DApp ecosystems with scalability and performance benefits. Cardano and Algorand are emerging as strong contenders with a focus on secure and efficient healthcare applications. Polkadot's cross-chain capabilities open up possibilities for innovative healthcare DApps. Stellar and Ethereum

Table 9.10 Comparison of systems by DApps

Blockchain platform	DApp support and ecosystem
Ethereum	Extensive DApp ecosystem; leading platform for diverse applications, including healthcare
Cardano	Developing DApp ecosystem; focus on high-assurance applications, suitable for healthcare
Binance Coin	Growing DApp ecosystem; compatible with Ethereum DApps, offering scalability benefits
Avalanche	Supports DApps with emphasis on customizability and scalability; growing healthcare DApp presence
Polygon	Enhances Ethereum DApps with scalability solutions; significant healthcare DApp development
Chainlink	Not a DApp platform but crucial for DApp functionality across platforms via oracle services
Stellar	Limited DApp capabilities; mainly focused on financial and transactional applications
Ethereum Classic	Similar DApp support to Ethereum but with a smaller ecosystem; less focus on healthcare
Polkadot	Robust DApp support with cross-chain interoperability; potential for innovative healthcare applications
Tron	Active DApp platform with a focus on content and entertainment; expanding into healthcare
Algorand	Growing DApp ecosystem; focus on efficiency and security, suitable for healthcare applications

Classic have more limited DApp capabilities, while Chainlink enhances DApp functionality with its oracle services. Tron and Avalanche are expanding their DApp ecosystems, including into healthcare.

9.5.3.11 Comparative analysis of blockchain solutions by time costs

Time efficiency in executing and processing smart contracts is a crucial factor in blockchain platforms, especially in healthcare applications where timely data processing can significantly impact patient care. Table 9.11 compares various blockchain platforms based on their time costs, focusing on transaction processing speeds and the efficiency of smart contract execution.

The time costs associated with these blockchain platforms vary, influencing their suitability for healthcare cybersecurity. Platforms like Avalanche, BSC, and Tron offer rapid transaction processing, suitable for time-critical healthcare applications. Ethereum and Ethereum Classic face challenges with slower transaction times, while Cardano and Polkadot aim to balance speed with security. Polygon enhances Ethereum's time efficiency, and Stellar provides fast processing for financial transactions. Algorand's speed and efficiency make it a strong contender for healthcare applications.

Table 9.11 Comparison of systems by time costs

Blockchain platform	Transaction processing speed	Smart contract execution efficiency
Ethereum	Around 13–15 seconds per block; can be slower during high congestion	Moderate; can be impacted by network congestion
Cardano	Approximately 20 seconds per block; aims for faster processing with upgrades	High; optimized for efficiency with formal verification
Binance Coin	Around 3 seconds per block; faster than Ethereum	High; benefits from BSC's high throughput
Avalanche	Sub-second finality; one of the fastest in the industry	Very high; optimized for rapid processing
Polygon	Varies; generally faster than Ethereum due to Layer 2 solutions	High; enhanced by Layer 2 scaling solutions
Chainlink	Not applicable (focuses on oracles)	Not applicable (depends on the underlying blockchain)
Stellar	3–5 seconds per transaction; optimized for fast financial transactions	Moderate; limited by simpler smart contract capabilities
Ethereum Classic	Similar to Ethereum; around 13–15 seconds per block	Moderate; similar to Ethereum
Polkadot	Varies; designed for fast and efficient processing	High; benefits from Polkadot's advanced architecture
Tron	Approximately 3 seconds per block; high throughput	High; optimized for speed and entertainment-focused DApps
Algorand	Under 5 seconds per block; very fast and efficient	High; optimized for speed with PPoS consensus

Figure 9.6 provides a visual comparison of the transaction processing speeds (measured in seconds per block) across different blockchain platforms. This metric is crucial for healthcare applications where timely data processing can significantly impact patient care and operational efficiency.

This comparative visualization underscores the importance of considering transaction processing speed when selecting a blockchain platform for healthcare applications, ensuring that the chosen technology aligns with the time-sensitive requirements of the healthcare sector.

9.5.3.12 Comparative analysis of blockchain solutions by financial costs

Financial costs associated with executing smart contracts are a critical consideration for blockchain platforms, especially in the healthcare sector where budget constraints are common. Table 9.12 compares various blockchain platforms based on their financial costs, focusing on transaction fees and the cost-effectiveness of smart contract execution.

The financial costs associated with these blockchain platforms vary, influencing their suitability for healthcare cybersecurity. Platforms like Ethereum face challenges with high transaction costs, while BSC, Avalanche, and Tron offer more cost-effective solutions. Cardano and Algorand provide predictability and

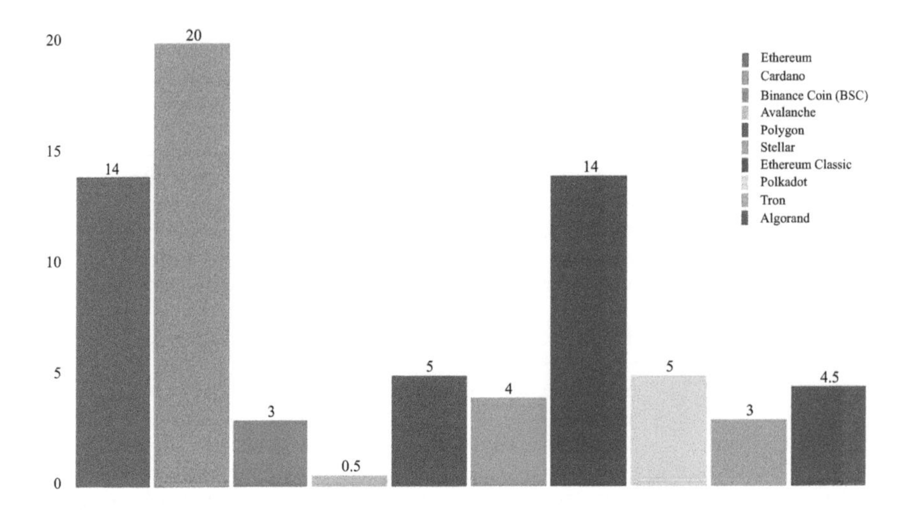

Figure 9.6 Transaction processing speeds across different blockchain platforms

Table 9.12 Comparison of systems by financial costs

Blockchain platform	Financial costs characteristics
Ethereum	High transaction fees during network congestion; variable costs based on gas prices
Cardano	Predictable and generally lower transaction costs; focus on cost-efficiency
Binance Coin	Lower transaction fees compared to Ethereum; cost-effective for high-volume transactions
Avalanche	Low transaction fees; emphasis on cost-efficiency and scalability
Polygon	Reduced transaction costs on Ethereum network through Layer 2 solutions
Chainlink	Costs associated with oracle services; varies based on data requirements
Stellar	Very low transaction fees; optimized for cost-effective financial transactions
Ethereum Classic	Similar to Ethereum; variable transaction costs based on network activity
Polkadot	Reasonable transaction fees; focus on efficiency and scalability
Tron	Generally low transaction fees; optimized for high throughput and cost-efficiency
Algorand	Low transaction fees; efficient consensus mechanism reduces operational costs

efficiency in costs, and Polygon enhances Ethereum's cost-effectiveness. Stellar stands out for its minimal transaction fees.

9.5.4 Comparative analysis of blockchain platforms for enhancing cybersecurity in healthcare: an application of the analytic hierarchy process

In the context of healthcare cybersecurity, the selection of an appropriate blockchain platform for smart contract processing is pivotal. This section employs the AHP, a structured technique for organizing and analyzing complex decisions, to compare the blockchain platforms based on the previously discussed criteria.

The AHP is a structured technique for organizing and analyzing complex decisions. Developed by Thomas L. Saaty in the 1970s, it involves decomposing a decision problem into a hierarchy of more easily comprehended sub-problems, each of which can be analyzed independently [46,47]. The steps in AHP include [47]:

1. Problem decomposition: Breaking down the decision problem into a hierarchy of interrelated criteria and sub-criteria.
2. Pairwise comparisons: Evaluating the elements of the hierarchy in a pairwise manner, using a scale of relative importance (from 1 to 9) to quantify the evaluators' subjective judgments.
3. Priority calculation: Deriving priority scales for the criteria and alternatives through the eigenvector method, which involves normalizing and averaging the pairwise comparison matrices.
4. Consistency check: Ensuring the consistency of the judgments through the calculation of a consistency ratio, which compares the consistency index of the matrix with the random index.
5. Synthesis of results: Aggregating the priorities across the hierarchy to determine overall priorities for the decision alternatives.

In the context of evaluating blockchain platforms for healthcare cybersecurity:

1. Evaluation of alternatives by criteria: This table involves pairwise comparisons of the blockchain platforms against each criterion. The scale from 1 to 9 reflects the relative superiority of one platform over another concerning each specific criterion.
2. Evaluation of criteria importance: This table assesses the relative importance of each criterion in the decision-making process. The scale from 1 to 9 is used to express how much more important one criterion is compared to another in the context of healthcare cybersecurity.

The final scores for each blockchain platform are calculated by multiplying the relative importance of each criterion by the platform's score for that criterion and then summing these products across all criteria. This process synthesizes the individual evaluations into an overall ranking of the platforms, considering both the importance of each criterion and the performance of each platform against those criteria.

Tables 9.13 and 9.14 provide a comprehensive framework for evaluating blockchain platforms in the context of healthcare cybersecurity. Table 9.13

Table 9.13 AHP-based evaluation of blockchain platforms

Criteria/Platform	Ethereum	Cardano	BSC	Avalanche	Polygon	Chainlink	Stellar	Ethereum Classic	Polkadot	Tron	Algorand
Programming languages	7	6	7	7	7	5	4	7	6	7	5
Execution environment	6	7	7	8	7	5	4	6	7	7	7
Resource management	4	7	8	8	7	5	9	4	7	8	8
Deployment and immutability	7	8	7	7	7	5	5	6	8	7	7
Interoperability and composability	7	6	7	7	7	5	4	6	8	6	6
Scalability and limitations	4	7	8	9	8	5	5	4	8	8	8
Security and governance	7	8	6	8	7	5	5	6	8	6	8
External data integration (Oracles)	8	6	7	7	7	9	4	6	7	6	6
DApps	9	6	7	7	8	5	4	6	7	6	6
Time costs	4	6	8	9	8	5	7	4	7	8	8
Financial costs	4	7	8	8	7	5	9	4	7	8	8

reveals the strengths and weaknesses of each platform across various criteria, highlighting areas where certain platforms excel or fall short. Table 9.14 reflects the prioritization of these criteria, emphasizing aspects like execution environment, scalability, and security as highly significant in healthcare cybersecurity.

Figure 9.7 provides a visual representation of the final AHP scores for various blockchain platforms, calculated for enhancing cybersecurity in healthcare. These scores are the result of a comprehensive evaluation based on multiple criteria, including programming languages, execution environment, resource management, and others:

Table 9.14 Evaluation of criteria importance

Criteria	Importance rating
Programming languages	8
Execution environment	9
Resource management	7
Deployment and immutability	8
Interoperability and composability	6
Scalability and limitations	9
Security and governance	9
External data integration (Oracles)	7
DApps	8
Time costs	7
Financial costs	6

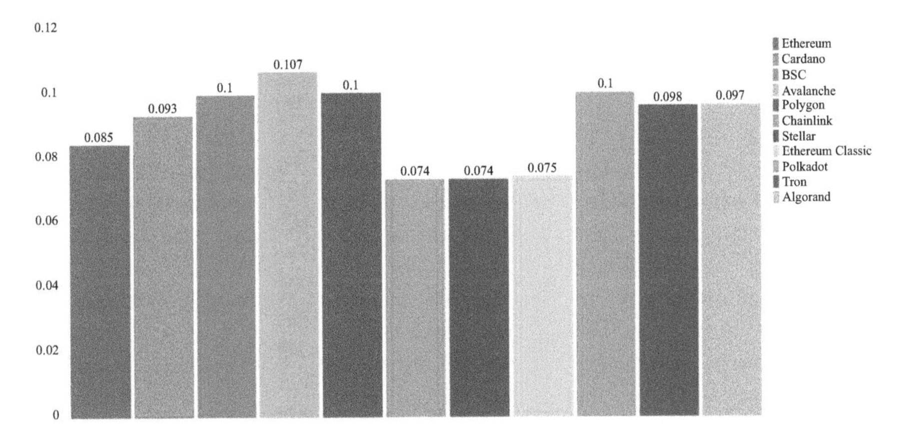

Figure 9.7 AHP scores for various blockchain platforms, calculated for enhancing cybersecurity in healthcare

- Avalanche emerges as the top-rated platform with the highest AHP score, indicating its strong alignment with the criteria deemed important for healthcare cybersecurity.
- Binance Coin and Polygon also score highly, reflecting their robust features and suitability for healthcare applications.
- Cardano and Algorand show strong performance, suggesting their potential in healthcare cybersecurity, particularly in terms of security and governance.
- Ethereum, despite being a pioneering platform, scores moderately. This is likely due to its current scalability and cost issues, though it remains a strong contender in areas like DApp support and programming languages.
- Tron, Polkadot, and Ethereum Classic exhibit good overall performance, each with unique strengths in the blockchain landscape.
- Chainlink and Stellar, while scoring lower, play specific roles in the blockchain ecosystem, with Chainlink excelling in oracle services and Stellar in financial transactions.

This visualization underscores the importance of a multi-criteria approach in selecting a blockchain platform for healthcare cybersecurity. It highlights that while some platforms may excel in certain areas, a comprehensive evaluation considering all relevant factors is crucial for making an informed decision. This analysis aids healthcare organizations in choosing a blockchain platform that best aligns with their specific cybersecurity needs and operational priorities.

9.5.5 Innovative applications of smart contracts in enhancing healthcare cybersecurity

The integration of smart contracts into healthcare cybersecurity represents a transformative shift, offering unprecedented opportunities for enhancing data privacy, streamlining processes, and ensuring compliance. This section delves into various pioneering applications of smart contracts in the healthcare domain, illustrating their potential to revolutionize the industry. Each example is explored in detail, highlighting the innovative approaches and the implications for healthcare cybersecurity.

1. The SAFE Project's Digital Health and Diagnostics Platform [48]. The SAFE project exemplifies the innovative use of smart contracts in healthcare. By generating unique health identifiers through a proprietary algorithm, patient privacy is meticulously preserved. These identifiers, while anonymized, maintain authenticity and verifiability, ensuring data integrity without compromising privacy. This approach addresses critical concerns in healthcare data management, such as maintaining confidentiality while allowing for accurate patient tracking and data analysis. The application of smart contracts in this context ensures that data access and sharing adhere to predefined rules, enhancing security and trust in digital health platforms.
2. IBM's Application in Clinical Trials [49]. IBM's implementation of smart contracts in clinical trials marks a significant advancement in healthcare

research. By automating consent verification and data collection processes, smart contracts reduce administrative errors, thereby increasing transparency and trust. This automation not only improves trial quality and patient safety but also leads to cost reductions, a crucial factor in large-scale clinical studies. The use of smart contracts in this setting exemplifies how blockchain technology can bring efficiency and reliability to complex healthcare processes.
3. Blockchain Product Traceability Solution by KPMG, Merck, Walmart, and IBM [50]. This collaboration highlights the power of blockchain in enhancing drug supply chain security. The developed solution demonstrates a remarkable reduction in the time required for medication recall notifications, streamlining what was once a days-long process into mere seconds. Such rapid response capabilities are vital in healthcare, where delays in recalls can have serious implications for patient safety. The integration of smart contracts in this solution ensures that recall processes are automatically triggered under specific conditions, showcasing an efficient and reliable approach to supply chain management.
4. IBM's Blockchain Network in Health Insurance [51]. IBM's application of blockchain in health insurance automates claim approval processes, significantly enhancing customer experience. Smart contracts in this context ensure the provenance and traceability of assets within the network, bringing transparency and efficiency to insurance operations. This automation not only streamlines administrative procedures but also reduces the potential for errors and fraud, crucial in the sensitive area of health insurance. The deployment of smart contracts here exemplifies their potential to transform traditional insurance processes, making them more user-friendly and secure.
5. Microsoft Azure's Integration in Healthcare Solutions [52]. Microsoft Azure's integration of IoT with healthcare solutions represents a significant step forward in data management and analysis. The connection of existing data sources, health record systems, and research databases through Azure facilitates the exchange of data in an interoperable format. Backed by advanced analytics and AI, this integration points to areas where smart contracts could be applied to ensure secure and efficient data management. The potential application of smart contracts in this integrated environment could automate data sharing agreements, ensuring compliance and enhancing data security.
6. Azure Blockchain Smart Contracts Application [25]. Researchers working with Azure Blockchain have applied the VeriSol tool to a diverse set of smart contracts within the Azure ecosystem. This includes governance applications for consortium members in Ethereum on Azure and Azure Blockchain Service. The use of VeriSol in validating and verifying smart contracts underscores the importance of ensuring their correctness and security, particularly in controlled enterprise environments. This application showcases the utility of smart contracts in ensuring compliance and governance in enterprise blockchain implementations, a critical aspect in healthcare settings.
7. Enterprise Smart Contracts on Azure [53]. Microsoft Azure's discussion on the evolution of enterprise smart contracts reflects significant technological

advancements. These contracts decompose the public smart contract approach, focusing on both contractual and technological aspects to deliver blockchain's promise in enterprise settings. For healthcare organizations, this evolution is particularly relevant, as it offers a way to integrate blockchain technology into their operations securely and efficiently. The application of enterprise smart contracts in healthcare could streamline various processes, from patient data management to supply chain operations, ensuring compliance and enhancing operational efficiency.

8. Oracle's Perspective on Smart Contracts [54]. Oracle recognizes the growing importance of smart contracts in various sectors, including healthcare. Their potential applications in managing complex processes and transactions in healthcare are significant, offering new ways to handle legal, business, and governance aspects. Oracle's perspective underscores the versatility of smart contracts, suggesting their applicability in diverse healthcare scenarios, from patient consent management to regulatory compliance. This recognition points to a broader trend of adopting blockchain technology in healthcare, with smart contracts playing a central role in this transformation.
9. Streamlining Healthcare Processes with Oracle [55]. Oracle notes that smart contracts can streamline the claim and payment process in healthcare, involving payers, providers, and patients. This application places patients in complete control of their medical data, a significant shift toward patient-centric healthcare models. By automating claims and payment processes, smart contracts can reduce administrative burdens and enhance the efficiency of healthcare financial transactions. The use of smart contracts in this context not only improves operational efficiency but also empowers patients, ensuring their data privacy and control.
10. Blockchain's Value in Healthcare According to Oracle [56]. Oracle emphasizes the value of blockchain in managing the vast volume of data in healthcare. The security, speed, and other benefits offered by blockchain are crucial in healthcare applications, where data integrity and accessibility are paramount. Smart contracts, as part of blockchain solutions, can automate and secure data-related processes, enhancing the overall effectiveness of healthcare systems. Oracle's emphasis on blockchain's value highlights the growing recognition of this technology's potential to revolutionize healthcare data management and security.

The practical applications of smart contracts in healthcare cybersecurity, as illustrated by these examples, demonstrate their versatility and transformative potential. From enhancing patient privacy and streamlining clinical trials to revolutionizing health insurance and supply chain management, smart contracts offer a range of solutions to longstanding challenges in healthcare. These examples underscore the growing importance of blockchain technology in healthcare, highlighting how smart contracts can be leveraged to improve cybersecurity, operational efficiency, and patient-centric care. As the healthcare industry continues to evolve, the integration of smart contracts is poised to play a pivotal role in shaping its future.

9.6 Discussion

- The investigation into the application of smart contracts in healthcare cybersecurity has yielded insightful results, underscoring the transformative potential of this technology in the sector. The discussion of these results is multifaceted, reflecting on the legal, technical, and practical aspects of smart contracts.
- Legal and regulatory insights. The study highlights the complex legal landscape that smart contracts must navigate, particularly in complying with stringent healthcare regulations like HIPAA and GDPR. The immutable and transparent nature of smart contracts presents both opportunities and challenges in this regard. While they offer a robust framework for enforcing compliance, their rigidity can conflict with regulations requiring data flexibility. This dichotomy underscores the need for innovative legal solutions and adaptive programming to reconcile smart contract technology with existing legal frameworks.
- Technical and security considerations. From a technical standpoint, the results indicate that while smart contracts offer enhanced security and efficiency, they are not without vulnerabilities. The potential for coding errors and the challenges in integrating with existing healthcare systems highlight the need for rigorous testing and validation processes. Furthermore, the study points to the necessity of ongoing technical development to address scalability and interoperability issues, ensuring that smart contracts can effectively support the diverse and complex needs of healthcare cybersecurity.
- Administrative efficiency and error reduction. One of the most promising findings is the potential of smart contracts to significantly reduce administrative burdens and minimize human error risks in healthcare. By automating routine tasks and compliance processes, smart contracts can streamline operations, allowing healthcare professionals to focus more on patient care rather than administrative duties. This automation also reduces the likelihood of human errors, which are common in manual processes, thereby enhancing the overall quality and reliability of healthcare services.
- Comparative analysis of blockchain platforms. The comparative analysis of various blockchain platforms supporting smart contracts reveals a diverse landscape with varying strengths and weaknesses. Platforms like Ethereum, while pioneering in the field, face challenges in scalability and cost. In contrast, newer platforms like Avalanche and BSC offer improvements in these areas but have their trade-offs in terms of security and decentralization. This analysis is crucial for healthcare organizations to make informed decisions when selecting a blockchain platform, balancing their specific needs with the capabilities and limitations of each platform.
- Innovative applications and future prospects. The exploration of innovative applications of smart contracts in healthcare cybersecurity demonstrates their versatility and potential for widespread adoption. From enhancing patient

privacy to streamlining clinical trials and supply chain management, smart contracts can be applied in various aspects of healthcare. Looking forward, the continued evolution of smart contract technology, coupled with advancements in blockchain platforms, is expected to further expand their applications and efficacy in healthcare cybersecurity.

In conclusion, the results of this study provide a comprehensive understanding of the role of smart contracts in healthcare cybersecurity. While there are challenges to be addressed, the potential benefits of smart contracts in enhancing compliance, efficiency, and security are clear. As the technology continues to mature, it holds the promise of significantly transforming healthcare cybersecurity practices.

9.7 Conclusion and future scope

This chapter has provided an in-depth exploration of the role of smart contracts in healthcare cybersecurity, revealing their significant potential to revolutionize the field. The critical analysis of legal, security, and technical aspects has highlighted both the opportunities and challenges inherent in integrating smart contracts into healthcare systems. The ability of smart contracts to automate compliance with regulations like HIPAA and GDPR, streamline administrative processes, and reduce human error presents a compelling case for their adoption in healthcare cybersecurity.

The comparative analysis of blockchain platforms supporting smart contracts has offered valuable insights into the strengths and limitations of various technologies in this space. It has become evident that while no single platform is universally superior, each offers unique attributes that can be leveraged in different healthcare contexts.

Looking ahead, the future of smart contracts in healthcare cybersecurity is poised for significant growth and evolution. Several key areas are identified for future development and research:

- Enhanced legal and regulatory frameworks: As legal and regulatory environments continue to evolve, there is a need for more adaptive and flexible smart contract frameworks that can seamlessly align with changing legal requirements.
- Advancements in technology: Ongoing technological advancements in blockchain and smart contract programming are essential to address current limitations in scalability, interoperability, and security. Future research should focus on developing more robust, efficient, and user-friendly platforms.
- Integration with emerging technologies: The integration of smart contracts with other emerging technologies like AI, IoT, and big data analytics presents exciting opportunities for innovation in healthcare cybersecurity. These integrations could lead to more sophisticated, predictive, and responsive healthcare security systems.
- Education and training: As smart contracts become more prevalent, there will be an increasing need for education and training programs to equip healthcare

professionals and IT staff with the necessary skills and knowledge to effectively implement and manage these technologies.

- Broader adoption and implementation studies: Future research should also focus on broader adoption strategies for smart contracts in healthcare, including pilot studies and implementation research to evaluate their practical impact in real-world settings.

In conclusion, smart contracts hold great promise for enhancing healthcare cybersecurity, offering solutions that are not only more efficient and secure but also more compliant with regulatory standards. As the technology continues to mature and overcome current challenges, it is poised to play a pivotal role in the digital transformation of healthcare cybersecurity. The ongoing collaboration between technologists, healthcare professionals, and legal experts will be crucial in realizing the full potential of smart contracts in this vital sector.

Acknowledgments

- This project has received funding from the European Union's Horizon 2020 research and innovation program under the Marie Skłodowska-Curie grant agreement No. 101007820 – TRUST.
- This publication reflects only the author's view and the REA is not responsible for any use that may be made of the information it contains.

References

[1] C. Gong and V. Ribiere, "Chapter 1 – A historical outline of digital transformation," in *Digital Transformation in Healthcare in Post-Covid-19 Times*, M. D. Lytras, A. A. Housawi, and B. S. Alsaywid, Eds., in *Next Generation Technology Driven Personalized Medicine and Smart Healthcare*, Academic Press, 2023, pp. 3–25. doi:10.1016/B978-0-323-98353-2.00016-2.

[2] P. Mccaffrey, "Chapter 1 – The healthcare IT landscape," in *An Introduction to Healthcare Informatics*, P. Mccaffrey, Ed., Academic Press, 2020, pp. 3–15. doi:10.1016/B978-0-12-814915-7.00001-6.

[3] J. Rosa-Bilbao and J. Boubeta-Puig, "Chapter 15 – Ethereum blockchain platform," in *Distributed Computing to Blockchain*, R. Pandey, S. Goundar, and S. Fatima, Eds., Academic Press, 2023, pp. 267–282. doi:10.1016/B978-0-323-96146-2.00006-1.

[4] H. Kim, H.-S. Kim, and Y.-S. Park, "Perpetual contract NFT as collateral for DeFi composability," *IEEE Access*, vol. 10, pp. 126802–126814, 2022, doi:10.1109/ACCESS.2022.3225884.

[5] S. Chakraborty, S. Aich, and H.-C. Kim, "A secure healthcare system design framework using blockchain technology," in *2019 21st International Conference on Advanced Communication Technology (ICACT)*, 2019, pp. 260–264. doi:10.23919/ICACT.2019.8701983.

[6] A. R. Iossifova and S. Meyer-Goldstein, “Impact of standards adoption on healthcare transaction performance: The case of HIPAA,” *International Journal of Production Economics*, vol. 141, no. 1, pp. 277–285, 2013, doi:10.1016/j.ijpe.2012.08.002.

[7] UCL, “GDPR – Glossary of terms and definitions,” Legal Services. Accessed: Nov. 07, 2021. [Online]. Available: https://www.ucl.ac.uk/legal-services/gdpr-glossary-terms-and-definitions

[8] N. Naik and P. Jenkins, “Your identity is yours: Take back control of your identity using GDPR compatible self-sovereign identity,” in *2020 7th International Conference on Behavioural and Social Computing (BESC)*, 2020, pp. 1–6. doi:10.1109/BESC51023.2020.9348298.

[9] S.-W. Lee, I. Singh, and M. Mohammadian, Eds., *Blockchain Technology for IoT Applications*. in Blockchain Technologies. Singapore: Springer, 2021. doi:10.1007/978-981-33-4122-7.

[10] P. Pawar, T. O. Edoh, M. Singh, and N. Parolia, “Hitching medical IoT devices to blockchain for personal health information management,” in *Blockchain Technology for IoT Applications*, S.-W. Lee, I. Singh, and M. Mohammadian, Eds., in Blockchain Technologies, Singapore: Springer, 2021, pp. 191–205. doi:10.1007/978-981-33-4122-7_10.

[11] I. Al-Dalati, “Chapter 10 – Digital twins and cybersecurity in healthcare systems,” in *Digital Twin for Healthcare*, A. El Saddik, Ed., Academic Press, 2023, pp. 195–221. doi:10.1016/B978-0-32-399163-6.00015-9.

[12] F. F. Alruwaili, B. Alabduallah, H. Alqahtani, A. S. Salama, G. P. Mohammed, and A. A. Alneil, “Blockchain enabled smart healthcare system using jellyfish search optimization with dual-pathway deep convolutional neural network,” *IEEE Access*, vol. 11, pp. 87583–87591, 2023, doi:10.1109/ACCESS.2023.3304269.

[13] D. K. Mukesh Varman, S. Kiran Shrinivaas, A. U. Rahul Karthick, and V. Vanitha, “Blockchain in healthcare data,” in *2023 2nd International Conference on Advancements in Electrical, Electronics, Communication, Computing and Automation (ICAECA)*, 2023, pp. 1–6. doi:10.1109/ICAECA56562.2023.10199723.

[14] J.-S. Lee, C.-J. Chew, J.-Y. Liu, Y.-C. Chen, and K.-Y. Tsai, “Medical blockchain: Data sharing and privacy preserving of EHR based on smart contract,” *Journal of Information Security and Applications*, vol. 65, p. 103117, 2022, doi:10.1016/j.jisa.2022.103117.

[15] F. Luh and Y. Yen, “Cybersecurity in science and medicine: Threats and challenges,” *Trends in Biotechnology*, vol. 38, no. 8, pp. 825–828, 2020, doi:10.1016/j.tibtech.2020.02.010.

[16] M. Sookhak, M. R. Jabbarpour, N. S. Safa, and F. R. Yu, “Blockchain and smart contract for access control in healthcare: A survey, issues and challenges, and open issues,” *Journal of Network and Computer Applications*, vol. 178, p. 102950, 2021, doi:10.1016/j.jnca.2020.102950.

[17] H. Szczepaniuk and E. K. Szczepaniuk, “Cryptographic evidence-based cybersecurity for smart healthcare systems,” *Information Sciences*, vol. 649, p. 119633, 2023, doi:10.1016/j.ins.2023.119633.
[18] Y. Nishat and S. Shahid, “Chapter 7 – Effects of smart-contract blockchain on smart healthcare center management,” in *Unleashing the Potentials of Blockchain Technology for Healthcare Industries*, M. M. Ghonge, N. Pradeep, A. Das, Y. Wu, and O. Pal, Eds., Academic Press, 2023, pp. 107–136. doi:10.1016/B978-0-323-99481-1.00008-0.
[19] J. C. Isichei, S. Khorsandroo, and S. Desai, “Cybersecurity and privacy in smart bioprinting,” *Bioprinting*, vol. 36, p. e00321, 2023, doi:10.1016/j.bprint.2023.e00321.
[20] M. Khalid, S. Hameed, A. Qadir, S. A. Shah, and D. Draheim, “Towards SDN-based smart contract solution for IoT access control,” *Computer Communications*, vol. 198, pp. 1–31, 2023, doi:10.1016/j.comcom.2022.11.007.
[21] I. Priyadarshini, R. Kumar, A. Alkhayyat, *et al.*, “Survivability of industrial internet of things using machine learning and smart contracts,” *Computers and Electrical Engineering*, vol. 107, p. 108617, 2023, doi:10.1016/j.compeleceng.2023.108617.
[22] S. Rani, A. Kataria, S. Kumar, and P. Tiwari, “Federated learning for secure IoMT-applications in smart healthcare systems: A comprehensive review,” *Knowledge-Based Systems*, vol. 274, p. 110658, 2023, doi:10.1016/j.knosys.2023.110658.
[23] S. Bistarelli, G. Mazzante, M. Micheletti, L. Mostarda, D. Sestili, and F. Tiezzi, “Ethereum smart contracts: Analysis and statistics of their source code and opcodes,” *Internet of Things*, vol. 11, p. 100198, 2020, doi:10.1016/j.iot.2020.100198.
[24] S. Ji, J. Wu, J. Qiu, and J. Dong, “Effuzz: Efficient fuzzing by directed search for smart contracts,” *Information and Software Technology*, vol. 159, p. 107213, 2023, doi:10.1016/j.infsof.2023.107213.
[25] L. LoPresti, “Bolstering Azure blockchain smart contracts with formal verification,” Microsoft Research. Accessed: Dec. 14, 2023. [Online]. Available: https://www.microsoft.com/en-us/research/blog/researchers-work-to-secure-azure-blockchain-smart-contracts-with-formal-verification/
[26] N. M. Thomasian and E. Y. Adashi, “Cybersecurity in the Internet of Medical Things,” *Health Policy and Technology*, vol. 10, no. 3, p. 100549, Sep. 2021, doi:10.1016/j.hlpt.2021.100549.
[27] M. Javaid, A. Haleem, R. P. Singh, and R. Suman, “Towards insighting cybersecurity for healthcare domains: A comprehensive review of recent practices and trends,” *Cyber Security and Applications*, vol. 1, p. 100016, 2023, doi:10.1016/j.csa.2023.100016.
[28] H. Arslanian, “Ethereum,” in *The Book of Crypto: The Complete Guide to Understanding Bitcoin, Cryptocurrencies and Digital Assets*, H. Arslanian, (eds.) Ed., Cham: Springer International Publishing, 2022, pp. 91–98. doi:10.1007/978-3-030-97951-5_3.

[29] Ethereum, "Ethereum Yellow Paper" in Ethereum Yellow Paper. ethereum, Dec. 06, 2023. Accessed: Dec. 08, 2023. [Online]. Available: https://github.com/ethereum/yellowpaper

[30] "Cardano is a decentralized public blockchain and cryptocurrency project and is fully open source," Cardano. Accessed: May 11, 2023. [Online]. Available: https://cardano.org/

[31] "Binance – Cryptocurrency Exchange for Bitcoin, Ethereum & Altcoins." Accessed: May 25, 2023. [Online]. Available: https://www.binance.com/en

[32] "Network Protocol | Avalanche Dev Docs." Accessed: May 04, 2023. [Online]. Available: https://docs.avax.network/specs/network-protocol

[33] PolygonScan.com, "Polygon PoS Chain (MATIC) Blockchain Explorer," Polygon (MATIC) Blockchain Explorer. Accessed: Dec. 17, 2023. [Online]. Available: http://polygonscan.com/

[34] "The Value Layer of the Internet." Accessed: Dec. 17, 2023. [Online]. Available: https://polygon.technology/

[35] "Chainlink: The Industry-Standard Web3 Services Platform." Accessed: May 11, 2023. [Online]. Available: https://chain.link/

[36] "Stellar – An open network for money." Accessed: May 11, 2023. [Online]. Available: https://stellar.org/

[37] "Ethereum Classic," Ethereum Classic. Accessed: Dec. 17, 2023. [Online]. Available: https://ethereumclassic.org/

[38] "Polkadot: Web3 Interoperability | Decentralized Blockchain," Polkadot Network. Accessed: May 11, 2023. [Online]. Available: https://polkadot.network/

[39] "TRON Network | Decentralize The Web." Accessed: Dec. 17, 2023. [Online]. Available: https://debug.tron.network

[40] "java-tron." tronprotocol, Dec. 16, 2023. Accessed: Dec. 17, 2023. [Online]. Available: https://github.com/tronprotocol/java-tron

[41] "Algorand | The Blockchain for FutureFi." Accessed: May 11, 2023. [Online]. Available: https://algorand.com/

[42] M. Iqbal, A. Kormiltsyn, V. Dwivedi, and R. Matulevičius, "Blockchain-based ontology driven reference framework for security risk management," *Data & Knowledge Engineering*, vol. 149, p. 102257, 2024, doi:10.1016/j.datak.2023.102257.

[43] S. Ahmadisheykhsarmast, S. G. Senji, and R. Sonmez, "Decentralized tendering of construction projects using blockchain-based smart contracts and storage systems," *Automation in Construction*, vol. 151, p. 104900, 2023, doi:10.1016/j.autcon.2023.104900.

[44] "Cryptocurrency Prices, Charts, and Crypto Market Cap," CoinGecko. Accessed: Dec. 17, 2023. [Online]. Available: https://www.coingecko.com/

[45] "Coinlib – Crypto Prices, Charts, Lists & Crypto Market News." Accessed: Dec. 17, 2023. [Online]. Available: https://coinlib.io/

[46] T. L. Saaty, "The analytic hierarchy process: Decision making in complex environments," in *Quantitative Assessment in Arms Control: Mathematical Modeling and Simulation in the Analysis of Arms Control Problems*,

R. Avenhaus and R. K. Huber, Eds., Boston, MA: Springer US, 1984, pp. 285–308. doi:10.1007/978-1-4613-2805-6_12.

[47] T. L. Saaty, "How to make a decision: The analytic hierarchy process," *European Journal of Operational Research*, vol. 48, no. 1, pp. 9–26, 1990, doi:10.1016/0377-2217(90)90057-I.

[48] "Smart Contracts in Healthcare," Hedera. Accessed: Dec. 14, 2023. [Online]. Available: https://hedera.com/learning/smart-contracts/smart-contracts-healthcare

[49] "Blockchain in healthcare and life sciences industries | IBM." Accessed: Dec. 14, 2023. [Online]. Available: https://www.ibm.com/blockchain/resources/healthcare/

[50] "Blockchain healthcare and life sciences solutions | IBM." Accessed: Dec. 14, 2023. [Online]. Available: https://www.ibm.com/blockchain/industries/healthcare

[51] R. Viswanathan, "Blockchain in a nutshell: Building enterprise solutions," IBM Blog. Accessed: Dec. 14, 2023. [Online]. Available: https://www.ibm.com/blog/blockchain-in-a-nutshell-building-enterprise-solutions/www.ibm.com/blog/blockchain-in-a-nutshell-building-enterprise-solutions

[52] "IoT in Healthcare Solutions | Microsoft Azure." Accessed: Dec. 14, 2023. [Online]. Available: https://azure.microsoft.com/en-us/solutions/industries/healthcare/iot/

[53] M. Gray, "Introducing Enterprise Smart Contracts," Microsoft Azure Blog. Accessed: Dec. 14, 2023. [Online]. Available: https://azure.microsoft.com/en-us/blog/introducing-enterprise-smart-contracts/

[54] G. Author, "Making Smart Contracts a Reality with Blockchain Technology." Accessed: Dec. 14, 2023. [Online]. Available: https://blogs.oracle.com/blockchain/post/making-smart-contracts-a-reality-with-blockchain-technology

[55] "Improve Your Healthcare Operations with Blockchain." Accessed: Dec. 14, 2023. [Online]. Available: https://www.oracle.com/in/blockchain/what-is-blockchain/blockchain-in-healthcare/

[56] "Managed Enterprise Blockchain Service." Accessed: Dec. 14, 2023. [Online]. Available: https://www.oracle.com/blockchain/cloud-platform/

Chapter 10

Cybersecurity computing in modern healthcare systems

Lateef Adesola Akinyemi[1,2,3,4], *Ernest Mnkandla*[1,4] *and Mbuyu Sumbwanyambe*[2,4]

Although the integration of digital technology into modern healthcare systems has revolutionised the administration of medical services, these systems are now susceptible to unprecedented cybersecurity vulnerabilities. In response to these challenges, machine learning-based algorithms have emerged as a powerful instrument for enhancing cybersecurity defences in the healthcare industry. This study explores the application of machine learning (ML) techniques such as K-nearest neighbours (KNN), random forest (RF), and linear regression (LR) for cybersecurity computing in emerging healthcare systems to solve cybersecurity problems in developing healthcare systems. This study provides a thorough analysis of the possible advantages of cybersecurity computing for enhancing healthcare systems. It focuses on how technology could change healthcare operations like drug development, customised medication, gene sequencing, health imaging, and so on. More significantly, this study uses ML-inspired algorithms to perform some data analytics on the security of data accessible in healthcare systems and includes a use case to illustrate the effectiveness of cybersecurity computing in emerging healthcare systems. The study begins by outlining the unique cybersecurity challenges and threats that nascent healthcare systems face, such as the abundance of networked medical devices, the complexity of healthcare information technology (IT) infrastructures, and the ever-changing landscape of threats. To anticipate the quantity of data and output file sizes needed to complete health-related tasks, LR, RF algorithms, and KNN

[1]Department of Computer Science, School of Computing, College of Engineering and Technology (CSET), University of South Africa, Florida Campus, South Africa
[2]Department of Electrical and Smart Systems Engineering, School of Engineering, College of Science, Engineering and Technology, University of South Africa, South Africa
[3]Department of Electronic and Computer Engineering, Faculty of Engineering, Lagos State University, Nigeria
[4]Centre for Augmented Intelligence and Data Science (CAIDS), University of South Africa, Florida Campus, South Africa

algorithms are employed. This allows for the identification of odd patterns or behaviours that may indicate security infractions. Mean square error (MSE), mean absolute error (MAE), and root mean square error (RMSE) are performance metrics used for the evaluation and comparison of ML algorithms. In general, the KNN algorithm in some cases outperforms other algorithms such as LR and RF when compared using MSE with numerical values of 833.6, 662.04, and 833.6, respectively.

Keywords: Cybersecurity; computing; healthcare systems; technology; machine learning; datasets

10.1 Introduction

Healthcare systems are rapidly becoming more digitally connected, which has completely changed how medical services are delivered and created previously unheard-of prospects for better treatment of patients, greater availability, and increased efficiency. However, with these developments also comes the growing threat of cyberattacks, which seriously jeopardise the confidentiality of patients, confidentiality of data, and healthcare equipment dependability. Strengthening healthcare cybersecurity measures is becoming more and more necessary therefore to these issues, especially in developing healthcare systems where the adoption of digital technology is speeding up. A subset of artificial intelligence (AI) called machine learning (ML) has become a formidable weapon in the security measures toolbox, with the ability to identify, stop, and react to cyberattacks more quickly and precisely than with more techniques that are conventional.

Healthcare companies may strengthen their defences and protect sensitive data by using AI techniques to analyse massive volumes of data and spot patterns suggestive of criminal behaviour. Tremendous breakthroughs in technological advancements have led to an enormous shift in the field of healthcare [1,2]. New computing and digital technologies have shown themselves to be potent drivers as well as enablers for creative thinking in the healthcare sector during the past several years. Several instances of technological advances that have quickly changed the healthcare industry are wearable devices, telemedicine, electronic records of healthcare, the Internet of Things (IoT) in healthcare, AI, and other emerging technologies, among others. Electronic medical records have simplified maintaining records and data sharing, wearable technology has allowed for continuous patient monitoring, telemedicine has made healthcare more accessible by permitting remote consultations, and AI has provided amazing insights for diagnosis and treatment.

The use of these technologies has increased the efficacy and efficiency of healthcare, but it has brought out new difficulties [1–3]. The use of technological advances in healthcare has unleashed a host of security flaws. Computer hacking can originate from connected gadgets, which are frequently equipped with insufficient security measures. Hackers frequently target information about patients, making it vulnerable to loss or illegal access. Sometimes, because of the quick speed of invention, security issues are neglected, leaving devices and systems vulnerable to changing threats. Furthermore, people including patients and healthcare workers can unintentionally create problems by exchanging passwords, falling for phishing frauds, or neglecting to update computer programmes and systems regularly. Therefore, it is imperative to respond to the vulnerabilities associated with growing computing and digital innovations in healthcare with vigilance and proactivity [4–6]. These dangers have repercussions that go beyond monetary losses; they also carry the risk of endangering the health and welfare of patients.

Healthcare organisations must prioritise cybersecurity since it can have negative legitimate and ethical effects. In the continuous endeavour to protect the healthcare sector from malevolent acts, it is imperative to comprehend these risks and their possible consequences [5–7]. It is critical to find an acceptable compromise between utilising the possible benefits of these technological developments and making sure, they do not spread harmful influences at a time when healthcare could undergo a revolution thanks to technology. By taking this action, we can create the conditions for a time in the future when new digital and accelerated computing healthcare technologies may be fully utilised to provide the best possible care for patients while protecting their information and well-being from constant cybersecurity threats.

Thus, it aims to offer an in-depth comprehension of the present state of the field, particularly to healthcare professionals. In contrast to prior research, papers that focused on specific technological topics related to emerging digital technologies, this article would explore the interlinked aspects of new digital innovations in cybersecurity and healthcare. Interested parties will learn more about the complex interplay between security and development in the healthcare industry by examining the advantages, risks, threats, and standards for excellence in healthcare cybersecurity. An in-depth discussion of the growing cybersecurity risks that healthcare organisations must contend with is presented in [8], with a focus on how the COVID-19 pandemic has made matters worse. The study emphasises how crucial strong cybersecurity measures are to protecting private patient information and guaranteeing the continuous provision of medical care. In light of the COVID-19 pandemic, the article attempts to do a preliminary assessment to investigate the cybersecurity issues and potential solutions unique to the healthcare industry.

Authors in [9] provide context for the increasing integration of digital technology in healthcare and the corresponding cybersecurity risks. The study emphasises how revolutionary technological advancements like smartphones and tablets, telemedicine, and electronic health records can enhance the treatment of patients and streamline business processes. More importantly, it draws attention to the weaknesses in these innovations and the necessity of strong cybersecurity defences to protect private medical information and maintain the reliability of healthcare providers. More so, by underlining the growing cybersecurity dangers that healthcare organisations around the world are facing, the study in [10] presents and captures the required details for cybersecurity in healthcare systems. It highlights how crucial cybersecurity is to protecting patient information, maintaining the trustworthiness of healthcare networks, and lowering the danger of intrusions. Hence, the purpose of the investigation in [10] is to compare cybersecurity experiences and maturity levels among international healthcare organisations to find efficient methods, typical problems, and areas for development. The acknowledgement of the growing complexity and regularity of cyberattacks on healthcare organisations opens the introductory section in [11].

The author in [11] presents the idea of a zero-trust approach to cybersecurity and emphasises the shortcomings of conventional perimeter-based security strategies in the face of changing cyber threats. Hence, the study in [11] aims to examine the tenets and practical applications of zero-trust principles in healthcare environments, with a focus on how it might improve the security environment and reduce threats from the internet. The significance of cybersecurity for the healthcare industry is the major feature in [12], which highlights the need to protect against digital hazards, maintain the security of medical infrastructure, and preserve patient data. It draws attention to the growing complexity and frequency of attacks against healthcare institutions, as well as their possible effects on patient safety and trust.

10.1.1 Motivation for the study

Given how quickly healthcare technology is developing, the incorporation of accelerated computing schemes into cybersecurity for developing healthcare systems is not just an academic pursuit but also rather a pressing requirement. Fortifying healthcare systems against advanced cyberattacks is becoming more and more important as these platforms undergo a revolutionary transition towards technological advancement, interdependent networks, and the sharing of large volumes of personally identifiable information about patients. This section addresses several important issues to encourage the use of powerful computing tools in healthcare cybersecurity. The most important thing is to prepare healthcare systems for the impending threat of adversaries. To protect patients' dignity and maintain the confidentiality of healthcare operations, it is necessary to safeguard private medical information. This is why it is important to investigate accelerated and powerful computing cybersecurity in emerging healthcare systems using ML algorithms as future possibilities. Another driving force is the possibility of creating a novel framework for safe communication in healthcare networks.

The flaws of conventional key transmission techniques could be addressed using powerful computing techniques, which improve the secrecy of health-related data communicated among healthcare providers by ensuring the sharing of cryptographic keys with the level of security. Therefore, the rationale also includes healthcare organisations' fundamental need to implement revolutionary innovations that protect the well-being of patients. In the long run, the need to safeguard the privacy of patients, strengthen vital medical facilities, and guarantee the moral obligation of healthcare institutions in the midst of developing cyber threats is the driving force underlying the investigation of computing for cybersecurity in developing healthcare systems.

Considering a rapidly developing cognitive-powered digital world, this chapter aims to illuminate the revolutionary potential of computing technologies by providing insights into a safe and robust future for medical systems. Therefore, the motivation for the study is as follows: The increasing reliance on digital technology for healthcare delivery is the driving force behind research on ML-based cybersecurity computing in upcoming healthcare systems. Healthcare organisations are growing increasingly linked and susceptible to cyberattacks as telehealth channels, IoT gadgets, and medical records that are electronic become more widely used. The research investigation uses machine-learning approaches to identify and reduce cyberattacks to meet the urgent need for strong cybersecurity safeguards in developing healthcare systems. The research work seeks to secure patient data, medical devices, and the accessibility and accuracy of medical services by improving security measures vulnerability.

10.1.2 Key contributions of the chapter

In brief, the noteworthiness of this study in terms of key contributions is outlined below:

- It offers the first thorough analysis of cybersecurity computing technologies for the medical field, encompassing the goals of the field, needs, uses, difficulties, architectures, and unresolved research questions.
- It talks about the computing enabling technologies that serve as the cornerstones for putting healthcare service delivery into practice.
- Examines the fundamental uses of computing and cybersecurity computing in healthcare systems with highlights how crucial they are to healthcare systems.
- It examines the body of research on cybersecurity computing that is currently available and how it relates to the creation of next-generation healthcare systems.
- It discusses, contrasts, and analyses the conclusion of the study based on an analysis of the data used in a healthcare system for fog-based computing. A cloud-fog-based detection scenario is utilised to predict the actual and prospective detection. This work is noteworthy because it emphasises the necessity of a cybersecurity mechanism based on cybersecurity computing in a healthcare system that is still evolving and can analyse data using machine-learning algorithms.
- Finally, the study addresses the problems of today, their causes, and the future concerning computing for cybersecurity in emerging technologies in healthcare systems.

Besides, we could not identify any study or investigation that applied or perhaps employed some ML algorithms to computing cybersecurity in emerging healthcare systems, making this study a key novel work.

10.1.3 Chapter organisation

Section 10.1 discusses the introductory section and contributions of the book chapter on computing for cybersecurity for emerging technologies in healthcare systems. Furthermore, Section 10.2 discusses the related work regarding computing for cybersecurity for emerging technologies in healthcare systems. The method

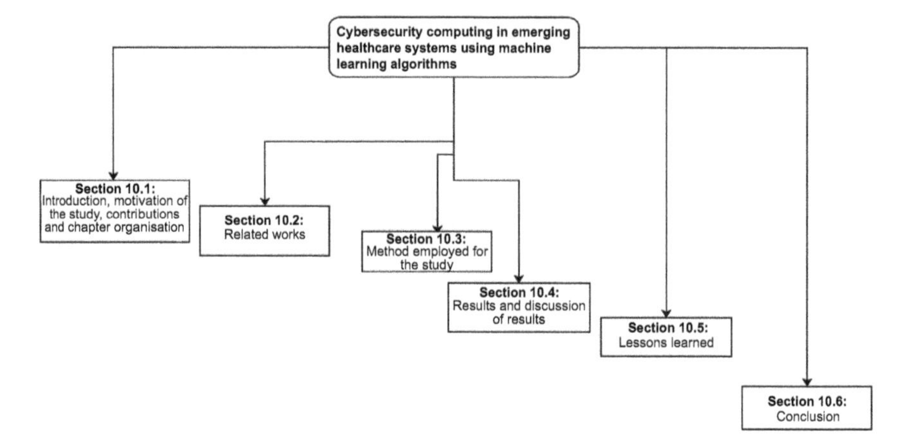

Figure 10.1 The organisational layout of the chapter

employed in this study for computing for cybersecurity for emerging technologies in healthcare systems is in Section 10.3. Preliminary results are presented and discussed in Section 10.4. More importantly, lessons that have been learned and summarily discussed in computing for cybersecurity for emerging technologies in healthcare systems are presented in Section 10.5. Section 10.6 completes the chapter by making conclusions regarding computing for cybersecurity for emerging technologies in healthcare systems. The organisational structure for this chapter is depicted in Figure 10.1.

10.2 Literature review

In this section, the relevant works are examined extensively regarding computing for cybersecurity in emerging healthcare systems. While Section 10.2.1 provides a clear overview of the methodologies now in use for healthcare systems, Section 10.2.2 presents computing applications in newly developing healthcare systems as discussed in Section 10.2.1. Additionally, this section of the chapter also includes Sections 10.2.3–10.2.6 that address applications of cybersecurity computing in emerging healthcare systems, cybersecurity threats in healthcare systems, cybersecurity in healthcare systems: technique in healthcare systems, and cybersecurity challenges in healthcare systems, respectively.

The study in [8] looks at the state-of-the-art regarding cybersecurity problems and approaches in the healthcare industry, with a particular emphasis on how the COVID-19 pandemic has changed things. The work in [8] combines the results of pertinent studies and papers, highlighting significant issues like the emergence of telemedicine, the dangers of remote labour, attacks caused by ransomware, and the function of laws and regulations. The review of the study as presented in [8] emphasises how critical it is to implement proactive cybersecurity measures to reduce risks and safeguard patient privacy and security. In addition, with an emphasis on cybersecurity issues, the scientific review in [9] offers a narrative synthesis of the body of research on emerging technological advances in healthcare. The work investigates the advantages and drawbacks of significant technological advancements, looking at how they may affect patient privacy, integrity of data, and legal compliance.

Moreover, the study in [10] by the authors, which draws from investigations, polls, and opinions from various geographic locations, offers a thorough synthesis of the body of knowledge regarding cybersecurity in healthcare. The study looks and examines at the state of cybersecurity in the healthcare industry, highlighting major issues such as ransomware attacks, data breaches, and legal compliance needs. It also discusses approaches and paradigms for evaluating the state of cybersecurity maturity and lists variables that affect resilience to attacks and adaptability. A recap of previous studies as well as business reports on cybersecurity issues in healthcare and the development of security paradigms is presented in [11]. The author in [11] talks about how network perimeter defences and other conventional security methods are not very effective in thwarting threats from within and persistent sophisticated adversaries (PSTs). It also looks at the fundamentals of Zero Trust, such as persistent verification, segmentation by category, and the concept of minimising advantage, emphasising its applicability and importance to healthcare environments.

Consequently, examining prior investigations on cybersecurity in healthcare and synthesising data from corporate reports, academic studies, and regulatory guidelines is the goal of the work carried out [12]. The work examines the different cybersecurity issues that healthcare companies deal with, including ransomware attacks, threats from within, and data breaches. The analysis also covers how rules are changing and what has to be done to comply with them, such as the General Data Protection Regulation in the European Union (EU) and the Health Information Privacy and in the United States. A thorough assessment of the state of cybersecurity in healthcare is presented in the study under the literature review section, which also highlights important trends, knowledge gaps, and potential research topics. Table 10.1 gives a summary view of some of the related works in this chapter stating the contributions, strengths, and weaknesses of each study.

10.2.1 Existing methods employed for healthcare systems

To thoroughly map the body of research on healthcare cybersecurity issues and solutions in the context of COVID-19, the work in [1] uses an in-depth review approach. The methodical identification and filtering of pertinent research from a variety of relational databases and the lack of clarity in the literature are part of the investigation approach employed in the study. The reviewed literature is analysed and categorised using information extraction and production procedures, which makes it easier to identify important themes and patterns. Additionally, to investigate how cybersecurity and developing digital technologies interface with healthcare, authors in [2] utilise a narrative review methodology. The review, which provides a qualitative examination of both the benefits and challenges provided by the rise of digital technologies, draws on a wide range of academic and industrial

Table 10.1 Summary of some of the reviewed works

Author (s)	Contribution(s)	Strengths	Weaknesses
He *et al.* [8]	The study in [8] adds to the body of knowledge on the subject by giving a thorough review of the problems and solutions related to healthcare cybersecurity in the COVID-19 age. It provides insightful information to cybersecurity experts, legislators, and healthcare organisations by highlighting new trends, vulnerabilities, and efficient procedures. The results guide the creation of focused interventions and tactics to improve healthcare cybersecurity vulnerability and adaptability to changing attacks.	The study uses an in-depth scoping methodology, which enables a thorough investigation into healthcare cybersecurity issues and solutions. By concentrating on the effects of coronavirus disease in 2019 (COVID-19), the study tackles a critical topic pertinent to the state of healthcare today. By strengthening cybersecurity safeguards and successfully mitigating risks, healthcare professionals can benefit from the lessons learned along with suggestions provided by the study.	The research could not include as much analysis as more targeted studies because of the scope of the scoping examination. The evaluation technique and the requirements for inclusion may create bias in the decision-making process, which could compromise the accurate representation and exhaustiveness of the material that is found.
Arafa *et al.* [9]	By offering a thorough analysis of the relationship between cybersecurity in healthcare and developing digital technologies, the work in [9] makes a significant contribution to the existing body of knowledge. It clarifies the potential that digital innovations offer to enhance the results of patients and healthcare delivery while emphasising how crucial cybersecurity is to reducing related dangers. The sequential assessment approach helps practitioners in cybersecurity, healthcare, and policymaking synthesise knowledge and offer practical insights [9].	All-encompassing viewpoint: Covering a wide variety of developments and considerations, the article provides an extensive analysis of the interaction between cybersecurity and digital technologies in healthcare. By permitting a detailed examination of significant issues and trends, the sequential assessment style offers stakeholders insightful information on the re-spective themes and trends. Considering urgent issues in the healthcare sector, the subject of cybersecurity and new technological developments in healthcare is both timely and important [9].	The narrative review approach has the potential to inject bias in the research selection as well as the interpretation process, which could affect the analysis of objectivity and comprehensiveness. Because of the inherently qualitative nature of the evaluation and the variety of sources used, the conclusions reached cannot be applied to a larger set of situations [9].
O'Brien *et al.* [10]	The study offers additional insights as information to the body of knowledge by providing a comparative examination of cybersecurity experiences and maturity across international healthcare institutions. Healthcare leaders,	To facilitate cross-national comparisons and provide insights into worldwide cybersecurity developments, the article employs a comparison and contrasting approach. Healthcare organisations looking to improve their defences	The sample used for the study could not be typical of the whole global healthcare system, which could restrict how broadly the results can be applied. The resilience of the comparison analysis may be impacted by variations in the preciseness

(Continues)

	legislators, and cybersecurity experts can benefit greatly from the study's identification of common concerns, best practices, and discrepancies in cybersecurity preparation. The results have the potential to improve cybersecurity resilience in the healthcare industry through the development of capacity, the distribution of resources, and strategic decision-making [10].	against cybersecurity threats and successfully reduce cyber risks should take note of the findings. By improving cybersecurity guidelines and procedures in the healthcare sector, legislation and regulations may be developed with the help of the research [10].	and reliability of the data gathered from healthcare organisations [10].
Vukotich [11]	The paper contributes to the body of knowledge by supporting the implementation of a zero-trust strategy for cybersecurity in the medical field. Healthcare organisations can improve the way they safeguard themselves and respond to changing cyber threats by using the research's explanation of Zero Trust's fundamental ideas and executing tactics. The results provide practical advice for cybersecurity experts, IT specialists, and leaders in the healthcare industry who want to apply Zero Trust concepts in their businesses [11].	The study presents a novel strategy for cybersecurity that questions established beliefs and pushes for a change in perspective in the direction of zero trust. The results offer healthcare organisations useful advice and efficient methods for putting non-trustworthy security frameworks into reality. As the value of Zero Trust security models in reducing cyber threats becomes increasingly apparent, the research findings are in line with these wider marketplace developments [11].	Theoretically beneficial as the concept of zero confidence may be, putting it into practice may present issues with organisational culture, resource availability, and compatibility with current systems. The report may not include research findings or empirical support for the practical efficacy of zero-trust methods in healthcare environments [11].
Weber and Kleine [12]	By offering insights into the state of cyberspace in healthcare today and outlining tactics for enhancing cybersecurity readiness and resilience, the article advances the profession. It provides healthcare organisations with useful advice on how to improve their defences against cybersecurity threats and successfully reduce cyber risks. The study may also emphasise how crucial it is for government organisations, cybersecurity experts, and participants in healthcare to work together to solve cybersecurity issues in the industry [12].	With intrusions against healthcare organisations becoming more frequent and severe, cybercrime in the industry is an important and timely topic. To help healthcare organisations strengthen their cybersecurity procedures and safeguard the information of patients, the report provides practical understanding and suggestions. Using a multidisciplinary strategy, the research may incorporate knowledge from technological innovation, cybersecurity, management of healthcare services, and other fields to deliver a thorough understanding of cybersecurity in the healthcare industry [12].	The findings presented in the paper might only apply to just a handful of healthcare organisations or a particular geographic area, which would limit its applicability in other situations. The robustness of the study and results may be impacted by variations in the quantity and quality of information collected on cybersecurity events and procedures in the healthcare industry [12].

literature to synthesise significant insights and trends. Because the process places a high value on narrative synthesis and thematic coherence, the subject can be explored comprehensively.

In [3], the study evaluates cybersecurity concerns and maturity levels among a sample of international healthcare organisations using a comparative assessment technique. Data from various sources, including interviews, questionnaires, and organisational assessments, are gathered and analysed for the study. Although qualitative perspectives add context and nuance to the investigation, quantitative metrics like cybersecurity maturity scores. This may be used to evaluate and compare the cybersecurity readiness of other organisations. Furthermore, in [4], the work utilises a conceptual analytic approach to investigate the tenets and tactics of Zero Trust in healthcare delivery. The study synthesises important ideas and recommendations related to Zero Trust security frameworks by drawing on a wide range of academic literature, industry publications, and expert comments.

Although qualitative research is the main focus of the procedure, statistical information can also be used to demonstrate how well Zero Trust techniques reduce cyber-related hazards. Considering the precise goals and parameters of the investigation, the authors in [5] proposed that certain issues may use a variety of research techniques to examine cybersecurity in healthcare. Common techniques to evaluate current cybersecurity practices, issues, and strategies include quantitative assessments or interviews with IT security specialists and healthcare professionals. Furthermore, industry publications, regulatory bodies, or cybersecurity threat intelligence databases may provide data for a quantitative assessment of cybersecurity occurrences and trends. The potential of the scheme to forecast the volume of data used to maintain patient and physician records has not been completely explored in any of the previous publications that have applied ML algorithms to healthcare-related data. Therefore, the goal of this research is to apply ML to cybersecurity computing in newly developed healthcare systems.

10.2.2 Computing applications in emerging healthcare systems

This subsection presents the computing applications in emerging healthcare systems via the following highlights and discusses briefly:

- Electronic Health Records (EHR): Digital platforms for safely archiving, organising, and exchanging patient medical data.
- Telehealth (TH): is the practice of providing healthcare remotely by using telecommunications technologies, such as videoconferencing, remote surveillance, and applications for mobile healthcare.
- Electronic tools called clinical decision support systems (CDSS) give evidence-based warnings and suggestions to help medical practitioners make clinical decisions.
- Health Information Exchange (HIE) refers to the cloud-based services that allow healthcare professionals to share health information, promoting transparency and integrated treatment.

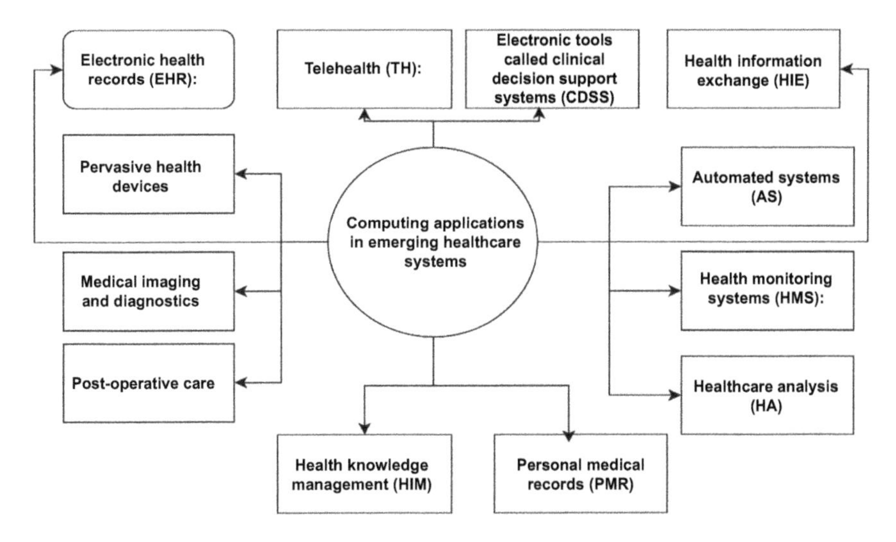

Figure 10.2 Computing applications in the emerging healthcare system

- Automated systems (AS) are used to take, store, and process medical pictures, such as those from MRIs, CT scans, ultrasounds, and X-rays.
- Pervasive health devices are gadgets that track vital signs including blood pressure, heart rate, and level of exercise. They are furnished with sensors and computational power.
- Health Monitoring Systems (HMS): These are autonomous monitoring systems that continuously record the breathing patterns and health condition of patients, allowing for proactively care management and early intervention.
- Healthcare analysis (HA): The use of data analytics technologies to examine vast amounts of medical data to spot patterns, gain new insights, and assist in administrative and therapeutic decision-making.
- Personal Medical Records (PMR) are online resources that give people the ability to view, control, and share their medical records, giving patients greater autonomy over their treatment.
- Health knowledge management (HIM) refers to systems that effectively and securely organise, store, and retrieve management and health-related patient data.

Hence, the computing applications in the emerging healthcare system are shown in Figure 10.2.

10.2.3 Applications of cybersecurity computing in emerging healthcare systems

This subsection presents the applications of cybersecurity computing in emerging healthcare systems via the following highlights and discusses briefly. In addition, some of the intelligent applications for cybersecurity in the healthcare system are depicted in Figure 10.3.

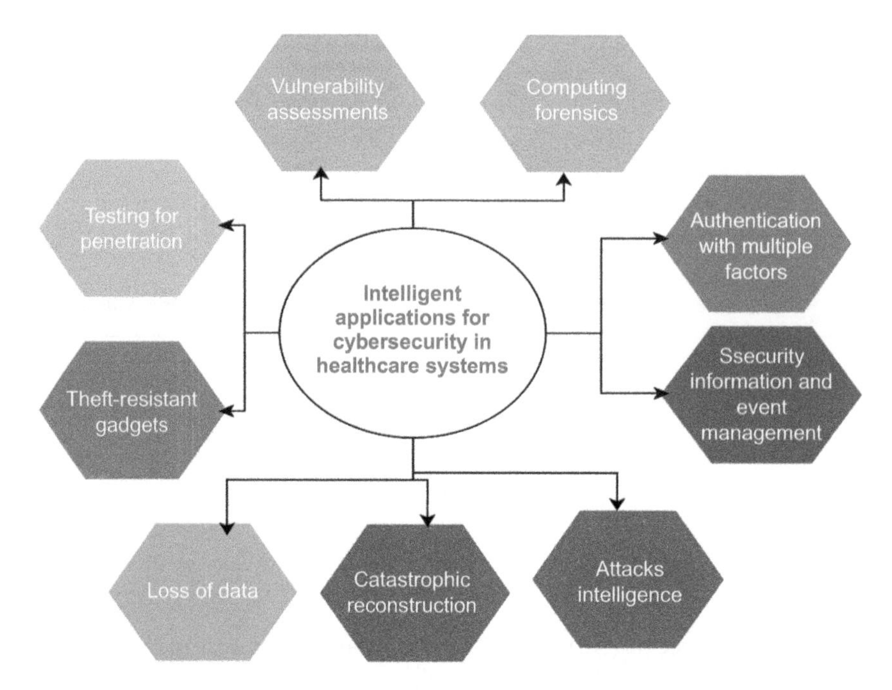

Figure 10.3 Some of the intelligent applications for cybersecurity in healthcare system

- Intrusion Detection Systems (IDS): computerised devices that monitor and react to infections with malware, illegal access attempts, and other security lapses.
- Security for endpoints refers to safety measures made to ward off cyberattacks on specific devices, like computers, smartphones, and healthcare supplies.
- Network safeguarding: The use of antivirus programmes, virtual private networks (VPNs), and encryption techniques to protect healthcare networks against cyberattacks, illegal accessibility, and data thefts.
- Information loss prevention (ILP): Techniques and guidelines designed to stop sensitive patient data from being accidentally revealed or leaked, both internally and outside the company.
- Systems for controlling the identities of users, responsibilities, and privileges to guarantee that only people with the proper authorisation can access confidential medical data and resources are known as identity and access management systems (AMS).
- Recovery from a catastrophe and emergency response are the plans and processes for handling cybersecurity events, recovering systems and data in the case of a breach, and minimising the effect on patient care.
- Systems for tracking, comparing, and evaluating security events and logs to identify and effectively address cybersecurity risks are known as security information and event management, or SIEM.

- Risk Intelligence: Information gathered, analysed, and shared on new and developing attacks and risks that are exclusive to the healthcare sector.
- Compliance with regulations refers to methods for making sure healthcare laws and guidelines such as The Health Information Technology for Economic and Clinical Health (HITECH), General Data Protection Regulation (GDPR), and Health Insurance Portability and Accountability Act (HIPAA) all about the safety of data, its confidentiality, and privacy are followed.
- Cybersecurity education and training: Activities aimed at educating end users and healthcare personnel about cybersecurity best practices, regulations, and guidelines to lower the risk of human mistakes and threats by insiders.

10.2.4 Cybersecurity threats in healthcare system

This subsection presents the cybersecurity threats in emerging healthcare systems via the following highlights and discusses briefly:

The lack of cybersecurity policies in healthcare institutions and practices puts the security of patients, the confidentiality of information, and healthcare administration at serious risk. Because health records are so valuable, fraudsters have found the healthcare industry to be a lucrative target.

- Data compromise: Financial information, insurance information, medical records, and personal identifiers are examples of compromised data. Medical institutions' reputations may suffer along with serious personal injury from the sale of stolen data to advertising companies, financial fraud, or identity theft [13–16].
- Risks in medical devices: Potential vulnerabilities are brought about by the growing usage of networked medical devices, such as pacemakers, medical imaging devices, and pumping infusions. These gadgets could be vulnerable to assaults because of out-of-date software or lax security measures [15–18].
- Phishing: Phishing assaults use phoney emails, texts, or telephone calls aimed at healthcare professionals. These attacks have the potential to cause data breaches by tricking people into disclosing private information or allowing unauthorised access [19–21].
- Dangers from insiders: Individuals represent a serious cybersecurity threat and can include workers, subcontractors, or partners. Insider risks might take the shape of deliberate acts, such as data theft or leaks, or accidental acts, like accidentally disclosing confidential data [22,23].
- Risks to third parties: Healthcare providers work with outside vendors, dealers, and partners more frequently, which broadens the attack surface. Hackers may use lax security procedures in these third-party platforms to gain unauthorised access to medical information networks [24,25].
- Attacks with ransomware: The potential danger of cyberattacks has grown significantly for healthcare establishments. The malicious software used in such attacks encodes data, making it unreadable unless a ransom is paid. Ransomware has the potential to seriously impair patient care, cause financial losses, and cause substantial disruptions in medical facilities [26,27].

10.2.5 Cybersecurity in healthcare system: technique in healthcare system

The following highlights and a brief discussion of the applications of computing are utilised in developing healthcare systems in this subsection:

- Create a thorough cybersecurity plan: Medical facilities need to have a strong cybersecurity plan with defined goals, guidelines, and protocols in place to safeguard patient information and vital infrastructure. To successfully manage possible cyber threats, this plan should include systems for prevention, detection, reaction, and recovery [13,14,28,29].
- Perform continual evaluations of risk: Frequent evaluations of risk assist in locating weak points and possible points of entry for cyberattacks. Healthcare organisations can proactively detect and reduce possible hazards and vulnerabilities by evaluating the security architecture of their networks, infrastructure, and applications [28,29].
- Put rigorous regulations for access in effect: Robust security measures are necessary to stop unwanted access to private patient information. Ensuring that only authorised personnel can access sensitive information is ensured by using authentication with multiple factors, role-based access management, and strong passwords [29].
- Data encryption: One essential precaution for safeguarding patient data is encryption. It guarantees that data will remain inaccessible and inaccessible even in the unlikely event that they are intercepted or stolen. Data at rest, in motion, as well as during safeguarding processes should all be encrypted [30,31].
- Training and empowering personnel: A major contributing element to cybersecurity incidents is still human mistakes. To inform staff members about cybersecurity threats, recommended procedures, and the significance of adhering to security guidelines, healthcare organisations ought to regularly hold awareness events and training sessions [32]. There are other ways to provide this instruction, such as through games, seminars, and lectures [33–35].
- Put secured networking segmentation into practice: Networking and devices in hospitals and other medical facilities are segmented to assist prevent breaches and restrict intruders' forward motion. Healthcare organisations can mitigate the effects of an effective cyberattack by dividing and enforcing stringent access rules between various portions of the computer network [36].
- Frequently store your information: To guarantee continuation and restoration from possible attacks involving ransomware or data loss incidents, data backups are essential. To ensure the confidentiality of information and efficacious data restoration, backups ought to be adequately encrypted, maintained safely, and subjected to routine testing [37].
- Track and find inconsistencies: Strong surveillance and detection mechanisms can be put in place to assist in quickly identifying and responding to cybersecurity events. Prompt threat identification and mitigation can be facilitated by systems that detect and avoid intrusions, security information and event monitoring tools, and instantaneous log analysis [29].

The healthcare-based model system is illustrated in Figure 10.4.

10.2.6 Cybersecurity challenges in the healthcare systems

In this section, the following is a list of cybersecurity issues/challenges that healthcare systems frequently deal with as shown in Figure 10.5.

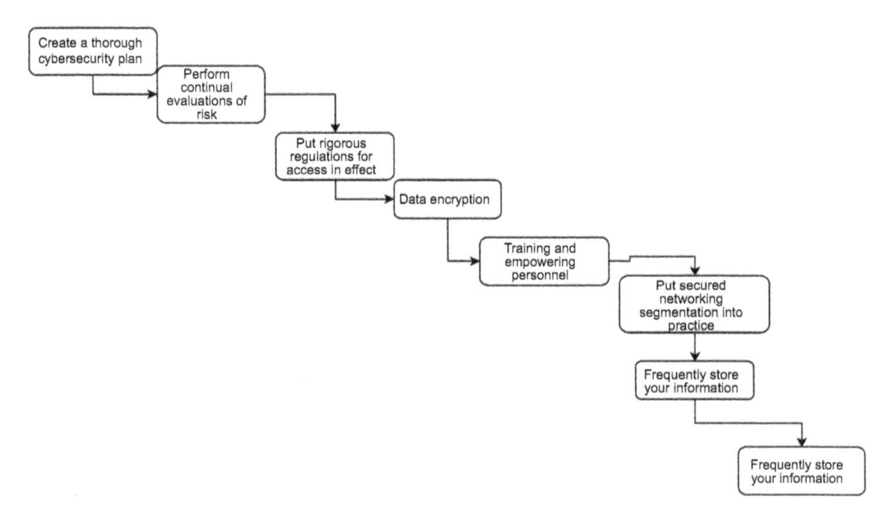

Figure 10.4 Cybersecurity mechanism in healthcare-based model system

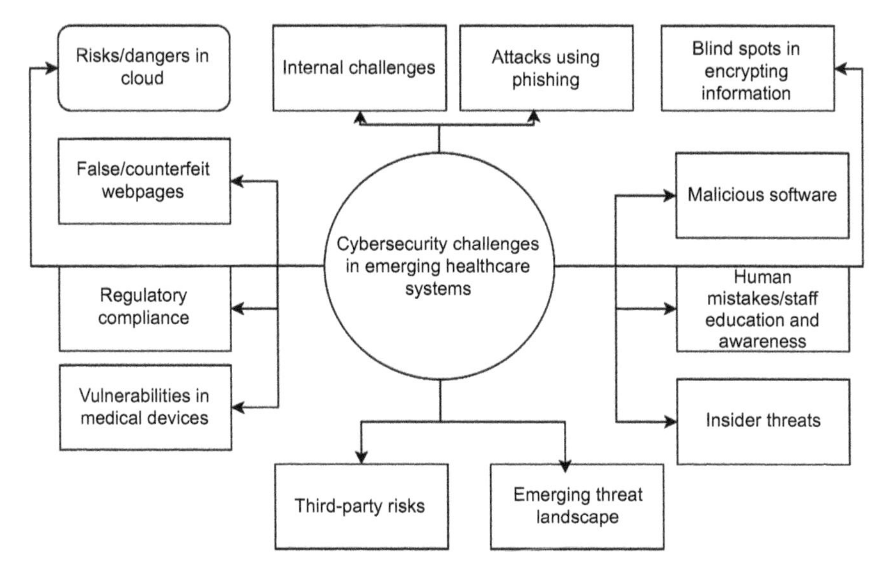

Figure 10.5 Cybersecurity challenges in the healthcare systems

- Information infringements: A serious risk to confidentiality and anonymity for patients is the theft or unauthorised access to patient health information (PHI), which includes individual markers, medical histories, and treatment data.
- Malware attacks: Malevolent software that encodes medical records and requests payment to unlock them; this can cause disruptions to medical procedures and jeopardise the quality of care provided to patients.
- Internal challenges: The possibility of information theft, tampering or illegal access by workers, subcontractors, or other dependable people within the healthcare company. This includes both deliberate insider fraud and unforeseen errors or carelessness.
- Medical equipment weaknesses: Due to their increasing level of complexity and connection, medical equipment including heart pacemakers, pumps for infusions and imaging technologies are vulnerable to cyberattacks, which could jeopardise the protection of patients and treatment results.
- Legacy computing and architecture: Cybercriminals can target outdated and unsupported software, hardware, and network infrastructure, posing security hazards owing to flaws that could not have been patched or updated. This leaves healthcare systems vulnerable.
- External risks: Because healthcare organisations depend on third-party suppliers and providers of services for a range of information technology systems and amenities, there are extra cybersecurity risks associated with vendor access, data-sharing bargains, and weaknesses in the supply chain.
- Enforcement conformity: Ensuring data security and privacy for healthcare organisations is a constant challenge when it comes to complying with healthcare standards and regulations, such as the General Data Protection Regulation (GDPR) in the European Union and the Health Insurance Portability and Accountability Act (HIPAA) in the United States.
- Staff education and awareness: One of the biggest cybersecurity challenges is still the human element. Healthcare personnel frequently lack knowledge of security best practices, become a target of social engineering scams, or unintentionally expose critical data by acting carelessly or ignorantly.
- Cyberspace resource limitations: Healthcare organisations face difficulties in establishing and maintaining effective security measures, such as security staff, training programmes, and tools, due to limited budgets, limited experience, and inadequate funds devoted to cybersecurity.
- Evolving risk environment: Healthcare companies face constant problems in keeping ahead of the curve and modifying their cybersecurity defences to counter emerging threats due to the ever-evolving nature of cyber threats, which include new attack vectors, tactics, and malware variants.

10.3 Methods, data collection, model training, and validation

This section presents the method, data collection, model training, and validation procedures in this work. Hence, in this study, the method employed is purely the

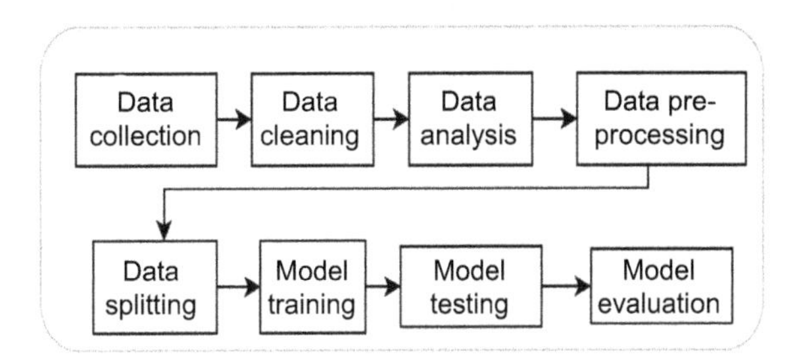

Figure 10.6 Summary of methods employed

application of some ML algorithms such as Random Forest (RF), Linear Regression (LR), and K-Nearest Neighbours to train a set of datasets for the analysis. These algorithms are employed because of their effectiveness on the available datasets used in this study to analyse the cloud-fog-based data computing for the prediction of output size in megabytes for the computing power required to process the level of detection of attacks on a given healthcare database management system. The illustration in Figure 10.6 presents a comprehensive summary of all the methods carried out throughout this study.

10.3.1 Data collection

For illustration, the datasets used in this study were obtained from Kaggle [38]. A ML system that used multiple ML algorithms to forecast the actual and predicted data sizes for cloud-fog computing in healthcare-based systems was fed certain attributes as inputs.

10.3.2 Data cleaning

One of the most important steps in removing anomalies from the dataset is data cleansing [26]. These anomalies can appear as duplicate rows, empty cells, or as a variety of other problems. The principal objective is to guarantee the provision of precise data to the ML model, thus augmenting the precision of the predictions generated by every ML algorithm.

10.3.3 Data analysis

Analysing data entails looking over a dataset to compile its most important features [27]. Understanding the connections between the several essential features and the target feature. That is, the feature that needs to be predicted is made easier by this method.

10.3.4 Model training

The ML models employed for the predictive task are as follows:

10.3.4.1 Linear regression (LR)

The link between the input variables is examined using this statistical technique. It seeks to locate the ideal line that best captures the relationship between the input variables. This statistical method uses approaches to calculate the best line intercept and slope for the model [39]. To enhance the model's performance, polynomial features are added.

10.3.4.2 Random forest (RF)

To do this, many decision trees are built, where "10 estimators" denotes the number of trees in the ensemble. The forecasts from these trees are then combined to get a final prediction. These trees are constructed using a combination of random factors and portions of the original dataset [40].

10.3.4.3 K-nearest neighbours (KNN)

Predicting continuous numerical values is done using this method. The number of nearest neighbours (K) that is taken into consideration is set to 5. The projected value is then calculated as the average or weighted average of the associated target values for the five training data points that are closest to the input [41]. This is how KNN operates.

10.3.5 Data pre-processing

Preparing the data for ML algorithms involves making the required changes to it beforehand. This procedure is known as data pre-processing. Furthermore, the idea of ML has also been shown in [42–46] for research focused on the following topics: telehealth system application, IoT in medical systems, testing and validation of AI and other technology-based models, and correspondingly resolving 6G security and privacy issues with AI. The flaws of the studies are that they do not take cybersecurity issues within the healthcare system into account. The steps in the pre-processing of data are shown in Figure 10.7. Initially, the dataset must be carefully examined for any missing values, as they could negatively affect the ML algorithms' performance. Furthermore, as ML algorithms operate on numerical values by nature, feature encoding is used to manage categorical attributes and convert them into numerical data. After that, the ML model receives the revised dataset for additional examination and forecasting.

10.3.6 Model validation and testing

This entails the application of diverse assessment criteria to appraise the efficacy of the computational models utilised in forecasting the true and anticipated dimensions of the data. It measures the discrepancy between the testing data's actual size in megabytes and the predicted size produced by each of the models used in this investigation. The following assessment metrics are used to do this.

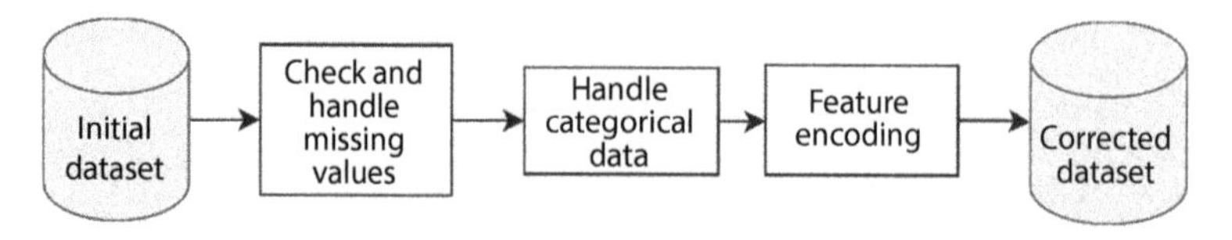

Figure 10.7 Data pre-processing stages

10.3.6.1 Mean absolute error (MAE)

This metric is employed to evaluate the accuracy of predictions made by computational models, specifically in predicting signal strength. It is computed by summing the absolute differences between the actual and predicted signal strengths and then dividing this sum by the total number of data points, as shown in Eq. (10.1). Lower MAE indicates superior prediction performance, signifying that the predictions made by the model closely align with the actual signal strength values. Conversely, a higher MAE suggests poorer model performance, indicating that the predictions by the model deviate more significantly from the actual signal strength values.

$$MAE = \frac{1}{N}\sum_{i=1}^{N}|z_i - z_a| \tag{10.1}$$

where z_i represents the predicted signal strength, z_a represents actual signal strength, and N represents the number of data points.

10.3.6.2 Mean squared error (MSE)

This statistical method is used to validate predictions. It is calculated by summing up the squared difference between predicted and actual signal strength values and dividing it by the total number of data points, as shown in Eq. (10.2). The lower the MSE value, the better the model is at prediction, while higher values imply that the model performs poorly.

$$MSE = \frac{1}{N}\sum_{i=1}^{N}|y_i - y_a|^2 \tag{10.2}$$

10.3.6.3 Root mean square error (RMSE)

This is calculated as the square root of the mean square error, as shown in Eq. (10.3). It not only considers the average discrepancy between predicted and actual values but also factors in the impact of significant errors.

$$RMSE = \sqrt{\frac{1}{N}\sum_{i=1}^{N}|y_i - y_a|^2} \tag{10.3}$$

10.4 Results and discussion of results

This section visualizes, explains, and compares the results obtained in this study based on the analysis of the data used and the predictive outcomes of the employed models for cloud-fog computing system Based on the examination of the data utilised for fog-based computing in a healthcare system, this section compares, illustrates, and explains the findings of the study. To anticipate the actual and projected detection, a cloud-fog-based detection scenario is used. Significantly, this work highlights the need for a cybersecurity mechanism based on cybersecurity computing in a developing healthcare system using some ML algorithms for analysis. In addition, Table 10.2 provides performance indicators including MAE, MSE, and RMSE as well as an overview of some of the ML methods that were employed in this investigation. It is noteworthy that the KNN regression scheme performs better than the other algorithms when looking at the MAE for the methods, with a numerical value of 26.20, compared to 24.7 and 23.08 for RF and LR, respectively.

The RF algorithm used the size of the input file, the number of instructions, and the amount of memory needed to forecast the output file sizes with exceptional speed. Interestingly, the RF model prediction and actual values match quite well for a variety of data points in the testing dataset shown in Figure 10.8. It demonstrated an impressive capacity for precise output file size estimation. Nonetheless, it is critical to recognise several subtleties in the model's operation. Predictions produced by the algorithm were often marginally higher than the actual values. It also had difficulties when trying to forecast numbers at the lower end of the range with accuracy. This raises the possibility that some extreme dataset variations may not be fully captured, especially those connected to extremely small output file sizes. A quantifiable indicator of the model's predicted performance is the MAE score of

Table 10.2 Performance metrics for different machine learning algorithms employed in this study

ML algorithms	MAE	MSE	RMSE
Random Forest	24.7	833.6	28.8
Linear Regression	23.08	662.04	28.87
KNN Regression	26.20	913.77	30.22

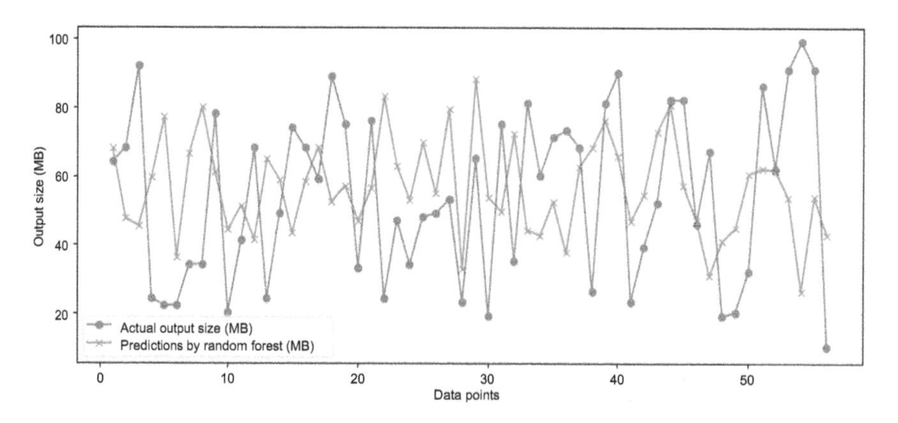

Figure 10.8 Predictions by Random Forest over the number of data points of the test data

23.08 from Table 10.2. Better accuracy is indicated by a lower MAE, and in this instance, the comparatively low MAE score highlights the RF algorithm's ability to produce reasonably accurate predictions. Nevertheless, additional investigation and improvement might be required to tackle the noted inclination towards more optimistic forecasts and the challenge of forecasting exceptionally low values.

LR exhibited moderate performance in predicting output file sizes. The model consistently generated predictions within the range of 45 to 60 MB, indicating a certain level of stability in its estimations. However, the model's effectiveness diminished when confronted with test data file sizes at both the higher and lower ends of the spectrum. In particular, LR struggled to make accurate predictions when the test data file size deviated significantly from the mid-range values as shown in Figure 10.9. This limitation is reflected in the model's inability to capture the nuances associated with extreme variations in input file sizes, leading to less precise predictions in these scenarios. The MAE score of 23.08, when compared to the RF algorithm in predicting output file sizes based on input file size and the number of instructions, suggests that LR falls short in achieving the same level of accuracy. While the model provides a baseline understanding of the relationship between input variables and output file size, its limitations in handling non-linearities and capturing complex patterns are apparent. Further exploration and consideration of alternative models may be beneficial for improving predictive performance in scenarios with varied and extreme data points.

K-Nearest Neighbours (KNN) exhibited a comparatively lower level of performance when contrasted with other algorithms, as evidenced by its predictions deviating significantly from the actual data points as depicted in Figure 10.10. The model's limitations became apparent, leading to predictions that were notably distant from the ground truth. Specifically, KNN struggled to accurately predict output file sizes based on input data and the number of instructions. This diminished predictive accuracy is reflected in the model for the MAE score of 26.02. A higher MAE score indicates a larger average discrepancy between predicted and

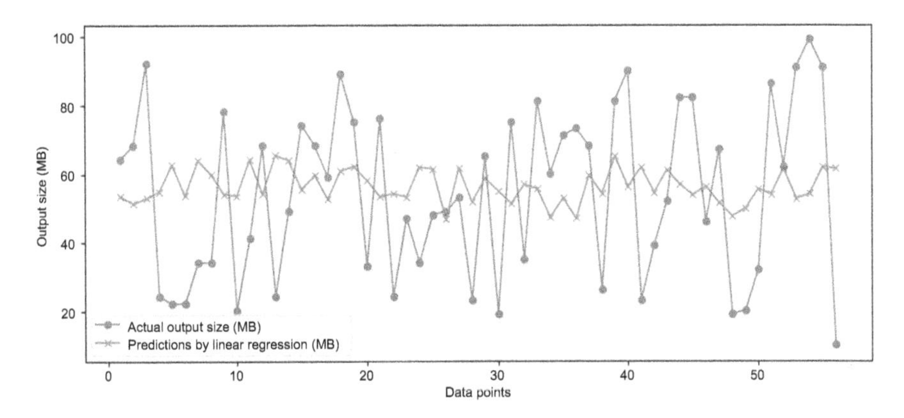

Figure 10.9 Predictions by Linear Regression over the number of data points of the test data

actual values, emphasising the challenges faced by KNN in capturing the underlying patterns and relationships within the dataset. The observed lower performance of KNN suggests that its reliance on proximity-based computations may not be well-suited for the complexities inherent in the given dataset. Exploring alternative algorithms that can better handle the nuances and intricacies of the data may be beneficial to improve predictive accuracy and bridge the gap between predicted and actual output file sizes.

Additionally, the MAE score of each algorithm, the MSE score of each algorithm, and the RMSE score of each algorithm are depicted in Figures 10.9, 10.10, and 10.11, respectively. In Figures 10.11–10.13, the size of data is plotted against the respective algorithms employed for this study for the sake of demonstration.

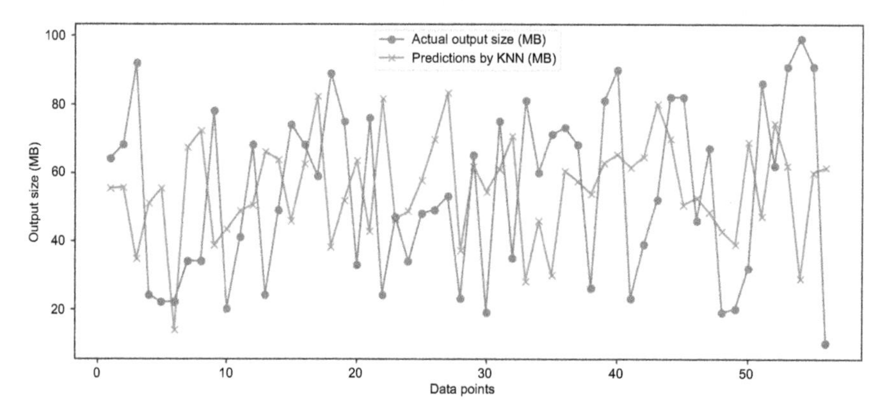

Figure 10.10 Predictions by KNN over the number of data points of the test data

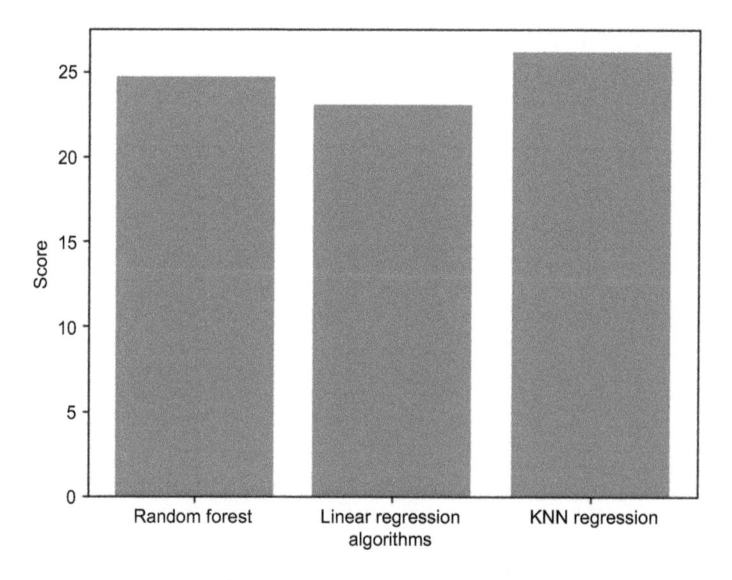

Figure 10.11 Bar chart showing the MAE score of each algorithm

Ultimately, Figures 10.11–10.13 demonstrate that the performance indicators of several ML algorithms exhibit notable improvements in terms of the RMSE. Figure 10.12 illustrates how the KNN algorithm performs better than other schemes in terms of MSE.

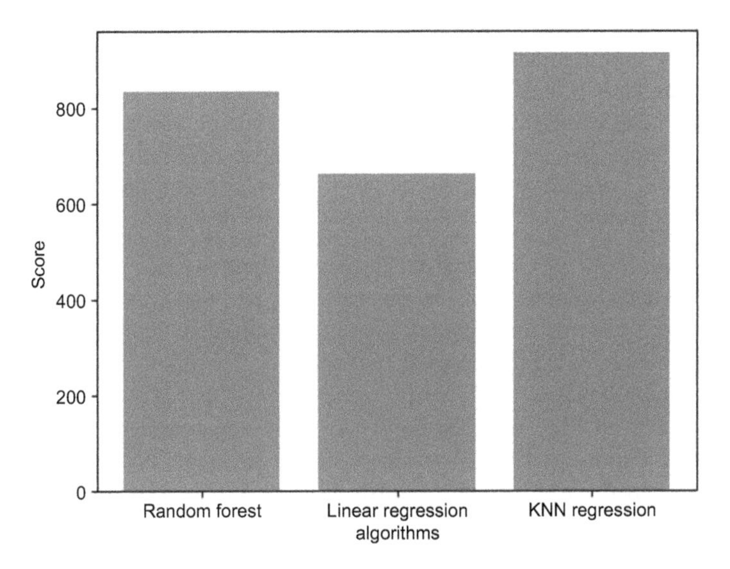

Figure 10.12 Bar chart showing the MSE score of each algorithm

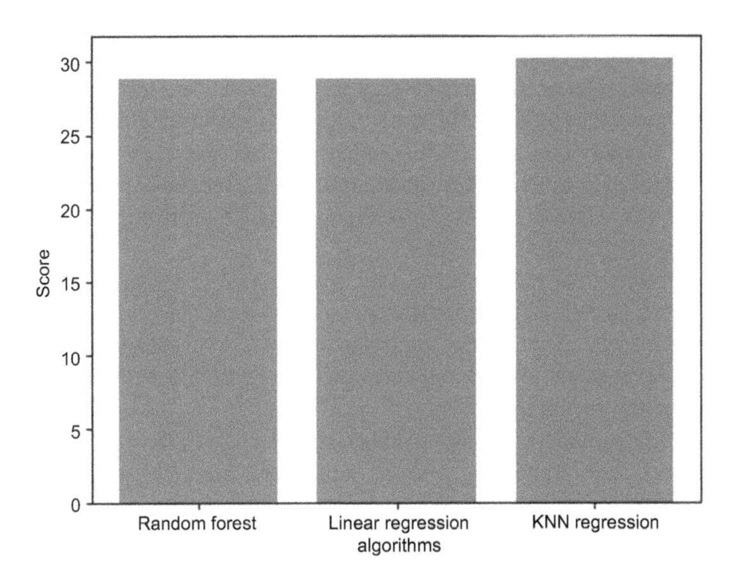

Figure 10.13 Bar chart showing the RMSE score of each algorithm

10.5 Lessons learned

This section highlights comprehensive lessons learned during the investigation of computing for cybersecurity in emerging healthcare systems. Even while massive, functional computers are still years away, and the field of computation is still in its infancy, there are valuable lessons to be learned about the potential convergence of cybersecurity and computing in the field of healthcare. The healthcare industry needs to stay alert, adjust cybersecurity procedures, and actively work with specialists to create and execute cognitive-resistant technologies as the field of computing develops. By taking proactive steps now, healthcare systems can be protected from computing risks in the not-too-distant future. Following are a few important takeaways:

- Cybersecurity Risk Complexity: The research emphasises the wide variety of cyber threats, such as ransomware, malware, and insider threats, that nascent healthcare systems must contend with. It emphasises how important it is to have systems for cybersecurity that are flexible enough to recognise and react to changing threats.
- Application of ML: With the ability to analyse vast amounts of data to spot unusual activity and pinpoint any security breaches, ML proves to be an effective instrument for cybersecurity in the healthcare industry. The investigation proves that ML methods are useful for improving identifying and responding to threats capacities.
- Incorporation issues: The analysis identifies difficulties in incorporating cybersecurity solutions through ML into the current healthcare infrastructure. These difficulties include problems with the interoperability of information, a lack of resources, and organisational opposition to change. Cooperation between cybersecurity specialists, medical practitioners, and information technology professionals is necessary to overcome these obstacles.
- Continuous enhancement: The study highlights how crucial it is to keep an eye on new dangers and adjust ML models regularly to keep up with changing healthcare environments. It draws attention to the recursive process involved in cybersecurity, where continued assessment and modification are required to preserve efficacy and pertinence.
- Implementation of conventional-safe specifications: Using robust-safe technologies is an innovative approach to cybersecurity. To guarantee that data is protected even if networks can defeat present cryptography techniques, healthcare systems should think about putting in place traditional-resistant cryptography regulations.
- Healthcare providers should evaluate how susceptible their cybersecurity equipment is to computing assaults and create tactics that are prepared for future developments in computing devices such as computers to reduce risks.
- Cooperation and information exchange: The cooperation of stakeholders is essential. To disseminate information and provide reliable solutions, healthcare organisations, cybersecurity professionals, and computational scientists

should work together. Mutually beneficial partnerships alongside business alliances can aid in addressing new risks.

- Investing in computing-safe technology: It is strategically necessary to make investments in computing-safe technology. To secure patient data over the long term, healthcare organisations should invest resources in computing-safe advancements in technology, studies, and applications.
- Teaching and learning: For cybersecurity experts, having accelerated computing consciousness is essential. To make well-informed choices and remain ahead of future risks, healthcare organisations should invest in providing their cybersecurity staff with training on the use of accelerated and powerful computers and their possible influence on current security procedures.
- The utilisation of accelerated computing cybersecurity in emerging healthcare systems leads to the safety and reliability of health data in the healthcare sector.
- Analysis of the dataset reveals how specific health parameters contribute to the detection of underlying ailments and forecasting of the amount of data used in the healthcare system for medical personnel and patients.
- ML algorithms can accurately be employed for predicting underlying medical ailments at its early stage such as stroke, chronic kidney disease, and so on.
- Evaluation metrics, which are utilised to gauge the performance of ML algorithms, reveal that KNN surpasses other algorithms in predicting the amount of data size used for cybersecurity computing systems in real-time applications such as cloud-fog computational processes.

10.6 Conclusion

ML approaches can improve the resilience of cybersecurity and defend against cyberattacks, as demonstrated by the study of cybersecurity computing in emerging healthcare systems. Healthcare organisations may efficiently manage risks and increase the level of their cybersecurity by utilising machine-learning algorithms for threat identification, recognition of anomalies, and predictive modelling. However, for the deployment to be effective, integration issues must be resolved, data privacy and legal compliance must be guaranteed, and cooperation and education about cybersecurity must be promoted. In summary, the research highlights the significance of pre-emptive cybersecurity protocols for preserving patient information, guaranteeing the accuracy of medical equipment, and upholding the faith and assurance of healthcare partners. Because computational and accelerated computing offers previously unthinkable speed, productivity, and dependability, it has completely changed conventional computer systems. Applications for healthcare with high computational efficiency can be developed by utilising these fundamental aspects of cybersecurity computing systems. To achieve this, we offer a thorough analysis of the body of research in this study that focuses on using computing to produce healthcare analysis and prediction of the amount of output data size for specific operations in the healthcare system. We specifically talk about the various ways that computing may be used in the healthcare industry. Additionally, we talked about several security considerations for applying cybersecurity computing to medical devices and various computing advancements and applications that can guarantee the security of those solutions. Lastly, we discussed the problems we face today, why they exist, and potential future study areas where computing could benefit. The scientific community keen on utilising and analysing different possibilities of computation in some healthcare-related applications might find a one-stop solution in this innovative study, which highlights every significant component of computation consequences in the healthcare framework.

References

[1] A.D. Stern, J. Brönneke, J.F. Debatin, *et al.*, "Advancing digital health applications: Priorities for innovation in real-world evidence generation," *Lancet Digit. Health*, 4, pp. e200–e206, 2022.
[2] Y. Ronquillo, A. Meyers, and S.J. Korvek, "*Digital Health*," StatPearls Publishing: Treasure Island, FL, USA, 2023.
[3] A.I. Stoumpos, F. Kitsios, and M.A Talias, "Digital transformation in healthcare: Technology acceptance and its applications," *Int. J. Environ. Res. Public Health*, 20, 3407, 2023.
[4] A.L. Neves, and J. Burgers, "Digital technologies in primary care: Implications for patient care and future research," *Eur. J. Gen. Pract.*, 28, pp. 203–208, 2022.
[5] D. Giansanti, "Ten years of telehealth and digital healthcare: Where are we?" *Healthcare*, 11, 875, 2023.
[6] B. Mesko, "Health IT and digital health: The future of health technology is diverse," *J. Clin. Transl. Res.*, 3 (Suppl. S3), pp. 431–434, 2018.
[7] M.S. Ibrahim, H.M. Yusoff, Y.I. Abu Bakar, M.M.T. Aung., M.I. Abas, and R.A. Ramli, "Digital health for quality healthcare: A systematic mapping of review studies," *Digit. Health*, 8, 20552076221085810, 2022.
[8] Y. He, A. Aliyu, M. Evans, and C. Luo, "Health care cybersecurity challenges and solutions under the climate of COVID-19: Scoping review," *Journal of Medical Internet Research*, 23(4), pp. e21747, 2021.
[9] A. Arafa, H.A. Sheerah, and S. Alsalamah, "Emerging Digital Technologies in Healthcare with a Spotlight on Cybersecurity: A Narrative Review," *Information*, 14(12), pp. 640, 2023.
[10] N. O'Brien, G. Martin., E. Grass, M. Durkin, A. Darzi, and S. Ghafur, "Cybersecurity in Healthcare: Comparing Cybersecurity Maturity and Experiences across Global Healthcare Organizations". 2020. Available at: https://dx.doi.org/10.2139/ssrn.3688885.
[11] G. Vukotich, "Healthcare and cybersecurity: taking a Zero Trust approach," *Health Services Insights*, 16, pp. 11786329231187826, 2023.
[12] K. Weber, and N. Kleine, "Cybersecurity in health care," *The Ethics of Cybersecurity*, 21, pp. 139–156, 2020.

[13] Y. He, A. Aliyu, M. Evans, and C. Luo, "Health care cybersecurity challenges and solutions under the climate of COVID-19: Scoping review," *J. Med. Internet Res.*, 23, e21747, 2021.

[14] S.T. Argaw, J.R. Troncoso-Pastoriza, D. Lacey, *et al.*, " Cybersecurity of hospitals: Discussing the challenges and working towards mitigating the risks," *BMC Med. Inform. Decis. Mak.*, 20, 146, 2020

[15] A.H. Seh, M. Zarour, M. Alenezi, *et al.*, "Healthcare data breaches: Insights and implications," *Healthcare*, 8, 133, 2020.

[16] W.W. Koczkodaj, J. Masiak, M. Mazurek, D. Strzałka, and P.F. Zabrodskii, "Massive health record breaches evidenced by the Office for Civil Rights data," *Iran. J. Public Health*, 48, 278–288, 2019.

[17] P.A. Williams, and A.J. Woodward, "Cybersecurity vulnerabilities in medical devices: A complex environment and multifaceted problem," *Med. Devices*, 8, 305–316, 2015.

[18] B. Ransford, D.B. Kramer, D.F. Kune, *et al.*, "Cybersecurity and medical devices: A practical guide for cardiac electrophysiologists," *Pacing. Clin. Electrophysiol.*, 40, 913–917, 2017

[19] W. Priestman, T. Anstis, I.G. Sebire, S. Sridharan, and N.J. Sebire, "Phishing in healthcare organisations: Threats, mitigation and approaches," *BMJ Health Care Inform.*, 26, e100031, 2019.

[20] M. Abdelhamid, "The role of health concerns in phishing susceptibility: Survey design study," *J. Med. Internet Res.*, 22, e18394, 2020.

[21] W.J. Gordon, A. Wright, R. Aiyagari, *et al.*, "Assessment of employee susceptibility to phishing attacks at US health care institutions," *JAMA Netw. Open 2019*, 2, e190393, 2019

[22] P. Chapman, "Are your IT staff ready for the pandemic-driven insider threat?" *Netw. Secur.*, 8–11, 2020.

[23] N. Khan, R. J. Houghton, and S. Sharples, "Understanding factors that influence unintentional insider threat: A framework to counteract unintentional risks," *Cogn. Technol. Work*, 24, 393–421, 2022.

[24] L.H. Yeo, and J. Banfield, "Human factors in electronic health records cybersecurity breach: An exploratory analysis," *Perspect Health Inf. Manag.*, 19, 2022.

[25] S. Nifakos, K. Chandramouli, C.K. Nikolaou, *et al.*, "Influence of human factors on cyber security within healthcare organisations: A systematic review," *Sensors*, 21, 5119, 2021.

[26] H.T. Neprash, C.C. McGlave, D.A. Cross, *et al.*, "Trends in ransomware attacks on US hospitals, clinics, and other health care delivery organizations," 2016–2021, *JAMA Health Forum.*, 3, e224873, 2022.

[27] C. Dameff, J. Tully, T.C. Chan, *et al.*, "Ransomware Attack associated with disruptions at adjacent emergency departments in the US," *JAMA Netw. Open*, 6, e2312270, 2023.

[28] S.T. Argaw, N.E. Bempong, B. Eshaya-Chauvin, and A. Flahault, "The state of research on cyberattacks against hospitals and available best practice recommendations: A scoping review," *BMC Med. Inform. Decis. Mak.*, 2019, 19, 10, 2019.

[29] J.M. Borky, and T.H. Bradley, "Protecting information with cybersecurity." *Eff. Model-Based Syst. Eng.*, 345–404, 2018.
[30] A. Almalawi, A.I. Khan, F. Alsolami, Y.B. Abushark, and A.S. Alfakeeh, "Managing security of healthcare data for a modern healthcare system," *Sensors*, 23, 3612, 2023.
[31] P. Sarosh, S.A. Parah, and G.M. Bhat, "An efficient image encryption scheme for healthcare applications," *Multimed. Tools Appl.*, 81, 7253–7270, 2022.
[32] M. Hijji, and G. Alam, "Cybersecurity Awareness and Training (CAT) framework for remote working employees," *Sensors*, 22, 8663, 2022.
[33] M.A. Arain, R. Tarraf, and A. Ahmad, "Assessing staff awareness and effectiveness of educational training on IT security and privacy in a large healthcare organization," *J. Multidiscip Health*, 12, 73–81, 2019
[34] J.L. Kamerer, and D.S. McDermott, "Cyber hygiene concepts for nursing education," *Nurse Educ. Today*, 130, 105940, 2023.
[35] F. Rubia, Y. Affan, L. Lin, and W. Jianmin, "How persuasive is a phishing email? A phishing game for phishing awareness," *J. Comp. Secur.*, 27, 581–612, 2019.
[36] D. Johansson, P. Jönsson, B. Ivarsson, and M. Christiansson, "Information technology and medical technology personnel's perception regarding segmentation of medical devices: A focus group study," *Healthcare*, 8, 23, 2020.
[37] M. Zarour, M. Alenezi, M.T.J. Ansari, *et al.*, "Ensuring data integrity of healthcare information in the era of digital health," *Health Technol. Lett.*, 8, 66–77, 2021.
[38] "Cloud-fog computing dataset": https://www.kaggle.com/datasets/sachin26240/vehicularfogcomputing?fbclid=IwAR3kmknuzvQycO23ji9KHtpzoCu0Khh_9k32-nWubjoy56I63NRGkqQcbM4 (accessed on January 20 2024).
[39] M. Huang, "Theory and Implementation of linear regression," 2020 International Conference on Computer Vision, Image and Deep Learning (CVIDL), Chongqing, China, 2020, pp. 210–217, doi:10.1109/CVIDL51233.2020.00-99.
[40] M. Aria, C. Cuccurullo, and A. Gnasso, "A comparison among interpretative proposals for Random Forests," *Machine Learning with Applications*, 6, p. 100094, 2021, doi:10.1016/j.mlwa.2021.100094.
[41] M. Mailagaha Kumbure, and P. Luukka, "A generalised fuzzy k-nearest neighbor regression model based on Minkowski distance," *Granular Computing*, 7(3), pp. 657–671, 2021, doi:10.1007/s41066-021-00288-w.
[42] A.L. Imoize, P.A. Gbadega, H.I. Obakhena, D.O. Irabor, K.V.N. Kavitha, and C. Chakraborty, "Artificial Intelligence-enabled Internet of Medical Things for COVID-19 pandemic data management," *Explain. Artif. Intell. Med. Decis. Support Syst.*, pp. 357–380, 2023.
[43] O.O. Shoewu, L.A. Akinyemi, and R. Edozie. "UAV cellular communication in 5G new radio wireless standards." In *Unmanned Aerial Vehicle Cellular Communications*, pp. 25–45. Cham: Springer International Publishing, 2022.
[44] L.A. Akinyemi, O.O. Shoewu, C.O. Folorunso, *et al.*, "Alleviating 6G security and privacy issues using artificial intelligence," *Book on Security*

and Privacy Schemes for Dense 6G Wireless Communication Network: doi.org/10.1049/PBSE021E_ch14, 2023.

[45] S.O. Oladejo, S.O. Ekwe, L.A. Akinyemi, and S.A. Mirjalili, "The deep sleep optimiser: A human-based metaheuristic approach," *IEEE Access*, 11, pp. 83639–83665, 2023

[46] A.L. Imoize, V.E. Balas, V.K. Solanki, C.-C. Lee, and M.S. Obaidat, Eds., *Handbook of Security and Privacy of AI-Enabled Healthcare Systems and Internet of Medical Things,* 1st ed., CRC Press, 2023. DOI:10.1201/9781003370321.

Chapter 11

Blockchain for secured cybersecurity in emerging healthcare systems

Abidemi Emmanuel Adeniyi[1], Rasheed Gbenga Jimoh[2], Joseph Bamidele Awotunde[2], Halleluyah Oluwatobi Aworinde[1], Peace Busola Falola[3] and Deborah Olufemi Ninan[4]

The integration of digital technology and the advent of networked healthcare systems are driving a transformational shift in the healthcare business. While this change offers greater patient care and improved medical processes, it also poses enormous cybersecurity and data protection problems. This study investigates the potential of blockchain technology as a strong and novel option for enhancing cybersecurity in the changing environment of healthcare systems. Blockchain, with its immutable ledger and decentralized design, provides a promising foundation for protecting sensitive healthcare data and crucial medical infrastructure. This study looks into the use of blockchain in healthcare cybersecurity, focusing on its capacity to provide tamper-proof data storage, effective access control mechanisms, and increased transparency. Blockchain reduces the dangers of data breaches, unauthorized access, and fraudulent activities by establishing a trust-based ecosystem, increasing patient trust and confidence in digital healthcare solutions. Furthermore, this chapter digs into real blockchain technology deployments within healthcare systems, spanning from electronic health record (EHR) administration to medication supply chain integrity and telemedicine platforms. It illustrates the benefits and drawbacks of each use case and provides real-world examples of blockchain adoption in healthcare cybersecurity. This study investigates the synergy between blockchain and developing technologies such as artificial intelligence (AI) and machine learning (ML) for predictive threat identification and

[1]Department of Computer Science, College of Computing and Communication Studies, Bowen University, Nigeria
[2]Department of Computer Science, Faculty of Communication and Information Sciences, University of Ilorin, Nigeria
[3]Department of Computer Sciences, Faculty of Pure and Applied Sciences, Precious Cornerstone University, Nigeria
[4]Department of Computer Science and Engineering, Obafemi Awolowo University, Nigeria

anomaly detection, in addition to blockchain. The combination of Blockchain secure data storage and AI-driven cybersecurity analytics provides a proactive method for recognizing and mitigating cyber risks, hence boosting healthcare systems' resilience. Ethical and regulatory concerns are also addressed in the context of blockchain deployment in healthcare cybersecurity, highlighting the need to adhere to healthcare data protection standards and ethical norms while managing sensitive patient information. Finally, this article emphasizes the crucial importance of blockchain technology in strengthening cybersecurity in new healthcare systems. Healthcare firms may develop a strong defense against cyberattacks while protecting patient privacy and data integrity by leveraging the capabilities of blockchain. Blockchain emerges as a cornerstone technology that assures both security and trust in the developing healthcare landscape as the healthcare sector embraces digital transformation.

Keywords: Information system; cryptographic algorithms; blockchain technology; healthcare sector; patients; medical records; electronic medical system

11.1 Introduction

Blockchain technology is crucial to cybersecurity. As efforts to develop huge electrical circuits continue, the most modern encryption techniques may be compromised. Because of the ethical and legal implications of a patient's health information, cybersecurity is both a critical and problematic issue in healthcare [1,2]. Image secrecy is highly sensitive to a range of challenges. As a result, building a cybersecurity model for healthcare applications demands special attention in terms of data safeguarding [3,4]. In the age of digital healthcare records, the industry creates and retains massive volumes of sensitive personal information [5,6]. This covers the patients' medical histories, diagnoses, medications, and financial information. While simple and economical, digitization has introduced a serious risk: cyberattacks. Healthcare organizations remain a popular target for cybercriminals due to the high value of patient data [7]. Breaches can lead to financial losses, reputational harm, and, most significantly, compromised patient privacy and care. According to the 2021 HIMSS Cybersecurity Survey, a startling 93% of healthcare businesses had experienced at least one hack in the last year.

Blockchain is a data structure made up of blocks that are ordered in time. The block is a collection of data including connected information and records, and it is the fundamental unit of blockchain [8,9]. The Blockchain data format consists mostly of a block header and a block body [10]. The block header primarily carries the preceding block's hash value, which is used to link the previous block and preserve the integrity of the blockchain; the block body provides the block's major content (such as transaction information). This information, along with the hash value of the previous block and the random number, makes up the hashed hash value of the current block. In the Bitcoin application scenario, each block data contains system transaction data information issued by participating nodes during a specific period. Transaction information consists of sender and recipient identities, transaction amount, transaction time, and various extra information [11]. Blockchain, the groundbreaking technology that powers cryptocurrencies, offers a promising alternative for improving healthcare cybersecurity. Its key qualities—decentralization, immutability, and transparency—provide significant benefits for safeguarding sensitive data and increasing overall cybersecurity posture.

A blockchain is simply a distributed ledger that stores transactions over a network of computers (nodes) rather than a single server. Each transaction is represented as a "block," which includes data and a unique identifier. New blocks are added in chronological order, resulting in an immutable chain. Blockchain key properties for healthcare cybersecurity include decentralization. Data is not stored in a single point of vulnerability, which makes it more difficult for hackers to attack the entire system.

Immutability: Once added, data cannot be changed or removed without impacting the following blocks, which ensures record integrity.

Transparency: Each network participant has access to a comprehensive and verifiable transaction record, which promotes trust and accountability.

Cryptography: Data is encrypted, providing an additional degree of protection.

Blockchain-based decentralized and unidentified diverse nodes facilitated data validation, and immutable data exchange methods were established for medical applications. Blockchain innovation is dependable and efficient. It verifies data and transfers it across known and unidentified nodes using an immutable algorithm. Three blockchain technologies are used for medical applications, including public, private, and communal systems. Numerous medical nodes provide extra amenities that are integrated into the procedure for comprehensive network operations [12,13].

Blockchain technologies have been extensively utilized in machine learning methods in IoMT-enabled wellness procedures, generating massive volumes of healthcare data from various bio-sensors and offloading it to the system for analysis. However, current blockchain-based ICPS has generated research issues for the IoMT, as seen by the research questions in these works [14–18].

We are reviewing the many research concerns amongst current investigations; the blockchain technology we have now needs to be better at preventing online assaults, which has created massive performance issues in medical applications. The blockchain techniques' consensus mechanisms could not identify known and unknown cyberattacks (e.g., malicious and benign) in linked actual nodes for examined workflows. The present machine learning-enabled blockchain solutions cannot manage malware threats during execution. The fundamental shortcoming of present public technologies is that they cannot spot real-time malware, which is quite fresh and does not follow any patterns. As a result, new techniques are needed to deal with runtime malware in ICPS for apps.

Safety and confidentiality are essential components of effective access control mechanisms in medical facilities. Additionally, the Internet has an impact on people's lifestyles and modes of interaction, as well as their professional and social ties [19]. The Internet of Things (IoT) is the use of small sensor-based technologies that connect the real and virtual worlds. The use of blockchain-based architectures enables tamper-proof and more decentralized communications between nodes. Blockchain is also known as a distributed, immutable ledger [20]. As a result, it delivers apps and services, functionality, management, and on-demand access [21]. However, suggestions and implementations of networking devices, among other things, continue to expand. As a result, most sectors are migrating toward IoT and the use of blockchain technology [22].

Furthermore, security and privacy concerns are critical for blockchain-based models, particularly those involving the incorporation of medical facilities. Security attacks include denial-of-service (DoS), structured query language (SQL) injections, tampering intercepting, and replay assaults, all of which pose a challenge to IoT-based systems. Such threats impact security applications and their permission, integrity, and privacy. As a result, it is critical to solve these concerns and develop a unique design framework that can secure IoT devices that use blockchain applications. Weak security at any node can result in access to patient health records. An electronic health record (EHR) is considered the most crucial and delicate type of data since it contains a large amount of confidential data about patients and diagnoses. However, the improvement and growth in digital healthcare systems have made EHR data increasingly sensitive to breaches [23], thus security and privacy must play an essential role in the case of decentralized and trustworthiness [24,25].

In an electronic medical system, a cross-domain architecture model can enable physicians and patients to access data that is scattered across many domains. Accessing data via a cross-domain business, on the other hand, necessitates increased security and more adjustable permission regulations. A policy establishes guidelines and rigorous restrictions for the characteristics of participants and data. Furthermore, data can be protected using cryptographic methods. In the literature, the methods of cryptography utilized by scientists are centered on ring and group identities [26]. These encryption approaches are specifically designed for established access control models such as role-based access control (RBAC), access control lists (ACL), discretionary access control lists (DAC), and trust-based access control (TBAC). For protecting data, the design proposed would combine attribute-based signatures (ABS) with an ABAC access control mechanism. We will take the model of Sahai and Water [27] as a baseline for our access management approach, which is fully based on ABAC.

11.1.1 Contribution of the chapter

This chapter makes substantial contributions to the current body of knowledge in various ways. It demonstrates Blockchain's transformational potential in tackling some of the most serious cybersecurity concerns confronting the healthcare industry today. The important contributions of this chapter are as follows:

(i) The chapter provides fundamental knowledge of Blockchain intrinsic qualities—decentralization, transparency, immutability, and security—and shows how these features are immediately applicable to protecting sensitive health data and systems.

(ii) The chapter emphasizes Blockchain importance in preserving data integrity, preventing illegal access, and enabling secure data sharing across several healthcare systems.
(iii) The chapter critically explores concerns such as scalability, energy consumption, regulatory compliance, and interaction with current healthcare IT infrastructure, offering a balanced view of the practical aspects of blockchain implementation.
(iv) The chapter points to continuing improvements in scaling solutions, energy-efficient consensus processes, legal frameworks, and interoperability protocols, presenting a forward-looking vision of how blockchain might grow to better fulfill the demands of the healthcare sector.
(v) The chapter helps to bridge the gap between technology innovation and healthcare demands. It underlines the significance of collaboration among tech developers, healthcare providers, regulatory agencies, and cybersecurity specialists to realize the full potential of blockchain for healthcare cybersecurity.

11.1.2 Chapter organization

The remaining chapter is divided into eleven sections; Section 11.2 discusses understanding cybersecurity threats in Emerging Healthcare Systems. Section 11.3 discusses the fundamentals of Blockchain Technology and the concept of blockchain. The applications of Blockchain Technology are thoroughly discussed in Section 11.4. Section 11.5 discusses the Security and Privacy of Blockchain. The Blockchain and Internet of Medical Things are discussed in Section 11.6. The various case studies used in Blockchain in Healthcare Security are discussed in Section 11.7. Section 11.8 discusses the challenges and limitations of implementing Blockchain, the key findings, and the future directions and innovations of the chapter while Section 11.9 concludes the chapter.

11.2 Understanding cybersecurity threats in emerging healthcare systems

The rapid adoption of emerging healthcare technologies, from artificial intelligence (AI) in diagnostics to wearable health sensors, has transformed the healthcare landscape [28]. While these advancements offer tremendous potential for improved patient care and efficiency, they also introduce new and evolving cybersecurity threats. This chapter delves into the specific vulnerabilities associated with these emerging systems, highlighting the latest threats and potential mitigation strategies. Emerging healthcare systems rely more on digital technology, such as EHRs and telemedicine, to enhance efficiency, patient care, and outcomes. However, this digital transition exposes healthcare to new cybersecurity dangers, making it an attractive target for cybercriminals. The sensitivity of personal health information (PHI), along with the crucial nature of healthcare services, emphasizes the significance of comprehensive cybersecurity safeguards (see Figure 11.1).

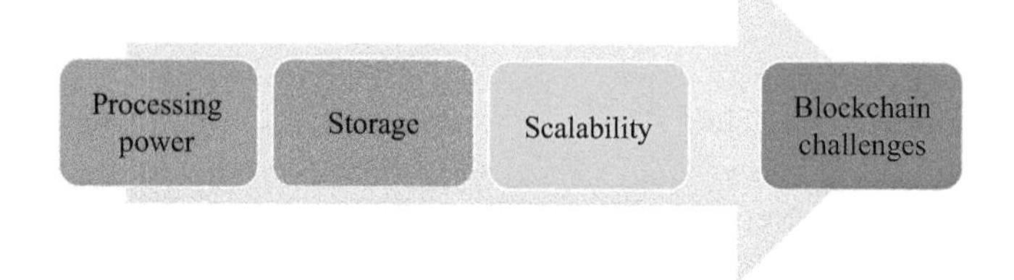

Figure 11.1 Blockchain computational complexity

Healthcare technology can save, lengthen, and improve lives. Technologies include those that store health information systems (HIS), gadgets that track health and administer medicines (including general-purpose gadgets and wearables, as well as equipment integrated within the human body), and technology for telemedicine that offers treatment remotely, even across borders [29]. Individuals increasingly utilize their smartphone apps, which may now be coupled with telemedicine or telehealth to establish the healthcare IoT for collaborative sickness treatment and care coordination [30].

Interconnected technologies beyond the clinical setting allow medical professionals to track and replace implanted devices without needing a hospital visit or invasive treatments. EHRs can improve patient care by making health information more readily available [3]. Unfortunately, interconnection introduces additional cybersecurity threats [31]. Cybersecurity focuses on safeguarding computer networks and the information they contain against intrusion and unintentional or purposeful interruption. Insufficient cybersecurity in healthcare has led to breaches of medical information confidentiality and data integrity [32].

Before the advent of EHRs, concerns about privacy breaches already existed. However, the interconnected nature of modern records introduces several new vulnerabilities: they can be accessed from remote locations, unlike paper records that were physically secured within hospital premises; there is a heightened risk of undetected data theft; and the consolidated nature of digital records makes them a richer target for potential attacks, in contrast to the previously fragmented health records across various hospitals and departments. In the past, the loss of paper records or a stolen laptop might have compromised the data of hundreds or thousands of patients [33]. Now, with this information digitized and stored across multiple networks, a single privacy breach has the potential to impact millions.

11.2.1 The expanding attack surface

The interconnected nature of emerging healthcare systems creates a vast attack surface, encompassing:

(i) **Medical devices:** Implantable devices, wearables, and connected medical equipment are susceptible to malware, data breaches, and manipulation.

(ii) **AI and machine learning (ML) algorithms:** Bias, data poisoning, and manipulation of model outputs can impact diagnosis, treatment recommendations, and research conclusions.
(iii) **Telehealth and remote patient monitoring:** Weak authentication protocols, insecure video conferencing platforms, and data leakage expose sensitive patient information.
(iv) **Electronic health records (EHRs) and health information exchanges (HIEs):** Integration complexities and access control challenges present opportunities for unauthorized access and data breaches.

11.2.2 Latest threat landscape

(i) **Ransomware attacks:** Targeting critical healthcare infrastructure like EHRs and medical devices, these attacks can disrupt patient care and extort hefty ransoms. Recent examples include the 2023 attack on Scripps Health and the 2022 attack on Mackay Regional Hospital.
(ii) **Supply chain attacks:** Compromising software vendors or third-party providers can inject malware into medical devices or manipulate software updates, impacting entire healthcare systems. The 2021 SolarWinds supply chain attack highlights this vulnerability.
(iii) **Insider threats:** Disgruntled employees or malicious actors with authorized access can steal data, sabotage systems, or manipulate patient records.
(iv) **Social engineering attacks:** Phishing emails targeting healthcare professionals and patients remain a prevalent threat, aiming to steal credentials or deploy malware.
(v) **Emerging threats:** Quantum computing advancements may pose future risks to current encryption methods used in healthcare systems.

11.2.3 Mitigating the risks

(i) **Proactive security measures:** Regularly update software, implement strong multi-factor authentication, and conduct vulnerability assessments.
(ii) **Security awareness training:** Educate healthcare professionals and patients on cybersecurity best practices and recognize phishing attempts.
(iii) **Zero-trust security models:** Grant least-privilege access, continuously monitor user activity, and segment networks to limit attack scope.
(iv) **Data encryption and anonymization:** Protect sensitive patient data at rest and in transit, considering privacy-preserving technologies like homomorphic encryption.
(v) **Collaboration and information sharing:** Establish industry-wide cybersecurity frameworks, share threat intelligence, and collaborate on incident response protocols.

11.2.4 Blockchain-integrated cybersecurity based on artificial intelligence

The medical sector utilizes blockchain-integrated cybersecurity (BICS)-AI for IoMT. End-to-end exchanges of information between unscrupulous parties have contributed to blockchain technology, and a completely decentralized blockchain is now available [34]. This cutting-edge idea has the potential to increase productivity and safety while managing property. Blockchain innovation may be defined as an autonomous peer-to-peer (P2P) network with a mirrored and distributed ledger [35]. Sensitive health information is frequently held in many places, which can cause delays in getting essential updates and impact patient outcomes [36]. Furthermore, there is an increasing demand for patients to have accessibility and handle their data as patient participation in health grows. Blockchain innovation could enhance medical outcomes since it is a private decentralized digital record that can be used to successfully manage EHRs.

Health information from IoMT and incorporated devices may be gathered and kept securely or disseminated using a traditional in-depth method paired with blockchain, making it suited for healthcare establishments such as medical centers, clinics, and the health sector, where data interchange is necessary [37]. Collaborative digital currencies emerge between private and public blockchains. In general, open digital currencies are less reliable than encrypted ones because cryptographic algorithms have a lower capacity, as measured by the number of operations validated per second. Collaborative digital currencies are less efficient than personal blockchains, but more efficient than public digital currencies (see Figure 11.2).

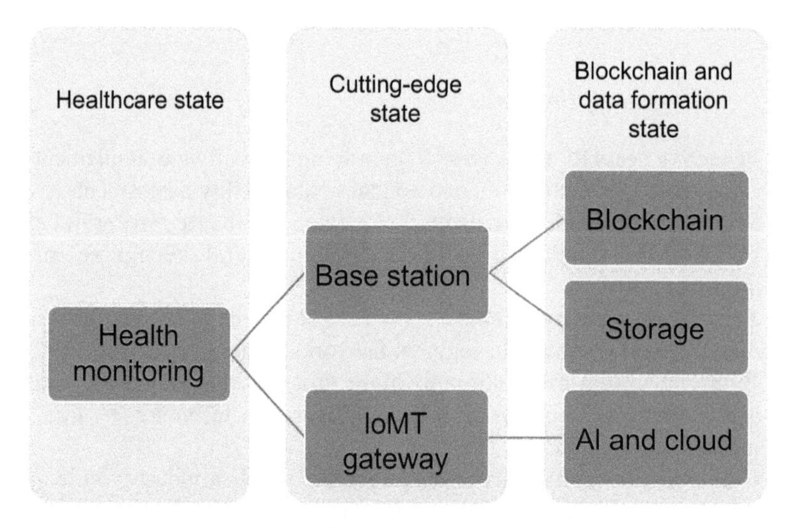

Figure 11.2 Framework of BICS using AI

11.3 Fundamentals of blockchain technology

Blockchain technology is a decentralized digital ledger that records transactions across several computers in such a way that they cannot be changed retrospectively. This technology forms the cornerstone of cryptocurrencies such as Bitcoin and Ethereum, but its potential uses are far-reaching [38]. Many promises are made in this period of new developing technologies, with a particular focus on blockchain technology. Blockchain has attracted numerous academics and practitioners from a variety of professions and fields because of the compelling reasons for using such technology [39]. Many scholars are interested in categorizing Blockchain-Based Software Systems (BBSSs) to have a better understanding of them. Recent advancements in blockchain technology and decentralized consensus systems provide new opportunities for creating untameable domain-specific ledgers without a central authority. Blockchains have been largely utilized for value transfers since Bitcoin's inception [40]. With the evolution of the Ethereum platform, the community recognized that by utilizing a chain of blocks and consensus rules, one may not only store currency and monitor its movement but also store some state and impose criteria under which this information can be updated. Table 11.1 provides a comparison table of consensus mechanisms, highlighting their key features, benefits, and drawbacks.

11.3.1 Core concepts of blockchain

(i) **Decentralization**: Unlike traditional ledgers or databases that are controlled by a central authority, a blockchain is distributed across a network of computers, often referred to as nodes.
(ii) **Immutability**: Once a transaction is recorded on a blockchain, it is extremely difficult to alter. This is due to the cryptographic hash functions used in the blockchain structure.
(iii) **Transparency**: While maintaining privacy through pseudonymous transactions, blockchain technology offers transparency as all transactions are visible to participants in the network.
(iv) **Consensus mechanisms**: These are protocols that ensure all nodes are synchronized with each other and agree on the validity of transactions. Examples include Proof of Work (PoW) and Proof of Stake (PoS).

11.3.2 Blockchain architecture

Figure 11.3 shows the blockchain architecture. It comprises the following components.

1. Blocks: Each block contains a collection of transactions, and every block is linked to the previous one through a cryptographic hash, forming a chain.
2. Transactions: The actions carried out by participants in the network, such as transferring cryptocurrency or data.

Table 11.1 Comparison table of consensus mechanism of blockchain

Feature	Proof-of-Work (PoW)	Proof-of-Stake (PoS)	Proof-of-Authority (PoA)	Byzantine Fault Tolerance (BFT)	Delegated Proof-of-Stake (DPoS)	Proof-of-Elapsed-Time (PoET)
Mechanism	Nodes solve complex mathematical puzzles to validate transactions.	Nodes validate transactions based on their stake in the network.	Pre-selected validators verify transactions.	Nodes use byzantine consensus algorithms to reach an agreement.	Staked nodes delegate voting power to elected validators.	Nodes are randomly selected based on waiting time to validate blocks.
Security	High due to computational difficulty.	Moderately high, dependent on stake distribution.	High due to limited validators.	Varies based on a specific BFT algorithm.	Moderately high, dependent on validator reputation.	Moderate, relies on randomness and verification by other nodes.
Scalability	She was limited due to energy consumption and complex calculations.	More scalable than PoW, but limited by stake distribution.	Highly scalable, but lacks decentralization.	Varies based on specific BFT algorithms, generally less scalable than PoS.	More scalable than PoW, but less than pure PoS.	Moderately scalable, limited by the number of nodes.
Energy Consumption	High, requires specialized hardware.	Low, minimal computational resources are needed.	Low, energy efficient.	Varies based on the BFT algorithm, generally higher than PoS.	Moderate, dependent on validator activity.	Low, no complex calculations involved.
Decentralization	Highly decentralized, open to anyone to participate.	Moderately decentralized, depends on stake distribution.	Less decentralized, and requires trusted validators.	Varies based on BFT algorithm, can be centralized or permissioned.	Moderately decentralized, depends on DPoS implementation.	Moderately decentralized, limited by random selection.
Cost	High due to energy consumption and hardware costs.	Lower than PoW, but can be dependent on staking requirements.	Low, no complex mining needed.	Varies based on BFT algorithm, can be expensive due to infrastructure needs.	Moderate, depends on DPoS implementation and staking requirements.	Low, no complex calculations or expensive hardware needed.
Suitable for	Public blockchains with high-security requirements (e.g., Bitcoin).	Public and private blockchains with the balance between security and scalability (e.g., Ethereum 2.0).	Permissioned blockchains with high efficiency and controlled access (e.g., Hyperledger Fabric).	Private blockchains requiring high fault tolerance and fast consensus (e.g., Hyperledger Burrow).	Public blockchains with efficient and scalable consensus (e.g., EOS).	Permissionless or permissioned blockchains with low energy consumption (e.g., Hyperledger Cactus).

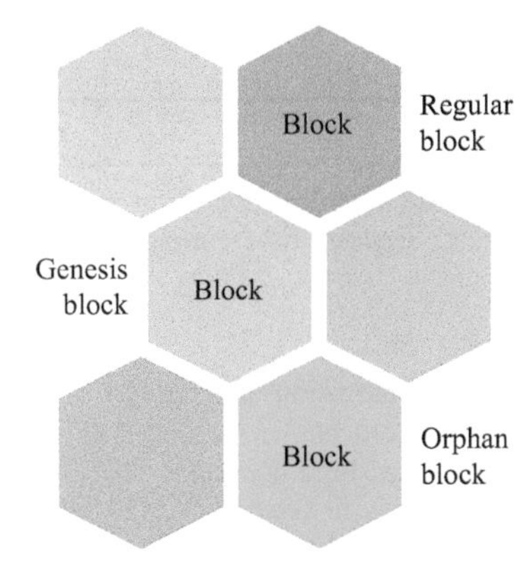

Figure 11.3 Blockchain architecture

3. Nodes: The individual computers connected to the blockchain network that validate and store the data.

11.4 Applications of blockchain technology

The emergence of blockchain may be divided into three periods. Blockchain 1.0 is characterized as a digital money system, with Bitcoin acting as its initial implementation. Blockchain 2.0 focuses on the financial system. Smart contracts emerged during Blockchain 2.0, and new types of assets were transformed using smart contracts, expanding blockchain applications outside the currency business [41]. The programmable society is blockchain 3.0's key differentiating characteristic. Based on existing networks such as the Internet and mobile communications, the use of blockchain is quickly spreading to many aspects of society and life, such as research, education, and culture, among others [42].

- (i) **Cryptocurrencies**: Digital or virtual currencies that use cryptography for security.
- (ii) **Smart contracts**: Self-executing contracts with the terms of the agreement directly written into lines of code.
- (iii) **Supply chain management**: Enhancing transparency and traceability of products from manufacture to distribution.
- (iv) **Voting systems**: Creating tamper-proof and transparent voting mechanisms.
- (v) **Identity verification**: Offering a secure and immutable system for digital identities.

The real effect of blockchain technology will be determined by a variety of factors, including legislative frameworks, technological breakthroughs, and user acceptance. Some applications are still in early development, and their long-term influence is unknown. Table 11.2 displays the various applications of blockchain technology.

Table 11.2 Application area of blockchain technology

Application area	Example	Potential impact
• Financial Services	• Secure digital payments (e.g., Bitcoin, Ethereum)	• Faster, cheaper, and more transparent transactions • Increased financial inclusion for unbanked populations
• Tokenized assets (e.g., fractional ownership of real estate)	• Democratization of access to investments • Increased liquidity and efficiency in asset markets	
• Decentralized finance (DeFi)	• Lending and borrowing platforms without intermediaries	• More accessible and transparent financial services
• Supply Chain Management	• Track the origin and movement of goods (e.g., IBM Food Trust)	• Enhanced transparency and traceability, reducing fraud and counterfeiting
• Improve efficiency and optimize logistics.	• Reduce food waste and ensure product safety	
• Healthcare	• Secure sharing of medical records (e.g., Medchain)	• Improved patient data privacy and control
• Streamline clinical trials and research data management.	• Enhance accuracy and transparency in healthcare research	
• Voting Systems	• Secure and transparent voting platforms (e.g., Voatz)	• Increase voter confidence and reduce fraud
• Improve accessibility and convenience of voting.	• Strengthen democratic processes	
• Identity Management	• Self-sovereign identity solutions (e.g., Sovrin)	• Secure and verifiable control over personal data
• Reduce the risk of identity theft and fraud.	• Enable easier access to online services	
• Energy	• Peer-to-peer energy trading (e.g., SunContract)	• Decentralize energy production and distribution
• Increase efficiency and sustainability of energy grids	• Empower consumers to participate in the energy market	

11.4.1 Applications of blockchain in enhancing cybersecurity

Blockchain is marketed as an innovation capable of providing a solid and powerful cybersecurity solution as well as high levels of privacy protection [43]. Proponents claim that this kind of equipment is secure by design. A blockchain concept eliminates the need to save information with third parties. The records are stored on many interconnected computers that contain similar information. If one computer's blockchain updates are compromised, the system rejects them [44]. Furthermore, multi-signature (multisig) safety, which requires more than one key to approve a transaction process, can increase safety and confidentiality. Even if a hacker infiltrates a network and attempts to steal money from an account, several redundancies and similar copies of the same ledger are maintained globally. If one is compromised, numerous others as backups can give payments for the hacked account [45]. In other words, data in blockchain is dispersed throughout a network of connected computers. For hacking attempts to be effective, more than half of the computer networks in the network must be infiltrated.

Many key systems in a variety of sectors rely on the "security through obscurity" approach to security engineering. The goal of this method is to keep a system's security measures and implementation hidden. However, one significant disadvantage of this strategy is that if someone finds the security mechanism, the entire system may fail. One such system may be the Society for Worldwide Interbank Financial Telecommunications (SWIFT), a secure messaging system used by financial organizations. Some contend that existing international payment systems, such as SWIFT, are obsolete and have questionable security [46]. Figure 11.4 shows the structural approach of blockchain to cybersecurity.

The usage of blockchain-based solutions is likely to help avoid assaults like those mentioned above [47]. Blockchain most likely lacks a single point of weakness or vulnerability. It is also worth mentioning that, while Bitcoin, the

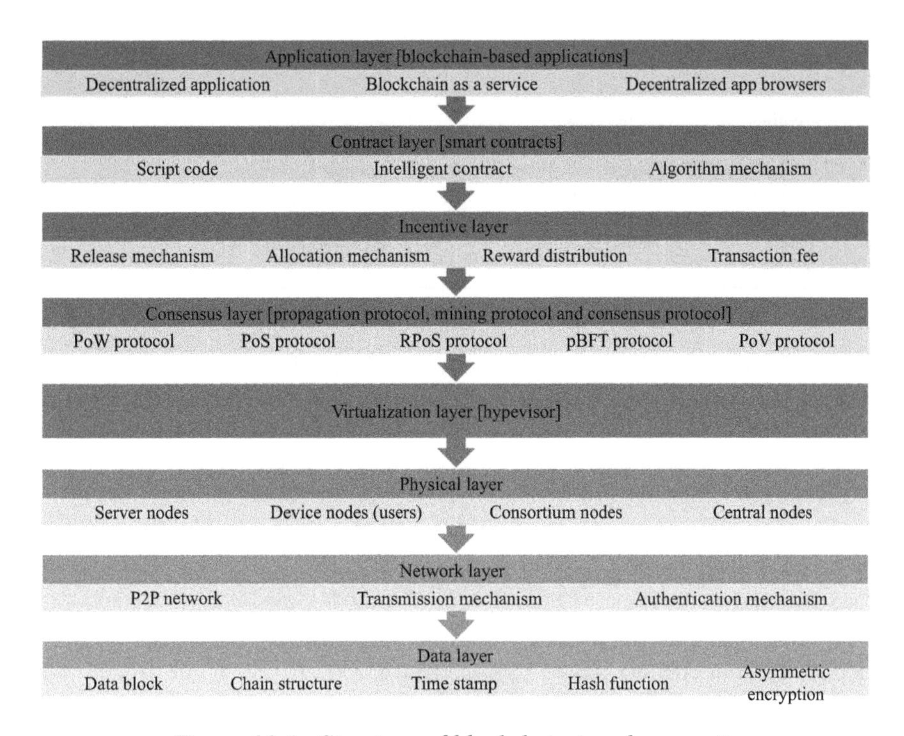

Figure 11.4 Structure of blockchain in cybersecurity

Table 11.3 Application of blockchain in enhancing cybersecurity

Application area	Example implementation	Security enhancement	Challenges
Secure Data Storage and Sharing:	– Medical record management (e.g., Medchain)	– Immutability and tamper-proof records	– Scalability for large datasets
– Supply chain provenance tracking (e.g., IBM Food Trust)	– Increased transparency and reduced counterfeiting	– Interoperability across different blockchain platforms	
– Secure identity management (e.g., Sovrin)	– Self-sovereign control over personal data	– Balancing privacy with regulatory compliance	
Access Control and Authorization:	– Role-based access control for sensitive data (e.g., Hyperledger Fabric)	– Granular control over data access and permissions	– Defining and enforcing complex access rules
– Decentralized authentication and authorization (e.g., uPort)	– Elimination of single points of failure and reduced trust dependence	– User adoption and integration with existing systems	
Auditing and Traceability:	– Event logs for software updates and transactions (e.g., Ethereum)	– Enhanced accountability and easier incident investigation	– Efficient data storage and query capabilities
– Proof-of-existence for digital assets (e.g., Filecoin)	– Verifiable proof of ownership and authenticity	– Scalability and cost-effectiveness for large data sets	
Cybersecurity Solutions:	– Decentralized identity verification (e.g., Civic)	– Reduced risk of identity theft and data breaches	– Integrating with existing identity management systems
– Secure voting systems (e.g., Voatz)	– Increased tamper-proofness and voter confidence	– Addressing regulatory hurdles and scalability concerns	
– Decentralized malware detection and mitigation (e.g., Cyberwatch)	– Enhanced threat intelligence sharing and collaborative defense	– Balancing privacy concerns with effective threat detection	

most well-known blockchain application, has a bad public image of security, the hacking attacks were restricted to other systems that attempted to preserve and store Bitcoin's secret keys [48,49]. Bitcoin transactions between parties are unlikely to be corrupted. Table 11.3 provides a valuable overview of how blockchain can contribute to improved cybersecurity across various domains.

11.5 Security and privacy in blockchain

A blockchain transaction often involves two separate ledgers [50]. Individually encrypted documents are stored in a content ledger. A transaction ledger stores encryption keys for accessing document files relating to the identification, health, academic qualifications, and other individual traits on a set of "key rings." The certifier adds digitally certified papers with varied properties to the subject's key rings. The certifier typically needs the subject's permission to do so. A law business, for example, may provide the subject with electronically signed copies of notarized documents [51]. A government organization may provide the individual in question with an electronically authenticated copy of her or his driver's license. After implementing the blockchain, certifiers no longer have access to the data. Inquisitors commonly rely on data stamped by a trusted third party [52]. Inquisitors can examine papers when the subject permits restricted keys use based on intelligent agreements. The system could restrict the number or duration of queries. All inquiries on the issue were properly recorded. A smart contract architecture allows other parties, such as banks and financial companies, insurance companies, and government organizations, to have access to documents. Commercial certifiers, such as municipal inspectors, accountants, attorneys, and notaries, may provide indemnities to investigators for a fee, such as validity assurance or home safety inspections. In this sense, documents stored on a blockchain are more likely to be valid. Blockchain technology has the potential to improve the privacy and security of information in the healthcare industry. This is a big worry because the healthcare data breaches totaled 112 million records in 2015.

It is stated that blockchain provides a fourth paradigm for securely sharing medical records between providers during a patient's lifetime [53]. Blockchain in EHR eliminates the need for an arrangement between the individual in question and the records. Blockchain does not function as a "new depository" or "safe bank box" for data. The time-stamped and configurable ledger in Bitcoin offers intelligent control over record access, eliminating the need to design specific features for each EHR provider. In a blockchain paradigm, all changes to a consumer's data are notified to the public ledger [54]. Blockchain-based healthcare solutions are being developed through corporate and public sector initiatives, as well as public–private partnerships (PPPs). Researchers at MIT Media Lab and Beth Israel Deaconess Medical Center suggested MedRec, a blockchain-based decentralized record management system for EHRs. MedRec is said to handle "authentication, confidentiality, accountability, and data sharing." Patients may have access to their medical records from numerous providers and healthcare venues. An irreversible history of every interaction containing the patient's data is created and delivered to the patient [55]. MedRec does not keep patient medical records. The system might save the record's signatures on a blockchain. Signing the record certifies that nothing has been altered. The patient will decide where the records can travel. In this method, the locus of control may shift from the facility to the patient. For individuals who do not prefer to handle their data, service companies may arise, and clients may transfer the responsibility to others [56,57].

11.6 Blockchain and Internet of Medical Things

Previous study suggests that the integration of blockchain and IoT has the potential to alter several sectors [58]. Smart IoT devices, for example, may be able to conduct autonomous transactions using smart contracts [59]. It's possible that merging blockchain and IoT with AI and big data solutions could result in a greater effect. At the same time, the IoT may provide significant security issues for enterprises. The issues mentioned above pose serious privacy and security threats. Criminals can, for example, determine whether someone is at home based on data collected from a Ubi device, such as the presence or absence of noise or light in the home. Attackers can exploit flaws in the Ubi or Wink Relay devices to turn on speakers and listen in on conversations. Vulnerabilities in the Chamberlain MyQ system enable robbers to identify whether the garage door is open or closed [60]. If an IoT device is hacked, the implications can be severe. Consider the widespread use of smart water meters and the attendant cybersecurity vulnerabilities.

As of early 2017, 20% of California residents have smart water meters, which gather data and send warnings about water leaks and usage to users' phones [61]. The Washington Suburban Sanitary Commission (WSSC) was also reported to be implementing IoT into its water supply system. Hackers and thieves can use water usage data to determine when people are not at home. Probably, the culprits may then burglarize residences when the inhabitants are away [61]. Blockchain may be especially relevant and promising for addressing the privacy and security issues related to the IoT. Some argue that blockchain might provide military-grade security for IoT devices [62–64] (see Figure 11.5). Below, there are essential procedures and methods, as well as various efforts that might help improve IoT security.

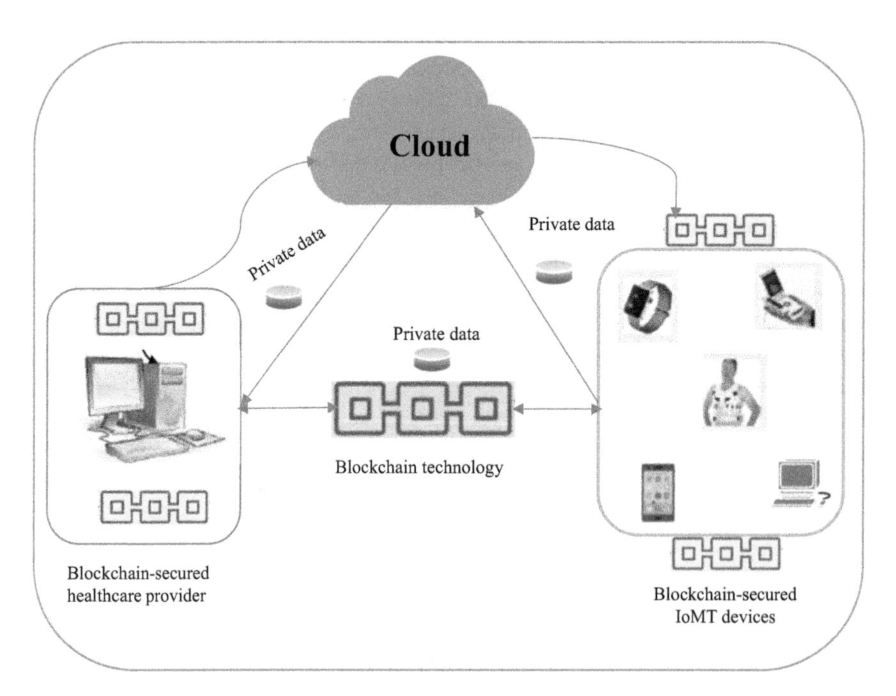

Figure 11.5 Blockchain enabling the security of IoMT devices and healthcare systems

11.7 Case studies: blockchain in healthcare security

The healthcare industry faces increasingly complex cybersecurity challenges, with patient data breaches and compromised medical devices posing significant threats. Blockchain, with its inherent features of immutability, transparency, and decentralization, offers promising solutions to enhance healthcare security. Here, are diverse case studies across various areas:

1. Secure medical record management:
   (i) Medchain: This platform leverages blockchain to create a tamper-proof and auditable record of medical data. Patients control their data access, granting permission to healthcare providers as needed. The immutable ledger ensures data integrity and simplifies compliance with regulations like HIPAA.
   (ii) HL7 FHIR on Blockchain: This initiative, led by HIMSS, explores deploying Health Level Seven's Fast Healthcare Interoperability Resources (FHIR) standard on blockchain. This enables secure and standardized data exchange between healthcare providers, improving patient data portability and access control.
2. Supply chain management for pharmaceuticals:
   (i) IBM Food Trust: This blockchain-based platform tracks the movement of pharmaceuticals throughout the supply chain, ensuring authenticity and combating counterfeiting. Recording timestamps and provenance data facilitates faster recalls and improves overall drug safety.
   (ii) MediLedger: This consortium, backed by pharma companies and technology providers, builds blockchain solutions for secure drug traceability and compliance management. Their platform automates regulatory reporting and streamlines supply chain processes, minimizing fraud and errors.
3. Decentralized clinical trials:
   (i) Triallink: This blockchain platform streamlines clinical trial data management, improving data integrity and transparency. Researchers, sponsors, and regulators can access an immutable record of trial data, enhancing trust and collaboration.
   (ii) Medishare: This platform uses blockchain to securely share and manage clinical trial data, ensuring patient privacy and compliance with GDPR. Patients retain control over their data and can choose to participate in specific research initiatives.
4. Decentralized identity management:
   (i) MedKey: This project enables patients to create self-sovereign identities on the blockchain, granting them complete control over their healthcare data. Doctors and researchers can access authorized data upon patient consent, streamlining data sharing and improving care coordination.
   (ii) Sovrin: This open-source, non-profit initiative builds a global infrastructure for self-sovereign identity. Healthcare institutions can leverage

Sovrin to implement secure and interoperable patient identity management solutions, reducing the risk of identity theft and improving data privacy.

5. Securing medical devices:
   (i) Medicalchain: This platform leverages blockchain to secure communication between medical devices and healthcare provider systems. Encrypting data and implementing access control mechanisms, minimizes the risk of unauthorized access and manipulation of device data.
   (ii) Chronicled: This company utilizes blockchain to track and authenticate medical devices throughout their lifecycle, reducing counterfeit devices and improving patient safety. Additionally, their platform simplifies device recalls and facilitates compliance with regulatory requirements.

11.8 Challenges and limitations of implementing blockchain

Blockchain technology is still in the testing phase, and its implementation has significant challenges that must be addressed when attempting to construct Blockchain-free, cryptographically safe systems. Implementing blockchain technology, while offering numerous benefits such as increased transparency, security, and efficiency, also comes with its set of challenges and limitations. These challenges can affect scalability, energy consumption, regulatory and legal issues, integration with existing systems, and more. Understanding these limitations is crucial for organizations considering blockchain adoption. This section delves into the details of these challenges.

Throughput problems: One restriction of Blockchain technology is its throughput. The present Bitcoin network executes 3–20 transactions per second (tps), with a potential throughput of 7 tps. In comparison, the VISA transaction network can process 2,000 tps (which was stress-tested in 2013 to handle 47,000 tps, and the Twitter network 5,000 tps.

Latency difficulties: One of the most important aspects of Blockchain deployment is the time component. Having requests handled on the Internet almost instantly impedes widespread technological adoption. To ensure the security of the Bitcoin transaction block, each transaction takes around 10 min to complete. For bigger transfers, the cost of a double-spend attack can last roughly an hour. The VISA transaction procedure takes no more than a few seconds.

Energy consumption: The energy consumption of blockchain networks, particularly those that rely on PoW, is another significant concern. The mining process, which involves solving complex mathematical problems to validate transactions and create new blocks, requires substantial computational power and, consequently, a large amount of electricity.

Example: The Bitcoin network's energy consumption rivals that of small countries, raising concerns about its environmental impact.

Regulatory and legal issues: The decentralized nature of blockchain poses regulatory and legal challenges. The lack of a central governing body means that it can be difficult to apply existing legal frameworks and regulations to blockchain transactions or smart contracts. Furthermore, the global nature of blockchain networks complicates jurisdictional issues. **Example:** Different countries have varied approaches to cryptocurrency regulation, ranging from outright bans to embracing them with open regulatory frameworks, affecting Blockchain adoption and use.

Interoperability: Interoperability between different blockchain systems is another challenge. With numerous blockchain networks in existence, the ability of these networks to communicate and exchange data seamlessly is limited. This lack of interoperability can hinder the adoption of blockchain technology across different sectors and applications. **Example:** A supply chain that utilizes one blockchain platform may have difficulty integrating with a financial services provider that uses a different blockchain platform.

Privacy concerns: While blockchain offers transparency, it also raises privacy concerns. Public blockchains store data across a network of computers, making the data accessible to anyone on the network. This can be problematic for sensitive personal or business data. **Example:** Transactions on a public blockchain, like Bitcoin, are visible to all users, potentially exposing user data or business transactions to competitors.

Security risks: Despite Blockchain security advantages, it is not immune to risks. Smart contracts, for instance, are prone to bugs and vulnerabilities that can be exploited. Additionally, the 51% attack, where a single entity gains control of the majority of a network's mining power, could allow them to manipulate transactions. **Example:** The DAO hack, where attackers exploited a vulnerability in a smart contract on the Ethereum blockchain, led to the theft of around $50 million worth of Ether.

Adoption and integration: The integration of blockchain technology into existing business processes and systems presents significant challenges. Organizations must consider the cost, complexity of implementation, and whether the benefits of blockchain outweigh these factors. Moreover, the lack of skilled blockchain professionals can hinder development and adoption. **Example:** Integrating blockchain with legacy banking systems requires substantial investment in technology and training, posing a barrier to widespread adoption.

Scalability: One of the most significant challenges facing blockchain technology is scalability. Blockchains, especially those utilizing Proof of Work (PoW) consensus mechanisms like Bitcoin, can handle only a limited number of transactions per second (TPS). This limitation arises from the need to maintain consensus across a vast network of nodes, which inherently slows down the processing speed compared to traditional centralized payment systems. **Example:** Bitcoin can process 4–7 tps, while Ethereum handles about 15–30. In contrast, Visa's payment network can process over 24,000 tps.

11.8.1 Key findings

The chapter findings highlight the transformational impact blockchain could have on securing sensitive health data and systems as well as hurdles that need to be overcome for its successful implementation. Here are the key findings distilled from this chapter:

1. Blockchain technology's inherent features, such as decentralization, immutability, and encryption, significantly enhance the security and integrity of healthcare data.
2. Blockchain enables more secure management of patient data, providing patients with greater control over their information.
3. The distributed nature of blockchain mitigates the risks associated with centralized data storage systems, which are vulnerable to cyberattacks and data breaches.
4. Innovations aimed at improving Blockchain scalability, energy efficiency, and interoperability are critical for its broader adoption in healthcare cybersecurity.

11.8.2 Future directions and innovations

Blockchain technology's future directions and advancements are positioned to solve its existing obstacles and limits, opening the path for more acceptance and more sophisticated applications. As we look ahead, many significant areas of development stand out, promising to improve scalability, reduce energy usage, improve regulatory compliance, protect privacy, and promote interoperability. These advances not only attempt to overcome current barriers but also to open up new opportunities for blockchain across a variety of industries.

11.8.2.1 Scalability enhancements

One of the most pressing issues with current blockchain technology is scalability. Future innovations are focusing on layer-2 solutions, such as Lightning Network for Bitcoin and Plasma and Sharding for Ethereum, which aim to significantly increase transaction throughput without compromising security or decentralization. These solutions operate on top of the blockchain, enabling faster and more cost-effective transactions.

11.8.2.2 Energy efficiency

The environmental impact of blockchain, especially networks that utilize Proof of Work (PoW), has prompted a search for more energy-efficient consensus mechanisms. Proof of Stake (PoS) and Delegated Proof of Stake (DPoS) are seen as viable alternatives that require significantly less energy. Additionally, innovations in cryptographic techniques, such as zero-knowledge proofs, offer ways to maintain network security and privacy with less computational effort.

11.8.2.3 Enhanced privacy

Privacy concerns associated with blockchain are being addressed through innovations such as confidential transactions and privacy-oriented cryptocurrencies. Technologies like zk-SNARKs (Zero-Knowledge Succinct Non-Interactive Arguments of Knowledge) allow for the verification of transactions without revealing any sensitive information, enabling both transparency and privacy.

11.8.2.4 Interoperability solutions

The future of blockchain lies in its ability to interoperate among diverse networks and systems. Projects like Polkadot and Cosmos are developing protocols that enable different blockchains to communicate and share information seamlessly. This interoperability is crucial for creating a unified blockchain ecosystem where diverse applications and services can interact without barriers.

11.8.2.5 Adoption and integration tools

To facilitate the integration of blockchain into existing business processes, future innovations will focus on developing user-friendly platforms, tools, and APIs that lower the barrier to entry for businesses and developers. Blockchain as a Service (BaaS) platforms are emerging, offering companies the ability to deploy blockchain technology without the need to develop their infrastructure from scratch.

The future of blockchain technology seems promising, with continuing research and development aimed at solving present hurdles and unlocking new possibilities. Scalability, energy efficiency, regulatory compliance, privacy, interoperability, and acceptance advancements are paving the way for blockchain to disrupt sectors far beyond its initial coin uses. As these advancements advance, blockchain is set to become a core technology for the digital era, allowing for more secure, transparent, and efficient transactions across the global economy.

11.9 Conclusion

The exploration of blockchain technology's application in enhancing cybersecurity within emerging healthcare systems reveals a promising horizon. The inherent features of blockchain, such as decentralization, transparency, and immutability, align well with the critical needs of healthcare information systems for security, privacy, and data integrity. As healthcare systems continue to evolve, incorporating digital records, telehealth services, and IoT devices, the security challenges they face become increasingly complex and demanding. Blockchain technology, with its unique attributes, stands out as a potent solution to address these challenges, offering a new paradigm in securing sensitive health data and ensuring the integrity of healthcare operations. Blockchain applications in healthcare cybersecurity can significantly enhance data security and privacy. By creating immutable records of healthcare transactions, blockchain ensures that once data is entered, it cannot be altered or tampered with. This attribute is invaluable for maintaining the integrity of medical records and protecting against data breaches, which are all too common in centralized data management systems. Moreover, the use of encryption and smart contracts adds a layer of security, ensuring that only authorized individuals can access sensitive information, thus preserving patient privacy. The decentralized nature of blockchain addresses another critical vulnerability in traditional healthcare systems: the risk of single-point failures and centralized data breaches. By distributing data across a network of nodes, blockchain reduces the potential impact of cyberattacks, making it exceedingly difficult for hackers to compromise the entire system. This decentralized approach not only enhances security but also improves the resilience of healthcare information systems, ensuring continuity of care even in the face of cyber threats. Blockchain technology also offers solutions to the challenges of interoperability and data integrity in healthcare systems. The ability to securely share patient data across different platforms and providers is crucial for the continuity and quality of care. Blockchain facilitates this through standardized protocols and secure data exchange mechanisms, ensuring that patient records are accurate, up-to-date, and accessible to authorized healthcare providers, regardless of the systems they use. Despite its potential, the adoption of blockchain in healthcare cybersecurity is not without challenges. Issues such as scalability, energy consumption of certain blockchain models, regulatory compliance, and integration with existing healthcare IT infrastructure need to be addressed. Future innovations in blockchain technology, including the development of more energy-efficient consensus mechanisms, enhanced privacy features, and interoperability solutions, are crucial for its successful implementation in healthcare. Moreover, as blockchain technology matures, the development of regulatory frameworks that support its use in healthcare, along with the training of a skilled workforce to implement and manage blockchain-based systems, will be essential. Collaboration between technology developers, healthcare providers, and regulatory bodies is necessary to realize the full potential of blockchain in enhancing cybersecurity in the healthcare sector. Blockchain technology presents a transformative approach to cybersecurity in emerging healthcare systems. Its applications in ensuring data security, privacy, and integrity are particularly relevant in the context of digital health records, telehealth, and IoT devices in healthcare. While challenges remain in the widespread adoption of blockchain, ongoing innovations, and collaborative efforts are paving the way for its integration into healthcare cybersecurity strategies. As we move forward, the potential of blockchain to secure sensitive health data and enhance the resilience of healthcare information systems against cyber threats cannot be underestimated. The future of healthcare cybersecurity, bolstered by blockchain technology, looks promising, offering a pathway to more secure, efficient, and patient-centered healthcare systems.

References

[1] R. Prakash, V. S. Anoop and S. Asharaf. (2022) Blockchain technology for cybersecurity: A text mining literature analysis. *International Journal of Information Management Data Insights*, 2(2), 100112.

[2] S. Gerke, T. Minssen and G. Cohen. (2020). Ethical and legal challenges of artificial intelligence-driven healthcare. In *Artificial intelligence in healthcare* (pp. 295–336). Academic Press.

[3] Abouelmehdi, K., Beni-Hessane, A., and Khaloufi, H. (2018). Big healthcare data: preserving security and privacy. *Journal of Big Data*, 5(1), 1–18.

[4] E. A. Adeniyi, R. O. Ogundokun, and J. B. Awotunde (2021). IoMT-based wearable body sensors network healthcare monitoring system. *IoT in*

Healthcare and Ambient Assisted Living. London: Springer Nature, pp. 103–121.

[5] R. O. Ogundokun, J. B. Awotunde, E. A. Adeniyi and F. E. Ayo. (2021). Crypto-Stegno based model for securing medical information on IOMT platform. *Multimedia Tools and Applications*, 80, 31705–31727.

[6] A. E. Adeniyi, K. M. Abiodun, J. B. Awotunde, M. Olagunju, O. S. Ojo and N. P. Edet. (2023). Implementation of a block cipher algorithm for medical information security on cloud environment: using modified advanced encryption standard approach. *Multimedia Tools and Applications*, 82(13), 20537–20551.

[7] J. Ibarra, H. Jahankhani and S. Kendzierskyj. (2019). Cyber-physical attacks and the value of healthcare data: facing an era of cyber extortion and organised crime. *Blockchain and Clinical Trial: Securing Patient Data*. Springer Nature, pp. 115–137.

[8] B. Zaabar, O. Cheikhrouhou, F. Jamil, M. Ammi and M. Abid. HealthBlock: A secure blockchain-based healthcare data management system. *Computer Networks*, 200, 108500.

[9] K. M. Abiodun, E. A. Adeniyi, J. B. Awotunde, *et al.* (2022). Blockchain and Internet of Things in Healthcare Systems: Prospects, Issues, and Challenges. In *Digital Health Transformation with Blockchain and Artificial Intelligence* (pp. 1–22). Boca Raton, FL: CRC Press.

[10] J. K. Adeniyi, S. A. Ajagbe, E. A. Adeniyi, *et al.* (2024). A biometrics-generated private/public key cryptography for a blockchain-based e-voting system. *Egyptian Informatics Journal*, 25, 100447.

[11] E. A. Adeniyi, R. O. Ogundokun, S. Misra, J. B. Awotunde and K. M. Abiodun. (2022). Enhanced security and privacy issue in multi-tenant environment of green computing using blockchain technology. In *Blockchain Applications in the Smart Era* (pp. 65–83). Cham: Springer International Publishing.

[12] A. Lakhan, M. A. Dootio, A. H. Sodhro, *et al.* (2021) Cost-efficient service selection and execution and blockchain-enabled serverless network for internet of medical things. *Mathematical Biosciences and Engineering*, 18(6), 7344–7362. doi:10.3934/mbe.2021363.

[13] M. A. Mohammed, A. Lakhan, D. A. Zebari, *et al.* (2024). Securing healthcare data in industrial cyber-physical systems using combining deep learning and blockchain technology. *Engineering Applications of Artificial Intelligence*, 129, 107612.

[14] M. A. Almaiah, A. Ali, F. Hajjej, M. F. Pasha and M. A. Alohali. (2022). A lightweight hybrid deep learning privacy preserving model for FC-based industrial internet of medical things. *Sensors*, 22(6), 2112.

[15] R. U. Rasool, H. F. Ahmad, W. Rafique, A. Qayyum, and J. Qadir. (2022). Security and privacy of internet of medical things: A contemporary review in the age of surveillance, botnets, and adversarial ML. *Journal of Network and Computer Applications*, 201, 103332.

[16] A. Lakhan, M. A. Mohammed, M. Elhoseny, M. D. Alshehri, and K. H. Abdulkareem. (2022). Blockchain multi-objective optimization approach-enabled secure and cost-efficient scheduling for the Internet of Medical Things (IoMT) in fog-cloud system. *Soft Computing*, 26(13), 6429–6442.

[17] Y. P. Chandra and T. Matuska (2022). Intelligent data systems for building energy workflow: Data pipelines, LSTM efficiency prediction and more. *Energy and Buildings*, 267, 112135.

[18] J. Yu, M. Gao, Y. Li, Z. Zhang, W. H. Ip and K. L. Yung. (2022). Workflow performance prediction based on graph structure aware deep attention neural network. *Journal of Industrial Information Integration*, 27, 100337.

[19] A. E. Adeniyi, R. G. Jimoh, and J. B. Awotunde. (2024). Securing healthcare data in industrial cyber-physical A systematic review on elliptic curve cryptography algorithm for internet of things: Categorization, application areas, and security. *Computers and Electrical Engineering*, 118, 109330.

[20] U. Rahardja, A. N. Hidayanto, N. Lutfiani, D. A. Febiani and Q. Aini (2021). Immutability of distributed hash model on blockchain node storage. *Sci. J. Informatics*, 8(1), 137–143.

[21] K. Zhang, and H. A. Jacobsen. (2018). Towards dependable, scalable, and pervasive distributed ledgers with blockchains. In *ICDCS* (pp. 1337–1346).

[22] J. B. Awotunde, A. L. Imoize, R. G. Jimoh, *et al.* (2024). AIoMT enabling real-time monitoring of healthcare systems: security and privacy considerations. *Handbook of Security and Privacy of AI-Enabled Healthcare Systems and Internet of Medical Things*. Taylor and Francis, pp. 97–133.

[23] A. H. Seh, M. Zarour, M. Alenezi, *et al.* (2020). Healthcare data breaches: insights and implications. *Healthcare* 8(2), 133.

[24] M. Chernyshev, S. Zeadally and Z. Baig. (2019). Healthcare data breaches: Implications for digital forensic readiness. *Journal of medical systems*, 43, 1–12.

[25] I. Keshta and A. Odeh. (2021). Security and privacy of electronic health records: Concerns and challenges. *Egyptian Informatics Journal*, 22(2), 177–183.

[26] M. N. S. Perera, T. Nakamura, M. Hashimoto, H. Yokoyama, C. Cheng and K. Sakurai (2022). A survey on group signatures and ring signatures: traceability vs. anonymity. *Cryptography*, 6(1), 3.

[27] S. F. Aghili, M. Sedaghat, D. Singelée and M. Gupta. (2022). MLS-ABAC: Efficient multi-level security attribute-based access control scheme. *Future Generation Computer Systems*, 131, 75–90.

[28] S. Shajari, K. Kuruvinashetti, A. Komeili and U. Sundararaj. (2023). The emergence of AI-based wearable sensors for digital health technology: A review. *Sensors*, 23(23), 9498.

[29] Kruse, C. S., Smith, B., Vanderlinden, H., and Nealand, A. (2017). Security techniques for the electronic health records. *Journal of Medical Systems*, 41, 1–9.

[30] J. B. Awotunde, R. O. Ogundokun, A. E. Adeniyi, *et al.* (2022). Cloud-IoMT-based wearable body sensors network for monitoring elderly patients during the COVID-19 pandemic. In *Biomedical Engineering Applications for People with Disabilities and the Elderly in the COVID-19 Pandemic and Beyond* (pp. 33–48). New York: Academic Press.

[31] A. K. Pandey, A. I. Khan, Y. B. Abushark, *et al.* (2020). Key issues in healthcare data integrity: Analysis and recommendations. *IEEE Access*, 8, 40612–40628.

[32] M. Zarour, M. Alenezi, M. T. J. Ansari, *et al.* (2021). Ensuring data integrity of healthcare information in the era of digital health. *Healthcare Technology Letters*, 8(3), 66–77.

[33] S. J. Blanke and E. McGrady. (2016). When it comes to securing patient health information from breaches, your best medicine is a dose of prevention: A cybersecurity risk assessment checklist. *Journal of Healthcare Risk Management*, 36(1), 14–24.

[34] M. Alshehri. (2023). Blockchain-assisted cyber security in medical things using artificial intelligence. *Electronic Research Archive*, 31(2), 708–728.

[35] A. Esmat, M. de Vos, Y. Ghiassi-Farrokhfal, P. Palensky and D. Epema. (2021). A novel decentralized platform for peer-to-peer energy trading market with blockchain technology. *Applied Energy*, 282, 116123.

[36] G. G. Dagher, J. Mohler, M. Milojkovic and P. B. Marella. (2018). Ancile: Privacy-preserving framework for access control and interoperability of electronic health records using blockchain technology. *Sustainable Cities and Society*, 39, 283–297.

[37] J. B. Awotunde, K. M. Abiodun, E. A. Adeniyi, S. O. Folorunso and R. G. Jimoh. (2021). A deep learning-based intrusion detection technique for a secured IoMT system. In *International Conference on Informatics and Intelligent Applications* (pp. 50–62). Cham: Springer International Publishing.

[38] I. E. Anika (2019). New technology for old crimes? The role of cryptocurrencies in circumventing the global anti-money laundering regime and facilitating transnational crime (Doctoral dissertation, University of British Columbia).

[39] D. Lizcano, J. A. Lara, B. White and S. Aljawarneh. (2020). Blockchain-based approach to create a model of trust in open and ubiquitous higher education. *Journal of Computing in Higher Education*, 32, 109–134.

[40] S. Khezr, M. Moniruzzaman, A. Yassine and R. Benlamri. (2019). Blockchain technology in healthcare: A comprehensive review and directions for future research. *Applied Sciences*, 9(9), 1736.

[41] B. Bhushan, A. Khamparia, K. M. Sagayam, S. K. Sharma, M. A. Ahad and Debnath, N. C. (2020). Blockchain for smart cities: A review of architectures, integration trends and future research directions. *Sustainable Cities and Society*, 61, 102360.

[42] U. Khalil, O. A. Malik, M. Uddin and C. L. Chen. (2022). A comparative analysis on blockchain versus centralized authentication architectures for IoT-enabled smart devices in smart cities: a comprehensive review, recent advances, and future research directions. *Sensors*, 22(14), 5168.

[43] N. Kshetri. (2017). Blockchain roles in strengthening cybersecurity and protecting privacy. *Telecommunications Policy*, 41(10), 1027–1038.

[44] S. Namasudra, G. C. Deka, P. Johri, M. Hosseinpour and A. H. Gandomi. (2021). The revolution of blockchain: State-of-the-art and research challenges. *Archives of Computational Methods in Engineering*, 28, 1497–1515.

[45] J. H. Huh and K. Seo. (2019). Blockchain-based mobile fingerprint verification and automatic log-in platform for future computing. *The Journal of Supercomputing*, 75, 3123–3139.

[46] E. F. Ahmet, D. Atakan and U. G. Altun. (2019). SWIFT attack via phishing against MIS of mobile banking security. *Yönetim Bilişim Sistemleri Dergisi*, 4(2), 24–48.

[47] Z. Shah, I. Ullah, H. Li, A. Levula and K. Khurshid. (2022). Blockchain based solutions to mitigate distributed denial of service (DDoS) attacks in the Internet of Things (IoT): A survey. *Sensors*, 22(3), 1094.

[48] A. Ghosh, S. Gupta, A. Dua, and N. Kumar. (2020). Security of Cryptocurrencies in blockchain technology: State-of-art, challenges and future prospects. *Journal of Network and Computer Applications*, 163, 102635.

[49] D. Dasgupta, J. M. Shrein and K. D. Gupta. (2019). A survey of blockchain from security perspective. *Journal of Banking and Financial Technology*, 3, 1–17.

[50] G. M. Riva. (2020). What happens in blockchain stays in blockchain. A legal solution to conflicts between digital ledgers and privacy rights. *Frontiers in Blockchain*, 3, 36.

[51] B. Biddle. (2017). Public Key Infrastructure and Digital Signature Legislation: Ten Public Policy Questions.

[52] N. Kshetri. (2023). Blockchain role in enhancing quality and safety and promoting sustainability in the food and beverage industry. *Sustainability*, 15 (23), 16223.

[53] T. F. Stafford, and H. Treiblmaier. (2020). Characteristics of a blockchain ecosystem for secure and sharable electronic medical records. *IEEE Transactions on Engineering Management*, 67(4), 1340–1362.

[54] B. Yu, J. Wright, S. Nepal, L. Zhu, J. Liu and R. Ranjan, R. (2018). IotChain: Establishing trust in the internet of things ecosystem using blockchain. *IEEE Cloud Computing*, 5(4), 12–23.

[55] A. G. M. Alzahrani, A. Alenezi, A. Mershed, H. Atlam, F. Mousa and G. Wills. (2020). A framework for data sharing between healthcare providers using blockchain. In *Proceedings of the 5th International Conference on Internet of Things, Big Data and Security*, SciTePress. vol. 1, pp. 349–358.

[56] B. Gbadamosi, R. O. Ogundokun, E. A. Adeniyi, S. Misra and N. F. Stephens. (2022). Medical data analysis for IoT-based datasets in the cloud using naïve Bayes classifier for prediction of heart disease. In *New Frontiers in Cloud Computing and Internet of Things* (pp. 365–386). Cham: Springer International Publishing.

[57] J. B. Awotunde, R. G. Jimoh, A. E. Adeniyi, E. F. Ayo, G. J. Ajamu and D. R. Aremu. (2023). Application of interpretable artificial intelligence enabled cognitive internet of things for COVID-19 pandemics. In *Explainable*

Machine Learning for Multimedia Based Healthcare Applications (pp. 191–213). Cham: Springer International Publishing.

[58] K. Christidis and M. Devetsikiotis. (2016). Blockchains and smart contracts for the internet of things. *IEEE Access*, 4, 2292–2303.

[59] B. Bhargava (2018). Technology Final Report Intelligent Autonomous Systems Based on Data.

[60] A. Allen, A. Mylonas, S. Vidalis and D. Gritzalis. (2024). Smart homes under siege: Assessing the robustness of physical security against wireless network attacks. *Computers & Security*, 139, 103687.

[61] R. Hackett. (2017). How blockchains could save us from another Flint-like contamination crisis. *Venturebeat*, Feb.

[62] J. Coward. (2016). Meet the visionary who brought blockchain to the industrial IoT. *IoT World News*, 14.

[63] M. AbdulRaheem, J. B. Awotunde, C. Chakraborty, E. A. Adeniyi, I. D. Oladipo, I. D. and A. K. Bhoi. (2023). Security and privacy concerns in smart healthcare system. In *Implementation of Smart Healthcare Systems using AI, IoT, and Blockchain* (pp. 243–273). New York: Academic Press.

[64] A. Sahai and B. Waters. (2005). Fuzzy identity-based encryption. In Advances in Cryptology–EUROCRYPT 2005: *24th Annual International Conference on the Theory and Applications of Cryptographic Techniques*, Aarhus, Denmark, May 22–26, 2005. Proceedings 24 (pp. 457–473). Berlin: Springer.

Chapter 12

The ethics of cybersecurity in emerging healthcare systems

Abubakar Aliyu[1], Emeka Ogbuju[1], Agbotiname Lucky Imoize[2], Ovye John Abari[1], Musa Muhammad Kunya[1], Godwin Sani[3], Folashade Aminat Salaudeen[1] and Francisca Oladipo[4]

This chapter delves into the ethics of cybersecurity in emerging healthcare systems, examining the complex relationship between ethical considerations and technological advancements. We begin by defining evolving healthcare systems and then highlight the significance of cybersecurity in preserving trust among patients. We examine the benefits and drawbacks of integrating technology while highlighting the delicate balance that must be drawn between innovation and data security. When it comes to patient autonomy, informed consent, and responsible data sharing for investigation, ethical considerations are crucial. A thorough analysis of the legal framework is conducted, with a focus on the challenges associated with enforcing cyber-security regulations in rapidly evolving healthcare systems. We analyse the ethical ramifications of AI and data breaches in the healthcare industry, promoting human oversight, fairness, and precautionary practices. In addition to providing a comprehensive road map for navigating this rapidly changing environment, the chapter concludes with a call to action that urges stake-holders to give ethical cybersecurity practices priority when creating and implementing new healthcare systems.

Keywords: Ethics; cybersecurity; healthcare systems; trust; confidentiality; privacy; security; transparency

[1]Department of Computer Science, Faculty of Science, Federal University Lokoja, Nigeria
[2]Department of Electrical and Electronics Engineering, Faculty of Engineering, University of Lagos, Nigeria
[3]Directorate of Information and Communication Technology, Federal University Lokoja, Nigeria
[4]Department of Computer Science, Faculty of Computing and Applied Science, Thomas Adewumi University, Nigeria

12.1 Introduction

Amidst the rapid growth of technology, modern healthcare systems signify a significant shift in the provision of patient-centred care [1]. The healthcare environment is evolving as a result of these systems, which are defined by the integration of cutting-edge technologies, data-driven decision-making, and networked infrastructures [2]. Now that innovation and healthcare are coming together [3], it is crucial to examine the ethical implications of these revolutionary advancements, particularly in the crucial area of cybersecurity [4]. Our investigation is centred on an advanced understanding of developing healthcare systems. These comprise a range of interconnected technologies, such as wearables, telemedicine, electronic health records, and artificial intelligence (AI), that are coming together to improve patient engagement, treatment modalities, and medical diagnostics [5]. A new era of healthcare marked by enhanced accessibility, personalised treatment, and effective healthcare delivery is heralded by the integration of various technologies [6]. Given this technological renaissance, cybersecurity in healthcare is crucial and cannot be overstated [7]. These interconnected devices communicate and retain enormous amounts of sensitive patient data, necessitating the construction of an impregnable fortress against potential cyber assaults [8]. Cybersecurity is essential for more than just protecting data [9], as it also plays a key role in maintaining patient confidence [10], guaranteeing the accuracy of medical records [10], and strengthening the fundamental principles of moral healthcare [11].

Complex ethical issues that require careful navigation are entwined in the relationship between cybersecurity and developing healthcare [12]. The ethical foundation of cybersecurity procedures in the healthcare industry is established by these ethical considerations, which range from protecting patient autonomy and gaining informed permission to finding a careful balance between the necessity of data sharing for research and the protection of individual privacy [13]. The choices taken in this arena have far-reaching effects, influencing patient trust, healthcare results, and the entire fabric of ethical healthcare delivery [14]. This chapter sets out on an extensive exploration, exploring the complex intersections between cybersecurity, ethics, and new healthcare systems. We seek to unravel the complex web that links advancements in technology with moral obligations in the field of healthcare by carefully examining terminologies, acknowledging the critical role that cybersecurity plays, and examining ethical issues.

12.1.1 Key contributions of the chapter

The chapter presents a thorough analysis of the complex interplay between ethics and cybersecurity in developing healthcare systems. To help stakeholders navigate the constantly changing nexus between healthcare and technology, the contributions made here aim to clarify the complex ethical issues. The key contributions of this are:

(a) The chapter makes a valuable contribution by providing a solid framework for comprehending the ethical aspects of developing healthcare systems. It explores the fundamentals of ethics and establishes the framework for further talks about the complex relationship with cybersecurity.

(b) Getting across the technological terrain of developing healthcare systems is crucial. The chapter unravels the incorporation of cutting-edge technology, highlighting the ethical challenges and prospects presented by breakthroughs such as telemedicine, AI, and data-driven healthcare.
(c) A significant amount of emphasis is placed on patient-centric ethics, which offers insightful information on maintaining patient confidentiality, protecting patient trust, and making sure ethical issues are at the centre of healthcare procedures. This assessment provides the basis for moral judgements made when providing patient care.
(d) The chapter significantly advances the conversation around the ethical governance of data. It focuses on methods for handling consent concerns, safeguarding patient data, and striking a balance between privacy concerns and the potential benefits of data sharing for public health and research.
(e) The chapter offers an in-depth examination and insights into the legal and regulatory frameworks controlling cybersecurity in the healthcare industry. It examines the rules that are in place, points out difficulties with their enforcement, and promotes the creation of regulations that are flexible enough to keep up with changes in technology.
(f) The chapter contributes by analysing ethical reactions to online occurrences. It highlights the necessity for responsibility and transparency when revealing cybersecurity breaches, examines the effect on patient trust, and describes ethical duties in incident response.
(g) The examination of the ethical ramifications associated with the use of AI in healthcare is a noteworthy highlight. The chapter explores ethical issues in decision-making, biases in AI algorithms, and the significance of retaining human oversight in AI-driven healthcare systems.
(h) By providing a framework for assuring ethical cybersecurity in developing healthcare systems, the chapter makes a significant contribution. These approaches operate as a road map for moral behaviour and include anything from making significant infrastructural investments to training healthcare personnel and giving ethical issues a top priority when designing systems.
(i) The chapter concludes with a summary of the major contributions and a discussion of future ethical requirements. The always-changing environment of developing healthcare systems, demands stakeholder collaboration, ongoing education, and an unrelenting commitment to giving ethical cybersecurity practices a top priority.

The contributions of the chapter shed light on the ethical foundation of developing healthcare systems by providing stakeholders with a forward-looking vision, practical insights, and nuanced viewpoints to help them navigate the moral challenges of healthcare cybersecurity.

12.1.2 Chapter organisation

We begin this chapter with a thorough introduction in Section 12.1, which highlights the critical role that ethics play in the dynamic interplay between cybersecurity and future healthcare systems. After that, the extensive review of relevant work in Section 12.2 offers a thorough investigation of extant literature, legal assessments, and empirical research, summarising important discoveries and pinpointing knowledge gaps. The approach used to examine the ethical landscape of healthcare cybersecurity is explained in the section on methodology that follows in Section 12.3. It provides details on the research methodology and synthesis process. Next, in Section 12.4, we examine the terrain of developing healthcare systems, exploring modern patterns, innovations in technology, and the changing role of cybersecurity in influencing healthcare provision. Section 12.5 lays forth the ethical underpinnings of healthcare cybersecurity by examining the fundamental ideas that guide moral behaviour in protecting patient information and guaranteeing the accuracy of medical technology. Section 12.6 discusses specific ethical concerns related to healthcare cybersecurity, including problems with patient privacy, informed consent, and the moral dilemmas associated with reliance on technology. Section 12.7 offers a summary of legal and regulatory aspects that provide light on current frameworks, difficulties with enforcement, and the requirement for legislation that is flexible enough to keep up with technological changes. Section 12.8 addresses the ethical issues of cybersecurity incidents, highlighting the significance of responsibility and openness as well as the influence these issues have on patient trust and the ethical duties associated with incident response. Section 12.9 of the chapter then delves deeply into the ethical ramifications of AI in healthcare, examining questions of prejudice, discrimination, and the moral concerns that arise when AI is used to make decisions. Section 12.10 outlines suggested approaches and best practices for moral cybersecurity in the healthcare industry. It covers the need for a strong cybersecurity infrastructure, outreach programmes, and ethical system design considerations. Section 12.11 presents a summary of the most important lessons discovered during the investigation of ethical issues, offering thoughtful observations and implications for upcoming advancements. In Section 12.12, the chapter wraps up by summarising the most important discoveries, highlighting the critical role ethics play in healthcare cybersecurity, and providing an outlook on the changing ethical situation.

12.2 Related work

This section delves into the complex topic of "The Ethics of Cybersecurity in Emerging Healthcare Systems," which is a critical nexus where ethical ideals in healthcare must be upheld and cutting-edge technology meets. A thorough evaluation of research works, which are summarised in Table 12.1, and each offers distinct viewpoints and insights to the conversation on ethical considerations within the changing field of healthcare cybersecurity, highlights the urgency of this investigation. Healthcare is undergoing a technical metamorphosis characterised by the incorporation of emerging technologies like blockchain, AI, and networked systems. This transition calls for a thorough analysis of the ethical concerns that go along with it. We embarked on a voyage through the ethical aspects of

Table 12.1 *Review of the related works*

Reference	Description of work done	Limitations of the work
[15]	Conducted a thorough examination of ethical issues, investigating the effect on patient data confidentially.	Limited to patient data; might not address more general cybersecurity issues.
[16]	Explored the relationship between patient trust and cybersecurity, focusing on consequences resulting from cybersecurity events.	Lacking empirical facts and mostly concentrating on the theoretical implications.
[17]	Provides insights into proactive cybersecurity measures regarding ethical hacking in the healthcare industry.	Limited use in practice and insufficient real-world case studies to support.
[18]	Examined how AI ethics relate to healthcare cybersecurity, with a particular emphasis on moral issues in AI applications.	Confined attention to AI, can leave out the larger cybersecurity scene.
[19]	Examined current healthcare cybersecurity legal system frameworks and gave a summary of regulatory contexts.	Restricted geographic reach, possibly failing to capture opinions on global cybersecurity.
[20]	Examined the challenges in implementing cybersecurity laws in the medical field, focusing on the regulatory elements.	Inadequate attention to new technology and a possible void in the mitigation of hazards in the future.
[15]	Examined the ethical consequences of healthcare data breaches, emphasising the effects above preventative measures.	Inadequate preventative measures and a possible void in tackling upcoming cybersecurity threats.
[21]	Suggested strategies for moral cybersecurity in the healthcare industry, including precautions to protect patient data.	Lacks empirical data demonstrating the efficacy of suggested tactics.
[22]	Analysed ethical issues with AI-driven diagnosis, focusing on applications of fairness and ethics in AI.	Little consideration is paid to the moral implications of AI in healthcare decisions.
[23]	Provided insight on cybersecurity education for medical workers, raising awareness, and advocating best practices.	Insufficient empirical evidence about the true influence of education on cybersecurity practices.
[24]	Examined the moral implications of blockchain technology in cybersecurity for healthcare.	Insufficient attention was paid to real-world implementation issues and industry adoption.
[25]	Investigated the moral fallout from ransomware assaults on medical networks.	Not a thorough examination of defences against new and developing cyber threats.
[26]	Examined the moral difficulties in preserving cybersecurity standards while guaranteeing interoperability.	Little consideration was paid to developing technologies other than compatibility problems.
[27]	Examined the moral implications of identifying patients in healthcare settings using biometric data.	May not fully examine the broader ethical issues of using biometrics.

(Continues)

Table 12.1 Review of the related works (Continued)

Reference	Description of work done	Limitations of the work
[28]	Published a framework with a focus on risk management for moral cybersecurity practices in the healthcare industry.	The usefulness of the concept in real-world circumstances has received limited empirical support.
[29]	Investigated the relationship between ethical issues in healthcare cybersecurity and data protection laws.	Insufficient information about the real-world difficulties in coordinating data protection regulations with changing cybersecurity requirements.
[30]	Examined the moral ramifications of utilising social media data for patient involvement in healthcare cybersecurity.	Lack of consideration paid to possible privacy issues and moral dilemmas arising from social media usage.
[31]	Examined the moral implications of cloud computing for the healthcare industry, putting a focus on compliance and data protection.	Failed to address new issues and developing moral dilemmas related to cloud computing.
[32]	Investigated the moral implications for outside suppliers in the field of healthcare cybersecurity.	Limited investigation of possible conflicts of interest and security issues related to collaborations with third parties.
[33]	Examined the moral ramifications of using health data in developing healthcare systems for research.	Possible omission in the discussion of developing ethical issues related to cutting-edge data analytics and research techniques.

cybersecurity, investigating how the swift advancements in healthcare systems necessitate a comparable development in ethical frameworks to guarantee patient data protection, privacy, and integrity. This section synthesises several viewpoints, utilising the collective knowledge and detailed analysis included in Table 12.1.

After a thorough analysis of relevant literature, it is clear that studying the Ethics of Cybersecurity in Emerging Healthcare Systems is not only a worthwhile academic endeavour but also a vital necessity. The literature that is now available, which includes legal analyses, comparative studies, and empirical research, emphasises how closely law and technology interact. This investigation is more than just a scholarly exercise; it also highlights how important it is to understand the complex dynamics guiding the ethical aspects of cybersecurity in the context of changing healthcare systems.

12.2.1 Gap analysis

As shown in Table 12.1, a comprehensive analysis of the ethics of cybersecurity in developing healthcare systems reveals several essential holes that must be filled immediately to strengthen the ethical framework at this crucial intersection of technology and healthcare. First, there is a clear disparity in the scant attention paid to developing technology. Although most of the evaluated literature explores well-established technologies such as AI and electronic health records, there is very little thorough investigation of newer technologies like edge computing, quantum computing, and blockchain. The swiftly changing technological environment presents distinct ethical obstacles that require immediate attention to guarantee ethical standards are maintained with advancements. The inadequate use of ethical concepts in practice is another significant shortcoming. There is a lack of solid empirical data or real-world case studies illustrating the actual application of suggested ethical frameworks, although numerous studies provide theoretical insights into ethical problems. To close this theory-to-application gap, theoretical ethical concepts must be translated into practical cybersecurity procedures, as this translation has not been well tested. The literature also clearly shows a regulatory and geographic mismatch. There is a major knowledge vacuum regarding global perspectives and heterogeneous regulatory environments because the majority of the attention paid to legal and regulatory frameworks is focused on certain geographic areas, especially the United States. Given the global nature of healthcare systems, a more comprehensive strategy to address cybersecurity issues and ethical considerations across regulatory environments is desperately needed.

Moreover, there is a significant void in the scant coverage of preventive measures. Healthcare systems are facing growing cybersecurity threats, and while the dangers and repercussions of cybersecurity breaches are acknowledged, preventive tactics and proactive measures are not well-analysed. This gap needs to be overcome to increase the resilience of healthcare systems against unanticipated cyberattacks. And last, there is glaringly little patient perspective included in the creation of ethical frameworks. The majority of the literature prioritises institutional and regulatory viewpoints over patient opinions. To create a cybersecurity strategy that is in line with patient values, a comprehensive ethical framework should take into account the viewpoints, worries, and expectations of patients. The investigation of emerging technologies, the empirical validation of ethical frameworks, international cooperation for regulatory alignment, the creation of strong preventive strategies, and the incorporation of patient-centric ethical considerations are among the areas that require immediate attention to close these gaps. By addressing these gaps, we can contribute to developing a strong, patient-centred digital healthcare ecosystem and reinforce the moral foundations of cybersecurity in emerging healthcare systems.

12.3 Methodology

In the context of the research work called "The Ethics of Cybersecurity in Emerging Healthcare Systems," a literature review methodology is a strong strategy. The study found important insights, trends, and gaps in the present body of knowledge by methodically going over, summarising, and synthesising the literature. The effectiveness of the literature review methodology is significant since it offers a thorough overview of cybersecurity ethics without requiring a lot of

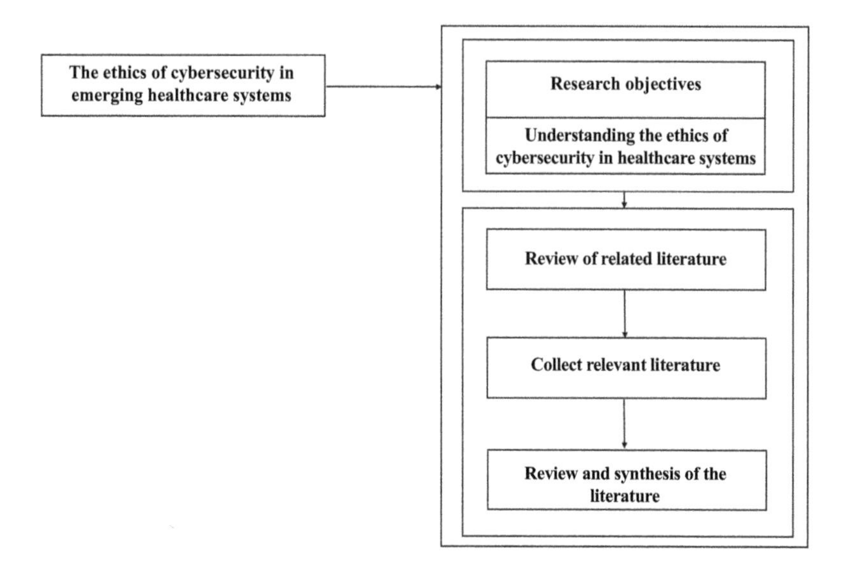

Figure 12.1 Review methodology

resources or laborious data collection procedures. This strategy is in line with expanding on the corpus of current research and advancing our understanding of the moral implications of the complex nexus of cybersecurity and healthcare systems. The suggested approach, as illustrated in Figure 12.1 for comprehending cybersecurity ethics in developing healthcare systems, begins with the specific goal of elucidating the ethical aspects involved in the intersection of cybersecurity and changing healthcare systems. The main component of this methodology is the literature review, which is a methodical process of gathering a large body of pertinent material, including books, papers, and scholarly articles. After the data is gathered, a thorough process of systematic review and synthesis takes place. To provide a coherent and thorough summary, every work of literature is examined, with significant insights, recurrent themes, and information synthesised from each one.

The outcome synthesises the current body of information regarding the moral issues in the ever-changing field where cybersecurity and healthcare collide. This method is selected due to its effectiveness and capacity to comprehensively comprehend without requiring substantial resources or drawn-out data-gathering processes. Figure 12.1 shows the sequential flow of the technique and emphasises the systematic literature review as the primary approach to achieving the study objectives.

12.4 The landscape of emerging healthcare systems

Technology breakthroughs, shifting demographics, and changing patient expectations are driving a radical change in the face of new healthcare systems. This ever-changing landscape includes a wide range of cutting-edge methods, tools, and techniques meant to improve healthcare service accessibility and delivery [34]. The terrain of developing healthcare systems is defined by several essential components, including:

(a) Digital transformation
Digital technology including wearables, telemedicine, electronic health records (EHRs), and Internet of Things (IoT) apps are seamlessly integrated into emerging healthcare systems. Real-time data interchange, remote monitoring, and individualised patient care are made possible by this connection [2].

(b) Patient-centric models
The environment highlights a move towards patient-centric models, in which the experience of the patient is prioritised. Personalised health applications, virtual clinics, and telehealth consultations enable people to take an active role in their healthcare journey [14].

(c) Data-driven healthcare
Healthcare decision-making has evolved as a result of the use of AI and big data analytics. Large-scale databases provide data-driven insights that support proactive disease prevention, individualised treatment regimens, and more precise diagnoses [18].

(d) Interconnected healthcare ecosystems
New healthcare systems place a strong emphasis on connectivity, encouraging networks of cooperation between payers, providers, researchers, and IT developers. This networked environment makes information interchange easy and encourages a patient-centred approach [16].

(e) Remote and decentralised care
The environment welcomes decentralised and remote care approaches, utilising telemedicine for online consultations and remote monitoring tools for the management of chronic illnesses. Access to healthcare services is improved by these developments, especially in rural or underserved areas [24].

(f) Blockchain for Security and Interoperability
The use of blockchain technology to improve the security and integrity of medical data is becoming more and more common. Its transparent and decentralised architecture promotes safe data exchange, interoperability, and defence against online attacks [26].

(g) Regulatory challenges and adaptations
Healthcare systems are facing regulatory problems as they adjust to new technology in this ever-changing landscape. Legislators are trying to create frameworks that strike a compromise between innovation and concerns about patient safety, privacy, and ethics [2].

(h) Personalised medicine
New healthcare systems place a high priority on personalised medicine, using biomarkers, genetic data, and predictive analytics to customise treatment plans based on the unique characteristics of each patient [30].

(i) Focus on preventive healthcare
Preventive healthcare is becoming more and more important, with technology-driven initiatives meant to advance well-being and health. Proactive health management is facilitated by wearable technology, health apps, and remote monitoring [14].

(j) Resilience to global health challenges
In light of global health concerns, the landscape recognises the significance of robust healthcare systems. Recent pandemic lessons have led to increased emphasis on readiness, quick action, and integrating digital technologies for crisis management [30].

Emerging healthcare systems are characterised by a dynamic interplay between patient-centred care, technological advancements, regulatory considerations, and a shared commitment to promoting an efficient, robust, and more accessible healthcare ecosystem. Integrating strong cybersecurity safeguards with ethical considerations is crucial as these systems develop to maintain the reliability and integrity of healthcare procedures in the digital era.

12.4.1 Benefits and risks of emerging healthcare systems

When navigating the terrain of developing healthcare systems, one finds a tapestry weaved with inherent dangers that require careful consideration [35], as described in Table 12.2. The benefits of the digital transformation of healthcare are highlighted in Table 12.3. The promises and potential traps [46], are clear; they include

Table 12.2 Benefits of emerging healthcare systems

Benefit	Description
Improved Access to Healthcare Services	New healthcare systems use technology to get over geographic limitations and give underprivileged and isolated communities more access to medical care, diagnosis, and consultations.
Enhanced Efficiency and Accuracy in Diagnosis	Medical practitioners can now diagnose patients more quickly and accurately, allowing them to tailor treatment regimens and make informed decisions. This is made possible by technological advancements like machine learning and artificial intelligence.
Personalised Medicine	New systems enable the provision of personalised healthcare by taking lifestyle factors, genetic information, and unique patient traits into account to customise treatment plans for improved results.
Remote Patient Monitoring	Giving healthcare practitioners access to real-time data, wearable technology and remote monitoring tools enables patients to take an active role in their care and promote the proactive management of chronic illnesses.
Efficient Health Information Management	Electronic health records, or EHRs, improve the overall efficiency of healthcare delivery by streamlining the management of health information, cutting down on paperwork, and minimising errors.

(Continues)

Table 12.2 Benefits of emerging healthcare systems (Continued)

Benefit	Description
Cost Savings	Because telemedicine and virtual healthcare models eliminate the need for physical infrastructure, travel costs, and needless hospital visits, they can save costs for both patients and healthcare providers.
Data-Driven Insights for Public Health	Big data analytics help with population health management by empowering medical professionals to recognise patterns, strategically distribute resources, and effectively address public health issues.
Accelerated Research and Development	Technology integration speeds up research procedures, including drug discovery and clinical trials, encouraging creativity and the creation of novel therapeutic approaches.
Enhanced Patient Engagement	Patients are involved in their healthcare journey through the use of digital tools and mobile applications, which also encourage adherence to treatment programmes, improve health literacy, and facilitate communication with healthcare practitioners.
Global Health Collaboration	New healthcare systems encourage cross-border cooperation by enabling medical practitioners to exchange knowledge, best practices, and skills around the world, advancing healthcare globally.

Table 12.3 Risk of emerging healthcare systems

Risk	Description
Data Security and Privacy Concerns	Concerns over the security and privacy of patient data are raised by an increased reliance on digital platforms, which leaves healthcare systems open to hacker attacks and illegal access.
Technological Reliability Issues	System malfunctions, downtime, or technical issues can interfere with the provision of healthcare services, thereby delaying patient care and jeopardising the dependability of medical technology.
Health Inequities and Accessibility Gaps	Even though technology makes things easier for many, it has the potential to exacerbate already-existing health disparities, especially for individuals who lack access to digital devices or dependable internet connectivity.
Ethical Concerns in Data Use	Huge volumes of health data are being collected and used, which raises ethical questions about permission, data ownership, and the possibility of discrimination based on medical information.
Overreliance on Technology	An over-reliance on technology could reduce the human element in healthcare, which could affect the standard of care coordination and patient-provider interactions.
Regulatory and Legal Challenges	Technology may progress more quickly than legal frameworks, making it difficult to create and implement regulations that protect patient rights and moral behaviour.
Digital Health Literacy Gaps	Some people lack the digital health literacy required to fully utilise and manage contemporary healthcare technologies, which may lead to inequities in health outcomes.

(Continues)

Table 12.3 Risk of emerging healthcare systems (Continued)

Risk	Description
Resistance to Change	The adoption of new technology by healthcare practitioners and organisations may encounter resistance, which could impede the smooth integration of emerging healthcare systems into current practices.
Interoperability Challenges	Inconsistencies among various healthcare systems and technologies could impede the smooth transfer of patient data, resulting in disjointed treatment and possible medical mishaps.
Lack of Standardisation	The integration of varied healthcare technology may be hampered by the lack of standardised procedures and interoperability standards, which could result in inefficiencies and communication hurdles within the healthcare ecosystem.

enhanced accessibility, personalised medication, streamlined operations, and international cooperation. On the other hand, the digital revolution poses hazards, such as worries about data security, moral conundrums, and the possibility of health disparities.

This section illuminates the complex relationship between technology progress and the ethical factors that will shape healthcare delivery in the future through a detailed examination of these advantages and concerns. The real promise of new healthcare systems emerges inside this narrow range, providing hitherto unheard-of prospects but also demanding a watchful eye to handle the difficulties that come with the digital transformation of healthcare.

12.5 Ethical foundations in healthcare cybersecurity

Ethical issues are the cornerstone that supports the integrity, efficacy, and trust of the healthcare and cybersecurity systems in this rapidly evolving environment [33]. The concepts of efficacy, integrity, and trust in the cybersecurity and healthcare systems are illustrated in Figure 12.2. Each of these ideas is vital to maintaining the stability and dependability of these interrelated domains.

(a) Integrity
The preservation and correctness of data, processes, and activities are referred to as integrity in the context of cybersecurity and healthcare systems. It guarantees that data inside the systems is kept unchanged, preserving its veracity and authenticity. The significance is in preventing unauthorised changes or tampering with patient data, treatment records, and general system operation.

(b) Efficacy
Efficacy is related to cybersecurity and healthcare systems' effectiveness and efficacy. It highlights the capacity of the system to provide precise and

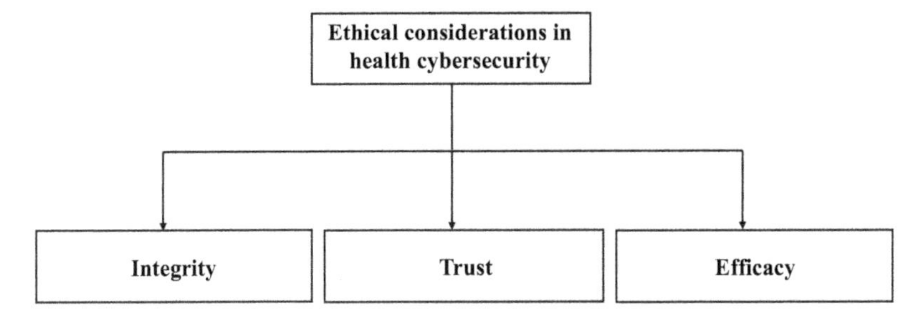

Figure 12.2 Ethical foundations in healthcare cybersecurity

prompt healthcare services while also putting strong cybersecurity safeguards in place. The illustration highlights how seamlessly technology is integrated to optimise healthcare procedures, guaranteeing that the systems function well without jeopardising patient care or data security.

(c) Trust
The trust and confidence that patients, healthcare providers, and system users have in healthcare and cybersecurity systems is known as trust. The foundation of this confidence is the guarantee of data privacy, system dependability, and moral behaviour.

Integrity, efficacy, and trust are all interconnected, and the illustration emphasises how important it is for these factors to work together to provide a safe and trustworthy healthcare environment.

This section explores the deep ethical underpinnings of healthcare cybersecurity, highlighting the critical role that ethical principles play in directing the creation, application, and continuous maintenance of strong cybersecurity procedures. These foundations are:

(a) Protection of patient privacy and confidentiality
The need to protect patient privacy and maintain the confidentiality of sensitive health information is at the heart of ethical healthcare cybersecurity. Ethical frameworks mandate strict precautions to avoid unauthorised access, data breaches, and potential misuse of the huge volumes of personal data handled by digital systems [47].

(b) Informed consent and patient autonomy
Respecting the privacy of patients and obtaining informed consent are essential components of ethical cybersecurity practices. As medical technology develops, it is critical to make sure patients understand the cybersecurity implications of their data and have a choice over how it is used [48].

(c) Balancing data sharing for research and privacy
Healthcare cybersecurity is an ethical tightrope walk that requires striking a careful balance between protecting patient privacy and promoting collaborative research through data exchange. To preserve ethical integrity, transparent frameworks that give priority to both imperatives must be established [49].

(d) Fairness and equity in access
Fairness and justice in access are important ethical considerations as healthcare institutions use technology to improve services. For cybersecurity in healthcare, addressing digital health inequities and reducing biases in technological applications become essential ethical objectives [50].

(e) Responsiveness to cyber incidents and transparency
Proactively reacting to cyber incidents is required by the ethical duty of patients and stakeholders. Ethics dictate that openness in communication, responsibility, and prompt reporting of violations are necessary to preserve public confidence in healthcare systems [51].

(f) Human oversight in AI-driven systems
The ethical underpinnings of AI in healthcare demand that the ethical implications of AI be carefully considered. Ensuring human supervision, responsibility, and openness in AI-driven choice- ensuring that procedures follow moral guidelines that put patients safety and well-being first [52].

(g) Educating healthcare professionals on cybersecurity ethics
Healthcare professional education is one area where ethical cybersecurity practices go beyond technology issues. Increasing knowledge of and proficiency with moral cybersecurity practices become crucial elements of career advancement [7].

(h) Integrating ethical considerations in system design
The design and implementation of healthcare cybersecurity systems should be deeply influenced by ethical considerations. Prioritising privacy, security, and ethical issues during the development stage guarantees that moral values are ingrained in the technological architecture [53].

The design and implementation of healthcare cybersecurity systems should be deeply influenced by ethical considerations. Prioritising privacy, security, and ethical issues during the development stage guarantees that moral values are ingrained in the technological architecture.

12.6 Legal and regulatory dimensions

A framework of laws and regulations aimed at safeguarding patient rights, maintaining data security, and regulating the moral application of technology has a significant influence on the dynamic landscape where cybersecurity and healthcare intersect [44,54,55]. This section explores the various legal and regulatory aspects that make-up healthcare cybersecurity. It looks at the frameworks that are currently in place, the difficulties associated with enforcing them, and the necessity of having comprehensive and flexible legislation in light of the rapidly changing healthcare landscape.

12.6.1 Existing laws and regulations in healthcare cybersecurity

A vast web of laws and regulations that are intended to protect patient information, guarantee data integrity, and preserve ethical standards tightly regulate the landscape of healthcare cybersecurity [44]. Table 12.4, which summarises this section, offers a detailed summary of the major legislation and regulations currently in effect that influence the legal environment surrounding healthcare cybersecurity.

This comprehensive overview highlights the varied legislative environment influencing healthcare cybersecurity across the globe. In an increasingly digitised healthcare ecosystem, the convergence of these laws and regulations creates a strong basis that supports the secure and moral management of healthcare information.

Table 12.4 Existing laws and regulations in healthcare cybersecurity

Regulation	**Description**
Health Insurance Portability and Accountability Act (HIPAA) [36]	A key component of healthcare data protection is HIPAA, which was implemented in the United States. It creates guidelines for the security and privacy of personally identifiable health information, requiring measures to protect electronic health records (EHRs) and guaranteeing patient data confidentiality.
General Data Protection Regulation (GDPR) [37]	GDPR imposes strict guidelines for data protection, including that of health-related data, and is being implemented throughout the European Union. It emphasises individual right to privacy by requiring clear consent, transparent processing, and strong security safeguards, with harsh consequences for noncompliance.
Health Information Technology for Economic and Clinical Health (HITECH) Act [38]	The HITECH Act is a piece of US legislation that encourages the use of health information technology and supplements HIPAA. By adding obligations to business associates, promoting the appropriate use of electronic health records, and enforcing penalties for data breaches, it enhances the rules of HIPAA.
Cybersecurity Information Sharing Act (CISA) [39]	Enacted in the United States, CISA makes it easier for the government and private sectors to share cybersecurity threat intelligence. It seeks to improve reaction capacities, cybersecurity awareness, and teamwork to lessen cyber threats in the healthcare industry.
NIST Cybersecurity Framework [40]	The National Institute of Standards and Technology (NIST) Cybersecurity Framework is a set of voluntary recommendations that are commonly used in the US healthcare industry, despite not being a legal requirement. It offers a methodical approach to cybersecurity risk management with a focus on risk assessment, mitigation, and ongoing development.
Data Protection Act 2018 (DPA 2018) [41]	DPA 2018 expands data protection legislation and integrates GDPR concepts in the United Kingdom. It governs how personal data, including health data, is processed in the healthcare industry and places a strong emphasis on the duties and rights of data controllers as well as data subjects.

(Continues)

Table 12.4 Existing laws and regulations in healthcare cybersecurity (Continued)

Regulation	Description
Personal Data Protection Act (PDPA) [42]	PDPA, which is in effect in Singapore, controls the gathering, utilising, and disclosing of personal data, including medical records. It promotes appropriate data management practices in the healthcare sector by emphasising consent, purpose limitation, and data accuracy.
Australian Privacy Principles (APPs) [43]	The Privacy Act 1988 in Australia governs the handling of personal information, including health information, through the APPs. They provide guidelines for the gathering, using, and disclosing of medical records, stressing the significance of data security and personal privacy.
Telemedicine Laws and Regulations [44]	Many nations have telemedicine-specific laws and rules, including those about licensure, reimbursement, and privacy standards. The objective of these rules is to maintain patient safety, data security, and ethical standards while balancing the advantages of telehealth.
Federal Risk and Authorization Management Program (FedRAMP) [45]	A government-wide initiative called FedRAMP is used in the United States to standardise the authorisation and security assessment process for cloud-based goods and services. FedRAMP standards must be followed by healthcare organisations using cloud technology to guarantee the security of patient information.

12.6.2 Challenges and solutions in enforcing cybersecurity regulations

The dynamic nature of cyber threats, resource limitations, and the rapidly changing technical landscape present numerous obstacles to the enforcement of cybersecurity legislation in the healthcare sector. This section examines important issues and suggests strategic solutions to strengthen cybersecurity laws in the healthcare industry. A succinct summary of the difficulties in implementing cybersecurity legislation in the healthcare industry is given in Table 12.5, along with relevant strategic recommendations.

Policymakers, cybersecurity specialists, healthcare organisations, and regulators must work together to develop a comprehensive strategy to tackle these issues and put strategic solutions into place. Through the reinforcement of enforcement mechanisms and the adaptation to the dynamic threat landscape, the healthcare industry may enhance its cybersecurity resilience and efficiently protect patient data.

Table 12.5 Challenges and solutions in enforcing cybersecurity regulations

Challenges	Solutions
Rapid Evolution of Cyber Threats [56]	Use proactive and adaptable tactics, such as training, cooperative research, and sharing of threat knowledge.
Resource Constraints and Budgetary Limitations [57]	Encourage public–private collaborations. Provide grants or tax advantages to encourage compliance and offer tools and cybersecurity resource packs as assistance.
Lack of Standardisation in Reporting and Assessment [40]	Create consistent reporting and evaluation frameworks. For uniformity, use international standards such as NIST or ISO.
Human Factor and Insider Threats [56]	Put user awareness and training initiatives into action. To identify and discourage insider threats, enforce stringent access controls, and perform regular audits.
Cross-Border Data Management and Jurisdictional Challenges [58]	Promote cross-border cooperation, global cybersecurity standardisation, and reciprocal regulatory framework recognition.
Lack of Cybersecurity Expertise [59]	Make investments in cybersecurity education and training initiatives, enable knowledge-sharing networks, and promote the recruitment of qualified personnel.
Inadequate Incident Response Planning [40]	Require comprehensive incident response strategies, organise frequent exercises and role-plays, and establish explicit communication guidelines.

12.6.3 The need for comprehensive and up-to-date regulations in emerging healthcare systems

In the ever-evolving setting of developing healthcare systems, where the demand for delivering intricate, patient-centred care meets with technological innovation, regulations play a crucial role.

This part looks at the need for comprehensive and up-to-date regulations to handle the complexities brought about by the rapid advancement of healthcare technologies. Figure 12.3 outlines the difficulties that arise when comprehensive and up-to-date regulations are required in developing healthcare systems. Table 12.6 provides a well-organised overview of the problems related to the need for comprehensive and up-to-date rules in emerging healthcare systems, along with suitable strategic solutions.

Regulatory frameworks must change as innovative solutions, like connected medical devices and AI, transform the healthcare industry to protect patient safety, maintain data integrity, and respect moral principles.

12.6.4 Accountability and liability in cyber incidents

Technological improvements and the necessity of establishing clear accountability and liability frameworks in the event of cyber incidents characterise the complex

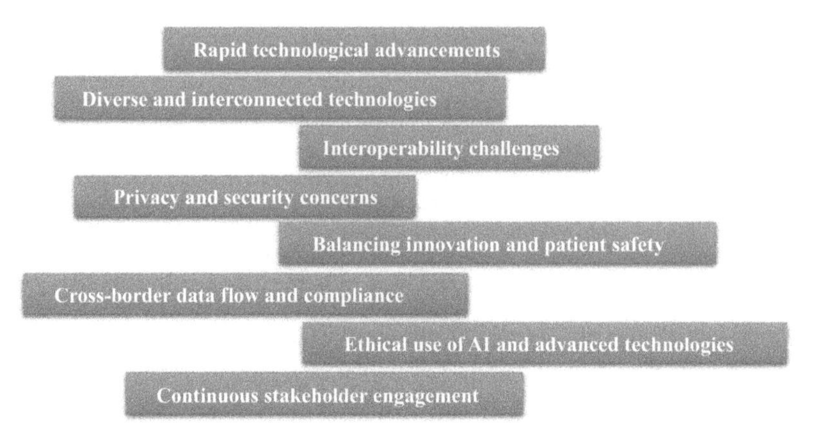

Figure 12.3 Challenges for comprehensive and timely regulations in developing healthcare systems

Table 12.6 Comprehensive and up-to-date regulations in emerging healthcare systems

Challenges	Solutions
Rapid Technological Advancements [60]	Establish regulatory agencies that can quickly adjust to advances in technology.
Diverse and Interconnected Technologies [60]	Provide adaptable regulatory frameworks that take into account a variety of new technologies and promote cooperation between industry stakeholders, regulatory agencies, and technology developers.
Privacy and Security Concerns [33]	Put the use of encryption, access controls, audits, and other measures front and centre in rules about data protection and cybersecurity. Update laws frequently to handle new privacy issues and cybersecurity dangers.
Interoperability Challenges [14]	Establish and implement interoperability standards to guarantee smooth system communication and promote the adoption of open standards to let different healthcare technologies work together more easily.
Balancing Innovation and Patient Safety [61]	Establish regulatory sandboxes to test and evaluate cutting-edge technology in safe settings. Adopt risk-based regulatory strategies, in which the degree of scrutiny is commensurate with the possible harm to patients.
Cross-Border Data Flow and Compliance [58]	Encourage international collaboration to standardise legal specifications for cross-border data management and create structures and agreements that allow data to flow seamlessly while guaranteeing privacy laws are followed.
Ethical Use of AI and Advanced Technologies [21]	Integrate ethical standards with regulatory frameworks that prioritise accountability, transparency, and equity. Promote the creation of moral AI standards and guidelines that are tailored to the needs of the healthcare industry.
Continuous Stakeholder Engagement [62]	Engage stakeholders in the regulatory process, such as patients, technology developers, and healthcare professionals. Make sure regulations are still relevant by conducting frequent evaluations and consultations to get opinions and thoughts.

junction of cybersecurity and healthcare [63]. The ethical obligation to patients is the foundation of cybersecurity accountability. Healthcare organisations should develop and uphold patient trust since they are the guardians of private health information. This trust is conditioned on a strong dedication to protecting privacy, safeguarding data, and acting morally when cyberattacks occur [23].

Legal frameworks, such as the General Data Protection Regulation (GDPR) [37] and the Health Insurance Portability and Accountability Act (HIPAA) [36], specify the duties and responsibilities of healthcare organisations for data protection and breach response. Establishing accountability requires an understanding of and adherence to these legal principles [44]. Accurately attributing a cyber incident to a particular actor or entity can be difficult in the complicated world of cybersecurity. Assigning responsibility and liability is affected by the challenges in locating the origin of cyber threats [63]. Patients demand a high degree of care when it comes to the safeguarding of their health information. This highlights the significance of coordinating accountability procedures with patient-centric principles and provides channels through which patients can seek compensation in the event of a data breach [14]. In the aftermath of a cyber event, leadership accountability becomes paramount for organisations to navigate. This entails duties including open communication, taking preventative action to lessen harm, and developing an organisation-wide culture of cybersecurity resilience [59].

In the wake of cyberattacks, insurance is essential since it provides financial security and facilitates the healing process. Organisational responsibility and the larger risk management plan are affected by the changing cybersecurity insurance market [64]. When cyber incidents entail illegal activity, law enforcement cooperation becomes essential. Ethical and legal problems arise when attempting to strike a fine balance between upholding patient confidentiality and assisting law enforcement [65]. International cooperation is necessary since cyber issues in the healthcare industry frequently cross national borders [66].

Through an examination of the complexities of responsibility and liability for cyber incidents in the healthcare industry, our goal is to shed light on the moral and legal issues that support patient-centred and ethical practices. It requires a thorough comprehension of these aspects to help healthcare organisations navigate the intricacies of the changing cybersecurity environment.

12.6.5 Patient rights and legal protections

When it comes to the area where cybersecurity and healthcare collide, protecting patient rights and creating strong legal frameworks become critical. Deeply ingrained in moral values, patient rights necessitate constant protection, particularly in light of emerging cyber threats [67]. This section delves into the intricate realm of patient rights and legal safeguards, encompassing the ethical duties, legal foundations, and protocols that safeguard the rights of people and fortify their legal path in the event of cyber incidents. The cornerstones of moral healthcare practices are informed consent and patient rights to privacy [68]. Maintaining patient data security becomes morally required in the digital age, as sensitive health information is susceptible to cyber assaults [69]. These values are codified by legal foundations like the General Data Protection Regulation (GDPR) [37] and the HIPAA [36], which set explicit standards for healthcare companies regarding the security of patient information. One of the rights enjoyed by patients in the event of a cybersecurity compromise is prompt and clear information [70]. People have a right to know when their health data is compromised so they can take the necessary precautions to keep themselves safe [71]. Legal safeguards specify how quickly healthcare organisations must tell impacted parties, highlighting the significance of openness in upholding confidence [72].

Access to individual health information is a fundamental right that enables people to take an active role in their care [73]. Legal frameworks require patients to have access to their medical records, encouraging openness and enabling people to make well-informed decisions about their health [74]. To maintain access security and protection, cybersecurity measures need to be in line with these rights [71]. Legal safeguards and patient rights interact in the framework of redress procedures. Following a cybersecurity event, people could look for redress for possible injuries or privacy violations. Legal frameworks define the channels by which patients can pursue compensation, highlighting the significance of responsibility and giving people a way to stand up for their rights [70].

The employment of developing technologies, such as AI in healthcare, raises ethical questions that are becoming more and more important as technology develops [21]. To prevent prejudice and preserve the ideals of equality and justice, patient rights require impartial and fair treatment, which calls for the establishment of moral standards and legal safeguards [51]. In the context of an international healthcare system, international collaboration becomes essential to protecting patient rights. Legal safeguards must be international, encouraging cooperation to standardise practices and guarantee uniform patient rights wherever patients may be found [58]. Global frameworks can manage the difficulties of cross-border healthcare data flow while preserving patient rights when they are compliant with ethical standards [74]. In the context of cybersecurity in healthcare, this section highlights how patient rights and legal safeguards are interwoven. It emphasises the moral requirements that shape these rights and the legal underpinnings that offer a structure for responsibility. To sustain patient-centred care in the digital era, healthcare establishments must consistently adapt their legal and ethical structures while respecting the rights of patients.

12.6.6 Telemedicine regulations

The ethical and legal foundation for remote healthcare delivery is significantly shaped by the regulatory environment around telemedicine [75]. The field of telemedicine, which includes remote monitoring, virtual consultations, and digital health technology, presents both revolutionary opportunities and difficulties [76]. Concerns about patient autonomy, privacy, and care quality give rise to ethical imperatives in telemedicine [44]. It becomes morally necessary to be able to give informed consent in a virtual environment, protect patient privacy, and uphold the same level of care as in-person consultations [77]. Maintaining the values that drive telemedicine techniques requires navigating these ethical challenges. Regulations about telemedicine are part of a complicated legal environment that differs between states. There may be unique regulations controlling telehealth practices in various nations, states, and regions [44]. Examining regional telemedicine legislation or legal underpinnings like the United States Health Insurance Portability and Accountability Act (HIPAA) can shed light on the regulatory landscape in which telehealth services must operate [38]. In telemedicine, the licencing issue becomes crucial, especially when patients and healthcare providers are spread across multiple jurisdictions [78]. This section examines how regulatory frameworks handle the intricacies of providing healthcare across borders, delving into the difficulties and developing solutions associated with telemedicine licensure. Policies regarding telemedicine reimbursement have a big influence on how widely used and long-lasting virtual care becomes. It is essential to comprehend the methods used by payers, such as commercial insurers and government health programmes, to remunerate for telehealth services [79].

Regulatory organisations must adjust to new horizons as telemedicine advances and incorporate cutting-edge technologies like AI and remote monitoring. An understanding of the changing telemedicine landscape can be gained by looking at how rules handle the ethical implications of wearable technology, AI-driven diagnostics, and other advances [51]. One essential component of regulatory frameworks is guaranteeing fair access to telemedicine services [21]. It is morally required to address access gaps based on variables like location, socioeconomic status, or technical literacy [58]. The worldwide uptake of telemedicine was expedited by the COVID-19 epidemic [77].

12.6.7 Emerging technologies and legal challenges

The symbiotic interplay between legal frameworks and technological technologies is changing the healthcare innovation landscape. Ethical issues are brought to the forefront when cutting-edge technologies like genomics, blockchain, and AI become essential. When implementing these technologies, privacy, bias, and patient autonomy are crucial ethical considerations that must be carefully considered [26].

Regulations are changing, especially when it comes to the application of AI in healthcare. To ensure the appropriate use of AI applications, regulations are changing to address issues like accountability, transparency, and bias reduction [21]. Genomic data, which is essential for customised treatment, presents new privacy and consent-related legal issues. To preserve informed consent and protect individual privacy, legal frameworks controlling the gathering and exchange of genetic data are investigated [80]. Blockchain technology brings legal ramifications for the healthcare industry despite its potential to improve data security and interoperability. As rules adjust to the decentralised nature of blockchain, factors including data ownership, smart contracts, and compliance must be taken into account [26]. Global events have sped up the adoption of telemedicine, posing legal issues with licensing, reimbursement, and privacy [81]. Legal frameworks are changing to make room for telehealth services and to address challenges like the delivery of healthcare across borders [58].

Strong cybersecurity protections are more important now that healthcare is digital. In the context of an interconnected health technology ecosystem, legal requirements for cybersecurity in healthcare, including data protection, incident response, and threat mitigation, are crucial [63]. Complex liability issues are raised by robotics in healthcare, from AI-assisted caring to surgical robots. Legal considerations examine questions of responsibility in the event of malfunctions, mistakes, or unfavourable results [23]. Although wearable technology gives people unparalleled access to health data, privacy, and data ownership laws provide obstacles [82]. Because developing technologies are global in scope, harmonised legal standards necessitate multinational collaboration. Coherent frameworks that guarantee ethical adoption, responsible adoption, and cross-border conformity with diverse legal requirements are being worked on [58]. This dynamic interplay between emerging technologies and legal considerations shapes the responsible and ethical integration of innovation in healthcare.

12.6.8 Cross-border implications and global cooperation in healthcare

The dynamics of healthcare systems beyond national boundaries offer opportunities as well as obstacles, highlighting the necessity of international cooperation [83]. Medical tourism brings to light the various regulatory environments that patients visiting other countries for treatment face, making cooperative efforts to standardise rules and guarantee uniform standards imperative [58]. Transnational patient data interchange is essential for providing informed medical treatment in the digital age. Establishing safe frameworks that regulate the moral exchange of patient data while resolving privacy issues requires international collaboration [84]. Pandemics and other global health emergencies highlight the need for coordinated planning and response. When it comes to exchanging information, organising reactions, and guaranteeing fair access to resources and treatments, international collaboration becomes essential [58]. Pharmaceutical businesses and healthcare providers face hurdles due to diverse regulatory frameworks [85]. The goal of international cooperation is to reduce regulatory heterogeneity, expedite approval procedures, and promote consistency in the effective and moral distribution of medical breakthroughs. The extensive use of telemedicine has cross-border ramifications, necessitating international collaboration to standardise laws, certification standards, and payment procedures for smooth telehealth delivery [86].

To improve healthcare results worldwide, health diplomacy is essential in promoting international cooperation through cooperative research projects, teamwork in tackling public health issues, and knowledge exchange. Trade agreements affect the availability and cost of medications on a worldwide scale. To achieve a balance between protecting intellectual property rights, guaranteeing equitable access to medications, and promoting innovation in pharmaceutical research, cooperation is crucial [87]. International cooperation is necessary to alleviate manpower shortages, maintain standardised training, and develop ethical recruitment processes to facilitate the mobility of healthcare workers across borders. Global collaboration is necessary for the surveillance of newly developing infectious illnesses to report, monitor, and contain possible outbreaks. Cooperation initiatives strengthen the capacity of nations to recognise and contain infectious diseases promptly [88].

Ethics, equitable access to healthcare resources, addressing health disparities, and cultural sensitivity are all fundamental components of global cooperation in healthcare. Due to the cross-border nature of healthcare, international collaboration is required to manage regulatory issues, promote information sharing, and cooperatively address common health risks. This cooperative strategy guarantees that everyone on the planet has access to high-quality healthcare.

12.6.9 Enforcement mechanisms and penalties

In the complex realm of healthcare regulation, enforcement mechanisms, and penalties serve as pivotal instruments to ensure compliance, protect patient rights, and maintain the integrity of healthcare systems. Regulatory agencies, whether at national or institutional levels, form the backbone of oversight, monitoring healthcare entities for adherence to established regulations [89].

Routine inspections and audits are fundamental components of enforcement, providing a proactive approach to assess compliance. Regulatory bodies conduct systematic examinations, scrutinising protocols, records, and practices to inform enforcement actions and contribute to ongoing quality improvement [90]. Legal sanctions and administrative penalties play a central role in enforcement, encompassing fines, license revocation, and punitive measures for regulatory violations. This range of penalties serves as a deterrent, fostering a culture of accountability within healthcare providers and institutions [91].

Enforcement mechanisms extend to civil and criminal actions, addressing violations through legal avenues that may involve fines, imprisonment, or both. Transparency is encouraged through public reporting of inspection results, performance metrics, and imposed penalties, enhancing public trust and promoting accountability. Corrective action plans and compliance assistance contribute to a collaborative approach in enforcement [89]. Regulatory bodies work with healthcare entities to address deficiencies, offering guidance and support for achieving and maintaining compliance. Licensing conditions and probationary measures provide additional tools for monitoring and ensuring adherence [92]. Whistleblower protections are integral to enforcement, fostering a culture of reporting and transparency. Legal safeguards for individuals reporting wrongdoing ensure that violations are exposed without fear of retaliation, reinforcing ethical standards [93].

In the globalised healthcare landscape, international cooperation is vital for effective enforcement. Collaborative efforts between regulatory bodies facilitate information exchange and enforcement actions across borders, harmonising strategies to address shared challenges [58]. Continuous improvement is essential in adaptive enforcement measures, refining strategies based on emerging risks, lessons learned, and technological advancements. This emphasis on adaptive enforcement aligns with the dynamic nature of the healthcare environment, ensuring the efficacy of regulatory efforts [94]. The effectiveness of healthcare regulations relies on robust enforcement mechanisms and penalties that encourage compliance, safeguard patients, and foster a culture of accountability. This multifaceted landscape of enforcement embraces a dual role in corrective action and deterrence, emphasising continuous improvement to meet the evolving demands of the healthcare sector.

12.7 Ethical challenges in cybersecurity incidents

Many ethical issues are raised by the convergence of cybersecurity and healthcare, especially in the wake of security breaches. Maintaining ethical standards and safeguarding patient information must be carefully balanced to successfully navigate these obstacles. The main ethical questions raised by cybersecurity incidents in the healthcare industry are examined in this section. An organised summary of the moral dilemmas raised by cybersecurity incidents in the healthcare industry may be found in Table 12.7.

Table 12.7 Challenges of ethics in cybersecurity incidents

Challenge	Description
Patient Trust Erosion [107]	Cybersecurity incidents have the potential to significantly erode patient confidence. Breach of private health information may have a long-term negative effect on the patient-provider relationship, which raises ethical issues about how these instances may influence public trust in healthcare institutions.
Ethical Obligations in Incident Response [63]	Healthcare institutions have ethical obligations when managing cybersecurity issues. Finding a balance between the need to secure patient data and the necessity of transparent and timely incident response is necessary to provide a principled approach to information security. This raises an ethical dilemma.
Transparency and Accountability [23]	Transparency and accountability are essential when disclosing cybersecurity vulnerabilities. Because of ethical considerations, all parties impacted must be informed as soon as practically possible and in a transparent manner, giving them complete details on the nature of the occurrence, any potential dangers, and the mitigation measures taken.
Navigating Privacy and Data Security [13]	To balance preserving robust data security with protecting patient privacy, complex ethical decisions must be addressed. It is imperative to prioritise ethical integrity to maintain confidence while implementing effective cybersecurity measures.

(Continues)

Table 12.7 Challenges of ethics in cybersecurity incidents (Continued)

Challenge	Description
Disparities in Impact [23]	Cybersecurity incidents may affect some groups disproportionately, which raises ethical concerns about equity. Vulnerable individuals may be more negatively impacted after incidents, so a proactive, ethical approach that reduces inequalities is required.
Ethical Challenges in Incident Investigation [63]	There are ethical challenges in examining and blaming cybersecurity events, particularly in identifying perpetrators and determining the root causes. Keeping the procedure for inquiry unbiased, avoiding unfounded accusations, and ensuring attribution accuracy are a few ethical considerations.
Balancing Security and User Convenience [33]	It takes balance to maintain user ease while implementing stringent cybersecurity measures. There are ethical challenges in striking the right balance between robust security and user-friendly interfaces; care must be taken to ensure that ethical considerations address both data protection and user satisfaction.
Informed Consent and Future Data Use [21]	Events related to cybersecurity may impact informed consent for future data use. Healthcare organisations have to handle post-event situations while respecting patient permission and handling privacy and data access issues.
Ethical Implications of Cybersecurity Insurance [30]	The introduction of cybersecurity insurance raises moral questions about organisational readiness. It becomes difficult to uphold ethical obligations to secure patient data while relying on insurance while also investing in strong cybersecurity solutions.
Ensuring Ethical Oversight in Cybersecurity Strategy [49]	Maintaining ethical oversight when developing cybersecurity plans is essential. In the dynamic landscape of healthcare cybersecurity, moral principles guide decision-makers to prioritise patient welfare, uphold openness, and foster a culture of responsibility.

The ethical issues raised by cybersecurity incidents in the healthcare sector emphasise how important it is to make ethical decisions to protect patient privacy, value transparency, and effectively manage the complexity of data security. Integrating ethical considerations into all facets of cybersecurity activities, including ongoing cybersecurity procedures and recovery efforts, guarantees the highest standards of patient care and ethical integrity.

12.8 Ethical implications of artificial intelligence (AI) in healthcare

The application of AI in healthcare brings up several ethical concerns that require careful consideration [19]. First, there are concerns about potential bias and discrimination in AI systems. Because these algorithms rely on historical data, there is a risk that they will perpetuate the demographically based healthcare disparities that exist today [22]. Ethical considerations require a dedication to justice and equity in the creation and application of AI to avoid exacerbating already-existing healthcare imbalances [26]. The main ethical concerns brought up by the application of AI to medical diagnostic and treatment decisions are accountability and responsibility [22]. Finding a balance between preserving human control and the benefits of AI-driven decision-making becomes essential. Understanding the roles and responsibilities of medical staff and AI systems is necessary to uphold ethical standards in patient care [31]. Ensuring human control and accountability in AI-enabled healthcare systems is at the core of ethical discussions [26]. When AI is given too much decision-making power without sufficient human input, ethical violations and unintended consequences in medical care become concerns [48]. Ethical considerations highlight the need for a harmonious integration of AI capabilities and human skills [52]. Patient data security and privacy become moral considerations when it comes to AI applications. Patient data security becomes crucial since AI systems rely so heavily on big datasets [44]. Ethical considerations include ensuring patient data integrity and confidentiality and implementing robust security measures to prevent unauthorised access and data breaches.

The idea of informed consent becomes more complex when it comes to AI-driven operations. It becomes an ethical challenge to convince patients to understand complex AI procedures and provide their informed permission [95]. Honest and open discussion is necessary to ensure that patients understand and consent to the use of AI in their diagnosis or treatment. Transparency is necessary to guarantee ethical integrity in AI algorithms. AI decision-making and recommendation systems must be understood by patients and physicians [80]. Ethical concerns state that transparency is essential for building trust, promoting prudent decision-making, and ensuring accountability in AI applications [81].

The application of AI in healthcare and its potential effects on employment and healthcare personnel raise ethical questions [19]. Ethics frameworks are essential for the adoption of AI technologies because of concerns about responsible AI deployment that complements human expertise rather than replaces it, workforce transformations, and professional upskilling. It is ethically right to distribute AI resources and advantages fairly [26]. Ensuring equitable access to the benefits of AI is critical to prevent concentration in specific healthcare settings or geographic locations. Ethical frameworks should prioritise diversity and accessibility while upholding the principles of justice in the healthcare industry [52]. Dealing with biases in AI training data is an important ethical concern. Biases in the dataset may lead to erroneous conclusions and even encourage unethical medical practices [48]. Ethical imperatives require actively striving to identify and remove biases in training data to guarantee that AI applications uphold the values of justice and equality [26]. The long-term societal repercussions of the broad usage of AI in healthcare necessitate ethical thought. Anticipating and mitigating potential repercussions, such as changes in healthcare dynamics and resource allocation, is crucial for ensuring the effective and ethical integration of AI into the larger healthcare ecosystem. Healthcare AI ethics demand a comprehensive approach that considers accountability, fairness, transparency, and the welfare of society.

12.9 Strategies for ethical cybersecurity in healthcare

Careful planning and implementation are necessary to address the difficult issue of ethical security in healthcare systems. Here, we outline the main tactics in Table 12.8 to support ethical cybersecurity practices in the healthcare industry.

A complex approach involving technology, education, proactive planning, adherence to ethical norms, and transparency is required for healthcare ethical cybersecurity. When used in combination, these strategies support patient privacy, confidence, and the ethical integrity of healthcare cybersecurity protocols.

Table 12.8 Techniques for addressing ethical issues in cybersecurity incidents

Strategy	Description
Investing in Robust Cybersecurity Infrastructure [96]	Implementing advanced cybersecurity infrastructure, including firewalls, intrusion detection systems, and encryption technologies, is a crucial tactic. Therefore, processing and storing patient data occurs in an encrypted setting.
Educating Healthcare Professionals about Cybersecurity Best Practices [11]	Providing periodic training sessions to healthcare personnel to teach them cybersecurity best practices. Emphasis is placed on the need to safeguard patient data and foster a cyberaware culture among medical staff.
Prioritising Ethical Considerations in System Design and Implementation [97]	Integrating ethical principles like patient consent, data security, and privacy into healthcare system design and implementation. This ensures that ethical considerations are considered from the outset while creating technological solutions.
Implementing Multi-Factor Authentication and Access Controls [98]	Strengthening access controls and using multi-factor authentication to provide an additional layer of security. By restricting unauthorised access to patient data, this strategy adheres to the ethical principles of confidentiality and data protection.
Conducting Regular Security Audits and Assessments [99]	Constantly performing regular security audits and evaluations to identify gaps and weak areas in the cybersecurity architecture. The outcomes of these assessments will determine how ethical cybersecurity practices are developed and monitored over time.
Establishing Incident Response Plans with Ethical Protocols [100]	Establishing comprehensive incident response plans that adhere to moral standards. Ensuring a swift and ethical reaction in the case of a security breach mitigates potential patient harm and maintains transparency throughout the process of resolving the issue.
Encouraging a Culture of Reporting Security Concerns [101]	Establishing a work environment where healthcare workers can freely express concerns about security without fear of reprisal. It is simpler to recognise potential cybersecurity issues early on and take swift action when transparency is encouraged.
Collaborating with Ethical Hackers for Penetration Testing [102]	Engaging ethical hackers to conduct penetration tests to identify vulnerabilities before malicious actors exploit them. This proactive strategy aligns with ethical cybersecurity norms by identifying and addressing vulnerabilities before they are exploited.

(Continues)

Table 12.8 Techniques for addressing ethical issues in cybersecurity incidents (Continued)

Strategy	Description
Ensuring Transparent Communication in the Event of Breaches [103]	Establishing clear channels of communication in the event of a cybersecurity crisis. Ethical cybersecurity standards include promptly informing affected parties on the nature of the issue, associated risks, and any mitigation actions implemented.
Regularly Updating Policies in Alignment with Ethical Standards [104]	Regulations related to cybersecurity should be routinely examined and revised to take into account evolving technological advancements and moral standards. Ensuring rules consider the latest ethical issues is essential to maintaining a robust cybersecurity framework.

12.10 Lessons learned

In this section, we examine the significant ideas that we learned while studying "The Ethics of Cybersecurity in Emerging Healthcare Systems." With a focus on stakeholder interaction, patient-centric ethics, and dynamic adaptation, the plot illustrates ethics vital role in controlling cybersecurity in healthcare. Open communication becomes morally required during cybersecurity events, and continuous education fosters the development of a resilient and morally strong culture. The lessons stress that to maintain moral integrity, preventative measures, regulatory flexibility, and ethical supervision of technology are essential. This concise overview establishes the foundation for distilling the collective understanding gained from the chapters and indicating the path towards an ethically-driven future in healthcare cybersecurity. The primary lessons to be learned from this chapter are:

(a) The chapter focuses on how ethics should be the basis for developing, implementing, and overseeing modern healthcare systems. It serves as a constant reminder that moral considerations should be given careful consideration and included in healthcare cybersecurity.
(b) Innovation in healthcare systems necessitates a delicate ethics and advancement balancing act, especially when incorporating new technologies. It is imperative to anticipate and address potential moral dilemmas that may arise from technology advancements.
(c) The call to action emphasises how important it is for different stakeholders—lawmakers, technologists, regulators, and healthcare professionals—to work together. The takeaway is that a cooperative commitment to moral cybersecurity practices requires collaboration and a multidisciplinary approach.
(d) It is driven by the outlook for the future to take the lead in transforming the ethical context. Stakeholders must address the ethical dilemmas of the present while also anticipating and planning for future challenges. The lesson is that anticipating future demands, remaining adaptable, and upholding continuous ethical oversight are all necessary components of being an ethical steward.

(e) The significance of patient-centric ethics is repeatedly emphasised throughout the chapter. Lessons learned include how important it is to uphold privacy, safeguard patient confidence, and prioritise the well-being of individuals within the digital healthcare ecosystem.
(f) Transparency in communication is morally necessary while handling cybersecurity incidents. The most crucial lessons emphasise the necessity of timely and open communication with affected parties, upholding accountability and transparency as the cornerstones of moral cybersecurity operations.
(g) Healthcare professionals should be proficient in cybersecurity best practices and have a basic education. The chapter highlights the lesson that continual instruction and training are necessary to foster a culture of cybersecurity awareness and moral behaviour.
(h) As AI and other technologies are increasingly incorporated into healthcare, ethical governance becomes increasingly important. The moral imperative should guide technology development and deployment to ensure transparency, accountability, and equity.
(i) The consideration of legal and regulatory frameworks emphasises the need for adaptability. The lesson is that laws must advance in step with technological advancements to effectively address and uphold ethical standards in evolving healthcare systems.
(j) Proactive policy modifications and penetration testing are emphasised in the chapter as instances of ethically pre-emptive measures. The lesson is that anticipating and addressing any ethical concerns before they arise is necessary to maintain the ethical integrity of healthcare cybersecurity.

The main takeaway from the lessons learned is that ethical issues are dynamic elements in the ever-changing landscape of healthcare systems that require ongoing attention, collaboration, and foresight.

12.11 Recommendations

Healthcare cybersecurity is a dynamic industry, therefore we must be proactive in addressing emerging ethical concerns as they come up. This section offers a number of suggestions for fortifying the moral underpinnings of evolving healthcare systems. The recommendations are meant to guide stakeholders towards a future where ethical concerns are seamlessly merged with technological advancements. They range from promoting transparent procedures and patient empowerment to collaborative frameworks. These recommendations are:

(a) Provide comprehensive training sessions to healthcare professionals in order to enhance their understanding of cybersecurity ethics. To foster a culture that is cognisant of cybersecurity, courses on data privacy, transparency, and incident response are offered.
(b) Establish cooperative frameworks that facilitate communication and collaboration amongst lawmakers, regulators, technologists, and healthcare professionals.

Promote interdisciplinary dialogue to ensure a thorough approach to cybersecurity governance and to collaboratively address ethical issues.

(c) Consider the ethical ramifications when creating and using new medical technology. Prioritise assessments that consider privacy issues, biases, and the overall ethical implications of emerging technologies.

(d) Establish and implement open channels of communication for cybersecurity emergencies. Make sure you promptly and openly communicate with individuals who are affected, emphasising the value of responsibility and openness as well as the actions done to mitigate the effects.

(e) Promote continuous modifications to the regulatory framework in order to keep up with new technologies. Collaborate with lawmakers to ensure that cybersecurity regulations in the healthcare industry adapt to emerging challenges and uphold moral standards.

(f) Establish guidelines and standards for the ethical management of AI in the medical domain. In particular, emphasises that algorithms used by AI must be open, fair, and responsible, with a focus on minimising prejudices and ensuring human oversight.

(g) Develop patient empowerment and education campaigns about the ethical ramifications of cybersecurity in healthcare. Provide resources to help individuals understand how important it is for them to safeguard the privacy and security of their health information.

(h) Provide funds for research projects that try to understand and address the ethical problems that modern medicine brings up. Promote studies that look at the sociological, cultural, and ethical effects of cybersecurity in the healthcare sector.

(i) Establish ethical review committees in medical facilities to evaluate the moral implications of new practices, policies, and technologies. To represent a wide range of ethical opinions, make sure there is a diverse presence on these boards.

(j) Encourage collaboration between vendors of technology, cybersecurity experts, and healthcare institutions. Promote the sharing of innovative concepts, insights gained, and optimal methodologies to enhance the ethical and technological standing of the healthcare industry in general.

Collectively, these recommendations aim to strengthen the ethical basis of evolving healthcare systems by emphasising collaboration, transparency, education, and adaptability of regulations. By implementing these actions, we can contribute to building a solid and ethically upright basis for cybersecurity in healthcare moving ahead.

12.12 Conclusion

"A patchwork of ethical issues and tactical needs emerges as we draw the curtains on this exploration of The Ethics of Cybersecurity in Emerging Healthcare Systems." This chapter embarked on a voyage by examining the intricate relationships between cybersecurity and healthcare ethics, dispelling any doubts, and suggesting a path forward for all stakeholders. Looking back reveals the intricate dance of moral dilemmas within the framework of evolving healthcare systems. The chapter covered the ethical ramifications of AI to the critical significance of patient privacy and data protection, weaving a thread across the moral fabric that underpins the intersection of cybersecurity and healthcare. The need to safeguard, the careful balancing act of transparency, and the call for fairness and equity resonated as core ethical principles in this developing story. A loud shout echoes through these discursive hallways after these inquiries. A request that all interested parties—lawmakers, techies, regulators, and medical professionals unite and resolve to prioritise ethical cybersecurity activities. This is not merely a suggestion; it is an ethical requirement. We are at the forefront of the digital transformation of healthcare, thus the need for action is critical. Establish morality as the cornerstone of emerging healthcare systems.

Finally, this chapter concludes with some thoughts on the future, where ethical issues will form the basis of the rapidly evolving field of healthcare cybersecurity. The future is dynamic, full with both technological advancements and moral conundrums. This chapter looks ahead, suggesting that instead of only reacting to moral quandaries, stakeholders can actively define the ethical path of healthcare cybersecurity. The ethical responsibility supporting the integration of cybersecurity and healthcare in emerging systems is demonstrated in this chapter. The journey cleared the way for a day when ethics will be the standard rather than merely a consideration while carefully navigating ethically challenging circumstances. The resounding moral symphony as the curtain goes up is a striking reminder that ethical principles must guide every decision made in the evolving healthcare systems.

References

[1] F. Frati, G. Darau, N. Salamanos, *et al.*, “Cybersecurity training and healthcare: the AERAS approach,” *International Journal of Information Security*, vol. 23, pp. 1527–1539, 2024.

[2] M. Henry and M. Maji, “Securing the Internet of Things (IoT): addressing cybersecurity challenges and implementing protective measures,” *EasyChair*, no. 11840, 2024.

[3] J. B. Wright and D. N. Burrell, “Cybersecurity leadership ethics in healthcare,” in *Handbook of Research on Cybersecurity Risk in Contemporary Business Systems*, pp. 137–148, IGI Global, 2023.

[4] A. Anyanwu, T. Olorunsogo, T. O. Abrahams, O. J. Akindote, and O. Reis, *et al.*, “Data confidentiality and integrity: a review of accounting and cybersecurity controls in superannuation organizations,” *Computer Science & IT Research Journal*, vol. 5, no. 1, pp. 237–253, 2024.

[5] L. Kasowaki and M. Kaan, “The evolving threatscape: understanding and navigating cybersecurity risks,” *EasyChair*, no. 11703, 2024.

[6] Z. Balani and N. I. Mustafa, “Enhancing cybersecurity against emerging threats in the future of cyber warfare,” *International Journal of Intelligent Systems and Applications in Engineering*, vol. 12, no. 2s, pp. 204–209, 2024.

[7] N. Jerry-Egemba, “Safe and sound: strengthening cybersecurity in healthcare through robust staff educational programs,” *Healthcare Management Forum*, vol. 37, no. 1, pp. 21–25, 2024.

[8] Y. Zhan, S. F. Ahmad, M. Irshad, *et al.*, "Investigating the role of cybersecurity's perceived threats in the adoption of health information systems," *Heliyon*, vol. 10, no. 1, 2024.
[9] A. S. George and A. H. George, "The emergence of cybersecurity medicine: protecting implanted devices from cyber threats," *Partners Universal Innovative Research Publication*, vol. 1, no. 2, pp. 93–111, 2023.
[10] S. D. Kale *et al.*, "PACS–building blocks of cyber security in medical data," *International Journal of Intelligent Systems and Applications in Engineering*, vol. 12, no. 9s, pp. 79–86, 2024.
[11] M. Waddell, "Human factors in cybersecurity: designing an effective cybersecurity education program for healthcare staff," *Healthcare Management Forum*, vol. 37, no. 1, pp. 13–16, 2024.
[12] R. Montasari, *Cyberspace, Cyberterrorism and the International Security in the Fourth Industrial Revolution: Threats, Assessment and Responses*, Springer Nature, 2024.
[13] A. I. Newaz, A. K. Sikder, M. A. Rahman, and A. S. Uluagac, "A survey on security and privacy issues in modern healthcare systems: attacks and defenses," *ACM Trans. Comput. Healthc.*, vol. 2, no. 3, pp. 1–44, 2021.
[14] A. N. Gohar, S. A. Abdelmawgoud, and M. S. Farhan, "A patient-centric healthcare framework reference architecture for better semantic interoperability based on blockchain, cloud, and IoT," *IEEE Access*, vol. 10, pp. 92137–92157, 2022.
[15] W. Roberts, S. A. McKee, R. Miranda Jr, and N. P. Barnett, "Navigating ethical challenges in psychological research involving digital remote technologies and people who use alcohol or drugs," *American Psychologist*, vol. 79, no. 1, pp. 24, 2024.
[16] M. N. AL-Nuaimi, "Human and contextual factors influencing cybersecurity in organizations, and implications for higher education institutions: a systematic review," *Global Knowledge, Memory and Communication*, vol. 73, no. 1/2, pp. 1–23, 2024.
[17] A. Alqudhaibi, A. Krishna, S. Jagtap, N. Williams, M. Afy-Shararah, and K. Salonitis, "Cybersecurity 4.0: safeguarding trust and production in the digital food industry era," *Discover Food*, vol. 4, no. 1, pp. 1–18, 2024.
[18] M. Alhasan and M. Hasaneen, "Digital imaging, technologies and artificial intelligence applications during COVID-19 pandemic," *Computerized Medical Imaging and Graphics*, vol. 91, p. 101933, 2021.
[19] S. Agarwal and A. Lyles, "Regulatory compliance of telemedicine platforms for remote diagnosis," *International Journal of Healthcare Information Systems and Informatics*, vol. 15, no. 2, pp. 1–15, 2020.
[20] A. B. Garcia, R. F. Babiceanu, and R. Seker, "Artificial intelligence and machine learning approaches for aviation cybersecurity: An overview," in *2021 Integrated Communications Navigation and Surveillance Conference (ICNS)*, pp. 1–8, April 2021.
[21] R. Montasari, "Exploring the imminence of cyberterrorism threat to national security," in *Cyberspace, Cyberterrorism and the International*

Security in the Fourth Industrial Revolution: Threats, Assessment and Responses, pp. 91–106, Springer International Publishing, 2024.

[22] Y. Wang and Z. Ma, "Ethical and legal challenges of medical AI on informed consent: China as an example," *Developing World Bioethics*, 2024.

[23] M. Jabar, E. Chiong-Javier, and P. Pradubmook Sherer, "Qualitative ethical technology assessment of artificial intelligence (AI) and the internet of things (IoT) among Filipino Gen Z members: Implications for ethics education in higher learning institutions," *Asia Pacific Journal of Education*, pp. 1–15, 2024.

[24] T. O. Abrahams, O. A. Farayola, S. Kaggwa, P. U. Uwaoma, A. O. Hassan, and S. O. Dawodu, "Cybersecurity awareness and education programs: a review of employee engagement and accountability," *Computer Science & IT Research Journal*, vol. 5, no. 1, pp. 100–119, 2024.

[25] N. Z. Bawany, T. Qamar, H. Tariq, and S. Adnan, "Integrating healthcare services using blockchain-based telehealth framework," *IEEE Access*, vol. 10, pp. 36505–36517, 2022.

[26] A. Oruc, N. Chowdhury, and V. Gkioulos, "A modular cyber security training programme for the maritime domain," *International Journal of Information Security*, vol. 23, no. 2, pp. 1–36, 2024.

[27] A. K. Tyagi, "Blockchain and artificial intelligence for cyber security in the era of internet of things and industrial internet of things applications," in *AI and Blockchain Applications in Industrial Robotics*, pp. 171–199, IGI Global, 2024.

[28] National Institute of Standards and Technology (NIST, 2023). Available at https://csrc.nist.gov/news/2023

[29] V. Sanchini and L. Marelli, "Data protection and ethical issues in European P5 eHealth," in *P5 eHealth: An agenda for the Health Technologies of the Future*, p. 173, 2020.

[30] C. Lieneck, M. McLauchlan, and S. Phillips, "Healthcare cybersecurity ethical concerns during the COVID-19 global pandemic: a rapid review," *Healthcare*, vol. 11, no. 22, p. 2983, MDPI, 2023.

[31] N. Liv and D. Greenbaum, "Cyberneurosecurity," in *Policy, Identity, and Neurotechnology: The Neuroethics of Brain-Computer Interfaces*, pp. 233–251, Springer International Publishing, 2023.

[32] N. Allahrakha, "Balancing cyber-security and privacy: Legal and ethical considerations in the digital age," *Legal Issues in the Digital Age*, vol. 4, no. 2, pp. 78–121, 2023.

[33] R. M. Caron, K. Noel, R. N. Reed, J. Sibel, and H. J. Smith, "Health promotion, health protection, and disease prevention: challenges and opportunities in a dynamic landscape," *AJPM focus*, vol. 3, no. 1, 2024.

[34] S. Ksibi, F. Jaidi, and A. Bouhoula, "A comprehensive study of security and cyber-security risk management within e-Health systems: synthesis, analysis and a novel quantified approach," *Mobile Networks and Applications*, vol. 28, no. 1, pp. 107–127, 2023.

[35] U.S. Department of Health & Human Services, "Summary of the HIPAA Security Rule," [Online]. Available: https://www.hhs.gov/hipaa/for-professionals/security/laws-regulations/index.html.

[36] European Commission, "General Data Protection Regulation (GDPR)," [Online]. Available: https://ec.europa.eu/commission/priorities/justice-and-fundamental-rights/data-protection/2019-reform-eu-data-protection-rules_en.
[37] S. Lincke, "Complying with HIPAA and HITECH," in *Information Security Planning: A Practical Approach*, pp. 345–365, Springer International Publishing, 2024.
[38] Cybersecurity Information Sharing Act (CISA). (2015). Procedures and Guidance. [Online]. Available: https://www.cisa.gov/resources-tools/resources/cybersecurity-information-sharing-act-2015-procedures-and-guidance
[39] NIST Cybersecurity Framework. (20). [Online]. Available: https://csrc.nist.gov/pubs/cswp/29/the-nist-cybersecurity-framework-20/ipd
[40] Data Protection Act 2018 (DPA 2018). [Online]. Available: https://www.legislation.gov.uk/ukpga/2018/12/contents/enacted
[41] Personal Data Protection Act (PDPA). [Online]. Available: https://www.pdpc.gov.sg/Overview-of-PDPA/TheLegislation/Personal-Data-Protection-Act
[42] Australian Privacy Principles (APPs). [Online]. Available: https://securiti.ai/solutions/australia-privacy-act/
[43] A. Aliyu, E. Ogbuju, T. Kolajo, I. Olalekan, and F. Oladipo, "Government regulatory policies on telehealth data protection using artificial intelligence and blockchain technology," in *Artificial Intelligence and Blockchain Technology in Modern Telehealth Systems*, 1st ed., The Institution of Engineering and Technology, London, United Kingdom, 2023, pp. 409–433.
[44] K. Kalra and B. Tanwar, "Cyber security policy in India: examining the issues, challenges, and framework," in *Cybersecurity Issues, Challenges, and Solutions in the Business World*, pp. 120–137, IGI Global, 2023.
[45] L. Judijanto, S. Anggo, T. P. Utami, D. Anurogo, and D. Ningrum, "The impact of the digital revolution on health research: a bibliometric review," *Journal of World Future Medicine, Health and Nursing*, vol. 2, no. 1, pp. 64–77, 2024.
[46] B. S. P. Thummisetti and H. Atluri, "Advancing healthcare informatics for empowering privacy and security through federated learning paradigms," *International Journal of Sustainable Development in Computing Science*, vol. 1, no. 1, pp. 1–16, 2024.
[47] J. Zhang and Z. M. Zhang, "Ethics and governance of trustworthy medical artificial intelligence," *BMC Medical Informatics and Decision Making*, vol. 23, no. 1, p. 7, 2023.
[48] L. Balcombe and D. De Leo, "Digital mental health challenges and the horizon ahead for solutions," *JMIR Mental Health*, vol. 8, no. 3, p. e26811, 2021.
[49] A. Palmer and D. Schwan, "More process, less principles: The ethics of deploying AI and robotics in medicine," *Cambridge Quarterly of Healthcare Ethics*, vol. 33, no. 1, pp. 121–134, 2024.
[50] A. Habbal, M. K. Ali, and M. A. Abuzaraida, "Artificial Intelligence Trust, Risk and Security Management (AI TRiSM): frameworks, applications, challenges and future research directions," *Expert Systems with Applications*, vol. 240, p. 122442, 2024.

[51] K. C. Rath, A. Khang, and D. Roy, "The role of internet of things (IoT) technology in Industry 4.0 economy," in *Advanced IoT Technologies and Applications in the Industry 4.0 Digital Economy*, CRC Press, pp. 1–28, 2024.

[52] B. Singh and C. Kaunert, "Integration of cutting-edge technologies such as internet of things (IoT) and 5G in health monitoring systems: a comprehensive legal analysis and futuristic outcomes," *GLS Law Journal*, vol. 6, no. 1, pp. 13–20, 2024.

[53] S. M. Williamson and V. Prybutok, "Balancing privacy and progress: a review of privacy challenges, systemic oversight, and patient perceptions in AI-driven healthcare," *Applied Sciences*, vol. 14, no. 2, p. 675, 2024.

[54] D. M. Mathkor, N. Mathkor, Z. Bassfar, *et al.*, "Multirole of the internet of medical things (IoMT) in biomedical systems for managing smart healthcare systems: an overview of current and future innovative trends," *Journal of Infection and Public Health*, vol. 17, no. 4, pp. 559–572, 2024.

[55] V. Patel, S. Saikali, M. C. Moschovas, *et al.*, "Technical and ethical considerations in telesurgery," *Journal of Robotic Surgery*, vol. 18, no. 1, p. 40, 2024.

[56] N. AllahRakha, "Rethinking digital borders to address jurisdiction and governance in the global digital economy," *International Journal of Law and Policy*, vol. 2, no. 1, 2024.

[57] O. Alshaikh, S. Parkinson, and S. Khan, "Exploring perceptions of decision-makers and specialists in defensive machine learning cybersecurity applications: The need for a standardized approach," *Computers & Security*, vol. 139, p. 103694, 2024.

[58] S. F. Ahmed, M. S. B. Alam, S. Afrin, S. J. Rafa, N. Rafa, and A. H. Gandomi, "Insights into Internet of Medical Things (IoMT): data fusion, security issues and potential solutions," *Information Fusion*, vol. 102, p. 102060, 2024.

[59] D. Greenbaum, "Striking the balance: harnessing machine learning's potential in psychiatric care amid legal and ethical challenges," *AJOB neuroscience*, vol. 15, no. 1, pp. 48–50, 2024.

[60] N. Haines, "Sustainable translation of digital health technologies," *Wellcome Open Res*, vol. 9, p. 19, 2024.

[61] R. Williams, V. Kemp, K. Porter, T. Healing, and J. Drury, *Major Incidents, Pandemics and Mental Health: The Psychosocial Aspects of Health Emergencies, Incidents, Disasters and Disease Outbreaks*. Cambridge University Press, 2024.

[62] S. Iftikhar, "Cyberterrorism as a global threat: a review on repercussions and countermeasures," *PeerJ Computer Science*, vol. 10, p. e1772, 2024.

[63] S. Bıçakcı and A. G. Evren, "Responding cyber-attacks and managing cyber security crises in critical infrastructures: a sociotechnical perspective," in *Management and Engineering of Critical Infrastructures*, pp. 125–151, Academic Press, 2024.

[64] C. A. Ezeigweneme, A. A. Umoh, V. I. Ilojianya, and A. O. Adegbite, "Review of telecommunication regulation and policy: comparative analysis USA and Africa," *Computer Science & IT Research Journal*, vol. 5, no. 1, pp. 81–99, 2024.

[65] Y. O. Okoro, O. Ayo-Farai, C. P. Maduka, C. C. Okongwu, and O. T. Sodamade, "A review of health misinformation on digital platforms:

challenges and countermeasures," *International Journal of Applied Research in Social Sciences*, vol. 6, no. 1, pp. 23–36, 2024.
[66] C. Golembeski, G. Eber, C. Sufrin, J. Lantsman, and H. Venters, "Discretionary ethics and governing public affairs in jails and prisons: upholding constitutional rights to health and safety," in *Empowering Public Administrators*, pp. 253–288, Routledge, 2024.
[67] J. B. Awotunde, A. L. Imoize, R. G. Jimoh, *et al.*, "AIoMT enabling real-time monitoring of healthcare systems: security and privacy considerations," in *Handbook of Security and Privacy of AI-Enabled Healthcare Systems and Internet of Medical Things*, pp. 97–133, 2024.
[68] A. G. Nienaber McKay, D. Brand, M. Botes, N. Cengiz, and M. Swart, "The regulation of health data sharing in Africa: a comparative study," *Journal of Law and the Biosciences*, vol. 11, no. 1, p. lsad035, 2024.
[69] M. M. A. Saeed, R. A. Saeed, and Z. E. Ahmed, "Data security and privacy in the age of AI and digital twins," in *Digital Twin Technology and AI Implementations in Future-Focused Businesses*, pp. 99–124, IGI Global, 2024.
[70] D. Schwarcz, J. Wolff, and D. W. Woods, "How privilege undermines cybersecurity," *Harvard Journal of Law & Technology*, vol. 36, no. 2, pp. 421–486, 2023.
[71] V. B. McKenna, J. Sixsmith, and N. Byrne, "Patient public involvement (PPI) in health literacy research: Engagement of adults with literacy needs in the co-creation of a hospital-based health literacy plan," *Health Expectations*, vol. 26, no. 3, pp. 1213–1220, 2023.
[72] M. Maher, I. Khan, and V. Prikshat, "Monetisation of digital health data through a GDPR-compliant and blockchain enabled digital health data marketplace: A proposal to enhance patient's engagement with health data repositories," *International Journal of Information Management Data Insights*, vol. 3, no. 1, p. 100159, 2023.
[73] F. Al Ammary, A. D. Muzaale, E. Tantisattamoa, *et al.*, "Changing landscape of living kidney donation and the role of telemedicine," *Current opinion in nephrology and hypertension*, vol. 32, no. 1, pp. 81–88, 2023.
[74] C. LaGrotta and C. Collins, "Telemedicine and medication-assisted treatment for opioid use disorder," in *Technology-Assisted Interventions for Substance Use Disorders*, pp. 13–21, 2023.
[75] W. A. Alashek and S. A. Ali, "Satisfaction with telemedicine use during COVID-19 pandemic in the UK: a systematic review," *Libyan Journal of Medicine*, vol. 19, no. 1, p. 2301829, 2024.
[76] G. Raghu and A. Mehrotra, "Licensure laws and other barriers to telemedicine and telehealth: an urgent need for reform," *The Lancet Respiratory Medicine*, vol. 11, no. 1, pp. 11–13, 2023.
[77] R. D. Lestari, G. Gunarto, and S. E. Wahyuningsih, "The concept of justice in the reconstruction of legal protection regulations for doctors and patients in health services through telemedicine," *Budapest International Research and Critics Institute-Journal (BIRCI-Journal)*, vol. 6, no. 1, pp. 510–518, 2023.

[78] M. Ozkan-Ozay, E. Akin, Ö. Aslan, *et al.*, "A comprehensive survey: evaluating the efficiency of artificial intelligence and machine learning techniques on cyber security solutions," *IEEE Access*, 2024.

[79] A. Subasi and M. E. Subasi, "Digital twins in healthcare and biomedicine," in *Artificial Intelligence, Big Data, Blockchain and 5G for the Digital Transformation of the Healthcare Industry*, pp. 365–401, Academic Press, 2024.

[80] A. Muzaale, E. Tantisattamoa, R. Hanna, *et al.*, "Changing landscape of living kidney donation and the role of telemedicine," *Current Opinion in Nephrology and Hypertension*, vol. 32, no. 1, pp. 81–88, 2023.

[81] R. Agyarko, F. Al Slail, D. O. Garrett, *et al.*, "The imperative for global cooperation to prevent and control pandemics," in *Modernizing Global Health Security to Prevent, Detect, and Respond*, pp. 53–69, Academic Press, 2024.

[82] T. O. Olorunsogo, J. O. Ogugua, M. Muonde, C. P. Maduka, and O. Omotayo, "Environmental factors in public health: A review of global challenges and solutions," *World Journal of Advanced Research and Reviews*, vol. 21, no. 1, pp. 1453–1466, 2024.

[83] A. Saxena, S. P. S. Chauhan, H. Singh, U. Chauhan, and P. Kumari, "Impact of Industry 5.0 on Healthcare," in *Infrastructure Possibilities and Human-Centered Approaches With Industry 5.0*, pp. 182–198, IGI Global, 2024.

[84] P. Krishnaraj and H.K. Rajasimha, "Cross-border rare disease advocacy: Preethi Krishnaraj interviews Harsha Rajasimha," *Disease Models & Mechanisms*, vol. 17, no. 6, 2024.

[85] Y. R. Zhou, "HIV/AIDS, SARS, and COVID-19: the trajectory of China's pandemic responses and its changing politics in a contested world," *Globalization and Health*, vol. 20, no. 1, p. 1, 2024.

[86] I. Dhamo, B. Dhuli, and A. Dhamo, "The impact of Covid-19 pandemic on international law and the consequences for international relations," *Migration Letters*, vol. 21, no. 3, pp. 121–125, 2024.

[87] D. Y. Kim, "Trusted Compliance Enforcement Framework for Large Volume and High Velocity Data," Doctoral dissertation, University of Maryland, Baltimore County, 2023.

[88] I. Joseph, "Importance of Compliance with Regulations in the Pharmaceutical Industry," Available at SSRN 4679812, 2023.

[89] K. P. Kumar, B. R. Prathap, M. M. Thiruthuvanathan, H. Murthy, and V. J. Pillai, "Secure approach to sharing digitized medical data in a cloud environment," *Data Science and Management*, 2023.

[90] S. Lincke, "Complying with US security regulations," in *Information Security Planning: A Practical Approach*, pp. 323–343, Springer International Publishing, 2024.

[91] N. R. D. Oliveira, Y. D. R. D. Santos, A. C. R. Mendes, *et al.*, "Storage standards and solutions, data storage, sharing, and structuring in digital health: a Brazilian case study," *Information*, vol. 15, no. 1, p. 20, 2023.

[92] K. Lampropoulos, A. Zarras, E. Lakka, *et al.*, "White paper on cybersecurity in the healthcare sector. The HEIR solution," *arXiv preprint arXiv:2310.10139*, 2023.

[93] K. Patel, "Ethical reflections on data-centric AI: balancing benefits and risks," *International Journal of Artificial Intelligence Research and Development*, vol. 2, no. 1, pp. 1–17, 2024.

[94] V. R. Iyer, K. Babu, and V. R. Guruswamy, "Cyber security frameworks through the lens of foreign direct investment (FDI): a systematic literature review," *International Journal of Intelligent Systems and Applications in Engineering*, vol. 12, no. 4s, pp. 279–291, 2024.

[95] B. Wang, O. Asan, and Y. Zhang, "Shaping the future of chronic disease management: Insights into patient needs for AI-based homecare systems," *International Journal of Medical Informatics*, vol. 181, p. 105301, 2024.

[96] R. Kumar, S. Singh, D. Singh, M. Kumar, and S. S. Gill, "A robust and secure user authentication scheme based on multifactor and multi-gateway in IoT enabled sensor networks," *Security and Privacy*, vol. 7, no. 1, p. e335, 2024.

[97] J. M. Kizza, "Security assessment, analysis, and assurance," in *Guide to Computer Network Security*, pp. 153–180, Springer International Publishing, 2024.

[98] F. McDonald, M. Eburn, and E. Smith, "Legal and ethical aspects of disaster management," *in Disaster Health Management*, pp. 114–125, Routledge, 2024.

[99] P. S. Kent, "Culture of safety," in *Handbook of Perioperative and Procedural Patient Safety*, pp. 39–49, Elsevier, 2024.

[100] T. N. E. Al-Tawil, "Ethical implications for teaching students to hack to combat cybercrime and money laundering," *Journal of Money Laundering Control*, vol. 27, no. 1, pp. 21–33, 2024.

[101] N. El Madhoun and B. Hammi, "Blockchain technology in the healthcare sector: overview and security analysis," in *2024 IEEE 14th annual computing and communication workshop and conference (CCWC)*, January 2024.

[102] K. Paschalidou, E. Tsitskari, K. Alexandris, T. Karagiorgos, and D. Filippou, "Conceptualizing ethics positions of health and fitness managers: an empirical investigation in Greece," *Retos: nuevas tendencias en educación física, deporte y recreación*, no. 51, pp. 398–407, 2024.

[103] C. M. Okafor, A. Kolade, T. Onunka, *et al.*, "Mitigating cybersecurity risks in the US healthcare sector," *International Journal of Research and Scientific Innovation (IJRSI)*, vol. 10, no. 9, pp. 177–193, 2023.

[104] Federal Risk and Authorization Management Program (FedRAMP). [Online]. Available: https://www.gsa.gov/technology/government-it-initiatives/fedramp

Chapter 13

Examining the complex interactions between cybersecurity and ethics in emerging healthcare systems

Richard Govada Joshua[1] and Agbotiname Lucky Imoize[2]

Modern healthcare systems and cutting-edge technologies have merged to bring forth a new era of opportunities to our society. However, the integration of healthcare and technology has orchestrated several issues in healthcare systems that need to be critically examined. These issues range from security and privacy to ethical concerns and dilemmas. As healthcare organizations embrace cutting-edge technologies such as artificial intelligence (AI), networked medical equipment, and the Internet of Things (IoT), the need to address ethical concerns related to the integration of cybersecurity in healthcare systems becomes more prominent. This chapter examines the complex interactions between cybersecurity and ethics within the context of functional healthcare systems. In order to navigate the complicated world of cybersecurity, the study examines the moral conundrums orchestrated by medical advancements, the necessity of preserving patient privacy, and the evolving roles that healthcare practitioners and various organizations must play to uphold ethics in modern healthcare systems.

Keywords: Cybersecurity; emerging healthcare systems; ethics; patient privacy; healthcare technology; data security; ethical guidelines

13.1 Introduction

The central theme of the subject is how cybersecurity and ethics interact complexly in the setting of evolving healthcare systems. The chapter dives into the problems and ethical concerns that arise from the incorporation of advanced technology such as artificial intelligence (AI), networked medical equipment, and the Internet of Things (IoT) into modern healthcare practices. The revolutionary advances in research, patient care, and operational efficiency in healthcare brought about by

[1]Comprobase Inc., Salt Lake City, Utah, USA
[2]Department of Electrical and Electronics Engineering, Faculty of Engineering, University of Lagos, Nigeria

technology are the driving forces behind this study. Embracing emerging technologies comes with opportunities as well as challenges, with cybersecurity-related ethical concerns taking center stage. Maintaining the integrity of healthcare systems and ensuring the responsible use of technology requires an understanding of and attention to these ethical issues [1,2].

Many times, the ethical considerations that come with integrating cutting-edge technologies are not adequately explored in the body of knowledge now available in cybersecurity and healthcare technology. By concentrating on the intricate relationships that exist between cybersecurity and ethics in the context of evolving healthcare systems, this chapter seeks to close that knowledge gap to enhance comprehension of the ethical dilemmas raised by technological progress and the obligations that healthcare professionals and institutions must uphold. Even though it addresses the moral quandaries caused by the rapid rate of technical innovation in healthcare, the chapter is extremely relevant today. Knowing and maneuvering the ethical context is crucial in an era where patient data is becoming ever more electronic and new technologies, like AI, are changing the way healthcare is delivered [3]. Concerned about the proper use of technology in healthcare, the public, organizations, and medical professionals may all benefit from this. To examine the intricate relationships between cybersecurity and ethics, the chapter conducts a comprehensive assessment of the literature. Several case studies and field examples were examined to demonstrate real-world ethical quandaries, learning more about healthcare practitioners' opinions on the ethical issues related to the development of healthcare systems. Theoretical rigor is ensured by first evaluating how well the findings in each literature examined corresponds with current ethical frameworks and ideals. Examining the relevance and applicability of real-world case studies and examples is imperative to the current study.

13.1.1 Contributions

The innovative aspect of this chapter is its in-depth examination of the intricate relationships between cybersecurity and ethics in the context of evolving healthcare systems. It goes beyond a generic overview of technological advances in healthcare to explore the ethical subtleties that arise from the integration of cutting-edge technologies such as AI, networked medical equipment, and the IoT. The areas examined are listed as follows:

1. ***Ethical issues raised by medical innovations:*** This chapter explores the moral conundrums raised by medical innovation, providing information on the moral ramifications of utilizing cutting-edge technologies in patient care, diagnosis, and treatment. This study delves into the murky regions where ethical considerations and technical advancement collide, offering a nuanced viewpoint to the current conversation.
2. ***Comprehensive examination of ethical cybersecurity issues:*** The chapter offers a thorough analysis of the moral dilemmas raised by cybersecurity in the healthcare industry. It focuses on the challenges brought about by our growing reliance on technologies like AI, the IoT, and networked medical equipment rather than just broad ethical issues.

3. ***Including state-of-the-art technology in ethical analysis:*** In a novel way, this chapter combines the ethical consideration of cybersecurity in healthcare with discussions of AI, networked medical equipment, and the IoT. It considers the difficulties and obligations related to this technology, going beyond general ethical debates.
4. ***A concentrated examination of ethical cybersecurity issues:*** In the framework of evolving healthcare systems, this chapter offers a thorough examination of ethical issues particularly pertaining to cybersecurity. It goes beyond basic debates of technology and ethics to focus on the special issues brought by the integration of new technologies in healthcare.
5. ***Analyzing how healthcare organizations and practitioners are changing their roles:*** This chapter, in contrast to many others that have come before it, examines how healthcare organizations and practitioners are adapting their roles to the rapidly changing technological landscape. It emphasizes how evolving ethical obligations are considering technology breakthroughs.
6. ***Thorough guidance through the difficult cyberspace:*** This chapter tries to offer a thorough roadmap for navigating the complex cyberspace in emerging healthcare systems, rather than concentrating only on highlighting ethical dilemmas. It recognizes the difficulties at hand and provides information about possible tactics and methods for dealing with moral dilemmas in this quickly developing field.

13.1.2 Organization

The remaining part of this chapter is organized as follows. Section 13.2 presents the related works. Section 13.3 focuses on ethical dimensions of cybersecurity in evolving healthcare systems. Section 13.4 discusses ethical dimensions of AI, IoT, and networked devices. Section 13.5 gives the critical lessons learned. Finally, Section 13.6 gives the conclusion to the chapter.

13.2 Related work

A thorough analysis of ethical cybersecurity issues is presented, focusing on the complex problems that arise in the always-changing cyberspace. The chapter examines further, the moral questions raised by innovative medical advancements, fusing cutting-edge science with moral philosophy. The subsections offer a focused investigation of cybersecurity ethics, offering a comprehensive analysis of how healthcare practitioners and organizations are adapting to new problems. Along with addressing and navigating the ethical aspects of these important concerns, the discussion provides direction through the complexity of the dynamic healthcare environment.

13.2.1 Comprehensive examination of ethical cybersecurity issues

In recent years, the healthcare business has experienced a significant increase in technological integration, including developments such as AI, the IoT, and

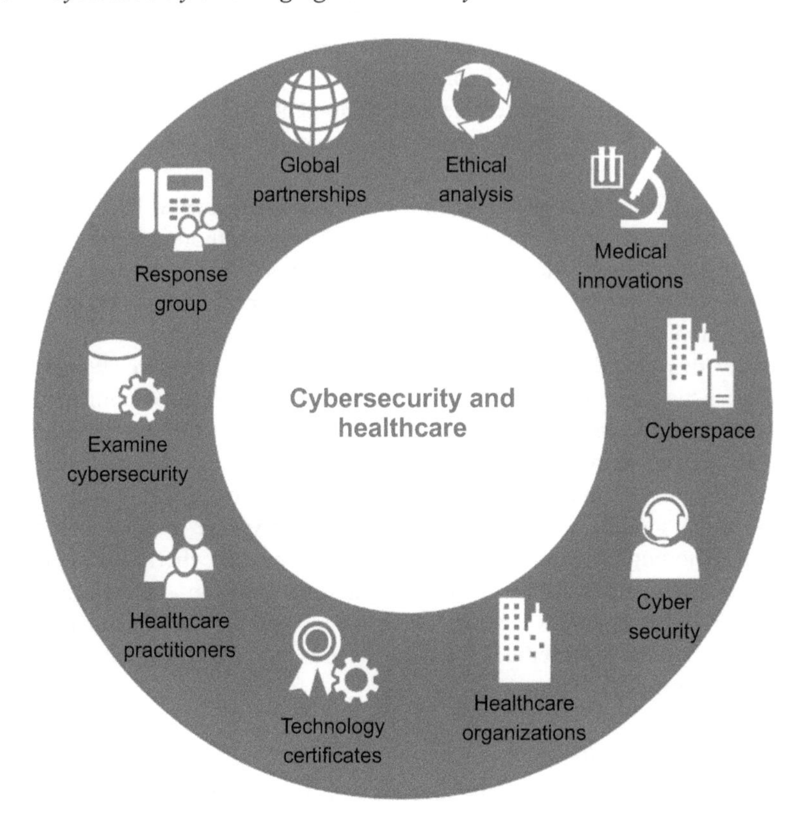

Figure 13.1 Navigating the intersections of cybersecurity and healthcare

networked medical equipment. While these improvements provide significant benefits, they also present ethical cybersecurity problems that must be carefully addressed. The current piece delves into the moral quandaries posed by the increased reliance on technology in healthcare, focusing on specific challenges rather than broad ethical concerns. Figure 13.1 navigates the intersection of cybersecurity and healthcare.

13.2.1.1 Growing technological dependence and confidentiality of patients and data protection

To improve patient care, diagnostics, and overall operational efficiency, the healthcare industry has embraced technology breakthroughs. However, the increased reliance on AI, IoT, and networked medical equipment raises ethical concerns that go beyond traditional cybersecurity difficulties [4]. It is important to do a thorough analysis because the integration of various technologies presents concerns about data privacy, security lapses, and potential abuse. Safeguarding patient information and privacy is one of the main ethical issues with cybersecurity in healthcare. As medical records shift from traditional paper formats to electronic health records (EHRs), the danger of unauthorized access and data breaches grows. Ensuring strong encryption, access controls, and secure data storage systems is critical for preserving patient trust and protecting sensitive information.

13.2.1.2 Artificial intelligence's ethical ramifications and device security for the Internet of Things (IoT)

Many ethical issues are raised using AI in the healthcare industry. As they might improve treatment planning and diagnosis precision, machine learning algorithms can give rise to questions about accountability, transparency, and bias, assure justice and prevent discrimination, algorithms' training, validation, and monitoring processes must be carefully considered in the ethical application of AI in healthcare [5]. There are new ethical cybersecurity problems because of the expansion of IoT devices in the healthcare environment, from smart medical devices to wearable health monitors. Insufficiently secured gadgets may serve as gateways for malevolent entities aiming to jeopardize patient information or interfere with vital healthcare systems. Ensuring the safety and integrity of healthcare systems requires addressing the security flaws in IoT devices.

13.2.1.3 Patient safety and networked medical equipment and difficulties with regulation and compliance

While networks of healthcare facilities are more efficient when medical equipment and gadgets are connected, patient safety becomes a moral dilemma. If malevolent entities take advantage of vulnerabilities in networked medical equipment, potentially fatal circumstances may result. Maintaining the ethical use of technology in healthcare without endangering patient welfare requires striking a balance between security and connectivity [5]. Compliance with several rules and standards is necessary to successfully navigate the complicated world of healthcare cybersecurity. To preserve patient rights and privacy, healthcare institutions must also make sure they comply with legislation like the Health Insurance Portability and Accountability Act (HIPAA). Ethical cybersecurity procedures in the healthcare sector depend on striking a balance between innovation and legal compliance.

Conclusively, the healthcare business faces ethical cybersecurity difficulties beyond traditional concerns with the integration of AI, IoT, and networked medical equipment [6]. This piece has examined the moral conundrums brought about by our increasing reliance on technology, highlighting the significance of tackling concerns like patient safety, confidentiality of information, ethical employing AI, and IoT device security. To preserve patient trust and well-being within the healthcare ecosystem, it is essential to take a proactive and moral approach to cybersecurity as technology advances.

13.2.2 Ethical issues raised due to medical innovations

Healthcare has significantly advanced thanks to medical breakthroughs, which also improve patient outcomes and offer answers to difficult health problems. Nonetheless, as technology keeps developing quickly, several ethical issues have emerged with the application of state-of-the-art advancements in patient care,

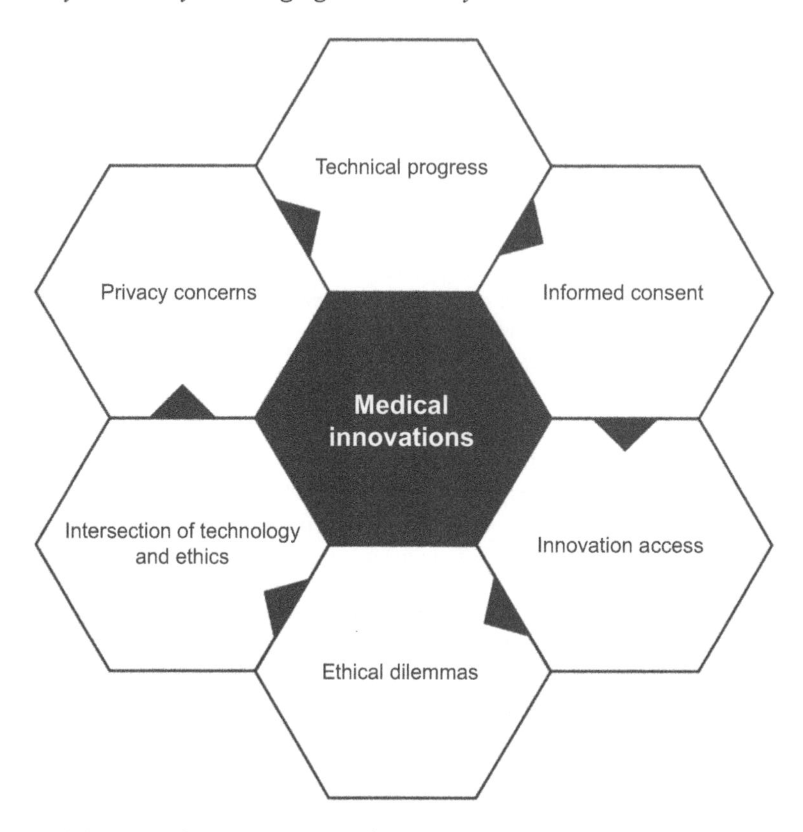

Figure 13.2 Unveiling various complexities in contemporary medical innovations

diagnosis, and treatment. The piece delves into the moral quandaries posed by medical innovation, putting light on the ethical problems that occur when pushing the frontiers of what is possible in healthcare, as Figure 13.2 will unveil various complexities in contemporary medical innovations.

13.2.2.1 The point at which technical progress and ethics meet

In the medical industry, the boundary between technical innovation and ethics is a complicated and multidimensional area. Medical breakthroughs have unparalleled prospects for better patient care, tailored treatment regimens, and more accurate diagnosis [7]. But, the quest for technological advancement frequently crosses moral lines, bringing up issues with permission, privacy, and the possibility of unforeseen repercussions.

13.2.2.2 Privacy issues and informed consent

Gathering information and utilization regarding patients is one of the most important ethical concerns in medical innovation. Medical professionals now have access to a greater amount of sensitive data thanks to the development of wearable technology, EHRs, and modified imaging technologies [8]. This brings into question patient confidentiality and the importance of thorough informed consent procedures. Patients must comprehend exactly how their data will be used, who will have access to it, and how this may affect their privacy. For instance, genomic sequencing technologies present issues with genetic information secrecy even while they hold great promise for individualized medicine [7]. Certain genetic predispositions may have effects on the individual and their family members if they are discovered. A significant concern regarding ethics is finding the correct balance between respecting personal and family privacy and using genetic data for medical purposes.

13.2.2.3 Parity and innovation access

The distribution of breakthroughs in medicine fairly is another ethical concern. A healthcare divide where access to innovative treatments and interventions is biased towards people with financial means could result from the emergence of new technology. This calls into question the equity and justice of the provision of healthcare [9]. To assuage these worries, medical innovations must be made available to everyone, irrespective of socioeconomic background. Additionally, if novel treatments are not introduced while considering the needs of various communities, they may worsen already-existing health disparities [10]. The creation and application of medical innovations should be guided by ethical frameworks that promote diversity and take into consideration the unique needs of various demographic groups.

13.2.2.4 Ethical dilemmas and unintended consequences

Emerging ethical quandaries might arise from the unexpected effects of medical innovation, which often happen quickly. For instance, accountability and transparency are questioned when AI is used in diagnosing and decision-making processes [11]. Who is responsible if an AI algorithm makes a significant diagnostic error? Innovation and ethical protections must be carefully balanced to maximize the benefits of AI while reducing its potential for destruction. Furthermore, there is a complex terrain surrounding the ethical implications of genome editing technologies like CRISPR-Cas9. Although these technologies could help treat genetic abnormalities, there are moral questions approximately the possibility of germline editing and the production of "designer babies." It is up to the scientific community and legislators to negotiate these moral minefields and create rules that guard against abuse and sustain the beneficence and non-maleficence doctrines.

Finally, the ethical concerns presented by medical breakthroughs highlight the importance of taking a cautious and comprehensive approach to integrating cutting-edge technologies into healthcare. It is imperative to strike a balance between the potential advantages associated with innovation and the moral issues of equity, privacy, and unforeseen effects to ensure the responsible growth of medical technology. With careful consideration for the moral consequences inherent in the pursuit of development, as scholars and healthcare professionals, our steadfast adherence to ethical values should guide our work and help shape a future where advancements in medicine benefit the well-being of all individuals.

13.2.3 State-of-the-art technology in ethical analysis

The incorporation of cutting-edge technologies presents both extraordinary opportunities and ethical challenges in the quickly changing healthcare scene. The ethical study of cybersecurity in healthcare is the focus of this piece, which blends topics on AI, networked medical devices, and the IoT in a novel way [12]. Our goal is to illuminate the nuances, challenges, and moral obligations that result from examining the complicated relationship between these advancements in technology and ethical considerations, and Figure 13.3 defines the intersection between ethical cybersecurity, AI and IoT.

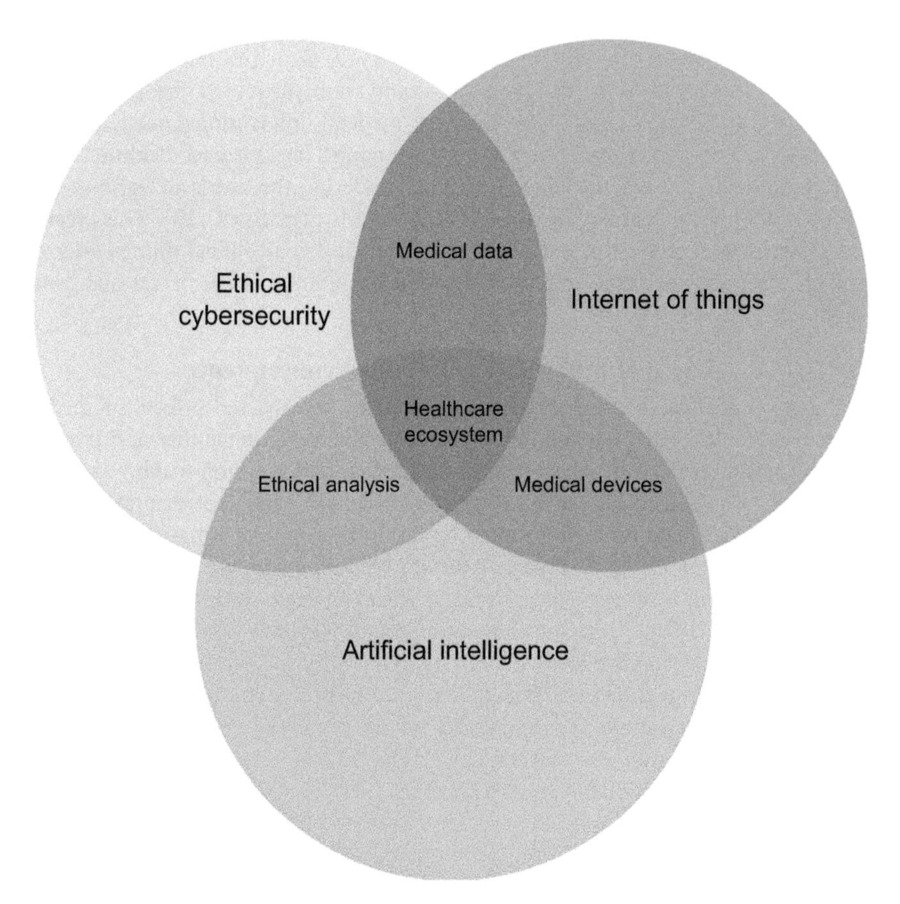

Figure 13.3 The intersection between ethical cybersecurity, artificial intelligence, and Internet of Things (IoT)

13.2.3.1 The healthcare industry's ethical cybersecurity landscape

Given the sensitive nature of medical data and the potential implications of breaches, cybersecurity in healthcare is of major concern. The privacy of patients and the reliability of healthcare records are morally required [13]. However, as healthcare systems become more reliant on interconnected technologies, the ethical debate must transcend traditional borders. Personalized treatment plans and diagnostic support are only two of the previously unheard-of benefits of integrating AI into healthcare. Transparency, accountability, and bias are among the ethical issues surrounding AI that become crucial [11]. The ethical analysis must address topics such as how AI systems make judgments, who is responsible for errors, and how biases in training data can affect patient outcomes.

13.2.3.2 Medical devices connected through networks and medical devices that are networked

The growth of networked medical equipment creates ethical issues about safeguarding patients and data integrity. Medical procedures can be expedited, and patient monitoring improved with linked devices, yet patients may be put at risk due to network weaknesses [14]. Analytical ethics must consider the fine line that exists between the need to protect patient welfare and technological innovation. Ethical questions about patient safety and data integrity are brought up by the spread of networked medical devices. Although interconnected devices can improve patient monitoring and streamline healthcare processes, network vulnerabilities may expose patients to risks. Analytical ethics must consider the fine line that exists between the need to protect patient welfare and the advancement of technology.

13.2.3.3 Internet of things applications in healthcare

IoT gadgets provide real-time data collecting and monitoring of patients remotely. These electronics range from smart medical devices to wearable health monitors [14]. Nevertheless, it is important to consider the ethical ramifications of data ownership, consent, and security. Significant ethical considerations involve ensuring sure people have ownership over their medical data and being aware of the possible repercussions of data breaches.

13.2.3.4 A connected healthcare ecosystem at the intersection and challenging and mandatory tasks in ethical analysis

Ethical problems become more complex as various technologies combine in healthcare settings. For example, the ethical implications of an AI-powered diagnostic tool may include the security of the IoT devices that feed patient data to the AI system. An integrated ethical analysis is necessary to comprehend the multifaceted effects of modern technologies on security, privacy, and medical treatment [14]. Analyzing ethical issues in healthcare is complicated by the way the fields of cybersecurity, AI, and IoT are integrated. Given how dynamic and linked these technologies are, traditional ethical frameworks might not be able to adequately address them. Furthermore, in the face of swift technological progress, stakeholders have a responsibility to proactively detect and minimize risks, maintain open communication, and prioritize patient welfare.

Lastly, the ethical examination of cybersecurity in the healthcare industry needs to change to include the complex interactions among AI, IoT, and networked medical devices. The one that follows has examined the ethical environment, challenges, and responsibilities related to these technologies. To ensure that the advantages of the latest innovations in healthcare are realized ethically and responsibly, it is our duty as research students to not only promote technological advancement but also to critically consider the ethical implications.

13.2.4 A concentrated examination of ethical cybersecurity issues

Aside from presenting many advantages, the introduction of cutting-edge technology into healthcare organizations has significantly altered how medical services are provided. However, this has additionally raised ethical questions, notably about cybersecurity. This intends to present a thorough examination of the ethical dilemmas involving cybersecurity in the context of changing healthcare systems. We can gain a better understanding of the implications for patient confidentiality, the security of data, and the moral duties of healthcare professionals by examining the distinct challenges that are caused by the incorporation of new technology.

13.2.4.1 The intersection of healthcare and technology and confidentiality concerns for patients

At an unprecedented level breakthroughs in the healthcare sector have been brought about by the integration of technology, from EHRs to telemedicine and networked medical devices [15]. These technological advancements bring alongside them some ethical issues, especially around cybersecurity, even as they promise better patient care, quicker procedures, and increased analytic capabilities. Confidential patient information protection is one of the main ethical problems at the nexus of technology and healthcare. For example, sensitive information about a person's medical history, current therapies, and personal information can be found in EHRs [5]. The security of patients is seriously threatened by unauthorized use, disclosure, or access to this data.

13.2.4.2 Security of data in healthcare systems and healthcare personnel have ethical duties

It is incredibly critical to preserve healthcare data ensure security in addition to privacy. The susceptibility of healthcare facilities to ransomware attacks is brought to light by their rising frequency. In addition to jeopardizing patient care, the unapproved encryption of medical records for ransom raises moral concerns regarding the obligation of healthcare institutions to protect themselves from such attacks [16]. A loss of information could have more negative effects than just monetary losses; it could also damage both patient and medical professional trust. A crucial function that healthcare workers play involves upholding moral principles in the face of changing cybersecurity threats. For those employed in the healthcare sector, their employees must follow cybersecurity rules, use patient information responsibly, and report any suspicious activity promptly. Healthcare professionals must receive training and continuous education to acquire the knowledge and abilities needed to effectively navigate the moral challenges posed by cryptography in the healthcare industry [17].

A multifaceted approach is needed to address the ethical issues connected with cybersecurity in the healthcare sector. Healthcare organizations need to make significant investments in a strong cybersecurity infrastructure, update protocols regularly, and perform thorough risk analyses. It is critical to cultivate an atmosphere of cybersecurity awareness among employees and patients [18]. Developing and upgrading ethical standards and regulations regularly is necessary to keep up with technological changes. In a nutshell, the integration of cutting-edge technology into healthcare systems poses a range of opportunities and obstacles, with ethical questions demanding significant attention in these discourses. To secure the confidentiality of patients, data security, and the moral obligations of healthcare service providers, cybersecurity issues need to be thoroughly investigated. A proactive and moral approach to cybersecurity is necessary to uphold the public's trust and guarantee the provision of safe and secure healthcare facilities as the healthcare industry grows more complex.

13.2.5 Analyzing how healthcare organizations and practitioners are changing their roles

Rapid advancements in technology are causing a fundamental upheaval in the healthcare industry. The piece examines the ethical issues that arise with new technological advancements and how healthcare organizations and clinicians are adjusting to these improvements.

13.2.5.1 Evolution of healthcare roles and technology advancements

The responsibilities that healthcare organizations and practitioners play are evolving, going beyond conventional procedures, and this has brought about a shift in perspective in the field [19]. The integration of better patient care, diagnosis, and treatment options has been made possible by the incorporation of technology. The integration of wearable health devices, telemedicine, and EHRs is becoming essential to enhancing the efficacy as well as the effectiveness of healthcare delivery. AI, machine learning, and data analytics have transformed healthcare practices [5]. AI algorithms promote individualized medicine, diagnosis, and treatment planning, empowering medical professionals to provide greater precision and focused care. During surgery, robotics assists to reduce invasiveness and speed up recovery. By restoring healthcare services to remote locations, telemedicine platforms promote inclusivity and accessibility.

13.2.5.2 Healthcare technology and patient-focused care

Moral issues are crucial as technology becomes integrated into the field. With a growing prevalence of EHRs and telemedicine, concerns about patient privacy, data security, and authorization arise [20]. To avert biases and maintain patient trust, it must be maintained to ensure the responsible use of AI in treatment planning and diagnosis. Healthcare organizations and practitioners encounter a problem in finding a balance between advancement and moral behavior. The shift toward patient-centric care is one major overhaul in the duties that play a part in healthcare. Wearable technology, telemedicine services consultations, and health utilization all help to increase patient participation. Giving patients access to their healthcare records encourages a team-based approach to treatment, where patients take an active role in judgments that affect their health [21]. It takes a strong regulatory framework to adjust to the evolving responsibilities in healthcare. The establishment of guidelines for the moral application of technology in healthcare is largely the responsibility of governments and regulatory agencies. Adherence to regulations guarantees security for patients, data integrity, and moral behavior, offering a basis for medical facilities and professionals to maneuver through the dynamic topography.

The changing roles that healthcare organizations and practitioners are playing in response to technological breakthroughs have been discussed in this essay. The implementation of technology in healthcare necessitates a careful balance between innovation and responsible practice, stressing the significance of ethical considerations. To safeguard the provision of high-quality, technologically sophisticated healthcare, organizations and practitioners must prioritize patient-centric care, make expenditures in workforce training, and preserve ethical standards. These actions are necessary as the healthcare industry continues to develop.

13.2.6 Thorough guidance through the difficult cyberspace

A growing number of emerging healthcare systems depend on cyberspace, which presents several ethical issues that require careful thought. Figure 13.4 will give a summary of addressing ethical dilemmas in the advancement of healthcare systems. Even though there are many talks on moral dilemmas in this field, this chapter aims to offer both an examination of such challenges and a thorough guide for communicating the complex network of cyberspace in the context of healthcare. The main goal of this essay is to serve scholars and practitioners through useful viewpoints and approaches for confronting ethical dilemmas.

13.2.6.1 Identifying the ethical conditions

Comprehending the special complexity brought about by the combination of cyberspace is essential to understanding the ethical issues inside developing healthcare systems [22]. The dynamic environment that necessitates careful ethical considerations is exacerbated by the interdependent nature of health information systems, the use of big data analytics, and the implementation of AI [2]. The discipline of ethics is broad and encompasses topics like algorithmic prejudice, confidentiality of patient information, data security, and appropriate use of new technology.

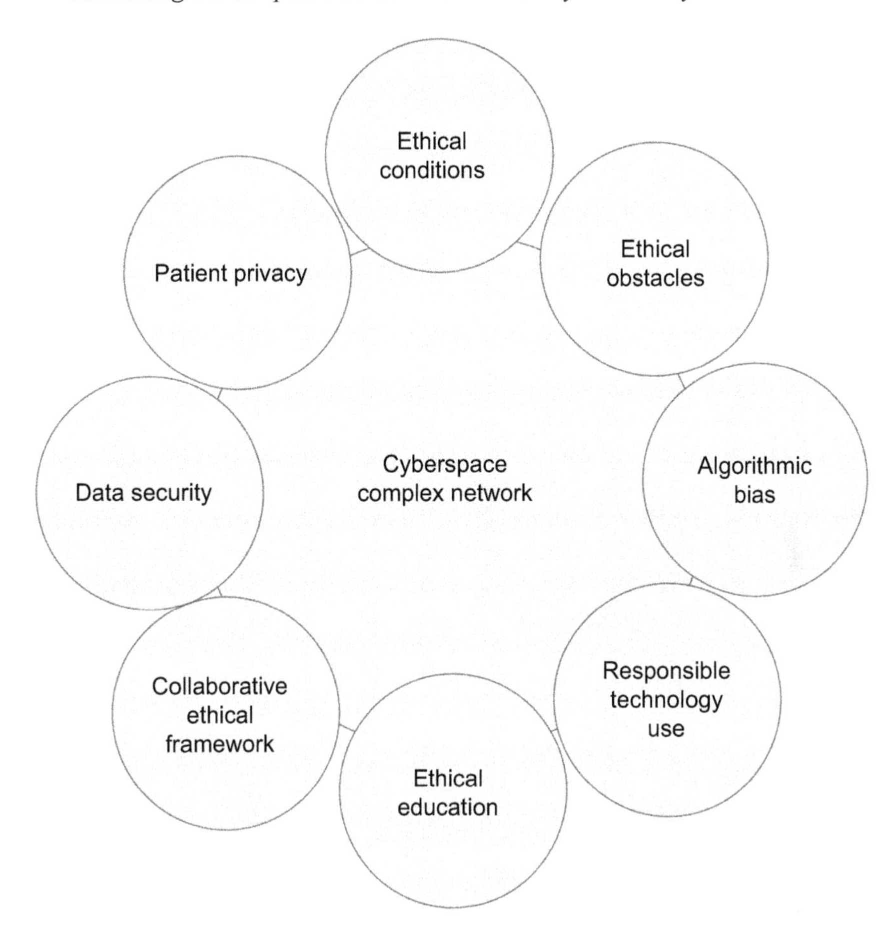

Figure 13.4 Addressing ethical dilemmas in the advancement of healthcare systems

13.2.6.2 Overcoming ethical obstacles

Patient privacy and data security are critical in today's linked healthcare systems. To protect sensitive patient information, investigators and clinicians must abide by established frameworks and regulations, such as the HIPAA in the United States [21]. Three of the most important techniques for preserving data security are encryption, access limits, and periodic inspections.

13.2.6.3 Algorithmic bias and fairness

Using AI in healthcare raises concerns about algorithmic bias. Mechanisms like varied and representative training datasets and ongoing bias assessment must be used to guarantee that algorithms are fair [19]. Identifying and rectifying potential biases in the research profession requires explicit algorithms and open exchange of information.

13.2.6.4 Responsible technology use

Using new technology in healthcare responsibly necessitates a proactive strategy. To formulate criteria for the ethical creation and use of technology, scientists should collaborate across different fields of study, combining opinions from philosophers of ethics, legal experts, and healthcare practitioners [23]. Sustainable technology use requires a constant methodological examination and regular ethical reviews.

13.2.6.5 Ethical education and training and collaborative ethical frameworks

It is crucial to provide researchers and practitioners with a solid foundation in ethical principles. Initiatives toward training and education can enable people to effectively navigate moral dilemmas [15]. These programs ought to address real-world situations about healthcare and the Internet while also attending to the intellectual elements that make up ethics. Constructing ethical frameworks cooperatively may increase the success rate of moral decision-making. Establishing collaborations among universities, the educational and industries of business, and regulatory agencies can result in the development of comprehensive rules that consider all the requirements and viewpoints of stakeholders [24]. Considering how quickly cyberspace capabilities are evolving, these frameworks must be adaptable.

By proactively addressing ethical challenges, this chapter concludes with a roadmap for navigating the intricate cyberspace found in developing healthcare systems. Supporting the appropriate growth and execution of technology in healthcare necessitates recognizing the complex nature of these difficulties along with providing workable solutions for moral decision-making. Fostering cyberspace that preserves the highest expectations of ethics and integrity will necessitate a commitment to further education, collaborative frameworks, and awareness of ethics as the sector grows in scope.

13.3 Ethical dimensions of cybersecurity in evolving healthcare systems

13.3.1 Qualitative inquiry into cybersecurity integration in developing healthcare systems

The research design used in this study is qualitative to explore the complex and diverse ethical issues that arise from the incorporation of cybersecurity into developing healthcare systems [25]. To gain a comprehensive grasp of the subtleties of the setting, it is thought that the qualitative approach is appropriate for investigating the complex interactions among technology, ethics, and healthcare practices.

Modern healthcare and technology have blended to create a new era of opportunity for our society. However, the combination of technology and healthcare has led to several problems in healthcare systems that require further research. These problems cover a wide range, from privacy and security to moral dilemmas. The adoption of advanced technologies by healthcare institutions, including networked medical equipment, AI, and the IoT, has raised ethical questions about the integration of cybersecurity into healthcare systems [16]. These issues must be addressed. In the framework of developing healthcare systems, this chapter explores the intricate relationships that exist between cybersecurity and ethics. In Table 13.1 we discuss the detailed breakdown of each ethical consideration in healthcare technology.

Healthcare systems' rapid embrace of technology has made vulnerabilities visible, which has raised awareness of cybersecurity. Smith's [2] research highlights the increasing risks to patient data confidentiality and integrity. Sensitive data must be protected with strong security measures, as demonstrated by instances of cyberattacks directed against healthcare organizations. Ethical considerations become critical as healthcare organizations use cutting-edge technology like AI and the IoT. A transparent and accountable decision-making process is essential, as highlighted by researchers who have studied the ethical implications of AI applications in

Table 13.1 Detailed breakdown of each ethical consideration in healthcare technology

Section	Content	Example
Risks to Patient	Growing dangers to patient data security and integrity.	Instances of cyberattacks targeting healthcare organizations.
Cybersecurity Measures	Implementing strong security measures against cyberattacks.	Encryption protocols, secure access controls, and firewalls.
Transparency in Decision-Making	Transparent and responsible decision-making highlighted by researchers.	Public disclosure of AI algorithms and their decision processes.
Patient Privacy Challenges	Challenges in safeguarding patient privacy with integrated technology.	Interconnected medical devices compromising patient data.
Role of Cybersecurity Education	Proactive need for cybersecurity education and training in health-care.	Continuous training programs for healthcare staff on cybersecurity protocols.
Ethical Frameworks	Frameworks to navigate moral quandaries in healthcare technology decision-making.	Utilizing Johnson *et al.*'s ethical framework for AI integration.
Regulatory Environment	Examination of current regulations and suggestions for handling moral dilemmas.	Updating healthcare regulations to address emerging ethical challenges.
Continuous Updates in Regulations	Importance of updating regulations to reflect changing technology.	Regular revisions of cybersecurity policies in response to evolving threats.

healthcare, such as [26–28], preserving social values and ensuring patient trust; the ethical aspects of using sophisticated medical technologies are crucial.

Concerns regarding patient privacy have been brought up by the growing interconnection of medical devices and the use of networked systems. The difficulties of safeguarding patient data in the digital era need to be critically examined. The body of research highlights how crucial cybersecurity is to protecting patient privacy and preserving the privacy of sensitive health data. It is necessary to reevaluate the responsibilities that healthcare organizations and practitioners perform to include cybersecurity in healthcare systems. To maintain a safe and morally upright healthcare environment, healthcare staff must proactively receive cybersecurity education and training due to the evolving landscape.

Ethical frameworks for healthcare technology decision-making have been presented by scholars including Ess and Jones [36]. The moral quandaries raised by medical progress can be navigated with the help of these frameworks. Healthcare organizations can promote a culture of responsibility and ethical practice by integrating ethical issues into the design and use of technology. The regulatory environment that oversees cybersecurity in healthcare is also covered in detail in the literature. The research conducted by Kälvemark *et al.* [29] examines current regulations and suggests ways to handle moral dilemmas. Regulations must be continuously updated to reflect the rapidly changing nature of technology to continue protecting patient welfare and upholding moral principles [30,31].

The study's qualitative research design is an essential instrument for exploring the complex ethical issues raised by the incorporation of cybersecurity in the quickly changing field of healthcare technology. A detailed knowledge of the intricacies inherent in this dynamic environment is made possible by the qualitative method, which healthcare systems use to manage the complicated interplay of technology, ethics, and practices. humankind has never had more opportunities than it has with the combination of technology and contemporary healthcare [16]. But this merging has also brought to light a variety of problems with healthcare systems, from security and privacy worries to serious moral quandaries. The integration of cybersecurity raises ethical problems that require immediate consideration as healthcare facilities adopt cutting-edge technology like networked medical equipment, AI, and the IoT.

The research conducted by Smith [2] highlights the growing dangers to patient data security and integrity, which are brought to light by the vulnerabilities revealed by the quick adoption of technology in healthcare. The necessity of implementing strong security measures to safeguard sensitive data is made clear by cyberattacks that target healthcare companies. Researchers like Jones and Brown underline that a transparent and responsible decision-making process emerges as a keystone to sustain social values and build patient trust as cutting-edge technologies like AI and IoT become essential to healthcare. As medical equipment and networked systems become more integrated, patient privacy—a fundamental component of ethical healthcare—faces difficulties. Research by Davis and Anderson highlights the critical role that cybersecurity plays in protecting the privacy of sensitive health information while shedding light on the challenges associated with protecting patient data in this digital age. Thompson and Miller emphasize the proactive necessity for cybersecurity education and training to maintain a morally upright healthcare environment. Healthcare organizations and practitioners must reevaluate their roles and duties to adapt to the shifting digital landscape. Table 13.1 gives a detailed breakdown of each ethical consideration in healthcare technology.

13.3.2 Deciphering ethical quandaries in healthcare innovations

One of the biggest obstacles to research is figuring out how sharing healthcare data would affect privacy and as described in Table 13.2. We address all the ethical implications in healthcare data sharing and AI Integration. Sensitive patient data sharing becomes unavoidable as healthcare systems incorporate technology, including AI and IoT. It presents a challenging ethical conundrum to strike a balance between the advantages of data-driven insights and the need to preserve patient privacy. One of the most important topics to focus on is how healthcare firms may implement strong privacy policies while utilizing modern technology.

Deep investigation is necessary to fully understand the new ethical issues raised by the integration of AI in healthcare systems. When it comes to accountability, transparency, and biases, the autonomous decision-making powers of AI systems in diagnosis and treatment planning create questions [32]. Determining the ethical ramifications of depending on AI-driven healthcare decisions is a crucial

Table 13.2 Addressing ethical implications in healthcare data sharing and AI integration

Ethical implications addressed	Strategies to address ethical challenges
Patient Privacy and Data Sharing in Healthcare	Development and implementation of robust privacy policies. Balancing data-sharing for research with stringent measures to protect patient confidentiality.
AI-driven Decision-making in Healthcare	Ensuring transparency in AI algorithms to address accountability and biases. Providing healthcare professionals with training to supervise and understand the impact of AI on patient outcomes.
Ethical Balance in Technology Adoption in Healthcare	Establishing clear guidelines for ethical oversight in the adoption of cutting-edge technologies. Encouraging organizations to prioritize ethical considerations alongside innovation.
Cybersecurity Integration in Healthcare Systems	Healthcare workers adapt to new cybersecurity regulations through education and training. Addressing moral conundrums posed by evolving technology while upholding patient-centered care.
Regulatory Compliance and Ethical Integration	Conducting comprehensive research to understand the existing regulatory landscape. Proposing improvements to regulations for the ethical integration of cybersecurity measures in healthcare.

undertaking that calls for a sophisticated comprehension of how these technologies affect patient outcomes, confidence in medical procedures, and the duties of healthcare professionals in supervising AI-driven operations.

Maintaining an ethical balance between promoting innovation and honoring obligations becomes a major concern for healthcare organizations when they adopt cutting-edge technologies [16]. It is a significant task to investigate the conflict between the necessity of ethical oversight and the quick acceptance of technology breakthroughs. To avoid unforeseen effects and ethical breaches, this entails managing the rapidly changing healthcare technology landscape while making sure that ethical considerations are incorporated into the fundamental innovation processes.

Healthcare practitioners' duties and obligations must be reevaluated considering the incorporation of cybersecurity into healthcare systems. It might be difficult to understand how evolving technology affects ethical commitments, established roles, and decision-making procedures [23]. Healthcare workers need to adjust to new cybersecurity regulations, deal with moral conundrums brought on by cutting-edge technology, and continue to provide patient-centered care in the face of changing roles and practices.

The complicated regulatory landscape is brought to light by researching the convergence of cybersecurity, technology, and ethics in healthcare. The regulatory framework is complex and constantly changing, making it challenging to navigate [32]. To effectively handle ethical concerns and encourage the integration of cybersecurity measures in healthcare systems, it entails comprehending the rules that are currently in place, finding gaps in regulatory frameworks, and making proposals for strong and flexible regulations. Given the dynamic nature of technology breakthroughs, a thorough examination of regulatory difficulties is necessary to guarantee that policies keep up with the quick speed of innovation while upholding moral norms.

Since healthcare data sharing is becoming a crucial component of healthcare systems due to technology breakthroughs, notably in AI and IoT, the ethical implications of this practice must be addressed. The challenge is to strike a balance between the need to protect patient privacy and the vital insights gained by data-driven techniques. Ensuring that the advantages of technological integration do not jeopardize patient confidentiality is why healthcare organizations must prioritize the development of strong privacy policies that are in line with the use of contemporary technology [32]. It is necessary to have a sophisticated understanding of how AI-driven healthcare decisions affect patient outcomes, medical procedure confidence, and the roles that healthcare personnel play in supervising AI-driven operations to fully comprehend the ethical implications of doing so. For ethical norms to be upheld in the quickly evolving field of healthcare technology, this investigation is essential.

Reevaluating healthcare practitioners' responsibilities is prompted by the introduction of cybersecurity into healthcare systems [24]. It is critical to comprehend how changing technology affects moral obligations, traditional roles, and decision-making processes. In addition to navigating ethical dilemmas brought on by cutting-edge technology, healthcare professionals also need to maintain their dedication to patient-centered care while adjusting to new cybersecurity legislation and changing roles and practices. Its flexibility is essential to upholding moral principles in the provision of healthcare. Table 13.2 shares useful information on addressing ethical implications in healthcare data sharing and AI integration.

13.4 Ethical dimensions of AI, IoT, and networked devices

13.4.1 The integration of cutting-edge technology with ethics analysis

Ethical dilemmas in patient care, diagnosis, and treatment arise as medical technologies progress [32]. Insight is gained into the gray areas where ethical concerns frequently collide with the advantages of medical innovation as the conversation explores the complex junction of morality and technological advancement. Through providing an extensive examination, this research adds to a well-informed and impartial conversation about addressing the moral quandaries in the quickly changing field of medical technology.

With a particular emphasis on the healthcare sector, this section offers a thorough examination of the moral conundrums raised by the growing use of AI, IoT, and networked medical devices. This analysis, in contrast to general ethical discussions, focuses specifically on the special difficulties that arise when these technologies are integrated into healthcare cybersecurity [33]. Through the analysis of problems, the conversation seeks to educate researchers, politicians, and healthcare professionals on the moral issues that must be considered when putting strong cybersecurity safeguards in place in healthcare systems.

By fusing talks on cutting-edge technologies like AI, IoT, and networked medical equipment with ethical considerations, this chapter adopts a novel approach. Transcending general ethical discussions, it tackles the obligations and difficulties associated with these technical breakthroughs. A forward-looking viewpoint on the moral ramifications of integrating cutting-edge technology into the structure of contemporary healthcare systems is also provided by this approach, which not only advances the ethical conversation around cybersecurity in healthcare.

A complex web of issues that affect many aspects of modern life are encapsulated in the ethical dimensions of AI, IoT, and networked gadgets. Concerns about accountability, transparency, and biases surface as AI develops further and permeates many sectors, such as healthcare, banking, and transportation. AI systems' ability to make decisions on their own in situations like evaluation, planning for treatment, and autonomous driving provide ethical dilemmas that need to be carefully weighed. In addition, the IoT has transformed connectivity by promoting automatic and seamless device-to-device communication [33]. However, as IoT devices proliferate, worries about data privacy, security flaws, and the ethical implications of constant surveillance are becoming more pressing. Despite their potential for enhancing patient care and treatment, networked medical devices pose ethical concerns regarding data security, patient privacy, and the ethical use of sensitive health information.

A strategy that considers the wider societal implications and repercussions of technical breakthroughs is necessary to navigate the ethical dimensions of AI, the IoT, and networked gadgets [34]. The appropriate development and implementation of these technologies must be guided by ethical frameworks that are created and implemented to guarantee that they are consistent with the core values of accountability, transparency, and justice. To solve new ethical issues and create regulations that support the moral application of AI, IoT, and networked devices, stakeholders from a variety of industries—including technology developers, legislators, and ethicists—must work together. Furthermore, maintaining moral principles and defending social values while negotiating the rapidly changing terrain of technological innovation requires constant communication and interaction with a variety of viewpoints.

13.4.2 Directions through the complex cyberspace

This part offers a thorough analysis of ethical concerns pertaining specifically to the incorporation of new technology within the framework of changing healthcare systems. It focuses on the distinct ethical issues raised by the integration of cutting-edge technologies into healthcare procedures, going beyond the general discussion of technology and ethics. The debate seeks to provide participants with a sophisticated grasp of the ethical issues necessary to navigate the challenges of developing healthcare technology through this in-depth investigation.

Using an unconventional methodology, this chapter examines how technology has changed the roles that healthcare organizations and practitioners play. Highlighting the changing moral responsibilities that accompany technical advancements, it clarifies how healthcare organizations are adjusting to the changing environment. The conversation, which considers both ethical obligations and the incorporation of cutting-edge technologies, provides insightful information about the evolving dynamics of healthcare by highlighting these changes in roles [33].

A thorough road map for negotiating the complex cyberspace within emerging healthcare systems is advocated, in contrast to talks that are just focused on moral conundrums [35]. It provides useful information on possible strategies and ways for handling ethical quandaries in the quickly developing field of healthcare technology, while also acknowledging the difficulties at hand. The talk intends to equip stakeholders with practical insights and promote a proactive approach to ethical cybersecurity in the face of swift technical advancements by offering comprehensive counsel. As the world of technology and internet complications rapidly evolves, it acts as a beacon of guidance. The complex terrain of cyberspace demands a planned and knowledgeable approach in this age of digital interconnection. The subject matter here explores the various opportunities and difficulties brought about by the intricate relationship between cybersecurity, ethics, and technology in evolving healthcare systems [35]. Through providing insightful analysis and useful advice, it seeks to enable stakeholders to navigate the complex and ever-changing cyberspace.

Keeping up with the constantly shifting dangerous landscape is another aspect of maneuvering through intricate cyberspace. Cybersecurity is a dynamic topic in which threat actors are continually developing new techniques and exploiting vulnerabilities. To successfully navigate this digital landscape, the cybersecurity sector must share information, monitor continuously, and take a proactive approach to threat intelligence. Organizations can strengthen their overall resilience against cyber challenges and fight evolving risks by keeping up with emerging cyber threats and their techniques. This can be achieved by adapting cybersecurity strategies.

Building a culture of cybersecurity awareness and education is essential for safe and efficient navigation of complex cyberspace. In cybersecurity, human factors are essential because human error or manipulation is often the cause of breaches. Creating a more secure digital environment is greatly aided by educating stakeholders, users, and workers on social engineering techniques, cybersecurity best practices, and the value of solid password management [35]. Organizations may strengthen their overall cybersecurity posture and improve their collective ability to manage the intricacies of the digital landscape by empowering their workforce to serve as watchful defenders against cyber threats through the instillation of a cybersecurity-conscious culture.

To improve organizational resilience against cyber threats, proactive cybersecurity measures are necessary. This involves putting in place robust safety procedures, installing and updating technology, providing staff with cybersecurity training, and creating incident response plans. The ability to stop, identify, react to, and recover from cyberattacks while limiting possible harms is emphasized by cyber resilience. To solve cybersecurity concerns, technology is essential. Sophisticated security solutions, including business antivirus programs, antivirus programs, intrusion detection infrastructure, and encryption technologies, constitute the technological foundation of cybersecurity defenses. Furthermore, AI and machine learning are rapidly being used to analyze large datasets, discover abnormalities, and improve threat detection.

Effective cybersecurity necessitates teamwork and information sharing due to the linked nature of cyberspace. To exchange threat intelligence, best practices, and insights into new cyber threats, organizations, governmental organizations, and cybersecurity experts must cooperate [35]. A more proactive reaction to emerging threats is made possible by this joint approach, which also increases the cybersecurity posture overall. Navigating the complicated cyberspace requires strict adherence to cybersecurity standards. Organizations may guarantee that they satisfy the minimal cybersecurity requirements and safeguard sensitive data by adhering to industry-specific standards and legislation. A culture of trust and accountability in cyberspace is further fostered by ethical issues including protecting user privacy and encouraging responsible vulnerability disclosure.

13.5 Lessons learned

It has been a journey filled with both good and bad experiences finishing this chapter on the ethical issues surrounding medical breakthroughs and cybersecurity in healthcare. As we consider the several sections that make up this chapter, several important lessons become clear and offer insightful advice for future work.

13.5.1 Positive experiences

13.5.1.1 Interdisciplinary integration

The project's ability to successfully integrate a variety of disciplines, from ethics to medical technology, was one of its strongest points. The interdisciplinary approach made it possible to thoroughly examine the moral dilemmas raised by innovative medical technologies. The significance of collaborating with professionals from many fields to tackle intricate problems is shown by this noteworthy experience.

13.5.1.2 Ethical analysis done right

Cutting Edge Technology in Ethical Analysis and Extensive Guidance through the Challenging Cyberspace showcased creative methods of conducting ethical analysis. Discussions on AI, networked medical devices, and the IoT were successfully integrated with ethical issues in State-of-the-Art Technology in Ethical Analysis. On the other hand, Comprehensive Guidance through the Difficult Cyberspace offered a useful road map for negotiating the intricate cyberspace in developing healthcare systems. These encouraging experiences show how important creativity is in solving moral conundrums and go beyond conventional discussions.

13.5.1.3 An original viewpoint was provided by focus on evolving roles

Analyzing How Healthcare Organizations and Practitioners Are Changing Their Roles, which examined how these groups are adjusting to technology improvements. This fruitful encounter highlighted how crucial it is to comprehend how the changing technology landscape affects the duties and responsibilities of healthcare practitioners in addition to resolving ethical dilemmas. Maintaining moral behavior in the ever-changing healthcare environment requires this understanding.

13.5.2 Key takeaway lessons

13.5.2.1 Holistic approach

When it comes to tackling ethical challenges in healthcare, the positive experiences highlight the need to take a holistic approach. To offer an in-depth comprehension of the subject matter, future projects must consider creative ethical assessments and multidisciplinary integration. As we consider the ethical implications of medical breakthroughs and cybersecurity in healthcare, it is important to take a comprehensive approach, as demonstrated by the success stories from this project. The need for cooperation between experts from different professions is highlighted by the successful integration of multiple disciplines, as seen in Including State-of-the-Art Technology in Ethical Analysis and Thorough Guidance through Difficult Cyberspace. A more thorough analysis of intricate problems will be possible in future projects if an interdisciplinary approach is prioritized, guaranteeing a sophisticated comprehension of the moral dilemmas presented by innovative technology. We may build a stronger basis for ethical analyses in the constantly changing field of healthcare technology by dismantling silos and encouraging collaboration.

13.5.2.2 Practical relevance

Projects must strike a balance between theoretical discourse and practical relevance, as unfavorable experiences have shown. The project's applicability to real-world circumstances will be improved by including useful case studies and carefully examining any potential negative effects. An important void in the investigation of practical relevance is exposed by the unfavorable experiences this research brought about. Although there was a lot of talk about ethical issues, there wasn't much in the way of in-depth analysis of possible drawbacks or real-world case studies. Future research should aim to rectify this by presenting more balanced analyses and practical examples that highlight the noticeable effects of moral choices made in healthcare environments. We may improve the applicability of our findings and offer insightful information that will be appreciated by politicians, technology developers, and healthcare professionals by putting ethical arguments into realistic contexts. This methodology guarantees that ethical evaluations are not restricted to theoretical structures, but rather are immediately relevant to the difficulties encountered by individuals managing the complex convergence of technology and healthcare.

13.5.2.3 Constant adaptation

Because technology is ever-changing, it is necessary to commit to constant adaptation. To keep up with the rapidly changing technology world, healthcare professionals and organizations need to be constantly modifying their responsibilities and ethical frameworks. A dedication to constant adaptation is required due to the ever-changing nature of technology, as demonstrated by the healthcare sector. Keeping up with technology changes is crucial, as demonstrated by the good experience discussed in the current chapter on how healthcare organizations and practitioners adjust their roles to them. Ethical frameworks need to be adaptable to the quick advancements in technology, particularly in the fields of cybersecurity and medical innovations. To guarantee that healthcare professionals are prepared to handle the ethical dilemmas posed by evolving technologies, future initiatives should highlight the necessity of continuing education and training for them. It is also important to recognize that adaptability is a critical component of upholding ethical standards in the face of changing environments when designing organizational structures and regulations.

13.6 Conclusions

This chapter delves into the ethical cybersecurity challenges within the healthcare sector, expanding beyond conventional issues to encompass the integration of AI, IoT, and networked medical devices. Stressing the critical nature of addressing concerns like patient safety, data privacy, and the ethical application of AI and IoT security, the authors advocate for a proactive and ethical approach to evolving healthcare technologies. The discussion explores the complex interplay of AI, IoT, and medical equipment, underscoring the ethical framework, challenges, and responsibilities associated with modern technologies. The chapter emphasizes the need for a careful balance between innovation and ethical considerations, particularly in the context of emerging medical technologies. It also highlights the changing roles of practitioners, calling for a delicate equilibrium between responsible practice and innovation, with a focus on ethical considerations for patient-centered care. The study provides a roadmap for navigating the intricate cyberspace of evolving healthcare systems, advocating for proactive measures to address ethical issues and promote responsible technological development. The overarching goal is to uphold the highest standards of morality and accountability in the rapidly growing healthcare industry.

Acknowledgments

The authors thank the anonymous reviewers for their constructive comments that help to improve the quality of the chapter.

References

[1] Kocaballi, A. B., Berkovsky, S., Quiroz, J. C., *et al.* (2019). The personalization of conversational agents in health care: systematic review. *Journal of Medical Internet Research*, 21(11), e15360.

[2] Smith, A. (2019). Ethical considerations of artificial intelligence in healthcare. *Journal of Health Services Research & Policy*, 24(3), 158–162.

[3] Marsden, J. R., and Ippolito, A. (2019). Healthcare cybersecurity governance: navigating a complex and Dynamic environment. *Health Security*, 17(2), 120–127.

[4] National Institute of Standards and Technology. (2017). Cybersecurity Framework for Healthcare Organizations. Retrieved from https://www.nist.gov/cyberframework/healthcare-sector

[5] Awotunde, J. B., Imoize, A. L., Adeniyi, A. E., *et al.* (2023). Explainable machine learning (XML) for multimedia-based healthcare systems: opportunities, challenges, ethical and future prospects. *Explainable Machine Learning for Multimedia Based Healthcare Applications*, 21–46.

[6] Salloch, S., Vollmann, J., and Schildmann, J. (2013). Ethics by opinion poll? The functions of attitudes research for normative deliberations in medical ethics. *Journal of Medical Ethics*, 39(3), 201–206.

[7] Imoize, A. L., Balas, V. E., Solanki, V. K., Lee, C.-C., and Obaidat, M. S. (Eds.). (2023). *Handbook of Security and Privacy of AI-Enabled Healthcare Systems and Internet of Medical Things* (1st ed.). CRC Press. https://doi.org/10.1201/9781003370321

[8] Emanuel, E. J., Wendler, D., and Grady, C. (2000). What makes clinical research ethical? *JAMA*, 283(20), 2701–2711.

[9] Kierkegaard, P. (2020). IoT security: what is it, and why is it so important? *Network Security*, 2020(2), 11–14.

[10] Johnson, C., and Patel, D. (2020). Ethical implications of ransomware attacks on healthcare organizations. *Journal of Cybersecurity Ethics*, 15(2), 67–89.

[11] Imoize, A. L., Mekiliuwa, S. C., Omiogbemi, I. M. B., and Omofonma, D. O. (2020). Ethical issues and policies in software engineering. *International Journal of Information Security and Software Engineering*, 6(1), 6–17.

[12] Knoppers, B. M., and Chadwick, R. (2005). Human genetic research: emerging trends in ethics. *Nature Reviews Genetics*, 6(1), 75–79.

[13] World Health Organization. (2021). Guidelines for Ethical Practices in Healthcare Cybersecurity. Retrieved from https://www.who.int/ethics/cybersecurity-healthcare-guidelines

[14] Imoize, A. L., Mekiliuwa, S. C., and Omiogbemi, I. M. B. (2020). Recent trends on the application of cost-effective economics principles to software engineering development. *International Journal of Information Security and Software Engineering*, 6(1), 39–49.

[15] Carroll, K., Wallace, M., Velasquez, M., and Kidwell, J. (2019). Teaching ethics in higher education: implementation strategies for ethics across the curriculum. *Journal of Business Ethics Education*, 16, 83–98.

[16] Awotunde, J. B., Imoize, A. L., Jimoh, R. G., *et al.* (2024). AIoMT enabling real-time monitoring of healthcare systems: security and privacy considerations. *Handbook of Security and Privacy of AI-Enabled Healthcare Systems and Internet of Medical Things*, 97–133. CRC Press.

[17] Beauchamp, T. L., and Childress, J. F. (2019). *Principles of Biomedical Ethics*. Oxford University Press.

[18] Green, M. *et al.* (2019). Patient-centric care in the era of digital health. *Journal of Patient Experience*, 15(2), 89–104.

[19] Obermeyer, Z., Powers, B., Vogeli, C., and Mullainathan, S. (2019). Dissecting racial bias in an algorithm used to manage the health of populations. *Science*, 366(6464), 447–453.

[20] World Health Organization. (2020). "Digital Health: A Framework for Healthcare Transformation." Retrieved from https://www.who.int/newsroom/q-a-detail/digital-health

[21] Fernández-Alemán, J. L., Señor, I. C., and Lozoya, P. Á. O. (2013). Security and privacy in electronic health records: A systematic literature review. *Journal of Biomedical Informatics*, 46(3), 541–562.

[22] Greenberg, M. (2018). The intersection of technology and healthcare ethics. *Journal of Bioethics in Technology*, 12(4), 231–256.

[23] Kluge, E. H. W., Rosenthal, M. J., and Foglia, M. B. (2021). Ethical considerations in artificial intelligence. *Annals of Internal Medicine*, 174(4), 576–578.

[24] Mittelstadt, B. D. (2019). Ethical guidelines for COVID-19 tracing apps. *Nature*, 582(7810), 29–31.

[25] Jones, B. *et al.* (2022). Ethical considerations in the use of telemedicine in mental health. *Journal of Healthcare Ethics*, 28(1), 67–82.

[26] Kasula, B. Y. (2024). Ethical implications and future prospects of artificial intelligence in healthcare: a research synthesis. *International Meridian Journal*, 6(6), 1–7.

[27] Schönberger, D. (2019). Artificial intelligence in healthcare: a critical analysis of the legal and ethical implications. *International Journal of Law and Information Technology*, 27(2), 171–203.

[28] Carter, S. M., Rogers, W., Win, K. T., Frazer, H., Richards, B., and Houssami, N. (2020). The ethical, legal and social implications of using artificial intelligence systems in breast cancer care. *The Breast*, 49, 25–32.

[29] Kälvemark, S., Höglund, A. T., Hansson, M. G., Westerholm, P., and Arnetz, B. (2004). Living with conflicts-ethical dilemmas and moral distress in the health care system. *Social Science & Medicine*, 58(6), 1075–1084.

[30] Assasi, N., Schwartz, L., Tarride, J. E., Campbell, K., and Goeree, R. (2014). Methodological guidance documents for evaluation of ethical considerations in health technology assessment: a systematic review. *Expert Review of Pharmacoeconomics & Outcomes Research*, 14(2), 203–220.

[31] Johnson, A. P., Sikich, N. J., Evans, G., *et al.* (2009). Health technology assessment: a comprehensive framework for evidence-based recommendations in Ontario. *International Journal of Technology Assessment in Health Care*, 25(2), 141–150.

[32] Kumar, R. L., Wang, Y., Poongodi, T., and Imoize, A. L. (Eds.). (2021). *Internet of Things, Artificial Intelligence and Blockchain Technology*. Cham: Springer. https://www.springer.com/gp/book/9783030741495

[33] Imoize, A. L., Adedeji, O., Tandiya, N., and Shetty, S. (2021). 6G enabled smart infrastructure for sustainable society: Opportunities, challenges, and research roadmap. *Sensors*, 21(5), 1709.

[34] Healthcare Information and Management Systems Society (HIMSS). (2021). “EHR Implementation and Data Security Guidelines.” Retrieved from https://www.himss.org/resources/ehr-implementation-and-data-security-guidelines

[35] Imoize, A. L., Hemanth, J., Do, D. T., and Sur, S. N. (Eds.). (2022). *Explainable Artificial Intelligence in Medical Decision Support Systems*. IET. https://digital-library.theiet.org/content/books/he/pbhe050e

[36] Ess, C., and Jones, S. (2004). Ethical decision-making and Internet research: Recommendations from the AOIR ethics working committee. In *Readings in Virtual Research Ethics: Issues and Controversies* (pp. 27–44). IGI Global.

Chapter 14

Securing modern insulin pumps with iCGM system: protecting patients from cyber threats in diabetes management

Lavanya Mandava[1], *Husam Ghazaleh*[2] *and Guilin Zhao*[3]

Managing diabetes is a demanding task that requires constant attention and effort. From monitoring blood glucose levels to administering insulin doses, individuals with diabetes face a daily regimen that can be particularly challenging. However, recent advancements in technology have introduced innovative solutions aimed at simplifying this process and improving the quality of life for those affected by the condition. One such advancement is the integration of continuous glucose monitoring (CGM) systems with insulin pumps, collectively known as integrated continuous glucose monitoring (iCGM) systems. These devices offer users the convenience of automated blood glucose monitoring and insulin administration, reducing the need for constant manual intervention. Moreover, modern iCGMs provide additional features such as connectivity with smart devices, allowing users to monitor their health data in real time. While these advancements undoubtedly offer numerous benefits, they also come with inherent risks, particularly concerning security vulnerabilities. The reliance on interconnected devices opens the door to potential exploitation, which could have serious consequences for individuals with diabetes. For instance, a security breach could lead to insulin overdose, resulting in severe hypoglycemia or even life-threatening complications such as severe brain injuries, coma, or even death. The architecture of iCGM systems has evolved rapidly in recent years, with a focus on compact, wearable designs that rely heavily on Bluetooth technology for connectivity. While Bluetooth provides basic security features, such as encryption, device authentication, and access control, the responsibility for implementing additional security measures such as user authentication falls on the device manufacturers. Unfortunately, this reliance on external security mechanisms and unavailable security features leaves iCGM systems vulnerable to cyber threats. Despite some efforts to address security concerns in iCGM systems,

[1]Department of Computer Science and Information Systems, Bradley University, USA
[2]Department of Computer Science, Quincy University, USA
[3]School of Computing and Artificial Intelligence, Southwest Jiaotong University, China

they have not undergone thorough scrutiny for practical implementation. Furthermore, existing recent works have not comprehensively covered all vulnerabilities, indicating a significant research gap in this area. This chapter outlines the modern architecture of insulin pumps, existing vulnerabilities, threats, and risks of iCGM systems, and provides insights on security measures, mitigation, and countermeasures. The goal is to bridge the research gap by identifying current architecture and threats while highlighting necessary security mechanisms. Furthermore, the chapter provides resources of open-source datasets for further research and testing to secure iCGM systems.

Keywords: iCGM systems; insulin pump (IP); blood glucose levels; insulin dosage; connected devices; wireless transmissions; Bluetooth; vulnerabilities; security services; security mechanisms

14.1 Introduction

Diabetes is a chronic, metabolic condition characterized by excess blood glucose levels, leading to significant damage over time to the heart, blood vessels, eyes, kidneys, and nerves [1]. Worldwide, approximately 422 million individuals suffer from diabetes [2]. In the United States, over 133 million people are affected by diabetes [3]. The three primary types of diabetes include type 1, type 2, and gestational diabetes. Type 1 diabetes is believed to result from an autoimmune reaction, where the body mistakenly attacks itself, hindering insulin (a crucial hormone for regulating blood sugar levels) production. Individuals with type 1 diabetes require daily insulin administration for survival. Type 2 diabetes occurs when the body's cells resist insulin signals and do not effectively absorb glucose from the bloodstream. Additionally, in some cases, the pancreas cannot produce sufficient amounts of insulin. Gestational diabetes occurs in pregnant women without a previous diabetes diagnosis, increasing the risk of health complications for the baby. Although gestational diabetes typically resolves after childbirth, it raises the risk of developing type 2 diabetes later in life [3]. Many individuals with advanced type 2 diabetes often require insulin supplementation [4].

Various types of insulin are available for diabetes treatment, and administration methods include injections, pumps, and inhalers. Research indicates that insulin pumps offer improved blood glucose level management with reduced insulin requirements [5]. Pumps deliver insulin more efficiently and accurately, and eliminate unpredictable effects [6]. Additionally, they provide greater flexibility in managing meals, exercise, and daily schedules, contributing to enhanced physical and psychological well-being.

A continuous glucose monitor (CGM) is used by individuals with diabetes to obtain readings at regular intervals throughout the day [7]. Typically attached to the arm or abdomen, the CGM enables real-time monitoring of glucose levels. Modern insulin pumps, equipped with integrated Continuous Glucose Monitoring Systems (iCGM), have revolutionized diabetes management [8–10]. These pumps with iCGM systems, offer features such as real-time glucose monitoring, compatibility with Bluetooth-enabled mobile apps, remote insulin dosage control, and automated insulin injection.

While these features enhance comfort and ease of use for individuals, they also introduce security concerns. Since the insulin pump relies on the iCGM for insulin dosage, securing the Bluetooth connections is of utmost importance. A breach or attack on these pumps could have serious consequences. In 2016, Johnson & Johnson, a leading vendor of insulin pump systems, issued a cautionary letter to its users, alerting them about potential vulnerabilities in the insulin pumps [11,12]. The letter raised concerns about unauthorized access and the susceptibility of the pumps to hacking.

In 2019, the U.S. Food and Drug Administration (FDA) issued a warning about certain Medtronic MiniMed insulin pumps due to cybersecurity risks, marking the first voluntary recall of a connected diabetes device for such vulnerabilities by a manufacturer [13,14]. The primary concern is the potential for hackers to wirelessly access nearby Medtronic MiniMed insulin pumps, manipulating their settings. This unauthorized access poses a risk of insulin overdose or insulin stoppage.

In 2021, Medtronic issued an update regarding a potential risk associated with the MiniMed Paradigm family of insulin pumps and their corresponding remote controllers [15]. Users were advised to immediately stop using and disconnect the remote controller. Additionally, they were instructed to disable the remote feature and return the remote controller to the company. These controllers, functioning similarly to key fobs, enable diabetes patients to self-administer insulin without physically accessing their insulin pump. A security concern was raised by an external researcher, indicating that an unauthorized individual in close proximity to the insulin pump user could capture wireless radio frequency (RF) signals emitted by the remote controller during bolus delivery [15]. These captured signals could potentially be replayed later to administer a malicious bolus to the pump user.

Identifying and addressing potential risks is crucial to safeguarding patients' health. Unauthorized access poses a significant threat, particularly in the context of insulin delivery systems, where it can lead to either excessive or insufficient insulin administration. An overdose of insulin may result in severe hypoglycemia [16], a condition associated with loss of consciousness, coma, irreversible brain injuries, or even fatality.

Conversely, the cessation of insulin delivery can trigger ketoacidosis [17], a serious complication in diabetes characterized by the excessive production of blood acids (ketones). This condition arises when there is an insufficient supply of insulin, often exacerbated by infections or other illnesses. Symptoms include thirst, frequent urination, nausea, abdominal pain, and weakness. In both cases, the patient's life is at imminent risk.

Therefore, it is imperative to intensify research efforts to address and rectify potential risks associated with insulin delivery systems. Despite the current focus on the security of medical devices, there is a noticeable gap in research pertaining to insulin pumps equipped with iCGM technology. This underscores the urgent need for comprehensive research in this specific domain to enhance the safety and reliability of insulin pumps with iCGM devices.

14.1.1 Key contributions of the chapter

The following are the significant contributions of this chapter:

(i) The chapter provides an overview of the modern architecture of insulin pumps with iCGM systems, detailing their security specifications.
(ii) An analysis of existing vulnerabilities, threats, and risks associated with iCGM systems is conducted, highlighting potential dangers and their implications.
(iii) Mitigation and countermeasures strategies are provided, emphasizing necessary security mechanisms to enhance the security of iCGM systems.
(iv) The chapter aims to bridge the research gap by identifying the current architecture and threats in iCGM systems, fostering a better understanding of their security landscape.
(v) Resources of open-source datasets are provided for further research and testing.

14.1.2 Chapter organization

Section 14.2 presents related works on cybersecurity standards, attack experiments, security issues, challenges, and research focusing on the security of insulin pumps with iCGM systems. The authors also provide their insights on existing works in this section. Section 14.3 depicts and describes the architecture of modern insulin pumps with iCGM systems. Section 14.4 provides details of iCGM Bluetooth security specifications. Section 14.5 analyzes existing vulnerabilities, threats, and associated risks of iCGM systems along with a discussion of the security challenges. Section 14.6 presents strategies for risk mitigation and countermeasures to enhance the security of iCGM systems. Section 14.7 presents a compilation of open-source datasets intended for researchers. These resources can be utilized by researchers to construct Artificial Intelligence (AI) or Machine Learning (ML) models aimed at bolstering the security of insulin pumps. Finally, Section 14.8 concludes the chapter.

14.2 Related work

This section presents a structured literature review divided into four subsections: works focusing on cybersecurity standards, studies conducting attack experiments, cybersecurity issues and challenges, and proposed approaches concerning the security of insulin pumps with iCGM systems. Following this, there is a section dedicated to the author's comments on the discussed and referenced related work.

14.2.1 Cybersecurity standards

A pivotal study by Klonoff in 2015 emphasized the necessity for a specialized set of rules (a cybersecurity standard) to protect devices that wirelessly manage diabetes [18]. These standards are crucial to ensure that the data and commands these devices handle remain private, accurate, and accessible when needed (Table 14.1).

Table 14.1 Literature review: cybersecurity standards

Paper	Year	Reference
Cybersecurity for Connected Diabetes Devices	2015	[18]
Now Is the Time for a Cybersecurity Standard for Connected Diabetes Devices	2016	[19]
Benefits of Conformity Assessment for Cybersecurity Standards of Diabetes Devices and Other Medical Devices	2021	[20]

Surprisingly, it is not just external hackers that we need to be concerned about. The study pointed out that even users themselves might attempt to extract additional information from the device beyond what it normally provides, without intervention [18]. This complexity in cybersecurity issues in healthcare technology underscores the importance of having clear and specific rules for these devices.

In response to these concerns, Klonoff and his team introduced the Diabetes Technology Society (DTS) Cybersecurity Standard, or DTSec for Connected Diabetes Devices, in 2016 [19]. This was a significant step toward establishing formal rules outlining the cybersecurity measures that these devices should adhere to. The authors argue that without such rules, the risks to patient safety increase, and the overall cost of cybersecurity across the medical device industry rises.

Underlining the significance of this effort, another study by T. Shang and colleagues in 2021 emphasized the need to verify if these cybersecurity rules are being followed [20]. They pointed out that neglecting this check in the medical device field is a missed opportunity to enhance the confidence of those who use these products.

14.2.2 Attack experiments

Li and team [21] addressed security and privacy concerns related to contemporary CGM and insulin delivery systems. The study discusses the vulnerabilities of such systems, emphasizing susceptibility to both passive and active attacks achieved through the reverse engineering of radio protocols, utilizing readily available hardware and software. Importantly, a comprehensive analysis of potential attack scenarios is presented, accompanied by the proposal of two distinct defense mechanisms.

Loboda and team [22] introduced two personalized insulin dose manipulation attacks—an overdose attack and an underdose attack. Additionally, an automated system for the detection of these intricate malicious insulin dose manipulations is designed and implemented. This detection system incorporates ML algorithms such as Logistic Regression, Random Forest, and ANN algorithms and employs advanced temporal pattern mining processes based on real data collected from insulin pumps and CGMs.

Another study [23] investigated the potential exploitation of unauthorized access to medical devices, focusing on subliminal harm inflicted on patients through alterations in clinical trials. The research delves into attacks against the performance of insulin treatments for type 1 diabetic patients over extended periods, revealing that adversaries may employ varied approaches to impact patients. The study emphasizes the risk of targeted integrity attacks leading to hypoglycemia or hyperglycemia without triggering conventional safety alerts. The results underscore the necessity for future research to prioritize the protection of drug administration processes using real-time data and patient-specific information, particularly in developing contingencies against process-aware attacks (Table 14.2).

14.2.3 Security issues and challenges

In 2011, Paul and team [24] addressed security issues in an insulin pump system, including embedded components such as the insulin pump, continuous glucose management system, blood glucose monitor, and associated devices like mobile phones or personal computers. This work aimed to bolster pump safety, focusing not only on escalating wireless communication threats in each component but also on additional threats related to availability and integrity (Table 14.3).

In review [25], the progress in Distributed Denial of Service (DDoS) attack detection using AI techniques was discussed. The features considered for detection include the number of packets, average packet size, time interval variance, packet size variance, number of bytes, packet rate, and bit rate. The recommendation is to utilize Random Forest Tree and Naive Bayes for classifying malicious and normal traffic due to their superior performance and accuracy. Additionally, the suggestion is made to combine multiple ML algorithms for enhanced accuracy and performance in detecting DDoS attacks.

Table 14.2 Literature review: attack experiments

Paper	Year	Reference
Hijacking an Insulin Pump: Security Attacks and Defenses for a Diabetes Therapy System	2011	[21]
Personalized Insulin Dose Manipulation Attack and Its Detection Using Interval-Based Temporal Patterns and Machine Learning Algorithms	2022	[22]
Process-Aware Attacks on Medication Control of Type-I Diabetics Using Infusion Pumps	2023	[23]

Table 14.3 Literature review: security issues and challenges

Paper	Year	Reference
A Review of the Security of Insulin Pump Infusion Systems	2011	[24]
DDoS Detection and Prevention Based on Artificial Intelligence Techniques	2019	[25]
Review of Security Challenges in Healthcare Internet of Things	2020	[26]

Another study [26] assessed major security issues in medical devices to identify risk factors, highlighting the insulin pump as the third most susceptible device to hijacking attacks, leading to a 45% fatality rate. The paper stated that DDoS attacks in the Internet of Medical Things (IoMTs) are more dangerous compared to other security issues. It also stated that authentication issues in wireless insulin pumps pose a significant risk at 55%.

14.2.4 Proposed security approaches

This section explores advancements in securing insulin pump systems, focusing on innovative approaches such as runtime verification, unsupervised anomaly detection, fingerprint-based security, deep learning, gesture recognition, and voiceprint-based access control (Table 14.4).

In a study by Ahmad *et al.* [27], a unique combination of deep learning and gesture recognition mechanisms was presented to secure the dosing process of insulin pumps. This approach enhances the accuracy of the dosing process and detects security attacks, showcasing the potential of advanced technologies.

Contributing to the field, Meneghetti *et al.* [28] explored unsupervised anomaly detection techniques to identify insulin pump faults. Their work aimed at improving safety in artificial pancreas systems, providing insights into detecting malfunctions through innovative algorithms, thus enhancing the overall reliability of insulin delivery.

Zheng *et al.* [29] in another study, proposed a Fingerprint-based Insulin Pump security (FIPsec) scheme. This scheme introduces a novel approach to access control by integrating a cancelable Delaunay triangle-based fingerprint matching algorithm. This extra layer of security mechanism prevents unauthorized access to the insulin pump, safeguarding it against potential serious attacks.

In a groundbreaking approach, Panda *et al.* [30] introduced the concept of runtime verification for an insulin infusion pump system using electrocardiogram (ECG) sensing. Emphasizing real-time detection of attacks on the insulin infusion system through a wearable device, this methodology represents a significant step forward in ensuring the integrity and safety of insulin delivery processes.

Table 14.4 Literature review: proposed security approaches

Paper	Year	Reference
Securing Insulin Pump System Using Deep Learning and Gesture Recognition	2018	[27]
Detection of Insulin Pump Malfunctioning to Improve Safety in Artificial Pancreas Using Unsupervised Algorithms	2019	[28]
Fingerprint Access Control for Wireless Insulin Pump Systems Using Cancelable Delaunay Triangulations	2019	[29]
A Secure Insulin Infusion System Using Verification Monitors	2021	[30]

14.2.5 Author's comments

All the works discussed above have demonstrated significant efforts in addressing the security issues of insulin pumps with iCGM, proposing valuable suggestions based on their findings. However, these recommendations or proposed works have not undergone thorough scrutiny for implementation. Considering the risk factors and the potential damage that could occur without proper studies, it is imperative to categorize the security areas that need attention for insulin pumps with iCGM.

More work is needed in this regard. Some of the proposed works and recommendations are over a decade old, and since then, the system components have undergone substantial changes. The latest proposed works lack sufficient study or verification with other algorithms. These critical issues must be addressed to ensure the effectiveness and reliability of security measures for insulin pumps with iCGM.

14.3 General architecture of modern insulin pump with iCGM system

Figure 14.1 depicts the architecture of a modern insulin pump featuring iCGM. The iCGM system consists of a sensor and a transmitter, typically placed on the arm or abdomen of the patient, continuously monitoring blood glucose levels and providing real-time or on-demand readings customizable to the user's preference. These readings are transmitted wirelessly to the Insulin Pump (IP) via Bluetooth.

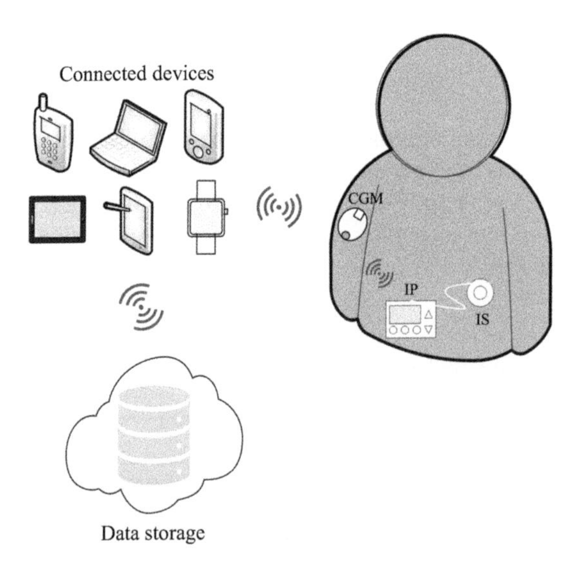

Figure 14.1 Insulin pump with iCGM

The IP, worn externally and powered by a battery, resembles a compact device similar to a small cell phone. It includes a reservoir for storing insulin, which is delivered through tubing to an infusion set (IS) attached to the body, usually in the stomach area or back of the upper arm. The IS delivers insulin through a thin plastic tube inserted semi-permanently into the subcutaneous fatty layer. Most insulin pumps administer insulin through tubing such as Medtronic Minimed 770G [31], Medtronic Minimed 780G [32], T:slimX2 [33], and Dana Diabecare IIS [34]. A few like Omnipod [35] administer insulin through a tubeless insulin pump called a Pod as shown in Figure 14.2.

Utilizing the readings provided by the iCGM, the IP calculates the necessary insulin dosage for the user at any given time, which is then administered via the reservoir-connected tubing. There are two main types of iCGM-insulin pump combinations: open-loop and closed-loop systems.

In an open-loop system, the user manually instructs the insulin pump based on iCGM readings, while a closed-loop system enables the pump to respond directly to iCGM readings without human intervention. These integrated systems have been demonstrated to deliver insulin more accurately, requiring less insulin dosage overall to maintain blood glucose levels, and offering greater flexibility in managing meals, exercise, and daily schedules, leading to potential improvements in both physical and psychological well-being.

Various additional accessories such as pump clips, activity guards, and skins enhance the accessibility of insulin pumps with iCGM, particularly for users like

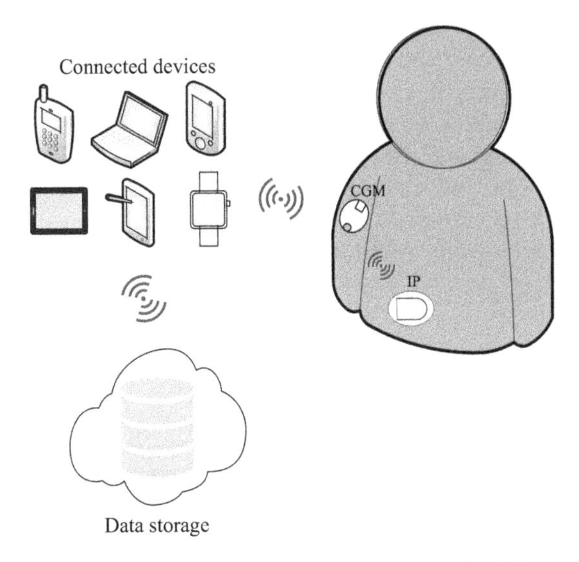

Figure 14.2 Tubeless insulin pump with iCGM

children and athletes. However, our focus remains solely on the primary architecture, without considering these supplementary accessories.

The iCGM's transmitter also enables wireless connectivity with various devices such as smartphones, Personal Diabetes Manager (PDM) devices, tablets, computers, and watches. These devices can further connect to or transmit readings to remote databases, such as hospital or cloud databases, facilitating user tracking, doctor review, and hospital record maintenance. The database serves to compile and organize the collected readings for analysis and reference.

14.4 iCGM Bluetooth security specifications

The evolution of iCGM technology has been closely intertwined with advancements in wireless communication, particularly Bluetooth technology [36]. In modern iCGM systems, transmitters play a crucial role in relaying data to users, employing Bluetooth 4.0 and later versions for connectivity. Notably, transmitters are designed with backward compatibility, ensuring seamless integration with existing devices.

Beyond the transmission of glucose readings, iCGM transmitters fulfill additional functions vital for seamless operation. This includes connection establishment and bond management tasks. Bond management encompasses actions such as removing connected devices and managing errors, ensuring the reliability of the system.

Utilizing Bluetooth 4.0 or later, iCGM devices and connected peripherals may operate in "dual mode," supporting both Basic Rate/Enhanced Data Rate (BR/EDR) and Bluetooth Low Energy (LE) [37]. While BR/EDR is utilized for bond management and primary functions, LE is favored for its low power consumption, making it ideal for continuous monitoring applications.

The specifications of Bluetooth BR/EDR and LE versions shown in Tables 14.5 and 14.6 delineate key features and improvements over time. For instance, BR/EDR in versions 4.0 and earlier supported a limited number of active and total piconet (a group of Bluetooth-connected devices) slaves, employing

Table 14.5 Bluetooth BR/EDR specifications

Characteristic	Version 4.0 and earlier	Versions 4.1, 4.2
Piconet slaves active	7	7
Piconet slaves total	255	255
Pairing algorithms	P-192 Elliptic Curve, HMAC-SHA-256	P-256 Elliptic Curve, HMAC-SHA-256
Encryption algorithms	E0/SAFER+	AES-CCM
Authentication algorithms	E1/SAFER	HMAC-SHA-256

Table 14.6 Bluetooth LE specifications

Characteristic	Version 4.1 and earlier	Version 4.2
Piconet slaves active	Unlimited	Unlimited
Piconet slaves total	Unlimited	Unlimited
Pairing algorithms	AES-128	P-256 Elliptic Curve, AES-CMAC
Encryption algorithms	AES-CCM	AES-CCM
Authentication algorithms	AES-CCM	AES-CCM

encryption and authentication algorithms tailored to that era's security standards. In contrast, subsequent versions like 4.1 and 4.2 expanded these capabilities, enabling unlimited active and total piconet slaves in LE mode while enhancing security through advanced algorithms such as AES-CCM and HMAC-SHA-256.

The concept of a piconet, comprising interconnected Bluetooth devices operating within proximity, is fundamental to iCGM systems. For instance, a piconet could be established between a PDM and the iCGM, facilitating seamless data exchange.

Bluetooth LE specifications evolved to support enhanced security and scalability. Version 4.1 and earlier iterations provided robust encryption and authentication algorithms like AES-128 and AES-CCM, while version 4.2 introduced further enhancements, including the adoption of P-256 Elliptic Curve and AES-CMAC for improved security measures.

14.5 iCGM system vulnerabilities, threats, and risks

14.5.1 Bluetooth vulnerabilities

The vulnerabilities in Bluetooth versions 4.0, 4.1, and 4.2, which are commonly used in iCGMs, are of particular concern. While older versions have additional vulnerabilities, this section focuses on these versions as they are prevalent in iCGM systems. It is important to note that the vulnerabilities, threats, and solutions discussed here apply not only to iCGMs with insulin pumps but also to any iCGM systems.

One significant vulnerability lies in bypassing authentication keys or being susceptible to Man-In-The-Middle (MITM) attacks. This occurs when connected devices share piconets or are paired with other devices. For instance, if a mobile phone connected to an iCGM is also connected to a headset, there is potential for the headset, lacking a keyboard or display, to join the same piconet without authentication. This opens up the possibility for other users or devices to be added to the piconet via these unauthenticated connections, making them vulnerable to MITM attacks, particularly in devices operating in LE mode.

Another concern involves the encryption algorithm used in the Bluetooth version 4.0 in BR/EDR mode. This mode of 4.0 uses the E0 stream cipher, which is considered relatively weak. Issues with backward compatibility further compound security challenges. When connecting to devices using older Bluetooth versions, iCGMs may need to compromise on certain security features, such as repeatable authentication attempts and a lack of waiting time for authentication challenge requests. This allows attackers to collect numerous challenge responses and conduct cryptanalysis to uncover the secret link key.

Additionally, all Bluetooth versions typically provide only device authentication without user authentication, and there is a lack of end-to-end security in terms of encryption and authentication. Bluetooth offers limited security services, including Data Confidentiality, Data Integrity, and Device Authentication. However, Bluetooth BR/EDR lacks device address privacy, while Bluetooth LE provides it through the use of Random Private addresses to protect device identity and prevent tracking by malicious third parties.

Notably, security services such as audits and non-repudiation are not part of the Bluetooth standard, further underscoring the need for robust security measures in iCGM systems beyond what Bluetooth alone can provide.

Exploitation of any such vulnerabilities by potential attackers may lead to severe loss. iCGM users blindly trust their devices for insulin dosage calculation and delivery. Any manipulation in dosage can have adverse effects and may also lead to death.

14.5.2 Other vulnerabilities

In addition to the vulnerabilities discussed in Section 14.5.1, iCGM systems face additional security challenges and vulnerabilities related to the transmission of data to remote database servers via connected devices. This data typically includes blood glucose readings, insulin dosages, and other relevant information intended for medical professionals, particularly doctors, to review.

These wireless connections pose risks to the security of the stored data on remote database servers, necessitating robust security measures to mitigate potential breaches or unauthorized access. While immediate health impacts may not be evident from these vulnerabilities, they could potentially affect future treatments based on the stored information.

14.5.3 Security challenges

Despite recent efforts to address security concerns in iCGM systems, such as proposals utilizing ML algorithms, these recommendations have not undergone thorough scrutiny for practical implementation. One major obstacle is the lack of comprehensive testing and validation of security algorithms specifically tailored for iCGM systems. Furthermore, existing works have not comprehensively covered all vulnerabilities, indicating a significant research gap in this area.

The rapid pace of technological advancement has outpaced the development of robust security protocols, leaving iCGM systems susceptible to emerging threats. Hardware limitations also pose challenges, as the compact nature of wearable devices may restrict the implementation of sophisticated security measures.

Moreover, the scarcity of clinical or trusted datasets necessary for testing these security algorithms further impedes progress in developing effective solutions. Although Section 14.7 provides some open-source datasets, the insufficient data for testing remains a significant challenge in enhancing the security of iCGM systems. These datasets ought to be utilized to build ML models aimed at safeguarding patients against abnormal insulin dosage calculations stemming from external attacks.

14.6 Enhancing security in iCGM systems: risk mitigation and countermeasures

This section explores key strategies for mitigating risks and implementing countermeasures to enhance the security of iCGM systems.

First and foremost, establishing robust foundational security measures is essential. This involves providing comprehensive security training to iCGM users and medical personnel, including doctors, nurses, and other staff with access to patient data. It is imperative to offer awareness-based education on the latest vulnerabilities and best practices. This fosters a culture of security consciousness, empowering stakeholders to effectively identify and mitigate potential threats. Training programs should be designed and structured to cater to different ages, backgrounds, and levels of technology literacy.

Addressing specific vulnerabilities inherent in Bluetooth-enabled devices is crucial. The Bluetooth specification lacks a mechanism to prevent unlimited authentication requests, leaving devices vulnerable to brute-force attacks. Implementing an exponentially increasing waiting interval between successive authentication challenge requests and upgrading to stronger encryption algorithms, such as Bluetooth 4.1 and above, bolster the security of communication channels. Additionally, enforcing user authentication at the application layer and ensuring end-to-end encryption prevent unauthorized access and data interception.

Mitigating the risk of MITM attacks during device pairing is paramount. Devices should incorporate MITM protection mechanisms and refuse unauthenticated link keys generated from non-keyboard devices. Employing unique, regularly changing key pairs and random passkeys for each pairing attempt enhances cryptographic resilience and mitigates the risk of unauthorized access.

Furthermore, minimizing exposure to potential adversaries is essential. Devices should be paired in secure environments to mitigate the risk of eavesdropping and MITM attacks. Devices operating in discoverable or connectable modes should limit exposure duration to reduce the window of opportunity for malicious actors.

Moreover, while audit and non-repudiation services are not inherent in the standard Bluetooth protocol, they can be implemented as overlay services by application developers. Incorporating these services enhances accountability and facilitates forensic analysis in the event of security incidents.

In conclusion, safeguarding the security and privacy of iCGM systems demands a multi-faceted approach encompassing user education, technological enhancements, and stringent security protocols. By implementing robust risk mitigation strategies and countermeasures, stakeholders can fortify the resilience of iCGM systems against evolving cyber threats, ensuring the integrity and confidentiality of user data.

14.7 Utilizing machine learning for enhanced security in iCGM systems: leveraging open-source datasets and architectural adaptations

This section emphasizes an additional strategy for safeguarding iCGM systems with insulin pumps using ML algorithms. Table 14.7 lists repositories that offer open-source datasets related to insulin pumps, blood glucose levels, iCGM, insulin levels, and insulin secretion in patients across various daily activities. These datasets contain diverse information, including insulin pump data, iCGM readings, and specifics about insulin administration through closed-loop systems. They serve as valuable resources for researchers aiming to develop predictive models to thwart potential attacks on insulin pumps. Notably, these datasets are relatively scarce [38].

These datasets will be leveraged to develop ML models intended to shield patients from abnormal insulin dosage calculations resulting from external attacks. Moreover, the fundamental architecture of IP and iCGM systems might undergo slight modifications to integrate these models. For instance, the IP may need to verify the validity of calculations by consulting the model. If discrepancies arise, the IP must notify the patient, who then must decide whether to approve or reject the calculated insulin dosage.

The DiaTrend dataset [38] includes iCGM and insulin pump data from 54 patients diagnosed with type 1 diabetes. The OhioT1DM dataset [39] provides 8 weeks' worth of data for each of the 12 individuals with type 1 diabetes it covers. Additionally, Anderson *et al.* [40] contributed a dataset comprising data collected over various phases, with each phase spanning 2 weeks, for 29 individuals with type 1 diabetes. Notably, all individuals in these datasets were undergoing insulin pump therapy with iCGM. The datasets includes insulin pumps that transmit life-event data via a custom smartphone application.

Moreover, Meneghetti *et al.* [28] introduced a dataset generated artificially using the Padova/UVA simulator, a popular diabetes simulator. This dataset contains simulated pump faults, offering insights into potential system failures and their impact on insulin delivery.

Table 14.7 Literature review: datasets

Dataset	Year	Reference
DiaTrend	2023	[31]
The OhioT1DM	2020	[32]
Anderson *et al.*	2018	[33]
Meneghetti *et al.*	2019	[34]

14.8 Conclusion

The integration of CGM devices with insulin pumps and various smart devices introduces security vulnerabilities, necessitating a thorough examination of technological and architectural changes and their associated risks. This chapter delves into the contemporary architecture of insulin pumps equipped with iCGM systems that establish wireless connections to smart devices. It outlines the features of iCGM systems and their current security specifications, followed by an analysis of existing vulnerabilities, threats, and associated risks, highlighting potential dangers and their consequences. Exploitation of these vulnerabilities can lead to severe consequences such as insulin overdose or underdose, posing risks of organ damage, seizures, unconsciousness, coma, or even death. To address these risks, the chapter provides strategies for mitigation, countermeasures, and essential security mechanisms aimed at enhancing the security of iCGM systems.

Given the recent incidents involving attacks on insulin pumps, emphasizing the importance of addressing current security needs is paramount. As the field of security is dynamic and constantly evolving, identifying and addressing new security requirements becomes increasingly challenging yet essential. This chapter addresses this gap in security research concerning iCGM systems and advocates for further exploration of future research avenues. Furthermore, the chapter provides resources, including open-source datasets, to facilitate the development of AI or ML models aimed at enhancing the security of insulin pumps. By shedding light on emerging research ideas and security aspects that demand attention, this chapter catalyzes advancing the understanding and fortification of iCGM system security.

References

[1] K. Kaul, J. M. Tarr, S. I. Ahmad, E. M. Kohner, and R. Chibber, "Introduction to Diabetes Mellitus," *Diabetes, Advances in Experimental Medicine and Biology*, vol. 771, pp. 1, Springer, New York, NY, 2013, doi:10.1007/978-1-4614-5441-0_1.

[2] World Health Organization, "Report of the WHO discussion group for people living with diabetes: virtual meeting, 30–31 March 2023," Geneva, Switzerland: World Health Organization, 2023. [Online]. Available: https://www.who.int/publications/i/item/9789240081451. Accessed: Feb. 15, 2024. [License: CC BY-NC-SA 3.0 IGO].

[3] Centers for Disease Control and Prevention, "Diabetes Basics," [Online]. Available: https://www.cdc.gov/diabetes/basics/index.html. Reviewed: Oct. 25, 2022. Accessed: Feb. 15, 2024.

[4] R. Kumar, P. Saha, Y. Kumar, S. Sahana, A. Dubey, and O. Prakash, "A Review on Diabetes Mellitus: Type1 and Type2," *World Journal of Pharmacy and Pharmaceutical Sciences*, vol. 9, no. 10, pp. 838–850, 2020, doi:10.20959/wjpps202010-17336.

[5] J. Kesavadev, B. Saboo, M. B. Krishna, and G. Krishnan, "Evolution of Insulin Delivery Devices: From Syringes, Pens, and Pumps to DIY Artificial Pancreas," *Diabetes Therapy*, vol. 11, pp. 1251–1269, 2020, doi:10.1007/s13300-020-00831-z.

[6] K. Ahmad, "Insulin Sources and Types: A Review of Insulin in Terms of Its Mode on Diabetes Mellitus," *Journal of Traditional Chinese Medicine*, vol. 34, no. 2, pp. 234–237, 2014, doi:10.1016/s0254-6272(14)60084-4.

[7] G. Freckmann, "Basics and Use of Continuous Glucose Monitoring (CGM) in Diabetes Therapy," *Journal of Laboratory Medicine*, vol. 44, no. 2, pp. 71–79, 2020, doi:10.1515/labmed-2019-0189.

[8] T. Martens, R. W. Beck, R. Bailey, *et al.*, "Effect of Continuous Glucose Monitoring on Glycemic Control in Patients with Type 2 Diabetes Treated with Basal Insulin: A Randomized Clinical Trial," *JAMA*, vol. 325, no. 22, pp. 2262–2272, 2021, doi:10.1001/jama.2021.7444.

[9] A. Haskova, L. Radovnicka, L. Petruzelkova, *et al.*, "Real-time CGM Is Superior to Flash Glucose Monitoring for Glucose Control in Type 1 Diabetes: The CORRIDA Randomized Controlled Trial," *Diabetes Care*, vol. 43, no. 11, pp. 2744–2750. 2020, doi:10.2337/dc20-0112.

[10] R. M. Bergenstal, D. M. Mullen, E. Strock, M. L. Johnson, and M. X. Xi, "Randomized Comparison of Self-monitored Blood Glucose (BGM) versus Continuous Glucose Monitoring (CGM) Data to Optimize Glucose Control in Type 2 Diabetes," *Journal of Diabetes Complications*, vol. 36, no. 3, pp. 108106, 2022, doi:10.1016/j.jdiacomp.2021.108106.

[11] L. Pycroft, and T. Z. Aziz, "Security of Implantable Medical Devices with Wireless Connections: The Dangers of Cyber-attacks," *Expert Review of Medical Devices*, vol. 15, no. 6, pp. 403–406, 2018, doi:10.1080/17434440.2018.1483235.

[12] D. Klonoff, and J. Han, "The First Recall of a Diabetes Device Because of Cybersecurity Risks," *Journal of Diabetes Science and Technology*, vol. 13, no. 5, pp. 817–820, 2019, doi:10.1177/1932296819865655.

[13] G. E. Hempel, "Do No Harm: Medical Device and Connected Hospital Security," In *Women Securing the Future with TIPPSS for Connected Healthcare: Trust, Identity, Privacy, Protection, Safety, Security*, pp. 49–61, Cham: Springer International Publishing, 2022.

[14] Food and Drug Administration (FDA), "Cybersecurity," Published: Dec. 29, 2022. [Online]. Available: https://www.fda.gov/medical-devices/digital-health-center-excellence/cybersecurity. Accessed: January 10, 2024.

[15] Security Bulletin, Medtronic Minimed MMT-500/MMT-503 Remote Controllers, Updated: Oct. 5, 2021. [Online]. Available: https://global.medtronic.com/xg-en/product-security/security-bulletins/minimed.html. Accessed: Feb. 15, 2024.

[16] S. Rzepczyk, K. D. Kaczmarek, A. Urusk, and C. Zaba, "The Other Face of Insulin-Overdose and Its Effects," *Toxics*, vol. 10, no. 3, p. 123, 2022, doi:10.3390/toxics10030123.

[17] B. Long, S. Lentz, A. Koyfman, and M. Gottlieb, "Euglycemic Diabetic Ketoacidosis: Etiologies, Evaluation, and Management," *The American*

Journal of Emergency Medicine, vol. 44, pp. 157–160, 2021, doi:10.1016/j.ajem.2021.02.015.

[18] D. C. Klonoff, “Cybersecurity for Connected Diabetes Devices,” *Journal of Diabetes Science and Technology*, vol. 9, no. 5, pp. 1143–1147, 2015. doi:10.1177/1932296815583334.

[19] D. C. Klonoff, and D. N. Kleidermacher, “Now Is the Time for a Cybersecurity Standard for Connected Diabetes Devices,” *Journal of Diabetes Science and Technology*, vol. 10, no. 3, pp. 623–626, 2016, doi:10.1177/1932296816647516.

[20] T. Shang, J. Y. Zhang, J. Dawson, and D. C. Klonoff, “Benefits of Conformity Assessment for Cybersecurity Standards of Diabetes Devices and Other Medical Devices,” *Journal of Diabetes Science and Technology*, vol. 15, no. 4, pp. 727–732, 2021, doi:10.1177/19322968211018186.

[21] C. Li, A. Raghunathan, and N. K. Jha, “Hijacking an Insulin Pump: Security Attacks and Defenses for a Diabetes Therapy System,” in *2011 IEEE 13th International Conference on e-Health Networking, Applications and Services*, Columbia, MO, USA, 2011, pp. 150–156, doi:10.1109/HEALTH.2011.6026732.

[22] T. L. Loboda, E. Sheetrit, I. F. Liberty, A. Haim, and N. Nissim, “Personalized Insulin Dose Manipulation Attack and Its Detection Using Interval-based Temporal Patterns and Machine Learning Algorithms,” *Journal of Biomedical Informatics*, vol. 132, pp. 104129, 2022, doi:10.1016/j.jbi.2022.104129.

[23] G. Stergiopoulos, P. Kotzanikolaou, C. Konstantinou, and A. Tsoukalis, “Process-Aware Attacks on Medication Control of Type-I Diabetics Using Infusion Pumps,” *IEEE Systems Journal*, vol. 17, no. 2, pp. 1831–1842, 2023, doi:10.1109/JSYST.2023.3236690.

[24] N. Paul, T. Kohno, and D. C. Klonoff, “A Review of the Security of Insulin Pump Infusion Systems,” *Journal of Diabetes Science and Technology*, vol. 5, no. 6, pp. 1557–1562, 2011, doi:10.1177/193229681100500632.

[25] D. Glavan, C. Racuciu, R. Moinescu, and N. F. Antonie, “DDoS Detection and Prevention Based on Artificial Intelligence Techniques,” *Scientific Bulletin of Naval Academy*, vol. 22, pp. 134–143, 2019, doi:10.21279/1454-864X-19-I1-018.

[26] R. Somasundaram, and M. Thirugnanam, “Review of Security Challenges in Healthcare Internet of Things,” *Wireless Networks*, vol. 27, pp. 5503–5509, 2021, doi:10.1007/s11276-020-02340-0.

[27] U. Ahmad, H. Song, A. Bilal, S. Saleem, and A. Ullah, “Securing Insulin Pump System Using Deep Learning and Gesture Recognition,” in *2018 17th IEEE International Conference on Trust, Security and Privacy in Computing and Communications/12th IEEE International Conference on Big Data Science and Engineering (TrustCom/BigDataSE)*, pp. 1716–1719, 2018, doi:10.1109/TrustCom/BigDataSE.2018.00258.

[28] L. Meneghetti, G. A. Susto, and S. D. Favero, “Detection of Insulin Pump Malfunctioning to Improve Safety in Artificial Pancreas Using Unsupervised Algorithms,” *Journal of Diabetes Science and Technology*, vol. 13, no. 6, pp. 1065–1076, 2019, doi:10.1177/1932296819881452.

[29] G. Zheng *et al.*, "Fingerprint Access Control for Wireless Insulin Pump Systems Using Cancelable Delaunay Triangulations," *IEEE Access*, vol. 7, pp. 75629–75641, 2019, doi:10.1109/ACCESS.2019.2920850.

[30] A. Panda, S. Pinisetty, and P. Roop, "A Secure Insulin Infusion System Using Verification Monitors," in *19th ACM-IEEE International Conference on Formal Methods and Models for System Design (MEMOCODE'21)*, 2021, doi:10.1145/3487212.3487342.

[31] Medtronic, "Medtronic MiniMed 770G System User Guide," [Online]. Available: https://www.medtronicdiabetes.com/sites/default/files/library/download-library/user-guides/MiniMed_770G_System_User_Guide.pdf. Accessed: Feb. 15, 2024.

[32] Medtronic, "Medtronic MiniMed 780G System User Guide," [Online]. Available: https://www.medtronicdiabetes.com/sites/default/files/library/download-library/user-guides/MiniMed-780G-system-user-guide-with-Guardian-4-sensor.pdf. Accessed: Feb. 15, 2024.

[33] Tandem Diabetes Care, "t:slimX2 User Guide," [Online]. Available: https://www.tandemdiabetes.com/docs/default-source/user-guide/aw-1007704_b-user-guide-mobile-bolus-tslim-x2-control-iq-7-6-mgdl-artwork-weba4e76d9775426a79a519ff0d00a9fd39.pdf?sfvrsn=18a507d7_231. Accessed: Feb. 15, 2024.

[34] SOOIL, "Dana Diabecare IISR User Manual," [Online]. Available: https://fcc.report/FCC-ID/VF9DANAIIS/821784.pdf. Accessed: Feb. 15, 2024.

[35] Insulet Corporation, "Omnipod 5 User Guide," [Online]. Available: https://www.omnipod.com/sites/default/files/Omnipod-5_User-guide.pdf. Accessed: Feb. 15, 2024.

[36] Bluetooth Special Interest Group (SIG), "Continuous Glucose Monitoring Profile 1.0.2," [Online] Available: https://www.bluetooth.com/specifications/specs/continuous-glucose-monitoring-profile-1-0-2/. Accessed: Feb. 15, 2024.

[37] NIST SP 800-121 Rev. 2, "Guide to Bluetooth Security," Updated: Jan. 19, 2022, [Online]. Available: https://doi.org/10.6028/NIST.SP.800-121r2-upd1. Accessed: Feb. 15, 2024.

[38] T. Prioleau, A. Bartolome, R. Comi, and C. Stanger, "DiaTrend: A Dataset from Advanced Diabetes Technology to Enable Development of Novel Analytic Solutions," *Scientific Data*, vol. 10, no. 1, p. 556, 2023, doi:10.1038/s41597-023-02469-5.

[39] C. Marling, and R. Bunescu, "The OhioT1DM Dataset for Blood Glucose Level Prediction: Update 2020," *CEUR Workshop Proceedings*, vol. 2675, pp. 71–74, 2020.

[40] Jaeb Center for Health Research, "Pilot Study 3 of Outpatient Control-to-Range: Safety and Efficacy with Day-and-Night In-Home Use (CTR3)," [Online] Available: https://clinicaltrials.gov/study/NCT02137512. Accessed: Feb. 15, 2024.

Chapter 15

Artificial intelligence and machine learning for DNS traffic anomaly detection in modern healthcare systems

Sarafudheen Muzaliamveettil Tharayil[1], *Abdullah Saeed Al-Ahmari*[1], *Abdallah Mohammad Baabdallah*[1] *and Uma Madesh*[2]

Domain Name System (DNS) is a critical component of the Internet infrastructure, responsible for resolving human-readable domain names into machine-readable IP addresses. However, DNS is also vulnerable to various types of attacks, such as denial-of-service, cache poisoning, domain hijacking, and malicious domain generation. These attacks can compromise the availability, integrity, and confidentiality of the DNS service and the network applications that rely on it. Therefore, it is essential to detect and mitigate DNS anomalies in a timely and accurate manner. One of the domains where artificial intelligence (AI) can play a crucial role in anomaly detection is DNS traffic. This chapter aims to provide an overview of the role of AI in DNS anomaly detection and to introduce the main AI techniques used in this field. By diving into the different studies and papers across the relevant contribution, this review chapter contributes by explaining the multifaceted landscape of the role of AI and machine learning (ML) in DNS traffic anomaly detection in modern healthcare systems It is trying to bridge knowledge gaps, weave together diverse perspectives, and offer a strong reference to navigate the field. In addition, the discussions in the chapter are bridging the gap to practice, translating insights into recommendations that are practical and can be implemented for tackling real-world scenarios. With critical questions and promising avenues for future research laid bare, this review serves as a foundation for advancing knowledge and shaping the future of AI, DNS, and the security of modern healthcare systems.

Keywords: Domain name systems (DNS); artificial intelligence; machine learning; anomaly detection, healthcare systems

[1]Saudi Aramco, Dhahran, Saudi Arabia
[2]Vidhya Nikethan Intel Public School, Sri Sakthi Institute of Engineering and Technology, Coimbatore, India

15.1 Introduction

The chapter introduces the concept of anomaly detection and explains its importance for various domains and applications. It discusses how AI can enhance anomaly detection performance and efficiency and presents some benefits and challenges of using AI for anomaly detection. Additionally, the chapter focuses on the role of AI in DNS anomaly detection and provides a detailed description of DNS anomalies, their impact on network security and performance, and how AI can help identify, classify, and mitigate them. The chapter also draws parallels with the healthcare domain, where anomaly detection can be used to diagnose and treat diseases and disorders. Moreover, it reviews the main AI techniques used in anomaly detection and explains how they can be applied to DNS anomaly detection, covering supervised learning, unsupervised learning, and semi-supervised learning methods, with examples and applications of each method. Following this, the chapter discusses recent developments in anomaly detection, such as the introduction of new datasets and methods. It also covers advancements in security models for DNS tunnel detection, a technique used by attackers to hide malicious data or commands in DNS traffic. Furthermore, the chapter explores innovations in anomaly detection using big data and ML, technologies that enable faster and more accurate analysis of large and complex data. In the same vein, the chapter describes progress in real-time detection techniques for DNS exfiltration and tunneling, methods used by attackers to steal or transfer sensitive data through DNS traffic. It then addresses the difficulties of identifying the scarcity of realistic and labeled DNS datasets as one of the main challenges and limitations of anomaly detection in DNS traffic, explaining why such datasets are difficult to obtain and use. Similarly, challenges in detecting encrypted DNS traffic are discussed, which is a technique used by legitimate users or applications to protect their privacy and security, but also by attackers to evade detection and analysis. Moreover, the chapter highlights the difficulties in detecting low-rate and distributed DNS attacks, types of attacks that use low volumes or frequencies of DNS traffic, or multiple sources or destinations, to avoid raising suspicion or triggering alarms. Finally, it addresses issues with false positives and false negatives in anomaly detection, errors that occur when an AI model incorrectly classifies a normal event as an anomaly or an anomaly as a normal event, respectively.

15.2 Artificial intelligence in anomaly detection

Anomaly detection is the process of finding patterns or events that deviate from the normal or expected behavior in a given dataset or system. Anomaly detection has many applications in various domains, such as cybersecurity, fraud detection, healthcare, industrial monitoring, and more. Anomaly detection can help identify potential threats, errors, faults, or opportunities for improvement in complex and dynamic environments. AI is a branch of computer science that aims to create machines or systems that can perform tasks that normally require human intelligence, such as reasoning, learning, decision-making, and problem-solving. AI can enhance anomaly detection performance and efficiency by providing scalable, adaptive, and robust solutions that can handle large and heterogeneous data, learn from feedback, and cope with uncertainty and noise.

15.2.1 What is anomaly detection and why is it important?

Anomaly detection is a fascinating field that focuses on finding patterns in data that do not conform to expected behavior. These non-conforming patterns, also known as anomalies, outliers, or exceptions, are often associated with problematic conditions or interesting events. For instance, an anomaly in credit card transaction data could indicate fraudulent activity.

Let's break it down further. Imagine you're a college student working part-time and managing your expenses with a credit card. You have a general idea of your spending habits—maybe you use your card for groceries, books, and the occasional treat. One day, you notice several high-priced items on your statement—purchases you don't recall making. This is where anomaly detection comes into play. Your bank, if it employs an anomaly detection system, can spot these unusual transactions as anomalies. These transactions deviate from your typical spending pattern, which makes them stand out. The system can then alert you to these suspicious activities, allowing you to take immediate action, such as blocking your card or reporting the issue to the bank. This example illustrates the importance of anomaly detection in our daily lives. It's not just about detecting fraud; anomaly detection systems are used in various fields and industries.

In computer networks, for example, anomaly detection plays a crucial role in maintaining security. It can help identify unusual network traffic patterns that could indicate a cyberattack or system compromise. A sudden increase in data transfer from a specific device might be an anomaly indicating that the device has been infected with malware. In Figure 15.1, we can see an example of data outliers that

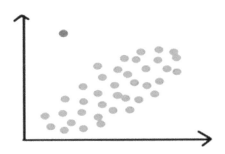

Figure 15.1 Example of data outlier [1]

shows the red point away from the clustering of the green points. The red point in this scenario would be considered an outlier or anomalous [1].

In healthcare, anomaly detection can be used to spot abnormal patterns in patient vital signs. These could be early warning signs of potential health issues. For instance, an unexpected increase in a patient's heart rate might be an anomaly that points to a possible heart condition. In essence, anomaly detection is about spotting the unexpected in data and alerting the relevant parties. It's a powerful tool that can prevent damage, save resources, and even save lives by identifying potential problems early on.

Whether it's safeguarding your credit card transactions from fraudsters, protecting computer networks from cyber threats, or monitoring patient health for early signs of disease, anomaly detection has a significant role to play. Its ability to spot anomalies in real-time allows for swift action to prevent further damage or loss [2].

Anomaly detection is an essential tool in data analysis that helps maintain safety and efficiency across various fields and industries. By identifying deviations from the norm, it allows us to spot potential problems early on and take appropriate action.

15.2.2 How AI can enhance anomaly detection performance and efficiency

AI has revolutionized many fields, including anomaly detection. Its ability to process and learn from large volumes of data quickly and accurately makes it a powerful tool for enhancing anomaly detection performance and efficiency.

Anomaly detection involves identifying data points or patterns that deviate significantly from the expected or "normal" behavior. These deviations, known as anomalies, can often indicate critical incidents, such as fraud in credit card transactions, faults in machines, or intrusions in network security. AI can significantly enhance the efficiency of this process. AI algorithms are capable of processing large volumes of data much faster than human analysts could. This speed is crucial in situations where timely anomaly detection can prevent significant damage or loss.

Moreover, AI models, especially those based on ML, can be trained to recognize complex patterns and dependencies in data. This ability allows them to detect anomalies that might be missed by traditional, rule-based systems, thereby increasing the accuracy of anomaly detection. Another advantage of AI is its adaptability. Unlike traditional systems that rely on predefined rules for detecting anomalies, AI models can learn from new data and adapt their anomaly detection strategies over time. This adaptability is particularly useful in dynamic environments where the definition of "normal" behavior can change rapidly.

AI also offers scalability, an essential feature in today's data-driven world. With the increasing volume and velocity of data generated by modern IT systems and IoT devices, it's crucial for anomaly detection systems to handle this growth without degrading performance. AI's ability to learn from large datasets ensures that its performance doesn't degrade as data grows. AI's ability to predict future anomalies based on historical data patterns is another significant advantage. This predictive capability enables proactive measures to prevent potential issues before they occur.

False positives, i.e., instances where normal behavior is incorrectly flagged as an anomaly, are a common challenge in anomaly detection. Through continuous learning and adjustment, AI can reduce the number of false positives, thereby improving the reliability of anomaly detection. In some cases, AI can not only detect anomalies but also initiate automated responses to mitigate their impact. For instance, in network security, an AI system could automatically block traffic from a source identified as anomalous.

AI brings a host of benefits to anomaly detection—from improving efficiency and accuracy to offering adaptability and scalability. Its ability to reduce false positives and initiate automated responses further enhances its value. By leveraging AI, organizations can significantly improve their ability to detect and respond to anomalies, thereby preventing potential damage and ensuring smooth operations.

15.3 Understanding the role of AI in DNS anomaly detection

What are DNS anomalies and how do they affect network security and performance?

15.3.1 What are DNS anomalies?

The Domain Name System (DNS) is a critical component of internet infrastructure, translating human-readable domain names into numerical IP addresses that computers use to communicate. As in Figure 15.2, the user is browsing Google.com and in the background the computer will query DNS for the IP address. After that, communication will be established using the IP addresses [3].

Like any system, DNS is not immune to anomalies or irregularities. DNS anomalies refer to patterns or activities in DNS traffic that deviate from what is considered normal. These anomalies can take various forms. For instance, a DNS query might contain invalid type or class values, or the Time to Live (TTL) value

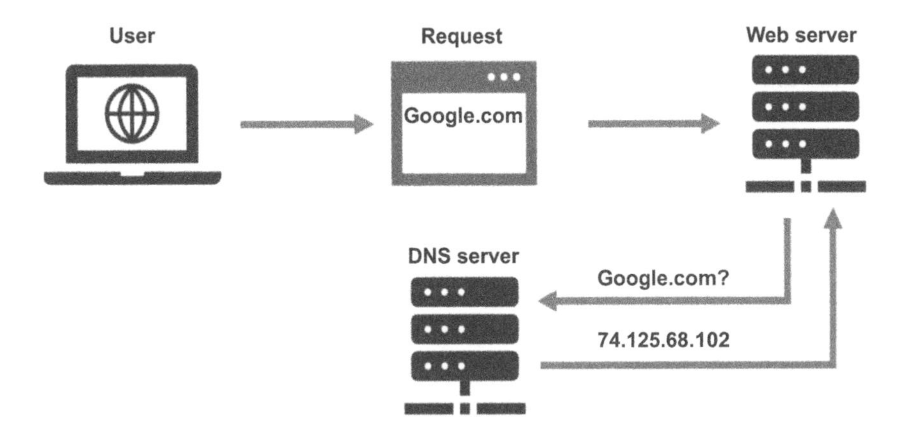

Figure 15.2 DNS protocol [2]

might be excessively long. Another example is a query or response packet containing excess data after valid DNS data, or a query/response with a null DNS name [4–6].

15.3.2 How do DNS anomalies affect network security and performance?

DNS anomalies can have significant implications for both network security and performance. From a security perspective, certain types of DNS anomalies can be indicative of malicious activities. For example, DNS Amplification and Reflection Attacks use open resolvers to increase the volume of an attack and hide its true source. This can result in Denial of Service (DoS) and Distributed Denial of Service (DDoS) attacks. Another type of attack, known as Resource Utilization Attack, tries to consume all available resources to negatively impact the operations of the open resolver. These attacks not only compromise the security of the network but can also disrupt its performance. Malware, for instance, can slow network speeds and disable devices and nodes installed on your network [4,7].

15.3.3 Parallels with healthcare

Interestingly, there are parallels between network security and healthcare when it comes to dealing with anomalies. In healthcare, anomaly detection is used to identify unusual patterns in patient vital signs, which could be early indicators of health issues. Similarly, in network security, anomaly detection identifies unusual traffic patterns that could indicate a cyberattack. Just as healthcare providers use advanced endpoint security platforms to validate patient data integrity and self-heal endpoint security, network administrators use AI and ML techniques to enhance anomaly detection performance and efficiency. Moreover, both fields face similar challenges. In healthcare, false positives (where a healthy patient is incorrectly identified as having a disease) can lead to unnecessary treatments and patient anxiety. Similarly, in network security, false positives (where normal network behavior is incorrectly flagged as an anomaly) can lead to unnecessary investigations and system downtime. DNS anomalies are irregularities in DNS traffic that deviate from the norm. They can significantly impact network security and performance by facilitating malicious activities and disrupting normal operations. The parallels between network security and healthcare highlight the universal importance of effective anomaly detection in maintaining system integrity and performance [8–10].

15.3.4 How AI can help identify, classify, and mitigate DNS anomalies

AI can help identify, classify, and mitigate DNS anomalies in the following ways:

- **Identify**: AI can use ML techniques to analyze DNS traffic and detect patterns that deviate from normal behavior. AI can also use historical data to learn the baseline of normal DNS activity and compare it with current data to identify anomalies.
- **Classify**: AI can use supervised or unsupervised learning methods to classify DNS anomalies into different types or categories, such as amplification

attacks, resource utilization attacks, malware infections, or configuration errors. AI can also use natural language processing to extract relevant information from DNS logs and provide context for the anomalies.

- **Mitigate**: AI can use reinforcement learning or rule-based systems to initiate appropriate actions to mitigate the impact of DNS anomalies. For example, AI can block malicious traffic, isolate infected devices, alert network administrators, or suggest solutions.

These are some of the ways that AI can enhance the process of detecting and dealing with DNS anomalies. By using AI, network administrators can improve their ability to protect and maintain their network systems.

15.4 AI techniques used in anomaly detection

15.4.1 Supervised learning: using labeled data to train AI models for anomaly detection

Supervised learning is a type of ML where an AI model is trained on a labeled dataset. In the context of anomaly detection, this means the model is provided with examples of both normal and anomalous data points so that it can learn to distinguish between the two [11,12].

One of the most popular applications of supervised learning in anomaly detection is the use of Support Vector Machines (SVMs). SVMs are frequently applied to classification problems, including anomaly detection. They work by finding the hyperplane that maximizes the margin between different classes of data points in a high-dimensional space. In the case of anomaly detection, these classes would be "normal" and "anomalous" data points. Another supervised learning technique used in anomaly detection is ensemble tree models, such as XGBoost. These models work by combining the predictions of multiple decision tree models to make a final prediction. They are particularly effective for anomaly detection because they can capture complex patterns and interactions in the data [11].

Deep learning models, such as Long Short-Term Memory (LSTM) networks, can also be used for anomaly detection. LSTM networks are a type of recurrent neural network that is capable of learning long-term dependencies in sequential data. This makes them well-suited for detecting anomalies in time-series data, such as network traffic logs or sensor readings. Autoencoders, a type of neural network, are another tool that can be used for anomaly detection. An autoencoder is trained to reconstruct its input data. During training, the autoencoder learns to encode the "normal" data points in a way that it can reconstruct them accurately. Then, when it encounters an anomalous data point, it will struggle to reconstruct it accurately, resulting in a high reconstruction error. This high reconstruction error can then be used as an indicator of an anomaly [11].

While supervised learning techniques can be very effective for anomaly detection, they do require labeled data for training. This means that you need examples of both normal and anomalous data points. Collecting and labeling this data can be a significant challenge, especially in domains where anomalies are rare or hard to define. However, once you have a labeled dataset, supervised learning techniques can provide several benefits. For one, they can result in more accurate and reliable anomaly detection models compared to unsupervised techniques. This is because they can learn directly from examples of anomalies, rather than having to infer what constitutes an anomaly based on the normal data points alone. Furthermore, supervised learning models can provide more interpretable results compared to unsupervised models. Because they are trained on labeled data, they can provide predictions that are directly tied to the labels in the training data. This means you can get a clear indication of whether a new data point is considered normal or anomalous according to the model [11–13].

Supervised learning provides powerful tools for anomaly detection. By training on labeled data, models can learn to accurately identify and classify anomalies. However, collecting and labeling this data can be challenging. Despite this challenge, the benefits of increased accuracy and interpretability make supervised learning an attractive option for many anomaly detection tasks.

15.4.2 Unsupervised learning: using unlabeled data to discover anomalies with AI models

Unsupervised learning is a branch of ML that deals with data that has not been labeled, classified, or categorized. Unlike supervised learning, where the model learns from a labeled dataset, unsupervised learning works with raw, unlabeled data. This approach is particularly useful in anomaly detection, where labeled data may be scarce or unavailable. In the context of anomaly detection, unsupervised learning algorithms are used to identify unusual patterns or outliers in the data. These algorithms work by learning the underlying structure of the data and then identifying data points that do not conform to this structure [14,15].

One common approach in unsupervised learning for anomaly detection is clustering. Clustering algorithms group similar data points together based on their distance in the feature space. Anomalies are typically data points that do not fit well into any of the clusters. Another approach is dimensionality reduction. Dimensionality reduction techniques, such as Principal Component Analysis (PCA) or autoencoders, transform the data into a lower-dimensional space. In this transformed space, anomalies often appear as data points that are far from most of the data [14].

Deep learning-based autoencoders have been particularly effective for anomaly detection. An autoencoder is a type of neural network that is trained to reconstruct its input data. During training, the autoencoder learns to encode the "normal" data points in a way that it can reconstruct them accurately. Then, when it encounters an anomalous data point, it will struggle to reconstruct it accurately, resulting in a high reconstruction error. This high reconstruction error can then be used as an indicator of an anomaly. Generative Adversarial Networks (GANs) are another powerful tool for anomaly detection. GANs consist of two neural networks: a generator that produces synthetic data, and a discriminator that tries to distinguish between real and synthetic data. In the context of anomaly detection, GANs can be trained on normal data and then used to generate new, synthetic normal data. Anomalies can then be detected as data points that the discriminator classifies as real with high confidence, but that are significantly different from the synthetic normal data produced by the generator [15].

Despite their potential, unsupervised learning techniques for anomaly detection also have their challenges. One major challenge is determining what constitutes an anomaly in the absence of labeled data. Another challenge is dealing with the high dimensionality of the data, which can make it difficult to visualize and interpret the results [14,16].

Unsupervised learning provides powerful tools for anomaly detection. By using unlabeled data to discover anomalies with AI models, we can overcome some of the limitations of supervised learning techniques and open up new possibilities for detecting and understanding anomalies in complex datasets.

15.4.3 Semi-supervised learning: combining labeled and unlabeled data to improve AI models for anomaly detection

Semi-supervised learning is a ML paradigm that leverages both labeled and unlabeled data during the training process. This approach is particularly beneficial in scenarios where obtaining labeled data is costly or time-consuming, such as in anomaly detection [17].

Semi-supervised learning can be highly effective. Anomalies are typically rare events, and therefore, it can be challenging to obtain sufficient labeled data for these events. By using both labeled and unlabeled data, semi-supervised learning can overcome this challenge and improve the performance of anomaly detection models. One common approach in semi-supervised learning for anomaly detection is to train a model on the labeled data (normal and anomalous instances) and then use this model to label the unlabeled data. The newly labeled data can then be used to retrain the model, improving its ability to detect anomalies. Another approach is to use the labeled data to learn a representation of the normal instances and then use this representation to score the unlabeled instances. Instances that deviate significantly from the normal representation are considered anomalies [18,19].

Deep learning techniques, such as autoencoders and GANs, can also be used in a semi-supervised manner for anomaly detection. For instance, an autoencoder can be trained on normal instances (labeled data) to learn a representation of the normal data. It can then score the unlabeled instances based on how well they fit this representation. Instances that do not fit well (i.e., that the autoencoder struggles to reconstruct) are considered anomalies. Similarly, a GAN can be trained on normal instances to generate synthetic normal data. The discriminator of the GAN, which is trained to distinguish between real and synthetic data, can then be used to score the unlabeled instances. Instances that the discriminator classifies as real with high confidence but that are significantly different from the synthetic normal data are considered anomalies [18,19].

Table 15.1 Comparing different ML mechanisms in DNS anomaly detection

Available technique	Summary of solution	Type of machine learning	Open challenges	Main features
SVM	A widely used classification method for anomaly detection that can handle linear and non-linear data	Supervised	Data scarcity, high dimensionality, non-linearity	Finds the optimal hyperplane that separates normal and anomalous data points
LOF	A density-based method for anomaly detection that can identify local outliers in complex data	Unsupervised	Parameter selection, noise sensitivity, scalability	Measures the local density deviation of a data point from its neighbors
LSTM	A deep learning method for anomaly detection that can capture temporal patterns and anomalies in time-series data	Supervised	Data scarcity, high complexity, interpretability	A type of recurrent neural network that can learn long-term dependencies in sequential data
GAN	A generative method for anomaly detection that can produce synthetic normal data and detect anomalies based on the discriminator's output	Unsupervised or semi-supervised	Mode collapse, training instability, evaluation difficulty	A type of neural network that consists of a generator and a discriminator that compete with each other

Despite their potential, semi-supervised learning techniques for anomaly detection also have their challenges. One major challenge is determining what constitutes an anomaly in the absence of sufficient labeled data. Another challenge is dealing with the high dimensionality of the data, which can make it difficult to visualize and interpret the results [20,21].

Semi-supervised learning provides powerful tools for anomaly detection. By leveraging both labeled and unlabeled data, these techniques can overcome some of the limitations of supervised and unsupervised learning techniques and open up new possibilities for detecting and understanding anomalies in complex datasets (Table 15.1).

15.5 Recent developments

15.5.1 Introduction of new datasets and methods for anomaly detection

There have been significant advancements in this area, particularly in the introduction of new datasets and methods for anomaly detection. These developments are paving the way for more effective and efficient detection of DNS anomalies, thereby enhancing the overall security of the internet.

One of the key developments is the introduction of a new labeled flow-based DNS dataset for anomaly detection, known as the PUF Dataset. This dataset is unique because it contains real and labeled DNS flows from a university campus network. This means that the data in the dataset closely mirrors the kind of DNS traffic that would be seen in a real-world scenario, making it an invaluable resource for researchers and cybersecurity professionals. The PUF dataset can be used to detect compromised hosts and sub-networks, providing a powerful tool for identifying potential security threats [22].

In addition to new datasets, there have also been advancements in the methods used for anomaly detection. One such method is a new, principled approach to anomaly detection. This approach defines an anomaly as an event with low probability and high impact. It uses probability theory to detect anomalies across different data sources, providing a more rigorous and robust method for identifying potential threats. Another significant development is the application of big data techniques to anomaly detection. By analyzing large volumes of DNS traffic, it is possible to identify patterns and trends that may indicate a potential security threat. For example, one approach uses three clustering algorithms: K-means, Self-Organizing Maps (SOMs), and Gaussian Mixture Model (GMM) to detect anomalous and suspicious patterns in DNS traffic [23].

ML is also being used to detect abnormal DNS traffic. Techniques such as K-means, GMM, Density-Based Spatial Clustering of Applications with Noise (DBSCAN), and Local Outlier Factor (LOF) are being applied to identify outliers in DNS traffic. These techniques can be particularly effective at detecting more subtle or complex anomalies that may be missed by other methods. Finally, there is the development of DNS-ADVP, a ML anomaly detection and visual platform designed to protect top-level domain name servers against DDoS attacks. This platform combines a visualization model and a ML algorithm to detect and mitigate DNS DDoS attacks on authoritative servers. This represents a significant step forward in the protection of critical internet infrastructure [24,25].

The recent developments in DNS anomaly detection represent significant advancements in the field of cybersecurity. The introduction of new datasets and methods for anomaly detection is enhancing our ability to detect and mitigate potential security threats, thereby making the internet a safer place for everyone.

15.5.2 Advancements in security models for DNS tunnel Detection

Due to DNS ubiquitous nature and lack of inherent security mechanisms, DNS has become a popular vector for cyberattacks. One such attack is DNS tunneling, where malicious actors use DNS queries and responses to covertly send data across a network. Detecting these tunnels is a challenging task, but recent advancements in security models have made significant strides in this area. As shown in Figure 15.3,

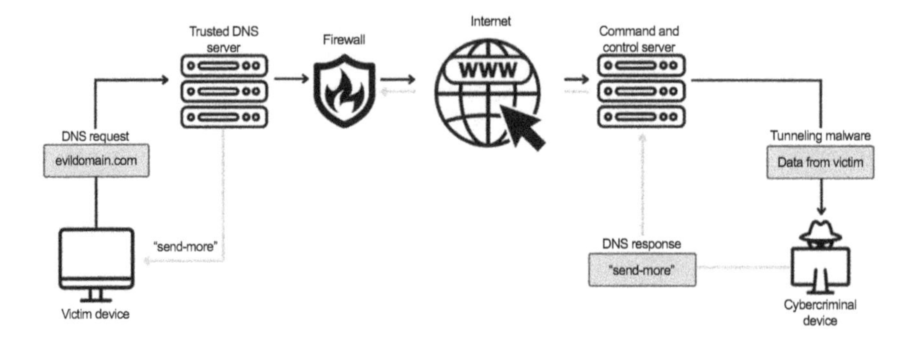

Figure 15.3 DNS tunneling [26]

the attacker would register its own domain on the internet and is expecting the victim that had been infected to query the malicious domain. Once the victim queries the malicious domain through the trusted DNS servers, the tunnel is established which can be used to exfiltrate data or for other malicious purposes [26].

One of the key advancements is the development of a security model for DNS tunnel detection on cloud platforms. As more organizations move their operations to the cloud, the need for robust security measures in these environments has become increasingly apparent. This model leverages the scalability and flexibility of cloud platforms to monitor DNS traffic and detect potential tunnels. It uses ML algorithms to analyze DNS query patterns and identify anomalies that may indicate a tunnel. This approach not only enhances the detection capabilities but also reduces the computational overhead, making it a viable solution for large-scale cloud environments. Another significant development is the application of big data analytics in DNS tunnel detection. With the exponential growth of internet traffic, traditional detection methods often struggle to keep up with the sheer volume of data. However, by applying big data analytics, it is possible to process and analyze large datasets in real time. This allows for more timely detection of DNS tunnels, thereby minimizing the potential damage caused by these attacks [27].

ML techniques have also been employed to improve DNS tunnel detection. These techniques can learn from past DNS traffic patterns and adapt to new and evolving threats. For instance, supervised learning algorithms can be trained on labeled datasets to classify DNS queries as either normal or anomalous. On the other hand, unsupervised learning algorithms can detect outliers in the DNS traffic, which may indicate a potential tunnel. The use of ML not only enhances detection accuracy but also enables the system to adapt to the ever-evolving threat landscape. In addition to these advancements, there has also been progress in the visualization of DNS traffic. Visualization tools can provide a graphical representation of DNS traffic, making it easier for security analysts to spot potential anomalies. These tools can also incorporate ML algorithms to automatically highlight potential threats, thereby reducing the manual effort required in the detection process [24].

The recent advancements in security models for DNS tunnel detection represent a significant step forward in the fight against DNS-based cyberattacks. By leveraging the power of cloud computing, big data analytics, ML, and visualization tools, these models provide a more effective and efficient means of detecting DNS tunnels. However, as the threat landscape continues to evolve, ongoing research and development in this area remain crucial.

15.5.3 Innovations in anomaly detection using big data and machine learning

The advent of big data and ML has brought about significant innovations in the field of anomaly detection. These technologies have enabled the development of more sophisticated and effective methods for identifying and mitigating potential threats in various domains, including cybersecurity, healthcare, finance, and more.

Big data refers to the vast amounts of data generated every second from various sources, such as social media, sensors, machines, and more. This data is characterized by its volume, velocity, variety, veracity, and value, collectively known as the 5Vs of big data. The sheer size and complexity of big data present unique challenges in terms of storage, processing, and analysis. However, it also provides unprecedented opportunities for extracting valuable insights and detecting anomalies that would otherwise go unnoticed. One of the key innovations in anomaly detection using big data and ML is the ability to process and analyze large volumes of data in real time. Traditional anomaly detection methods often struggle to keep up with the sheer volume and velocity of big data. However, by leveraging big data technologies such as Hadoop and Spark, it is now possible to process and analyze data at scale in near real-time. This allows for more timely detection of anomalies, thereby enabling quicker response and mitigation. The combination of big data and ML has also enabled the development of more robust and adaptive anomaly detection systems. These systems can learn and evolve with the data, allowing them to adapt to new and emerging threats. For instance, they can use reinforcement learning to continuously improve their detection performance based on feedback from the environment [28].

The innovations in anomaly detection using big data and ML represent a significant leap forward in our ability to detect and mitigate potential threats. However, as the volume and complexity of data continue to grow, ongoing research and development in this area are crucial to keep up with the evolving threat landscape.

15.5.4 Progress in real-time detection techniques for DNS exfiltration and tunneling

Recent advancements in real-time detection techniques for DNS exfiltration and tunneling have leveraged ML algorithms to differentiate between normal and anomalous

DNS requests. These techniques analyze stateless attributes extracted from DNS queries, such as query names, lengths, and frequencies. By employing algorithms like Isolation Forest, researchers have developed systems capable of identifying suspicious DNS activities with high accuracy and low false alarm rates. These systems have been evaluated using live traffic streams from operational networks, demonstrating their effectiveness in detecting injected malicious queries [28].

One notable contribution to this field is the development of DNS-ADVP, a ML anomaly detection and visual platform designed to protect top-level domain name servers against DDoS attacks. This platform integrates visualization models and one-class classifiers to continuously learn typical traffic patterns and alerts upon detecting anomalies. The architecture of DNS-ADVP has been tested using artificial attacks, yielding promising results in terms of classification accuracy [25].

Another significant advancement is the proposal of a hierarchical anomaly-based detection system for distributed DNS attacks on enterprise networks. This system employs a dynamic graph structure to monitor DNS activity at various levels, including host, subnet, and autonomous system. The approach has been validated using both benign and synthetic attack traffic, achieving detection accuracies exceeding 99% [29].

Furthermore, researchers have explored the use of deep learning models for generalized classification of DNS over HTTPS (DoH) traffic. These models aim to distinguish between benign and malicious DoH traffic, addressing the challenges posed by encrypted DNS requests. The use of LSTM and Bi-directional LSTM models has shown effectiveness in classifying DoH traffic with high accuracy and low latency [30].

The progress in real-time detection techniques for DNS exfiltration and tunneling is marked by the integration of ML and deep learning algorithms into detection systems. These systems can analyze vast amounts of DNS traffic in real time, distinguishing between legitimate and malicious activities. As cyber threats continue to evolve, further research is necessary to enhance the detection capabilities and adapt to new attack patterns.

15.5.5 Safeguarding healthcare data and systems using anomaly detection

Healthcare organizations juggle the critical responsibility of safeguarding sensitive patient data while maintaining reliable and accessible systems. Traditional security measures are often overwhelmed by the evolving sophistication of cyberattacks, necessitating the adoption of proactive and innovative approaches. In this context, DNS anomaly detection emerges as a promising tool to strengthen healthcare cybersecurity.

Addressing the security challenges of smart healthcare systems (SHSs) is another area of focus. A paper presents HealthGuard, a data-driven security framework that uses ML to detect malicious activities in SHSs. HealthGuard monitors the vital signs of different connected devices in an SHS and correlates them to understand the changes in body functions of the patient and distinguish benign and malicious activities [31].

In the realm of healthcare IoT systems, a significant body of work has been dedicated to the development of efficient anomaly detection frameworks. One such study proposes a novel framework that utilizes a combination of deep learning and optimization techniques for detecting anomalies in data collected from healthcare devices. This framework aims to improve the quality, reliability, efficiency, and security of IoT services, and its performance has been evaluated using a disease dataset [32].

In parallel, there has been considerable interest in the use of DNS traffic monitoring techniques for protecting Internet of Healthcare Things (IoHT) networks from various attacks. A survey paper reviews various methods and tools for DNS traffic monitoring and evaluates them based on factors such as scalability, accuracy, security, ease of use, integration, and cost. As shown in Figure 15.4, the chapter suggests utilizing an architecture with a four-layer approach: sensors gather data, a network transmits it, a middle layer analyzes and prepares it (located in gateways or the cloud), and the topmost application layer houses various IoT applications accessible to user programs in the cloud. This layered approach promotes modularity, scalability, and efficient data flow, making it a robust and flexible foundation for IoT implementations. In addition, the paper also explores the potential of AI techniques for enhancing DNS traffic monitoring in IoHT networks [33].

The importance of anomaly detection in IoT healthcare analytics has been highlighted. Anomaly detection can aid in early diagnosis and prevention of diseases, as well as improving the quality and affordability of healthcare services. Future research directions using AI techniques for anomaly detection have also been suggested. These studies collectively contribute to the ongoing efforts to enhance the security and efficiency of healthcare IoT systems [34]. leveraging DNS anomaly detection offers a valuable addition to the healthcare cybersecurity arsenal. By

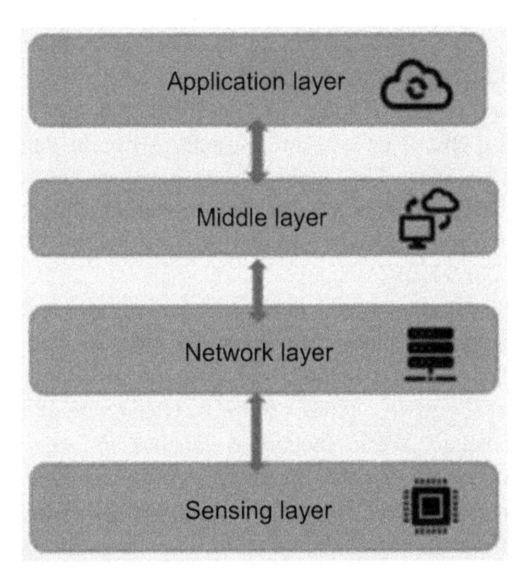

Figure 15.4 IoHT-layered architecture

analyzing the fundamental layer of network communication, healthcare organizations can gain valuable insights into potential threats targeting their sensitive data and systems. Recent research demonstrates the promising results of DNS-based anomaly detection in healthcare, providing evidence for its potential to safeguard patient information and ensure the uninterrupted operation of critical healthcare systems. However, careful implementation and integration with existing security measures are essential to maximize the effectiveness of this approach while ensuring data privacy and regulatory compliance. Moving forward, continuous research and development efforts are needed to refine DNS anomaly detection algorithms and optimize their application in the ever-evolving healthcare cybersecurity landscape.

15.6 Challenges and limitations

15.6.1 Scarcity of realistic and labeled DNS datasets

The scarcity of realistic and labeled DNS datasets poses a significant challenge in the field of DNS attack detection. This issue has far-reaching implications for both research and practical applications in DNS security.

The lack of realistic DNS data is a major hurdle. Most existing DNS datasets are either synthetic, outdated, or incomplete, limiting the applicability and validity of detection methods. For instance, Sharma *et al.* point out that available flow-based DNS datasets often lack typical traffic, DNS flows, or plausible scenarios [35]. Similarly, Ahmed *et al.* note that public DNS datasets fail to reflect the diversity and complexity of real-world DNS traffic [36].

The absence of labeled DNS data further compounds the problem. Most existing DNS datasets are either unlabeled or poorly labeled, hindering the development and evaluation of detection methods. DNS dataset labeling often relies on unreliable sources, such as blacklists or heuristics, which may introduce errors and biases. In addition, DNS dataset labeling is often done manually, which can be time-consuming and inconsistent [37,38].

The implications of this scarcity are manifold. For one, the lack of realistic DNS data makes it difficult to test and compare different detection methods in a fair and consistent manner. This lack of data hampers the ability to accurately assess the performance of various detection methods. Furthermore, the lack of labeled DNS data makes it challenging to train and validate ML models for DNS anomaly detection [24,39,40].

In addition to these challenges, the dynamic nature of DNS traffic adds another layer of complexity. DNS traffic patterns can change rapidly, making it difficult for static models to keep up. This necessitates the use of adaptive models that can learn and evolve with the changing traffic patterns. Moreover, the increasing use of encrypted DNS traffic presents another challenge. While encryption enhances privacy and security, it also makes it harder to analyze DNS traffic for anomalies. This necessitates the development of new techniques that can detect anomalies in encrypted DNS traffic [40,41].

The scarcity of realistic and labeled DNS datasets poses significant challenges in DNS attack detection. Overcoming these challenges requires concerted efforts from researchers and practitioners alike. This includes the creation of more realistic and well-labeled DNS datasets, the development of adaptive models that can handle the dynamic nature of DNS traffic, and the invention of new techniques for analyzing encrypted DNS traffic. By addressing these challenges, we can enhance the security of DNS and make the internet a safer place for everyone.

15.6.2 Challenges in detecting encrypted DNS traffic

The detection of encrypted DNS traffic, such as DoH and DNS over TLS (DoT), presents a unique set of challenges. These protocols were developed to enhance user privacy and security by encrypting plaintext DNS, thereby preventing eavesdropping and manipulation of DNS data by man-in-the-middle attacks. However, this encryption also poses significant hurdles for network administrators and security analysts [42].

One of the primary challenges is the lack of visibility into the DNS traffic. Encrypted DNS traffic prevents network operators from inspecting or filtering DNS queries and responses. This lack of visibility can pose security risks as it can potentially allow malicious activities to go undetected. For instance, attackers can use these protocols to bypass enterprise firewalls and exfiltrate private data through the establishment of DNS tunnels [40,42].

Another challenge is the complexity of analyzing encrypted DNS traffic. Since the traffic is encrypted, it requires additional steps and tools to decrypt and analyze it. This can increase the computational cost and latency of detection. Moreover, traditional DNS tunnel detection methods based on packet inspection are no longer applicable because of DNS encryption. The diversity of sources from which encrypted DNS traffic can originate also adds to the challenge. Encrypted DNS traffic can come from various sources, such as browsers, applications, operating systems, or devices. This diversity can make it difficult to identify and isolate malicious traffic. Furthermore, encrypted DNS traffic can use different techniques to evade detection. For example, it can change ports, domains, or servers, or use obfuscation or tunneling methods. This makes the detection even more challenging [40,42].

Despite these challenges, researchers have been exploring various methods to detect anomalies in encrypted DNS traffic. For instance, some studies propose using ML techniques to automatically learn feature representations and detect anomalies via reconstruction error. While encrypted DNS protocols like DoH and DoT enhance user privacy and security, they also present significant challenges in detecting malicious activities. Overcoming these challenges requires the development of new techniques and tools that can effectively analyze encrypted DNS traffic and detect anomalies. By doing so, we can ensure the security of DNS and protect users from potential threats [40].

15.6.3 Difficulties in detecting low-rate and distributed DNS attacks

Detecting low-rate and distributed DNS attacks presents a unique set of challenges. These types of attacks are particularly insidious because they are designed to fly under the radar, making them difficult to detect and mitigate. Low-rate DNS attacks involve sending intermittent bursts of malicious traffic at a rate that is low enough to avoid detection by traditional security measures. Because the traffic volume is low, these attacks can easily blend in with normal network traffic, making them hard to distinguish from legitimate DNS queries. Distributed DNS attacks, on the other hand, involve multiple compromised systems (often part of a botnet) targeting a single system. The distributed nature of these attacks makes it difficult to identify a single source of the attack, further complicating detection efforts [29].

One of the main challenges in detecting these types of attacks is the lack of effective detection methods. Traditional detection methods, such as threshold-based detection, are often ineffective against low-rate and distributed attacks. These attacks can easily evade detection by staying below the detection threshold or by distributing the attack traffic across multiple sources [29].

The dynamic nature of DNS traffic also poses a challenge. The constantly changing traffic patterns can make it difficult for static detection models to keep up. This necessitates the use of adaptive models that can learn and evolve with the changing traffic patterns. Despite these challenges, researchers have been exploring various methods to detect low-rate and distributed DNS attacks. For instance, some studies propose using ML techniques to automatically learn feature representations and detect anomalies via reconstruction error. Other studies suggest analyzing the communication behavior of the IPs to infer service intentions [29].

While low-rate and distributed DNS attacks pose significant challenges in terms of detection, ongoing research and advancements in ML and anomaly detection hold promise for the development of more effective detection methods. However, it is clear that a multi-faceted approach that includes not only advanced detection methods but also robust security policies and practices will be necessary to effectively combat these types of attacks [29].

15.6.4 Issues with false positives and false negatives in anomaly detection

Anomaly detection in DNS traffic is a critical task for maintaining network security, as it helps identify potential threats and breaches. However, one of the significant challenges in this domain is the issue of false positives and false negatives. False positives occur when benign activities are incorrectly flagged as anomalies, leading to unnecessary alerts and potential disruption of legitimate operations. Conversely, false negatives represent actual anomalies that go undetected, allowing malicious activities to persist undeterred.

The occurrence of false positives can be attributed to the dynamic nature of DNS traffic, where legitimate variations in patterns may be mistaken for anomalies. For instance, a sudden increase in DNS requests could be a sign of a DDoS attack or simply a spike in legitimate user activity. ML models, such as those based on clustering algorithms like K-means, SOMs, and GMM, are employed to discern these patterns. However, the effectiveness of these models can be hindered by the inherent noise and variability in the data, leading to a higher rate of false positives [23].

On the other hand, false negatives pose a severe threat to network security, as they allow malicious activities to go unnoticed. This can occur due to the sophisticated techniques employed by attackers, such as the use of Domain Generation Algorithms (DGAs) or DNS tunneling, which can mimic normal traffic patterns. ML techniques, including unsupervised methods like DBSCAN and LOF, are utilized to detect such sophisticated attacks. However, the challenge lies in the model's ability to learn and adapt to the evolving tactics of attackers, which requires continuous updating and tuning of the algorithms [24].

To address these challenges, researchers have proposed various solutions, such as the development of hierarchical anomaly-based detection systems that monitor DNS activity at multiple levels, including host, subnet, and autonomous system (AS). These systems aim to identify critical properties that can signal unusual behavior and reduce the incidence of false negatives. Additionally, the implementation of ML models that can automatically learn feature representations, such as those based on variational autoencoders (VAEs), offers a promising direction for reducing false positives by focusing on reconstruction errors rather than preset attributes [40].

While ML provides powerful tools for anomaly detection in DNS traffic, the issues of false positives and false negatives remain significant challenges. Ongoing research and development of more sophisticated models and techniques are essential for improving the accuracy and reliability of anomaly detection systems (Table 15.2).

Table 15.2 Summary of the issues and challenges and their impact

Challenge/Issue	**Explanation**	**Impact**
Scarcity of Realistic and Labeled DNS Datasets	Refers to the lack of DNS datasets that can capture the diversity and complexity of DNS traffic and anomalies.	Hindering the development and evaluation of anomaly detection methods and models.
Challenges in Detecting Encrypted DNS Traffic	Refers to the difficulties in analyzing and filtering DNS traffic that is encrypted using protocols like DoH and DoT.	Reduces the visibility and control of network operators and security analysts over DNS traffic.
Difficulties in Detecting Low-Rate and Distributed DNS Attacks	Refers to the problems in identifying DNS attacks that are designed to evade detection by sending intermittent or distributed bursts of malicious traffic.	Attacks can blend in with normal traffic and cause significant damage.
Issues with False Positives and False Negatives in Anomaly Detection	Refers to the errors in anomaly detection that occur when benign activities are flagged as anomalies (false positives) or when actual anomalies are missed (false negatives).	These errors can affect the accuracy and reliability of anomaly detection systems.

15.7 Multi-model approaches and future direction

Anomaly detection for DNS is an important and challenging task that aims to identify and mitigate various types of attacks that target or exploit the DNS service. Some of the future directions of anomaly detection for DNS are:

- Developing more realistic and labeled DNS datasets that can capture the diversity and complexity of DNS traffic and anomalies. Such datasets can help evaluate and compare different anomaly detection methods and improve their performance and generalization.
- Designing more robust and adaptive AI models that can handle the challenges and limitations of anomaly detection in DNS traffic, such as data scarcity, encryption, low-rate and distributed attacks, and false positives and false negatives.
- Integrating more domain knowledge and human feedback into the anomaly detection process, such as using expert rules, active learning, or explainable AI techniques. This can help enhance the accuracy, interpretability, and usability of the anomaly detection models.

Neural networks, multi-model, and generative AI are some of the technologies that can be used to enhance the anomaly detection capabilities for DNS. Some of the benefits and applications of these technologies are:

- Neural networks can learn complex and high-dimensional patterns from DNS traffic data and detect anomalies based on the reconstruction error, the prediction error, or the adversarial loss. Different types of neural networks, such as convolutional, recurrent, or attention-based, can be used to capture the spatial, temporal, or contextual features of DNS traffic.
- Multi-model can combine different types of data sources or models to improve anomaly detection performance and robustness. For example, multi-model can fuse the DNS traffic data with other network data, such as IP flows or packets, to obtain a more comprehensive view of the network behavior. Alternatively, multi-model can ensemble different anomaly detection models, such as generative, discriminative, or hybrid, to leverage their strengths and reduce their weaknesses.
- Generative AI can simulate the normal distribution of DNS traffic data and generate synthetic data for minor or rare anomalies. This can help address the data imbalance problem and improve anomaly detection performance. Generative AI can also be used to generate adversarial examples or perturbations to test the robustness and security of the anomaly detection models.

15.8 Implementation framework in healthcare systems

Based on the different studies and contributions in the field, the framework shown in Figure 15.5 summarizes the collective knowledge and expertise, outlining a multi-pronged approach to building robust defenses, from crafting diverse datasets to

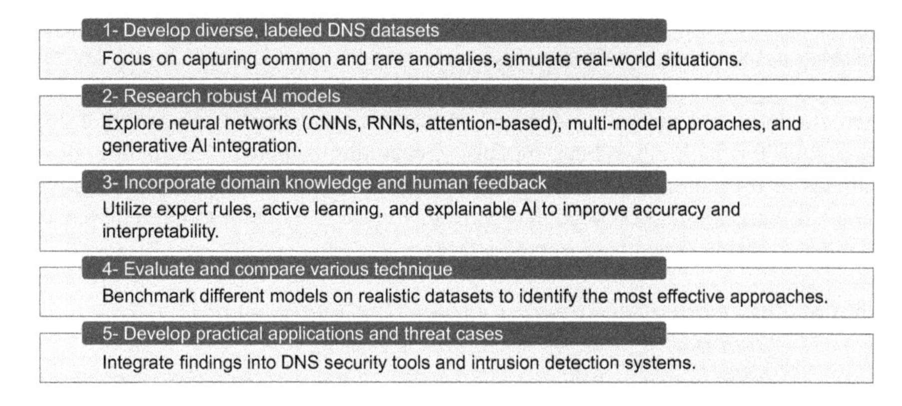

Figure 15.5 Summary of the implementation framework steps

unleashing the power of AI and human-in-the-loop insights. This shall help healthcare to increase cybersecurity level and maturity by utilizing DNS anomaly detection as the digital detective that keeps our systems healthy, both physically and digitally.

15.8.1 Building diverse, labeled DNS datasets

The foundation of robust anomaly detection lies in accurate and diverse data. Healthcare systems must collaborate with cybersecurity experts to identify common and rare DNS-based attacks targeted toward their sector, like domain shadowing or hijacking. Analyzing historical attack data and simulating real-world scenarios through tools like honeypots can further enrich the dataset with realistic examples. This data should encompass various healthcare sub-sectors and regions to account for geographical variations in threat patterns. Labeling strategies involve a blend of automation and human expertise. While advanced algorithms can identify potential anomalies, manual refinement by cybersecurity analysts and healthcare professionals ensures accuracy and domain-specific insights. Semi-supervised learning can then automate labeling on larger datasets, reducing manual effort. Additionally, temporal variations like daily, seasonal, and event-based fluctuations must be considered for realistic network behavior. Patient privacy is vital; anonymization or data aggregation techniques should be implemented to preserve relevant features for anomaly detection while protecting sensitive information.

15.8.2 Researching robust AI models

Neural networks offer great potential for healthcare anomaly detection. Convolutional Neural Networks (CNNs) can analyze the spatial patterns in DNS data, like sequences of domain names, to identify abnormal network behavior. Recurrent Neural Networks (RNNs) excel at analyzing temporal dynamics, such as sudden spikes in queries, to detect malicious activity. Attention-based models focus on specific features within DNS data, like suspicious domain names, for heightened accuracy. Beyond individual models, multi-model approaches can exploit synergy by fusing DNS traffic with other network data like IP flows or packet analysis, offering a more comprehensive view of network activity. Ensemble learning combines different models, like neural networks and statistical models, to leverage their strengths and mitigate individual weaknesses. Generative AI can be a powerful tool for building robust models. Generating synthetic anomalies allows training in diverse scenarios and improves generalizability. Additionally, adversarial training, where AI models face carefully crafted, malicious DNS queries, can test their robustness against targeted attacks.

15.8.3 Incorporating domain knowledge and human feedback

Expert rules based on healthcare cybersecurity expertise can be invaluable guides for anomaly detection. Defining specific patterns or rules based on domain names, IP addresses, or query behavior can help flag malicious activity. Integrating these rules with AI models adds valuable context and improves interpretability. Active learning allows human experts to interactively refine the training data for AI models. By querying experts on ambiguous anomalies identified by AI, healthcare systems can reduce false positives and improve the overall accuracy and efficiency of anomaly detection. This transparency fosters trust and empowers human analysts to make informed decisions in healthcare cybersecurity.

15.8.4 Evaluating and comparing techniques

Robust evaluation is crucial for selecting the most effective models for healthcare environments. Standardized datasets containing realistic healthcare-related DNS anomalies should be used as benchmarks for rigorous model comparison. Performance metrics like accuracy, precision, recall, and F1-score provide essential insights into the effectiveness of different models in detecting anomalies. However, healthcare applications demand interpretability and explainability as well. Understanding why models flag anomalies is crucial for informed decision-making and building trust among human analysts. Analyzing false positives and negatives helps identify model limitations and refine training data to mitigate unintended consequences.

15.8.5 Developing practical applications and threat cases

The ultimate goal is to translate insights into practical safeguards for healthcare systems. Plugins or extensions for existing DNS security tools can leverage anomaly detection models for real-time threat identification. Integration with intrusion detection systems can trigger alerts and initiate incident response protocols upon detecting malicious DNS activity. Finally, creating platforms or communities for sharing DNS anomaly data and threat intelligence across healthcare organizations can foster collaboration and strengthen collective defenses against cyber threats.

By diligently pursuing these action points, healthcare organizations can build tailored and robust DNS anomaly detection systems. This proactive approach empowers them to safeguard sensitive patient data and ensure the uninterrupted operation of critical healthcare systems in the face of evolving cyber threats. Continuous research, development, and adaptation remain crucial for staying ahead in this ongoing battle against malicious actors targeting the healthcare sector.

15.9 Conclusion

This chapter has discussed the role of AI in DNS anomaly detection, which is a vital task for ensuring network security and performance. DNS anomalies are diverse and complex phenomena that require advanced and intelligent methods to detect, classify, and mitigate. The chapter has presented the main AI techniques used in this field, such as supervised, unsupervised, and semi-supervised learning, and has shown how they can be applied to various types of DNS anomalies, such as tunneling, exfiltration, hijacking, and more. The chapter has also highlighted some of the recent developments and innovations in anomaly detection, such as new datasets, methods, models, and technologies. Furthermore, the chapter has identified some of the challenges and limitations of anomaly detection in DNS traffic, such as data scarcity, encryption, low-rate and distributed attacks, and false positives and false negatives. The chapter has concluded that AI is a powerful and promising tool for DNS anomaly detection, but also that there is still room for improvement and further research in this domain. The chapter has suggested some possible directions for future work, such as developing more realistic and labeled DNS datasets, designing more robust and adaptive AI models, and integrating more domain knowledge and human feedback into the anomaly detection process. By addressing these challenges and exploring these opportunities, AI can help enhance the security and performance of the DNS service and the Internet as a whole.

References

[1] GeeksforGeeks, "Types of Outliers in Data Mining," GeeksforGeeks, 4 May 2023. [Online]. Available: https://www.geeksforgeeks.org/types-of-outliers-in-data-mining/.

[2] Rehman, "What is Domain Name Server (DNS) with Example," IT Release. [Online]. Available: https://www.itrelease.com/2021/11/what-is-domain-name-server-dns-with-example/

[3] E. Esther, "What Happens When You Type https://www.google.com in Your Browser and Press Enter," Medium, 13 October 2023. [Online]. Available: https://medium.com/@ejimofor81/what-happens-when-you-type-https-www-google-com-in-your-browser-and-press-enter-7887966fdda4.

[4] I. Shakeel, "Detection and Prevention of DNS Anomalies," 16 August 2016. [Online]. Available: https://resources.infosecinstitute.com/topics/malware-analysis/detection-prevention-dns-anomalies/.

[5] M. Čermák, P. Čeleda and J. Vykopal, "Detection of DNS Traffic Anomalies in Large Networks," *Meeting of the European Network of Universities and Companies in Information and Communication Engineering*, p. 215–226, 2014.

[6] Fortinet, "DNS Anomalies Feature Control tab," [Online]. Available: https://help.fortinet.com/fddos/4-7-0/fortiddos/Configuring_SPP_settings_DNS_anomaly_feature_controls.htm.

[7] D. Hein, "Best Network Monitoring Vendors, Software, Tools and Performance Solutions," 31 May 2019. [Online]. Available: https://solutionsreview.com/network-monitoring/network-security-and-performance-monitoring-the-basics/.

[8] G. W. Brown, G. Bridge, J. Martini, *et al.*, "The role of health systems for health security: a scoping review revealing the need for improved conceptual and practical linkages," *Globalization and Health*, p. 18, 2022.

[9] S. Argaw, J. Troncoso-Pastoriza, D. Lacey, *et al.*, "Cybersecurity of hospitals: discussing the challenges and working towards mitigating the risks," *BMC Medical Informatics and Decision Making*, p. 146, 2020.

[10] L. Columbus, "5 Strategies Healthcare Providers Are Using to Secure Networks," 20 October 2019. [Online]. Available: https://www.forbes.com/sites/louiscolumbus/2019/10/20/5-strategies-healthcare-providers-are-using-to-secure-networks/?sh=3b3ca4174b40. [Accessed 11 November 2023].

[11] K. Gülen, "Finding Loopholes with Machine Learning Techniques," 10 October 2022. [Online]. Available: https://dataconomy.com/2022/10/10/machine-learning-anomaly-detection/. [Accessed 4 November 2023].

[12] AI & Insight, "Anomaly Detection with OpenAI API: How to Train AI Models for Outlier Detection," 2 March 2023. [Online]. Available: https://medium.com/muthoni-wanyoike/anomaly-detection-with-openai-api-how-to-train-ai-models-for-outlier-detection-a8bff0588af7.

[13] "What Is Anomaly Detection?," Deepai, 17 May 2019. [Online]. Available: https://deepai.org/machine-learning-glossary-and-terms/anomaly-detection. [Accessed 4 November 2023].

[14] "Unsupervised Learning for Anomaly Detection," Centum, 16 September 2021. [Online]. Available: https://centum.com/en/unsupervised-learning-for-anomaly-detection/. [Accessed 16 November 2023].

[15] K. Young, "Learn How to Build Applications of AI for Anomaly Detection," NVIDIA, 2 August 2021. [Online]. Available: NVIDIA Technical Blog. [Accessed 4 November 2023].

[16] A. Zewe, "Using Artificial Intelligence to Find Anomalies Hiding in Massive Datasets," MIT News, 25 February 2022. [Online]. Available: https://news.mit.edu/2022/artificial-intelligence-anomalies-data-0225. [Accessed 4 November 2023].

[17] M. Frąckiewicz, "Semi-Supervised Learning: Combining Labeled and Unlabeled Data for AI Model Training," TS2 Space, 6 May 2023. [Online]. Available: https://ts2.space/en/semi-supervised-learning-combining-labeled-and-unlabeled-data-for-ai-model-training/. [Accessed 5 November 2023].

[18] H. Zhang, Z. Xiao, J. Gu and Y. Liu, "A Network Anomaly Detection Algorithm Based on Semi-supervised Learning and Adaptive Multiclass Balancing - The Journal of Supercomputing," SpringerLink, 15 June 2023.

[Online]. Available: https://link.springer.com/article/10.1007/s11227-023-05474-y. [Accessed 4 November 2023].

[19] L. Ruff, R. Vandermeulen, N. Görnitz, *et al.*, "Deep Semi-Supervised Anomaly Detection," DeepAI, 6 June 2019. [Online]. Available: https://deepai.org/publication/deep-semi-supervised-anomaly-detection. [Accessed 4 November 2023].

[20] S. Larsen and P. Hooper, "Deep Semi-supervised Learning of Dynamics for Anomaly Detection in Laser Powder Bed Fusion," SpringerLink, 23 September 2021. [Online]. Available: https://link.springer.com/article/10.1007/s10845-021-01842-8. [Accessed 4 November 2023].

[21] DataRobot Docs, "Anomaly detection," DataRobot, 15 September 2023. [Online]. Available: https://docs.datarobot.com/en/docs/modeling/special-workflows/unsupervised/anomaly-detection.html. [Accessed 4 November 2023].

[22] R. Sharma, R. K. Singla and A. Guleria, "A New Labeled Flow-based DNS Dataset for Anomaly Detection," in *International Conference on Computational Intelligence and Data Science*, 2018.

[23] K. S. B. Kai, E. Chong and V. Balachandran, "Anomaly detection on DNS traffic using big data," *CEUR Workshop Proceedings*, vol. 2622, p. 14, 2019.

[24] T. Q. Nguyen, R. Laborde, A. Benzekri and B. Qu'hen, "Detecting Abnormal DNS Traffic Using Unsupervised Machine Learning," in *4th Cyber Security in Networking Conference (CSNet)*, Lausanne, Switzerland, 2020.

[25] L. A. Trejo, V. Ferman, M. A. Medina-Pérez, F. M. Arredondo Giacinti, R. Monroy and J. E. Ramirez-Marquez, "DNS-ADVP: a machine learning anomaly detection and visual platform to protect top-level domain name servers against DDoS attacks," *IEEE Access*, vol. 7, pp. 116358–116369, 2019.

[26] "Why You Should Pay Attention to DNS Tunneling," BlueCat Networks, 1 May 2023. [Online]. Available: https://bluecatnetworks.com/blog/why-you-should-pay-attention-to-dns-tunneling/.

[27] L. de Souza Bezerra Borges, R. Oliveira Albuquerque and R. de Sousa Júnior, "A Security Model for DNS Tunnel Detection on Cloud Platform," *2022 Workshop on Communication Networks and Power Systems (WCNPS)*, pp. 1–6, 2022.

[28] J. Ahmed, H. H. Gharakheili, Q. Raza, C. Russell and V. Sivaraman, "Real-Time Detection of DNS Exfiltration and Tunneling from Enterprise Networks," *IFIP/IEEE Symposium on Integrated Network and Service Management*, pp. 649–653, 2019.

[29] M. Lyu, H. H. Gharakheili, C. Russell and V. Sivaraman, "Hierarchical anomaly-based detection of distributed DNS attacks on enterprise networks," *IEEE Transactions on Network and Service Management*, vol. 18, no. 1, pp. 1031–1048, 2021.

[30] L. F. Gonzalez Casanova and P.-C. Lin, "Generalized Classification of DNS over HTTPS Traffic with Deep Learning," *Asia-Pacific Signal and Information Processing Association Annual Summit and Conference (APSIPA ASC)*, pp. 1903–1907, 2021.

[31] A. I. Newaz, A. K. Sikder, M. A. Rahman and A. S. Uluagac, "HealthGuard: A Machine Learning-Based Security Framework for Smart Healthcare Systems," in *2019 Sixth International Conference on Social Networks Analysis, Management and Security (SNAMS)*, Granada, Spain, 2019.

[32] S. Kumar and H. N. Champa, "Anomaly Detection Framework for Efficient Sensing in Healthcare IoT Systems," in *2022 International Conference on Computing, Communication, and Intelligent Systems (ICCCIS)*, Greater Noida, India, 2022.

[33] M. Weqar, M. Shabana and G. Dhawal, "DNS Traffic Monitoring to Access Vulnerability in the Internet of Healthcare Things Networks: A Survey," in *2023 International Conference on Recent Advances in Electrical, Electronics & Digital Healthcare Technologies (REEDCON)*, New Delhi, India, 2023.

[34] A. Ukil, S. Bandyoapdhyay, C. Puri and A. Pal, "IoT Healthcare Analytics: The Importance of Anomaly Detection," in *2016 IEEE 30th International Conference on Advanced Information Networking and Applications (AINA)*, Crans-Montana, Switzerland, 2016.

[35] R. Romero-Gomez, Y. Nadji and M. Antonakakis, "Towards Designing Effective Visualizations for DNS-based Network Threat Analysis," *IEEE Symposium on Visualization for Cyber Security (VizSec)*, pp. 1–8, 2017.

[36] J. Ahmed, H. Gharakheili, Q. Raza, C. Russell and V. Sivaraman, "Monitoring Enterprise DNS Queries for Detecting Data Exfiltration from Internal Hosts," *Transactions on Network and Service Management*, vol. 17, no. 1, pp. 265–279, 2020.

[37] D. Lambion, M. Josten, F. Olumofin and M. De Cock, "Malicious DNS Tunneling Detection in Real-Traffic DNS Data," *2020 IEEE International Conference on Big Data (Big Data)*, pp. 5736–5738, 2020.

[38] S. Ding, D. Zhang, J. Ge, X. Yuan and X. Du, "Encrypt DNS Traffic: Automated Feature Learning Method for Detecting DNS Tunnels," *2021 IEEE Intl Conf on Parallel & Distributed Processing with Applications*, pp. 352–359, 2021.

[39] Z. Wang and M. Zhang, "The Research of DNS Anomaly Detection Based on the Method of Similarity and Entropy," *2010 International Conference on Intelligent Computation Technology and Automation*, pp. 905–909, 2010.

[40] H. Jha, I. Patel, G. Li, A. K. Cherukuri and S. Thaseen, "Detection of Tunneling in DNS over HTTPS," *7th International Conference on Signal Processing and Communication (ICSC)*, pp. 42–47, 2021.

[41] J. Ruohonen and V. Leppänen, "Investigating the Agility Bias in DNS Graph Mining," *IEEE International Conference on Computer and Information Technology (CIT)*, pp. 253–260, 2017.

[42] S. Mahdavifar, N. Maleki, A. H. Lashkari, M. Broda and A. H. Razavi, "Classifying Malicious Domains Using DNS Traffic Analysis," *IEEE Intl Conf on Dependable, Autonomic and Secure Computing*, pp. 60–67, 2021.

Chapter 16

Harnessing edge computing for real-time cybersecurity in healthcare systems

Oleksandr Kuznetsov[1,2,3], *Emanuele Frontoni*[1,4], *Natalia Kryvinska*[5], *Sarychev Volodymyr*[6] *and Tetiana Smirnova*[7]

This book chapter presents an in-depth exploration of the integration of Edge Computing with cybersecurity within healthcare systems, a critical development in the era of digital healthcare transformation. As the Internet of Medical Things (IoMT) continues to expand, generating vast amounts of data, traditional cloud-centric models are becoming increasingly insufficient. These models, while once groundbreaking, now struggle to meet the urgent demands for low-latency and high-security data processing essential in healthcare applications. The chapter advocates for a paradigm shift toward Edge Computing architectures. Unlike conventional models, Edge Computing processes data at the network's edge, closer to where it is generated. This proximity significantly reduces response times and bandwidth usage, crucial for real-time medical data analysis and prompt decision-making in patient care. The chapter meticulously dissects the design, implementation challenges, and potential of edge-based cybersecurity frameworks. It emphasizes how these frameworks can leverage distributed data processing to enhance threat detection and mitigation, ensuring robust protection against cyber threats. In-depth case studies are presented, illustrating successful implementations of Edge Computing in enhancing cybersecurity in healthcare settings. These real-world examples serve as a blueprint for future implementations, demonstrating practical applications and the tangible benefits of Edge Computing in healthcare. Furthermore, the chapter delves into

[1]Department of Political Sciences, Communication and International Relations, University of Macerata, Italy
[2]Department of Information and Communication Systems Security, V. N. Karazin Kharkiv National University, Ukraine
[3]Faculty of Engineering, eCampus University, Italy
[4]Department of Information Engineering, Marche Polytechnic University, Italy
[5]Department of Information Management and Business Systems, University of Comenius, Slovakia
[6]Department of Economics and Economic Security, University of Customs and Finance, Ukraine
[7]Department of Cyber Security and Software, Central Ukrainian National Technical University, Ukraine

the broader implications of this technological shift. It discusses the evolving landscape of healthcare infrastructure, the need for adaptive strategies to accommodate these advanced technologies, and the role of Edge Computing in facilitating secure, efficient, and patient-centric healthcare services. By highlighting the synergies between Edge Computing and cybersecurity, the chapter underscores the critical need for healthcare systems to evolve and adapt. It presents Edge Computing not just as a technological innovation but as a strategic necessity to address modern healthcare challenges, particularly in cybersecurity and data management.

Keywords: Edge computing; cybersecurity; digital healthcare; Internet of Medical Things (IoMT); threat detection; cloud computing; healthcare infrastructure

16.1 Introduction

In the rapidly evolving landscape of healthcare technology, the integration of Edge Computing and cybersecurity emerges as a critical area of focus [1,2]. This convergence is driven by the increasing reliance on digital technologies, particularly the Internet of Medical Things (IoMT), which has revolutionized patient care but also introduced complex challenges and vulnerabilities.

The subject area of this research encompasses the application of Edge Computing in healthcare, specifically its role in enhancing cybersecurity measures. The proliferation of IoMT devices has led to an exponential increase in healthcare data, necessitating real-time processing and robust security protocols [3,4]. However, traditional cloud-based models often fall short in meeting these demands, leading to concerns over data latency, network dependency, and vulnerability to cyber threats.

There exists a significant research gap in understanding the full potential and implications of integrating Edge Computing with cybersecurity in healthcare. While there is an acknowledgment of the need for advanced computing solutions, comprehensive studies detailing the implementation, challenges, and outcomes of such integrations are scarce [5]. This research aims to bridge this gap by providing an in-depth analysis of Edge Computing's role in enhancing cybersecurity in healthcare settings.

The primary objective of this research is to elucidate the impact of Edge Computing on cybersecurity in healthcare, exploring its benefits, challenges, and future potential. To achieve this, the research is structured around several key tasks:

1. Analyzing the current state: Examining the existing healthcare infrastructure and the role of traditional computing models in managing healthcare data.
2. Identifying challenges and vulnerabilities: Investigating the cybersecurity challenges and vulnerabilities inherent in current healthcare systems, particularly in the context of IoMT.

3. Exploring edge computing solutions: Delving into the specifics of Edge Computing technologies and how they can address the identified challenges, enhance data processing speeds, and improve cybersecurity measures.
4. Assessing implementation and outcomes: Evaluating real-world applications of Edge Computing in healthcare, including case studies and quantitative data, to understand its impact on cybersecurity.
5. Predicting future trends: Forecasting future developments in Edge Computing and cybersecurity within healthcare, including potential innovations and emerging threats.

By addressing these tasks, this research aims to provide a comprehensive understanding of the intersection between Edge Computing and cybersecurity in healthcare. It seeks to offer valuable insights for healthcare providers, policy-makers, and technology developers, guiding them in making informed decisions about integrating Edge Computing solutions to create more secure, efficient, and patient-centric healthcare systems.

16.1.1 Key contributions of the chapter

1. Highlighting edge computing in healthcare: Presents a comprehensive analysis of Edge Computing's role in revolutionizing data processing and cybersecurity in healthcare systems.
2. Shift from cloud-centric to edge architectures: Emphasizes the transition to Edge Computing for improved data processing efficiency, crucial for real-time medical applications.
3. Exploration of edge-based cybersecurity frameworks: Offers an in-depth examination of the design and challenges of cybersecurity frameworks in Edge Computing, focusing on enhancing threat detection and mitigation.
4. Real-world case studies: Provides practical examples demonstrating the successful implementation and benefits of Edge Computing in healthcare cybersecurity.
5. Integration of IoMT and cybersecurity: Addresses the unique challenges and solutions in combining the IoMT with Edge Computing for enhanced security.
6. Strategic insights for infrastructure evolution: Discusses the necessary adaptations in healthcare infrastructure to support Edge Computing and advanced cybersecurity measures.
7. Future trends and predictions: Explores potential future developments in Edge Computing within healthcare, highlighting its role as a key driver in technological advancement.
8. Filling research gaps: Contributes new insights by focusing on less-explored areas such as specific cybersecurity frameworks suitable for healthcare Edge Computing environments.

16.1.2 Chapter organization

This chapter methodically unfolds the narrative of Edge Computing and cybersecurity in healthcare, beginning with a thorough literature analysis to set the foundational understanding. It then progresses to examining the limitations of traditional cloud models in healthcare, particularly focusing on latency and bandwidth challenges in critical medical applications. The discussion shifts to the paradigm of Edge Computing, exploring its principles and advantages for cybersecurity in healthcare.

Further, the chapter delves into the development of Edge-Based Cybersecurity Frameworks, detailing their design principles, functionalities, and the orchestration of responses in IoMT environments. This includes an in-depth look at the stateful dynamics, architectural blueprint, and deployment strategies of these frameworks.

The application of Edge Computing in healthcare is analyzed through successful examples and their quantitative impact, followed by an assessment of global adoption and risk. The chapter concludes with future trends and predictions in Edge Computing and cybersecurity, emphasizing the need for adaptive healthcare infrastructure. This structure provides a comprehensive and cohesive understanding of the interplay between Edge Computing, cybersecurity, and healthcare technology.

16.2 Related work

Aceto *et al.* [6] provide a comprehensive overview of how Industry 4.0 technologies, particularly the Internet of Things (IoT), Cloud and Fog Computing, and Big Data, are revolutionizing eHealth and moving toward Healthcare 4.0. Their work systematically surveys the adoption of these technologies in healthcare, discussing their applications, benefits, and cross-disciplinary challenges. However, their analysis primarily focuses on the broader implications of these technologies without delving into the specific cybersecurity challenges and solutions within Edge Computing environments.

Akkaoui *et al.* [7] introduce EdgeMediChain, a hybrid Edge Blockchain-based framework for health data exchange. Their work emphasizes the potential of combining Edge Computing and blockchain to enhance performance and security in healthcare data management. While their architecture demonstrates significant improvements in execution time and scalability, it does not extensively explore the integration of advanced cybersecurity measures within the Edge Computing framework.

Pascarella *et al.* [8] discuss the application of risk assessment matrices in healthcare, aligning with the ISO 31000 framework. Their methodological approach provides valuable insights into risk management in healthcare settings. However, their focus is more on general risk management rather than the specific cybersecurity risks associated with Edge Computing in healthcare.

Tawalbeh *et al.* [9] present an IoT model for secure healthcare, emphasizing latency and energy efficiency. Their model is significant in showcasing the integration of Edge Computing for data security in healthcare. However, their analysis primarily focuses on the technical performance of the system, with less emphasis on the strategic implementation of cybersecurity measures.

Unal *et al.* [10] investigate the security risks in big data platforms within healthcare and explore how machine learning (ML) can mitigate these risks, especially in edge computing-based applications. Their focus on privacy protection in open and sensitive communication channels is crucial. However, their chapter primarily addresses big data security without an in-depth exploration of the specific cybersecurity frameworks for Edge Computing in healthcare.

Liu and Li [11] propose a permissioned blockchain and deep reinforcement learning (DRL)-empowered Healthcare IoT (H-IoT) system to address security and energy efficiency. Their research is pivotal in demonstrating how blockchain and DRL can be utilized in H-IoT. However, the study primarily focuses on the balance between security and energy efficiency without a detailed analysis of the specific cybersecurity frameworks suitable for Edge Computing in healthcare.

Mahbub and Shubair [12] provide an extensive survey on Multi-Access Edge Computing (MEC), covering its fundamentals, architecture, technologies, and deployment cases in healthcare. Their work significantly contributes to understanding MEC's role in reducing transmission latency in e-healthcare applications. However, their survey primarily focuses on the technological aspects of MEC, leaving a gap in the exploration of specific cybersecurity strategies within MEC frameworks.

Yao *et al.* [13] provide a comprehensive study on differential privacy (DP) in edge computing-based smart city applications, including smart health. They discuss various privacy-preserving methods and focus on resource consumption for data privacy in edge computing environments. While their study is a significant contribution to understanding DP in smart city applications, it lacks a detailed focus on healthcare-specific challenges in Edge Computing.

Hazra *et al.* [14] discuss the integration of blockchain with Edge Computing for cybersecurity in various applications, including healthcare. They highlight the scalability challenges of blockchain and the decentralized security benefits it brings to Edge Computing. However, their discussion is more general and does not specifically address the unique cybersecurity challenges in healthcare Edge Computing.

Table 16.1 provides a concise overview of the current state of research in Edge Computing and cybersecurity within the healthcare sector, highlighting the key contributions of each work and identifying the existing gaps that our research aims to address.

Each of these studies contributes valuable insights into the evolving field of Edge Computing and cybersecurity in healthcare. However, there remains a need for focused research on comprehensive cybersecurity frameworks and specific challenges within Edge Computing frameworks in healthcare. Our research aims to bridge this gap, offering a comprehensive analysis of cybersecurity strategies and solutions tailored to the unique requirements of healthcare Edge Computing environments.

Table 16.1 Brief overview of the current state of research in edge computing and cybersecurity in the healthcare sector

Reference	Key contributions	Existing gaps
Aceto *et al.* [6]	Comprehensive overview of Industry 4.0 technologies in eHealth.	Lacks specific focus on cybersecurity challenges in Edge Computing.
Akkaoui *et al.* [7]	Introduction of EdgeMediChain, a hybrid Edge Blockchain framework for health data exchange.	Limited exploration of advanced cybersecurity measures within the Edge Computing framework.
Pascarella *et al.* [8]	Discussion on the application of risk assessment matrices in healthcare.	Focuses more on general risk management rather than specific cybersecurity risks associated with Edge Computing.
Tawalbeh *et al.* [9]	Presentation of an IoT model for secure healthcare emphasizing latency and energy efficiency.	Analysis primarily on technical performance, with less emphasis on strategic cybersecurity implementation.
Unal *et al.* [10]	Investigation of security risks in big data platforms in healthcare and the role of machine learning.	Addresses big data security without exploring specific cybersecurity frameworks for Edge Computing.
Liu and Li [11]	Proposal of a permissioned blockchain and DRL-empowered H-IoT system.	Focuses on the balance between security and energy efficiency, lacking detailed Edge Computing cybersecurity analysis.
Mahbub and Shubair [12]	Extensive survey on Multi-Access Edge Computing in healthcare.	Focuses on technological aspects of MEC, lacking exploration of specific cybersecurity strategies.
Yao *et al.* [13]	Comprehensive study on differential privacy in edge computing-based smart city applications.	Lacks a detailed focus on healthcare-specific challenges in Edge Computing.
Hazra *et al.* [14]	Discussion on the integration of blockchain with Edge Computing for cybersecurity.	General discussion, lacking specific focus on unique cybersecurity challenges in healthcare Edge Computing.

16.3 Traditional cloud models and their limitations

The advent of cloud computing has been a cornerstone in the evolution of healthcare technology, offering scalable, flexible, and cost-effective solutions for data storage and processing [1,6]. However, as the healthcare industry increasingly adopts digital technologies, particularly the IoMT, the limitations of traditional cloud-centric models are becoming more pronounced. These models, while revolutionary at their inception, now face challenges in meeting the burgeoning demands for real-time data processing and stringent cybersecurity in healthcare environments [13,15]. This section aims to critically analyze traditional cloud models in healthcare, highlighting the inherent limitations that necessitate the shift toward more dynamic and responsive computing paradigms like Edge Computing.

16.3.1 Analysis of traditional cloud models in healthcare

- Centralization of data processing. Traditional cloud models are characterized by their centralization of data processing and storage in remote data centers. This centralization, while beneficial for aggregating and managing large volumes of data, introduces significant latency issues. In healthcare, where real-time data analysis is often crucial for patient monitoring and emergency response, any delay in data processing can have critical implications.
- Network dependency and bandwidth constraints. Cloud-centric models are heavily reliant on network connectivity and bandwidth availability. In healthcare settings, where IoMT devices continuously generate large amounts of data, the bandwidth required for transmitting this data to and from the cloud can be substantial. This reliance not only strains network resources but also poses risks of network congestion and potential data transmission delays.
- Security and privacy concerns. While cloud computing offers robust security measures, the transmission of sensitive healthcare data across networks to centralized cloud servers poses inherent security risks. The risk of data breaches and cyberattacks is amplified due to the increased exposure of data during transit. Additionally, the centralized nature of cloud storage creates a single point of failure, which can be a significant vulnerability in terms of data privacy and security.
- Scalability and flexibility limitations. Although cloud computing is inherently scalable, the scalability in traditional cloud models is often limited by the capacity of the central data centers and the network infrastructure. As the volume of data generated by IoMT devices grows exponentially, scaling up cloud resources to match this growth can be challenging and costly. Furthermore, the one-size-fits-all approach of traditional cloud models may not adequately address the diverse and specific needs of various healthcare applications.
- Compliance and regulatory challenges. Healthcare data is subject to stringent regulatory standards, such as HIPAA in the United States and GDPR in Europe. Ensuring compliance with these regulations in a cloud-centric model can be complex, given the trans-border nature of cloud services and the varying legal jurisdictions involved in data storage and processing.

Figure 16.1 provides a clear overview of the key challenges associated with traditional cloud computing models in the healthcare sector, including issues related to data centralization, network dependency, security concerns, scalability limitations, and regulatory challenges.

In summary, while traditional cloud models have laid the foundation for digital transformation in healthcare, their limitations in terms of latency, network dependency, security, scalability, and regulatory compliance are becoming increasingly

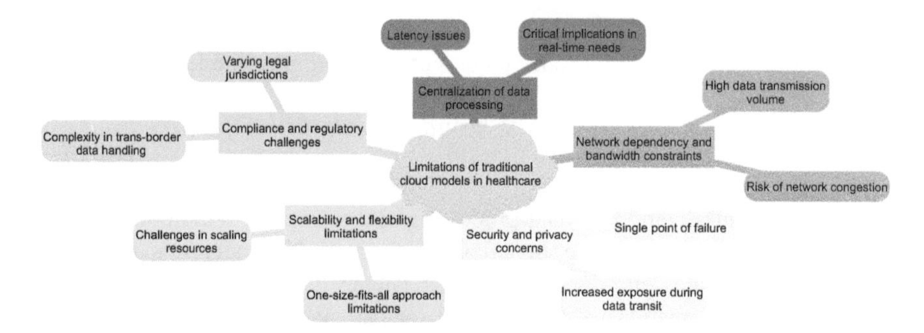

Figure 16.1 Limitations of traditional cloud models in healthcare

apparent [13,15]. These challenges underscore the need for more innovative computing solutions, such as Edge Computing, which can address the unique demands of modern healthcare systems.

16.3.2 Latency and bandwidth issues in critical medical applications

The reliance on traditional cloud models in healthcare has brought to the forefront significant challenges related to latency and bandwidth, particularly in critical medical applications [2,9]. This subsection delves into these issues, elucidating their implications and the pressing need for more efficient computing solutions.

- Latency in medical data processing. Latency, the delay before a transfer of data begins following an instruction, is a critical concern in healthcare applications. In scenarios such as remote patient monitoring, telemedicine, and emergency response systems, any delay, even milliseconds, can be detrimental. Traditional cloud models, where data must travel to distant servers for processing, inherently introduce latency. This delay can hinder the real-time analysis of patient data, potentially delaying critical medical decisions and interventions.
- Impact on patient monitoring systems. In patient monitoring systems, continuous real-time data analysis is essential for detecting life-threatening conditions like heart attacks or strokes. Latency in these systems can lead to delayed alerts, reducing the window for timely medical intervention. For instance, in a cardiac monitoring system, a delay in processing electrocardiogram (ECG) data could result in a missed or delayed diagnosis of a potentially fatal arrhythmia.
- Challenges in telemedicine. Telemedicine relies heavily on real-time data exchange between patients and healthcare providers. Latency issues can disrupt the quality of video consultations, the accuracy of remote diagnostics, and the effectiveness of telesurgery applications. In telesurgery, even a slight delay in data transmission can affect the surgeon's ability to perform precise movements, potentially leading to adverse patient outcomes.

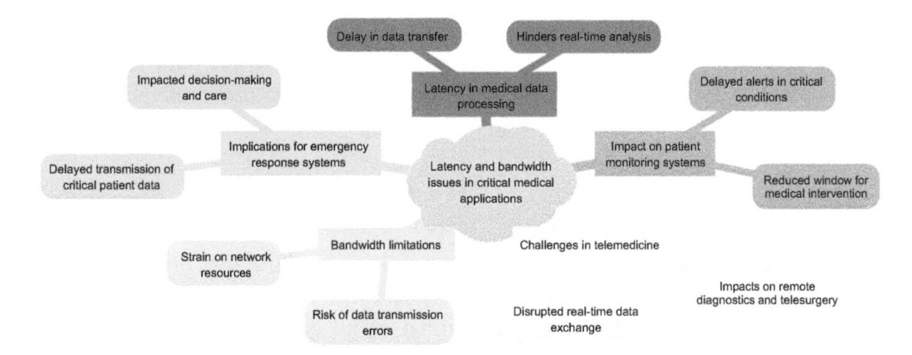

Figure 16.2 Latency and bandwidth issues in critical medical applications

- Bandwidth limitations. The bandwidth requirement for transmitting large volumes of medical data to the cloud is substantial. As the number of connected IoMT devices grows, the data generated increases exponentially, placing a significant strain on network bandwidth. This can lead to network congestion, further exacerbating latency issues and potentially leading to data transmission errors or loss. In critical healthcare applications, where data integrity and timely delivery are paramount, such bandwidth limitations pose a substantial risk.
- Implications for emergency response systems. In emergency response systems, where every second counts, latency and bandwidth issues can impede the swift transmission of critical patient data to emergency personnel. Delays in receiving this data can hinder the ability of first responders to make informed decisions and provide timely care, potentially impacting patient survival rates.

Figure 16.2 succinctly captures the various challenges associated with latency and bandwidth in critical healthcare settings, highlighting their impact on medical data processing, patient monitoring systems, telemedicine, network resources, and emergency response systems.

In conclusion, the latency and bandwidth challenges inherent in traditional cloud computing models pose significant risks in critical medical applications [9]. These issues underscore the necessity for more efficient computing paradigms, such as Edge Computing, which can provide real-time data processing and reduced latency essential for modern healthcare systems.

16.4 The paradigm of edge computing

In the evolving landscape of digital healthcare, the integration of Edge Computing represents a significant paradigm shift [10,16]. This transition is driven by the growing demand for real-time data processing and the need for robust cybersecurity measures in healthcare systems [10]. As the IoMT continues to expand, generating vast amounts of data, the limitations of traditional cloud-centric models become increasingly apparent. Edge Computing emerges as a pivotal solution, addressing these challenges by bringing computational power closer to the data source [16]. This subsection aims to elucidate the definition and fundamental principles of Edge Computing, setting the stage for understanding its critical role in enhancing cybersecurity in healthcare environments.

16.4.1 Definition and key principles of edge computing

Edge Computing refers to a distributed computing paradigm that brings computation and data storage closer to the location where it is needed, to improve response times and save bandwidth. Unlike traditional cloud computing models that centralize data processing in distant data centers, Edge Computing processes data at or near the source of data generation [1]. This approach is particularly beneficial in healthcare settings, where real-time data analysis and immediate action are paramount.

Key principles of edge computing (Figure 16.3):

- Proximity to data sources: At its core, Edge Computing is about minimizing the physical and network distance between data generation and data processing. This proximity enhances the ability to process data in real-time, crucial for time-sensitive applications in healthcare.
- Decentralization: By decentralizing data processing, Edge Computing reduces the reliance on central data centers. This not only decreases latency but also distributes the computational load, leading to more efficient system performance.
- Scalability and flexibility: Edge Computing allows for scalable and flexible deployment of applications. Healthcare providers can tailor the computing resources to specific needs of different IoMT devices and applications, ensuring optimal performance.
- Enhanced security and privacy: Processing data locally reduces the risk of data breaches during transmission. Edge Computing also enables more granular

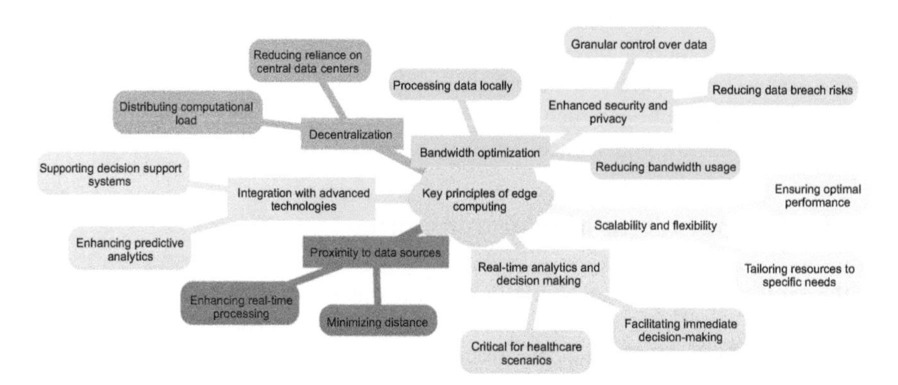

Figure 16.3 Key principles of edge computing

control over data, which is vital for complying with healthcare privacy regulations.

- Bandwidth optimization: By processing data locally and sending only relevant information to the cloud, Edge Computing significantly reduces bandwidth usage. This is essential in healthcare settings where network resources are often limited.
- Real-time analytics and decision-making: Edge Computing facilitates real-time data analysis, enabling immediate decision-making. This is critical in healthcare scenarios where delays can have serious consequences.
- Integration with advanced technologies: Edge Computing seamlessly integrates with other advanced technologies like Artificial Intelligence (AI) and ML, enhancing the capabilities of IoMT devices in predictive analytics and decision support systems.

Figure 16.3 provides a clear and structured overview of the fundamental principles that underpin Edge Computing, highlighting its relevance and application in the context of healthcare cybersecurity.

In summary, Edge Computing represents a transformative approach in managing and processing data in healthcare systems. Its principles align closely with the needs of modern healthcare environments, particularly in enhancing cybersecurity and ensuring timely response to medical situations [17].

16.4.2 Advantages of edge computing for cybersecurity in healthcare

The integration of Edge Computing into healthcare cybersecurity frameworks offers numerous advantages, addressing the unique challenges posed by the healthcare sector's increasing reliance on digital technologies [12]. This subsection explores the key benefits of Edge Computing in enhancing cybersecurity measures within healthcare systems (Figure 16.4).

1. Enhanced data security and privacy. Edge Computing strengthens data security and privacy by processing sensitive patient information closer to its source.

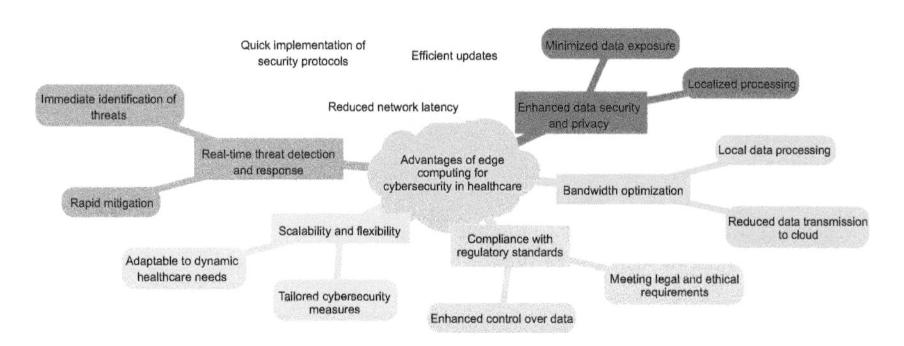

Figure 16.4 Key benefits of edge computing for cybersecurity in healthcare

This localized processing minimizes the exposure of data to potential threats during transmission to distant cloud servers. By reducing the distance data travels, Edge Computing inherently decreases the attack surface, making it more difficult for cyberattackers to intercept sensitive information. Additionally, Edge Computing allows for the implementation of robust, localized encryption and security protocols, providing an added layer of protection for patient data.

2. Real-time threat detection and response. In healthcare, where seconds can be critical, Edge Computing enables real-time threat detection and response. By processing data at the edge, healthcare providers can immediately identify and mitigate potential cybersecurity threats. This rapid response capability is crucial in preventing the escalation of security breaches, which can have dire consequences in medical environments. Edge Computing facilitates the deployment of advanced analytics and ML algorithms at the edge, enhancing the system's ability to detect anomalies and respond to them swiftly.
3. Reduced network latency. Edge Computing significantly reduces network latency by processing data near its source, rather than relying on a central data center. In the context of cybersecurity, this reduced latency means that security protocols and updates can be implemented more quickly and efficiently. This is particularly important in healthcare settings, where IoMT devices require constant, real-time monitoring and updates to ensure their security and functionality.
4. Scalability and flexibility. Healthcare systems are dynamic, with varying computational and security needs. Edge Computing offers scalability and flexibility, allowing healthcare providers to tailor cybersecurity measures to specific requirements of different devices and applications. This adaptability ensures that each component of the healthcare system receives the appropriate level of security attention, based on its risk profile and functionality.
5. Bandwidth optimization. By processing data locally, Edge Computing reduces the volume of data that needs to be transmitted to the cloud. This bandwidth optimization is crucial in healthcare settings, where network resources are often limited. It ensures that critical systems and communications remain functional and are not compromised by bandwidth constraints, especially during peak usage times.
6. Compliance with regulatory standards. Healthcare data is subject to stringent regulatory standards, such as HIPAA in the United States. Edge Computing facilitates compliance with these regulations by providing enhanced control over where and how patient data is processed and stored. Localized data processing and storage can be tailored to meet specific regulatory requirements, ensuring that healthcare providers remain compliant with legal and ethical standards.

Figure 16.4 succinctly captures the various benefits that Edge Computing brings to cybersecurity in healthcare settings, highlighting its role in enhancing data security, real-time threat response, network efficiency, scalability, bandwidth optimization, and regulatory compliance.

In conclusion, Edge Computing offers a suite of advantages that significantly bolster cybersecurity in healthcare systems. Its ability to provide real-time, localized, and scalable security solutions makes it an indispensable component in the modern healthcare cybersecurity landscape [10,11]. As healthcare continues to evolve with the integration of more digital technologies, Edge Computing will play a pivotal role in safeguarding patient data and ensuring the resilience of healthcare systems against cyber threats.

16.5 Development of edge-based cybersecurity frameworks

The shift toward Edge Computing in healthcare cybersecurity is not just a technological upgrade but a strategic reorientation [10,14]. This section focuses on the development of Edge-Based Cybersecurity Frameworks, a critical component in safeguarding healthcare data and systems in the era of IoMT. As healthcare organizations increasingly adopt Edge Computing, the need for robust, scalable, and efficient cybersecurity frameworks becomes paramount. These frameworks must not only address the unique challenges posed by Edge Computing but also leverage its advantages to enhance overall security.

16.5.1 Principles of designing edge-based cybersecurity systems

This subsection will explore the principles of designing cybersecurity systems based on Edge Computing, highlighting their significance in the context of healthcare [14].

1. Data localization and protection. One of the foundational principles of Edge-Based Cybersecurity is the localization of data processing and storage. By keeping data on or near the device that generates it, the risk of data breaches during transit is significantly reduced. This approach necessitates the implementation of strong encryption protocols and access controls at the edge, ensuring that data is securely stored and processed.
2. Real-time threat detection and response. Edge Computing enables real-time monitoring and analysis of data, which is crucial for immediate threat detection and response. Designing cybersecurity systems with integrated, advanced analytics and ML capabilities at the edge allows for the rapid identification of potential security breaches. This immediate response capability is vital in preventing the escalation of threats and minimizing their impact.
3. Decentralized security management. In contrast to traditional centralized security models, Edge-Based Cybersecurity emphasizes decentralized security management. This involves distributing security responsibilities across various

edge nodes, making the system more resilient to attacks. Each edge node operates independently in terms of security, ensuring that a breach in one node does not compromise the entire network.

4. Scalability and flexibility. Cybersecurity frameworks based on Edge Computing must be scalable and flexible to accommodate the growing number of IoMT devices and their varying security needs. The design should allow for easy integration of new devices and technologies, as well as the ability to scale security measures up or down based on real-time risk assessments.
5. Compliance with regulatory standards. Given the sensitive nature of healthcare data, Edge-Based Cybersecurity systems must be designed in compliance with relevant regulatory standards, such as HIPAA and GDPR. This includes ensuring patient data privacy, secure data handling processes, and transparent data governance practices.
6. Continuous monitoring and maintenance. Continuous monitoring and regular maintenance are essential in Edge-Based Cybersecurity systems. This involves not only the monitoring of network traffic and device behavior but also the regular updating of security protocols and software to address new threats and vulnerabilities.
7. Integration with existing systems. Finally, Edge-Based Cybersecurity frameworks should be designed to integrate seamlessly with existing healthcare IT systems. This integration ensures a unified approach to security, where edge computing complements and enhances the existing security measures rather than operating in isolation.

In summary, the design of Edge-Based Cybersecurity systems in healthcare requires a comprehensive approach that addresses the unique challenges and leverages the strengths of Edge Computing [10,14]. By adhering to these principles, healthcare organizations can develop robust cybersecurity frameworks that protect against modern cyber threats while enabling the efficient and safe use of IoMT devices.

16.5.2 Key functions and interactions in edge-based cybersecurity for healthcare

In the rapidly evolving domain of healthcare technology, the implementation of Edge-Based Cybersecurity Frameworks marks a significant stride toward robust data protection and efficient threat management [18]. This subsection delves into the intricate web of functionalities and interactions that constitute these frameworks. By dissecting the roles and responsibilities of various stakeholders and system components, we gain insights into the holistic approach required to safeguard sensitive healthcare data in the era of IoMT.

Figure 16.5 presents a comprehensive view of the interactions and functionalities within Edge-Based Cybersecurity Frameworks in healthcare. This diagram serves as a pivotal tool for understanding the complex network of roles, responsibilities, and processes that ensure the security and integrity of healthcare data in the context of IoMT.

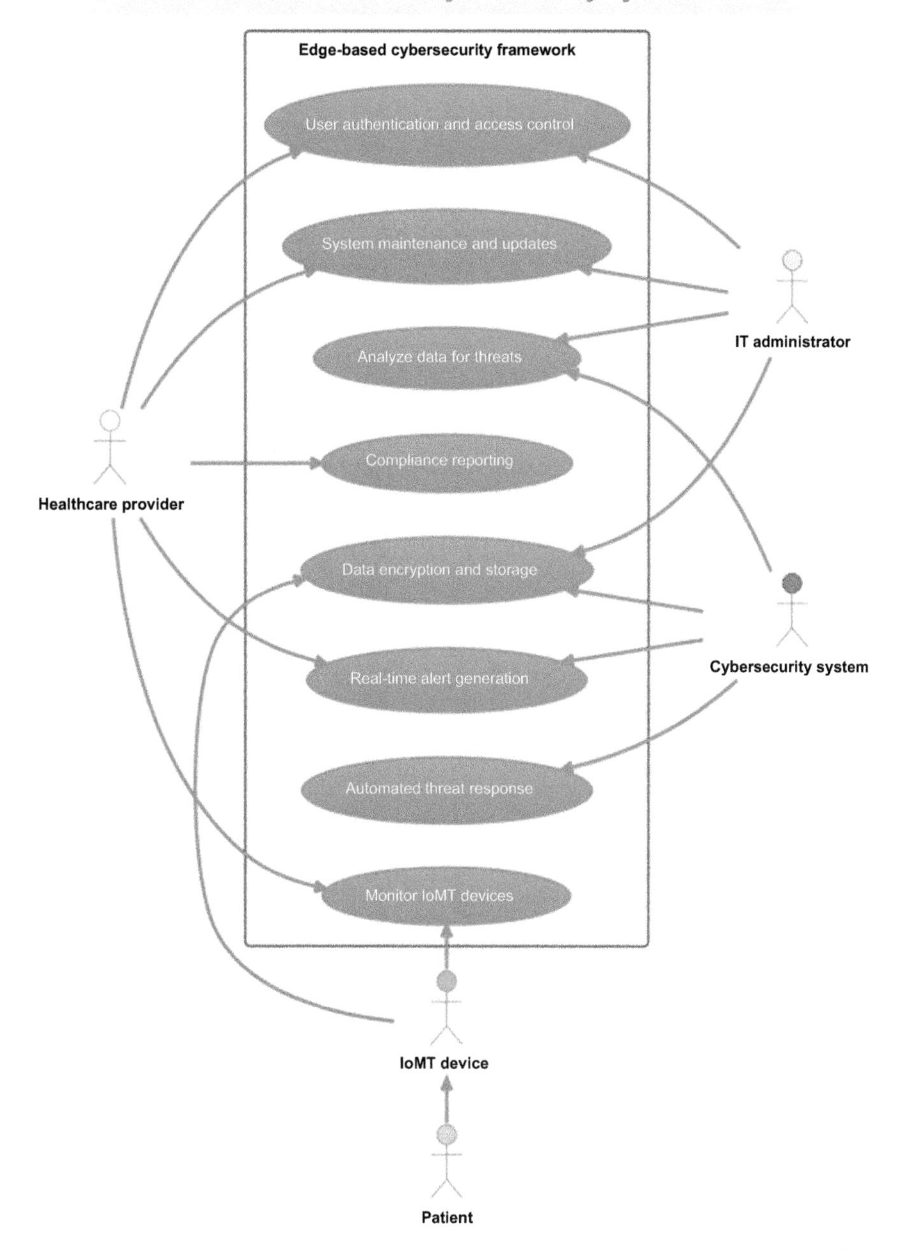

Figure 16.5 Healthcare cybersecurity ecosystem

Figure 16.5 effectively illustrates these interactions, depicting a network where each actor plays a specific role in maintaining the cybersecurity ecosystem. The use cases are strategically positioned to reflect their relevance to each actor, providing a clear understanding of how different components of the system interact and contribute to the overall security and efficiency of healthcare data management.

Actors and their roles:

1. Healthcare provider: This actor represents medical professionals and staff who utilize the cybersecurity system to monitor patient health through IoMT devices. They are the primary users of the system, responsible for interpreting data and responding to alerts.
2. IT administrator: This role involves managing the technical aspects of the cybersecurity system, including system configuration, maintenance, and updates. IT Administrators ensure the smooth operation of the cybersecurity infrastructure.
3. Cybersecurity system: Representing the automated, intelligent aspect of the framework, this actor is crucial for real-time threat detection, data analysis, and initiating automated responses to identified threats.
4. Patient: Patients are indirect users of the system, whose health data is collected and monitored through IoMT devices. They are the primary beneficiaries of the secure and efficient functioning of the system.
5. IoMT device: These devices are the sources of medical data and are integral to the system. They include wearable devices, monitors, and other medical equipment connected to the network.

Use cases and interactions:

1. Monitor IoMT devices: Healthcare Providers continuously monitor data from IoMT devices. This use case is crucial for real-time health monitoring and early detection of medical issues.
2. Analyze data for threats: The IT Administrator and Cybersecurity System collaboratively analyze data from IoMT devices to identify potential security threats, using advanced algorithms and ML techniques.
3. Real-time alert generation: Upon detecting a threat, the Cybersecurity System generates real-time alerts to Healthcare Providers, enabling swift response and mitigation of potential risks.
4. Automated threat response: This use case involves the Cybersecurity System automatically responding to identified threats, ensuring immediate action to protect data and system integrity.
5. Data encryption and storage: IoMT Devices encrypt and store patient data locally, minimizing the risk of data breaches during transmission. This use case is vital for maintaining patient privacy and data security.
6. Compliance reporting: Healthcare Providers are responsible for ensuring that the system complies with regulatory standards like HIPAA. This use case involves generating reports and documentation to demonstrate compliance.

7. System maintenance and updates: Managed by the IT Administrator, this use case ensures that the cybersecurity system is up-to-date and functioning optimally, safeguarding against emerging threats.
8. User authentication and access control: This use case, overseen by Healthcare Providers and IT Administrators, involves managing access to the system, ensuring that only authorized personnel can view or manipulate sensitive data.

In summary, Figure 16.5 is a vital tool for visualizing the complex interplay of actors and functionalities within Edge-Based Cybersecurity Frameworks. It underscores the collaborative nature of cybersecurity in healthcare, highlighting the importance of each actor and use case in the broader context of patient data protection and healthcare service delivery [2,6].

16.5.3 Orchestrating cybersecurity responses in IoMT environments

In the realm of healthcare cybersecurity, particularly within the framework of the IoMT, the orchestration of responses to potential security threats is a critical aspect [8]. Figure 16.6 provides a detailed depiction of the interactive processes involved

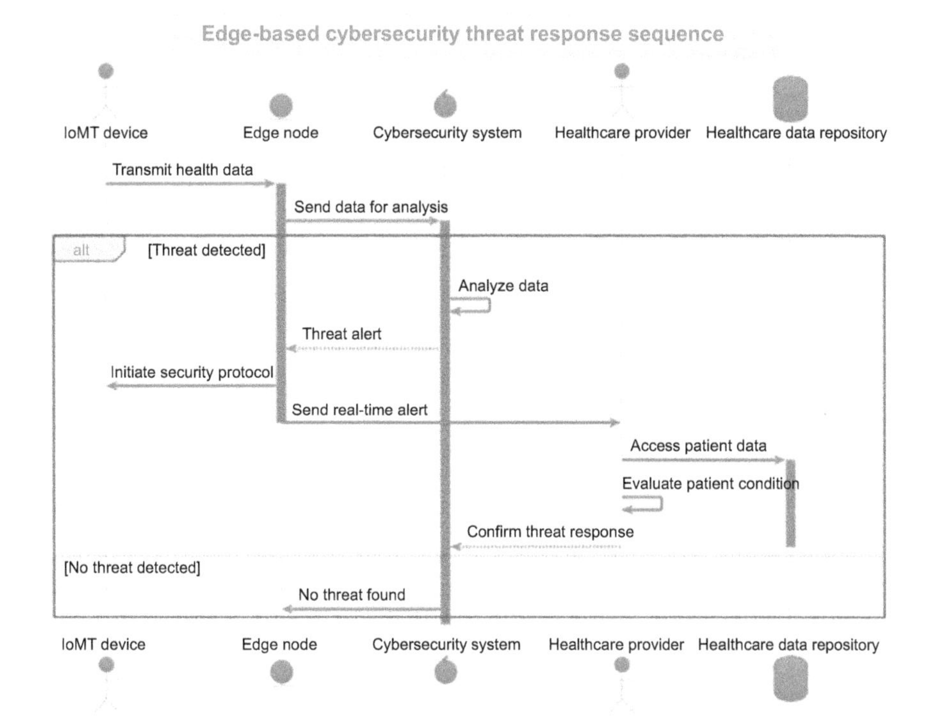

Figure 16.6 Real-time cybersecurity response in IoMT-enabled healthcare

in identifying and responding to cybersecurity threats in a healthcare setting equipped with IoMT devices.

1. Initiation of data transmission: The sequence commences with an IoMT Device, such as a wearable health monitor or a connected medical instrument, transmitting vital health data to an Edge Node. This Edge Node acts as a local processing hub, ensuring rapid data handling and analysis.
2. Analysis of health data: Upon receiving the data, the Edge Node forwards it to the Cybersecurity System. This system, equipped with advanced analytical capabilities, scrutinizes the data for potential security threats, employing algorithms that can detect anomalies indicative of cyberattacks or system malfunctions.
3. Threat detection and alert mechanism: In scenarios where a threat is detected, the Cybersecurity System undertakes a deeper analysis of the data. Subsequently, it generates an alert that is relayed back to the Edge Node. This alert signifies the identification of a potential security breach or a data integrity issue.
4. Activation of security protocols: The Edge Node, upon receiving the threat alert, initiates predefined security protocols on the IoMT Device. These protocols may include steps to isolate the device, secure the data, or initiate countermeasures to mitigate the threat.
5. Alerting the healthcare provider: Concurrently, the Edge Node dispatches a real-time alert to the Healthcare Provider. This alert is crucial as it informs the medical staff of the potential threat, enabling them to take appropriate actions, which may range from clinical decisions to technical interventions.
6. Healthcare provider's role:
   - The Healthcare Provider accesses the patient's health records and related data from a centralized Healthcare Data Repository. This step is pivotal for contextualizing the alert within the patient's health history and current condition.
   - The Provider assesses the patient's condition in light of the alert, determining the clinical implications of the reported data anomaly or security threat.
   - Subsequently, the Healthcare Provider communicates with the Cybersecurity System to confirm or refine the response to the detected threat, ensuring patient safety and data integrity.

7. Handling non-threat scenarios: In instances where the Cybersecurity System does not detect a threat, it communicates this status to the Edge Node. This communication marks the end of the sequence, indicating that the data transmitted by the IoMT Device is secure and free from any immediate cyber threats.

Figure 16.6 effectively encapsulates the dynamic and multi-layered approach required in modern healthcare cybersecurity frameworks. It underscores the importance of swift, coordinated actions among IoMT Devices, Edge Nodes,

Cybersecurity Systems, and Healthcare Providers [10]. This orchestrated response mechanism is vital for ensuring the security of sensitive health data and the uninterrupted functionality of critical medical devices in the face of evolving cyber threats.

16.5.4 Stateful dynamics of edge-based cybersecurity in IoMT

The intricate nature of cybersecurity in the context of the IoMT necessitates a comprehensive understanding of the various states and transitions that a system undergoes in response to potential threats [3]. Figure 16.7 provides a detailed visualization of these dynamic processes, illustrating how an Edge-Based Cybersecurity System transitions between different states based on specific triggers and conditions:

1. Idle state: The system begins in an "Idle" state, where it is operational but not actively processing data. This state represents the system's readiness to receive and process data from IoMT devices.
2. DataReceiving state: Upon initiation of data transmission from an IoMT device, the system transitions to the "DataReceiving" state. Here, it actively receives health data from the IoMT devices for analysis.
3. Analyzing state: Once the data is received, the system moves to the "Analyzing" state, where it employs algorithms to analyze the data for potential security threats or anomalies.
4. ThreatDetected state: If an anomaly or threat is detected during analysis, the system enters the "ThreatDetected" state. This state triggers the system's security protocols to respond to the identified threat.
5. Responding state: In the "Responding" state, the system executes predefined response protocols to mitigate the detected threat. This may include isolating affected devices or systems, initiating countermeasures, or other security actions.
6. Reporting state: Following the response, the system transitions to the "Reporting" state, where it generates reports and logs for compliance and review purposes. This state ensures that all actions and data are documented for regulatory compliance and future analysis.
7. Alerting state: Simultaneously, in the case of a detected threat, the system may also enter an "Alerting" state, where it sends real-time alerts to healthcare providers or IT administrators, informing them of the threat and the actions taken.
8. Return to idle: After completing the necessary actions in the "Responding," "Reporting," and "Alerting" states, the system returns to the "Idle" state, ready to process new data transmissions.

Figure 16.7 effectively illustrates the dynamic nature of an Edge-Based Cybersecurity System within a healthcare IoMT context. It highlights the system's ability to transition between various states in response to data inputs and detected

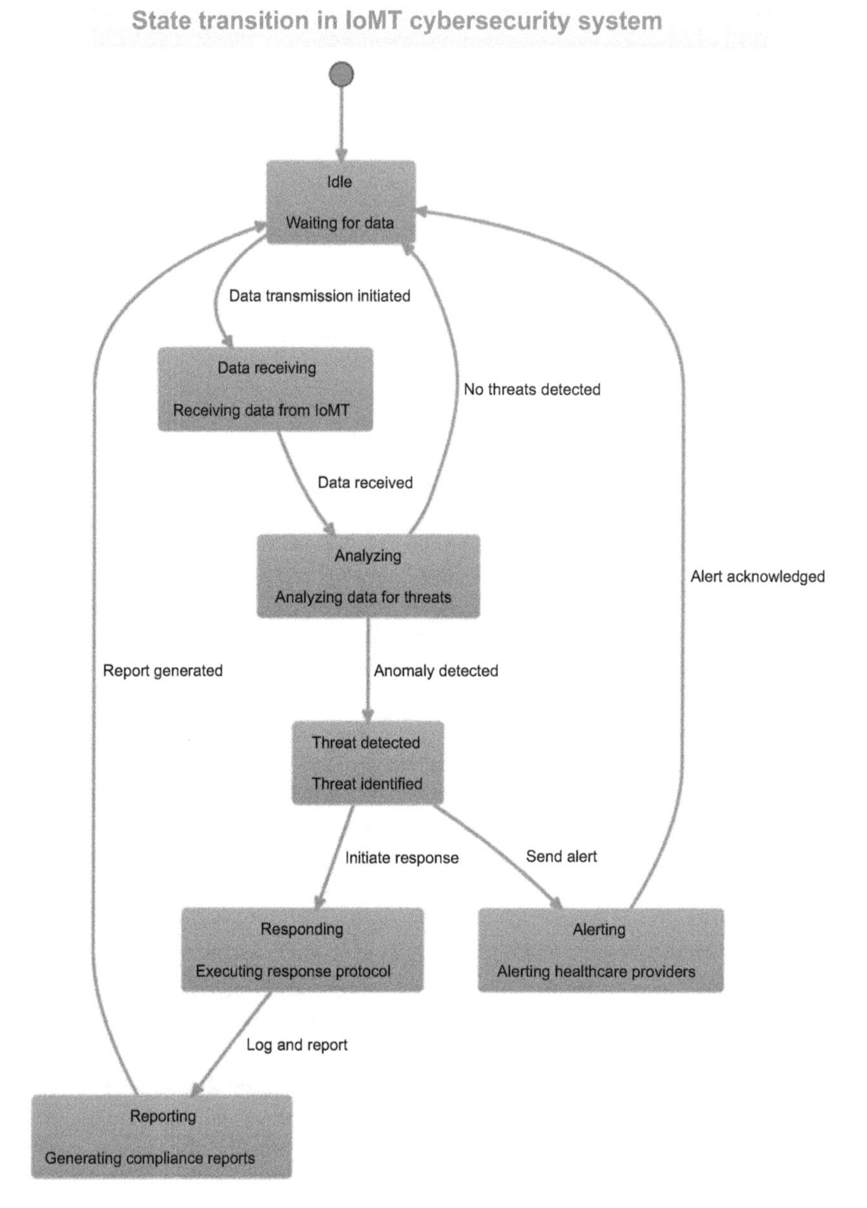

Figure 16.7 State transition in IoMT cybersecurity system

threats, showcasing the agility and responsiveness required for effective cybersecurity in healthcare [5,14]. This stateful approach ensures that the system remains vigilant and proactive in protecting sensitive health data, adapting to emerging threats, and maintaining the integrity of the healthcare IoMT ecosystem.

16.5.5 Architectural blueprint of edge-based cybersecurity in IoMT

Figure 16.8 is a comprehensive representation of the modular structure of an Edge-Based Cybersecurity Framework within the IoMT environment. This diagram delineates the key components and their interconnections, providing a clear overview of the system's architecture and the collaborative functionality of its parts [7,17]:

1. IoMT devices: This component represents various medical devices and sensors that collect health data from patients. These devices are integral to the IoMT ecosystem, providing real-time health monitoring.

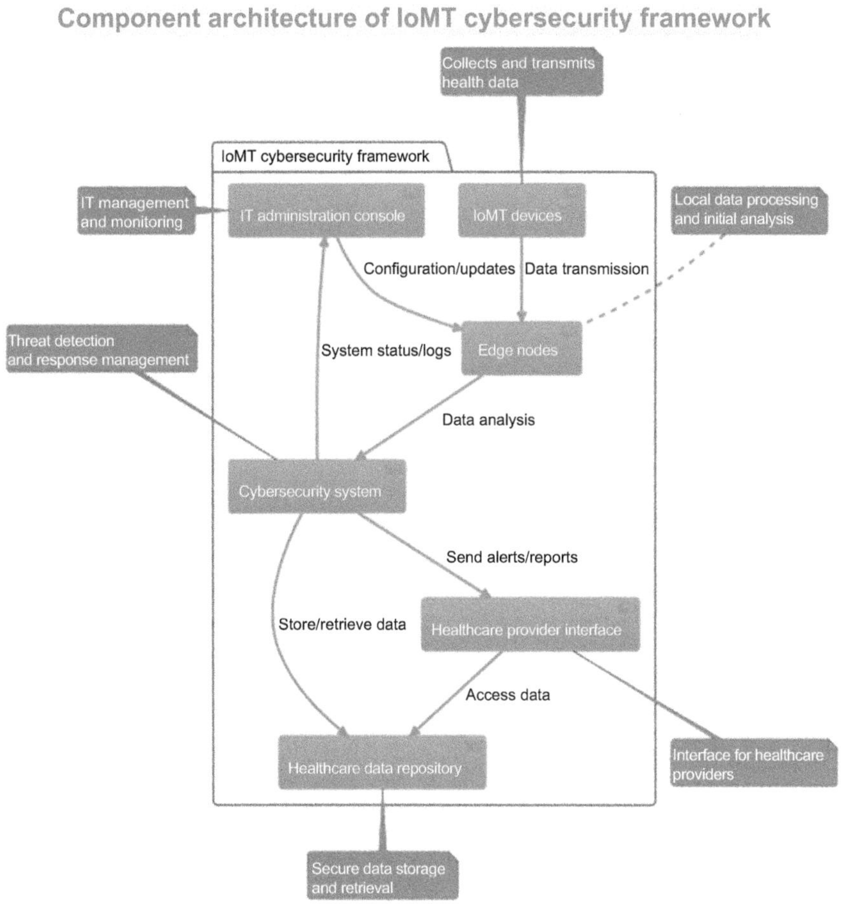

Figure 16.8 Component architecture of IoMT cybersecurity framework

2. Edge nodes: Serving as local processing hubs, Edge Nodes receive data from IoMT Devices. They perform initial data processing and analysis, reducing latency and bandwidth usage by handling data close to its source.
3. Cybersecurity system: This central component is responsible for advanced data analysis, threat detection, and response management. It employs sophisticated algorithms to identify potential security threats and coordinates the system's response to these threats.
4. Healthcare data repository: A secure storage component, the Data Repository, is where patient data and system logs are stored. It ensures data integrity and compliance with healthcare regulations.
5. Healthcare provider interface: This interface allows healthcare providers to access patient data, receive alerts, and review reports generated by the Cybersecurity System. It is designed for ease of use, ensuring that medical professionals can quickly respond to potential issues.
6. IT administration console: This component provides IT administrators with tools for system configuration, monitoring, and maintenance. It allows for the management of Edge Nodes and the overall cybersecurity infrastructure.

Interconnections and collaborative functionality:

- Data flow: Data flows from IoMT Devices to Edge Nodes for initial processing. The processed data is then sent to the Cybersecurity System for advanced analysis.
- Alerts and reporting: The Cybersecurity System communicates with the Healthcare Provider Interface to deliver real-time alerts and reports, ensuring prompt response to any detected threats.
- System management: The IT Administration Console interacts with both the Edge Nodes and the Cybersecurity System, facilitating system configuration, updates, and monitoring.

Figure 16.8 provides a clear and structured view of the system's architecture, highlighting the interplay between its various components. This architectural blueprint is crucial for understanding how different parts of the system work together to provide a comprehensive cybersecurity solution in the IoMT landscape [12,15]. It underscores the importance of each component in ensuring the security and efficiency of healthcare services, reflecting the complexity and collaborative nature of modern healthcare cybersecurity systems.

16.5.6 Deployment strategy for edge-based cybersecurity in IoMT

Figure 16.9 provides a strategic view of the deployment architecture for an Edge-Based Cybersecurity Framework within the IoMT environment. This diagram illustrates the physical and logical distribution of system components, highlighting how they are interconnected across different locations and networks to ensure a robust cybersecurity posture [7,19].

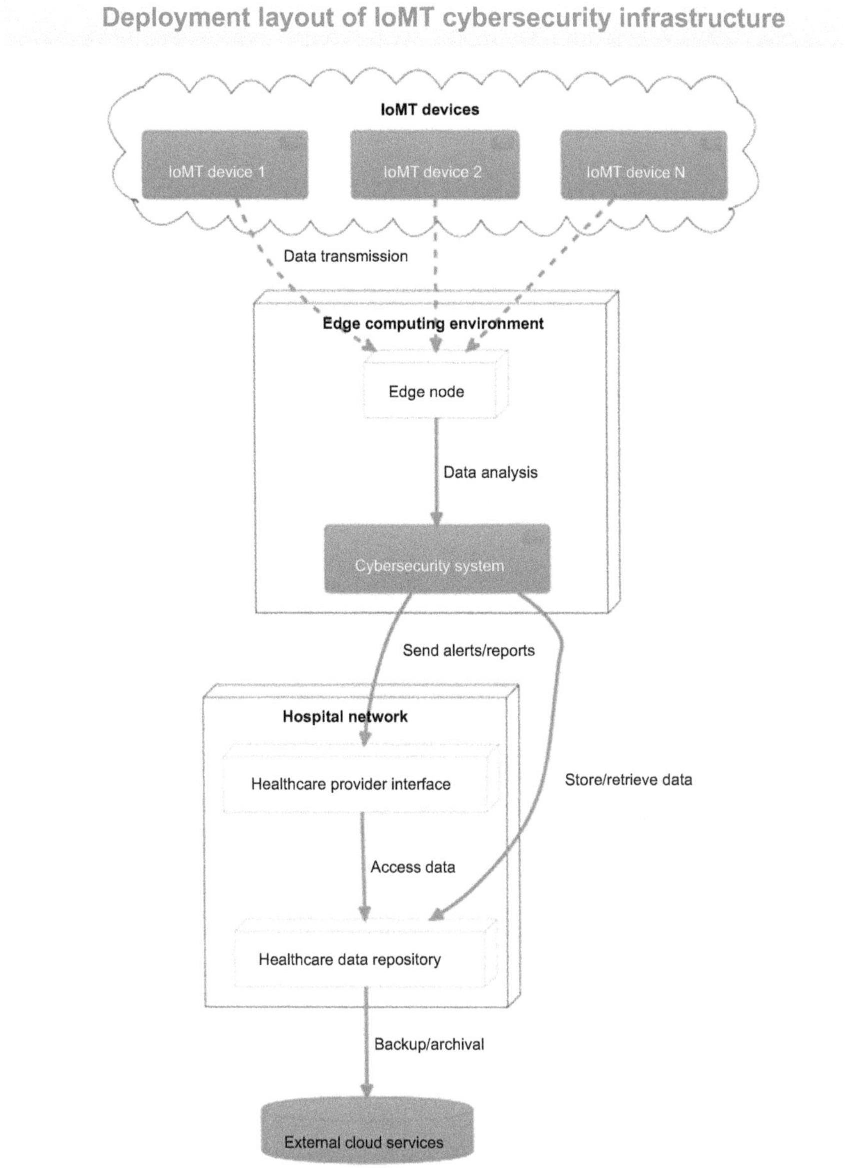

Deployment layout of IoMT cybersecurity infrastructure

IoMT devices
IoMT device 1
IoMT device 2
IoMT device N
Data transmission
Edge computing environment
Edge node
Data analysis
Cybersecurity system
Send alerts/reports
Hospital network
Healthcare provider interface
Store/retrieve data
Access data
Healthcare data repository
Backup/archival
External cloud services

Figure 16.9 Deployment layout of IoMT cybersecurity infrastructure

Detailed description of the deployment diagram:

1. IoMT devices: Represented as a cloud, this component includes various IoMT devices (IoMT Device 1, 2, …, N) such as wearable health monitors and connected medical instruments. These devices are deployed within patient environments and are responsible for collecting health data.

2. Edge computing environment: This node encapsulates the Edge Node and the Cybersecurity System. The Edge Node receives data from IoMT devices, performing initial processing and analysis. The Cybersecurity System, co-located with the Edge Node, conducts advanced data analysis for threat detection.
3. Hospital network: Within this network, two critical components are deployed:
   - Healthcare data repository: A secure database that stores and manages patient data and system logs.
   - Healthcare provider interface: An interface used by healthcare professionals to access patient data, receive system alerts, and review reports.
4. External cloud services: This database represents cloud-based services used for additional data backup and archival purposes, ensuring data redundancy and recovery capabilities.

   Interconnections and data flow:

- Data transmission: IoMT devices transmit health data to the Edge Node for initial processing.
- Data analysis and reporting: The Edge Node sends processed data to the Cybersecurity System for further analysis. Detected threats and reports are then communicated to the Healthcare Provider Interface in the Hospital Network.
- Data storage and backup: Processed and analyzed data is stored in the Healthcare Data Repository, with additional backups maintained in External Cloud Services.

Figure 16.9 elucidates the deployment architecture of an Edge-Based Cybersecurity Framework in a healthcare setting. It demonstrates the strategic distribution of components across patient, edge, and hospital environments, ensuring efficient data processing, robust security, and seamless communication. This deployment strategy is pivotal in achieving a comprehensive and resilient cybersecurity infrastructure, capable of protecting sensitive health data in the increasingly interconnected world of IoMT [9].

16.5.7 Realizing an integrated edge-based cybersecurity framework in IoMT

The development of an Edge-Based Cybersecurity Framework for the IoMT represents a significant advancement in healthcare technology. Through a series of meticulously designed diagrams—Use Case, Sequence, State, Component, and Deployment—we have systematically constructed a blueprint for a robust cybersecurity system. Each diagram serves as a cog in the intricate machinery of this framework, collectively providing a comprehensive understanding of its functionality, architecture, and deployment strategy.

The integration of this cybersecurity framework with IoMT devices is a cornerstone of its design. IoMT devices, ranging from wearable health monitors to sophisticated medical equipment, are the primary data sources in this ecosystem. The Edge-Based approach ensures that data from these devices is processed in real-time, minimizing latency and enhancing the responsiveness of the system [9,12]:

1. Real-time data processing: At the Edge Nodes, data from IoMT devices undergoes initial processing. This proximity to data sources allows for swift analysis, crucial for timely threat detection and response. The real-time processing capability is vital in healthcare settings, where delays can have serious implications for patient care.
2. Seamless integration: The framework's architecture is designed to seamlessly integrate with a wide array of IoMT devices. This integration is facilitated through standardized communication protocols and interfaces, ensuring compatibility and interoperability across different devices and systems.
3. Advanced threat detection and response: The Cybersecurity System, equipped with sophisticated algorithms, analyzes data from Edge Nodes to detect potential threats. Upon detection, it initiates immediate response protocols, including real-time alerts to healthcare providers and automated countermeasures to mitigate risks.
4. Data security and compliance: Throughout this process, data security and compliance with healthcare regulations such as HIPAA are maintained. Data encryption at the edge, secure data storage, and compliance reporting are integral components of the framework, ensuring the protection of sensitive patient information.

The Edge-Based Cybersecurity Framework for IoMT is not just a solution for current challenges but also a foundation for future advancements. As IoMT continues to evolve, this framework can adapt and scale, incorporating new technologies and addressing emerging threats. The integration of AI and ML into this framework could further enhance its analytical capabilities, paving the way for predictive cybersecurity measures [3].

In conclusion, the development of this Edge-Based Cybersecurity Framework marks a significant step forward in securing the IoMT landscape. By prioritizing real-time data processing, seamless integration with IoMT devices, and robust threat detection and response mechanisms, this framework stands as a testament to the potential of modern cybersecurity solutions in healthcare. It embodies a proactive approach to cybersecurity, ensuring that healthcare providers can deliver safe and uninterrupted care in an increasingly digital world.

16.6 Application of edge computing in healthcare

The integration of Edge Computing into healthcare systems has emerged as a transformative approach to enhance cybersecurity and operational efficiency. This section delves into the successful applications of Edge Computing in healthcare, analyzing how this technology has been instrumental in fortifying cybersecurity measures, optimizing data processing, and improving overall healthcare delivery.

16.6.1 Analysis of successful examples of edge computing in enhancing cybersecurity

1. General use in hospitals [20]:
    - On-premise computing: Hospitals have increasingly adopted Edge Computing for on-premise computing through distributed servers, sensors, and micro data centers. This localized approach allows for immediate data analysis at the source, significantly enhancing the detection and mitigation of cybersecurity threats.
    - Benefits: The primary benefits include substantial bandwidth savings, real-time processing of local data, and reduced operational expenses. Moreover, Edge Computing facilitates network segmentation within hospitals, isolating systems like power management, HVAC, and medical equipment. This segmentation is crucial as it confines cybersecurity breaches to subnetworks, thereby limiting their overall impact.
    - Case study: A notable example is a metropolitan hospital that implemented Edge Computing to segregate its patient data processing from its general IT network. This segregation not only improved data processing speeds but also significantly reduced the risk of widespread data breaches.
2. Remote monitoring software [21]:
    - EcoStruxure TM IT by Schneider electric: This software exemplifies the effective management of Edge Computing systems in healthcare. It collects sensor data from critical infrastructure and transmits it to a centralized cloud-based data lake. This data is crucial for generating predictive reports and understanding the root causes of system issues, which is vital for maintaining robust cybersecurity.
    - Impact: The implementation of EcoStruxure TM IT in a network of clinics resulted in improved uptime and enhanced security, with predictive analytics enabling proactive responses to potential cybersecurity threats.
3. Managed service providers (MSPs) [22]:
    - Role of MSPs: With the scarcity of skilled IT staff, particularly in smaller and rural hospitals, MSPs have become essential. They remotely monitor Edge Computing IT, power, and cooling systems, implementing predictive maintenance to pre-emptively address issues before they lead to system downtime.
    - Cybersecurity enhancement: MSPs play a pivotal role in enhancing cybersecurity by ensuring continuous monitoring and maintenance of Edge Computing systems, thereby reducing the risk of cyberattacks and data breaches.
4. Secure development life cycle (SDL) [23–25]:
    - Selection of edge products: When choosing edge software and hardware products, it is crucial to opt for solutions developed with an SDL approach. This approach encompasses secure architecture reviews, threat modeling, secure coding practices, and rigorous security testing of each product.

- Enhanced security: Products developed under SDL are inherently more resilient against cyberattacks, as they are designed with security as a foundational element.

5. AT&T's cybersecurity insights report [26]:
   - Adoption trends: According to this report, nearly three-quarters of healthcare industry respondents were either planning to or had already implemented Edge Computing use cases. The surge in virtual and at-home care has been a significant driver of this adoption.
   - Popular use cases: The most prevalent use case involves consumer virtual care or "care anywhere." The report also highlights that 65% of respondents implementing Edge use cases sought the expertise of third-party trusted advisors for implementation, underscoring the importance of expert guidance in deploying Edge Computing solutions effectively.

Table 16.2 encapsulates the diverse applications of Edge Computing in enhancing cybersecurity within the healthcare sector. It highlights the multifaceted benefits ranging from operational efficiencies to improved cybersecurity measures.

Thus, the application of Edge Computing in healthcare has demonstrated substantial benefits in enhancing cybersecurity, optimizing data processing, and

Table 16.2 Edge computing applications in healthcare cybersecurity

Application	**Key features**	**Description**
General Use in Hospitals	On-Premise Computing	Hospitals utilize edge computing for localized data processing, enhancing speed and security.
	Benefits	Includes bandwidth savings, real-time data processing, and reduced operational expenses.
	Case Study	Example of a hospital improving data processing and security through network segmentation.
Remote Monitoring Software	EcoStruxure TM IT	Software by Schneider Electric for managing edge computing systems, enhancing predictive maintenance and cybersecurity.
	Impact	Improved system uptime and enhanced security in clinics through predictive analytics.
Managed Service Providers (MSPs)	Role of MSPs	MSPs monitor edge computing IT and infrastructure, addressing the shortage of skilled IT staff.
	Cybersecurity Enhancement	Implement predictive maintenance to enhance cybersecurity and system reliability.
Secure Development Life Cycle (SDL)	Selection of Edge Products	Emphasizes choosing products developed with SDL for increased resilience against cyber-attacks.
	Enhanced Security	Products developed under SDL are more secure due to rigorous security testing and design.
AT&T's Cybersecurity Insights Report	Adoption Trends	Reports a significant trend in healthcare toward adopting edge computing for virtual care.
	Popular Use Cases	Most popular use case involves consumer virtual care, with many seeking third-party expertise for implementation.

improving patient care. Through examples ranging from hospital network segmentation to remote monitoring software, and the involvement of MSPs and SDL-based product development, Edge Computing has proven to be a pivotal technology in modern healthcare. Its ability to process data at the source and its integration with advanced cybersecurity measures have set a new standard in protecting sensitive health information and ensuring the reliability of healthcare services.

16.6.2 Quantitative impact of edge computing in healthcare

- Enhancing algorithm performance [27]. One of the most significant impacts of Edge Computing in healthcare is the enhancement of algorithm performance. A notable example is GE Healthcare's use of the Intel® Distribution of OpenVINO™ toolkit. This technology enabled a significant acceleration in the detection of pneumothorax, a critical condition, on the Optima XR240amx X-ray system. The implementation of Edge Computing technologies facilitated a more than threefold increase in processing speed. This acceleration is not just a technical achievement; it translates into faster diagnosis and treatment, potentially saving lives by enabling healthcare providers to respond more rapidly to critical conditions.
- Reduction in hospital readmissions [27]. A 2015 study highlighted the impact of Edge Computing in reducing hospital readmissions. The study focused on patients receiving remote medical care, a field where Edge Computing plays a pivotal role. The findings were remarkable: there was a 50% reduction in 30-day hospital readmissions and a 19% reduction in 180-day readmissions among patients under remote care. These statistics underscore the effectiveness of Edge Computing in enhancing remote patient monitoring systems, leading to better patient outcomes and reduced healthcare costs.
- Early sepsis detection by HCA healthcare [28]. HCA Healthcare's implementation of the SPOT (Sepsis Prediction and Optimization of Therapy) system, developed in collaboration with Red Hat, is another testament to the power of Edge Computing. The SPOT system leverages Edge Computing to analyze patient data in real-time, enabling the early detection of sepsis symptoms. Remarkably, this system has been able to detect signs of sepsis up to 20 hours earlier than traditional methods. This early detection is crucial, as sepsis is a time-sensitive condition where each hour can significantly impact patient outcomes. The SPOT system's success in early sepsis detection demonstrates how Edge Computing can be a lifesaver in critical care scenarios.

These examples provide concrete evidence of the transformative impact of Edge Computing in healthcare. By enhancing algorithm performance, reducing hospital readmissions, and enabling early detection of critical conditions like sepsis, Edge Computing is not just improving healthcare operations but also saving lives. Its ability to process data rapidly and locally translates into real-world benefits: faster diagnoses, more effective treatments, and improved patient care. As Edge Computing continues to evolve, its role in healthcare is poised to become even more significant, driving innovations that cater to the ever-growing needs of modern medicine.

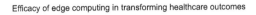

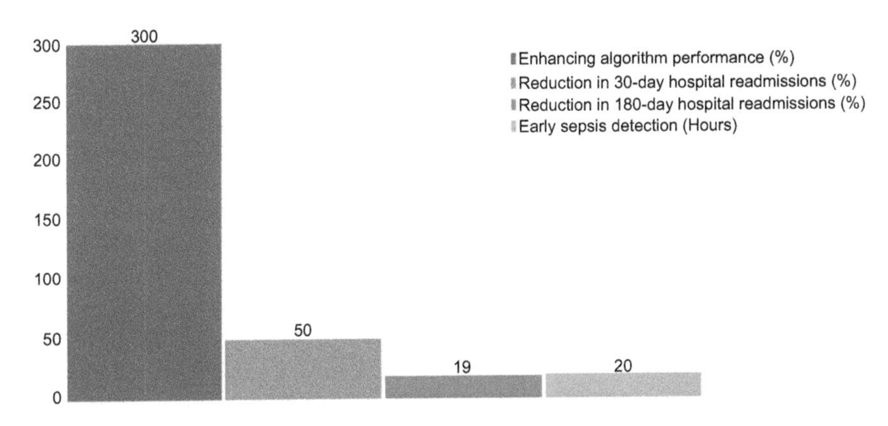

Figure 16.10 Efficacy of edge computing in transforming healthcare outcomes

Figure 16.10 elucidates the significant advancements in healthcare outcomes attributed to edge computing. It quantifies the enhancement in algorithm performance and the reduction in hospital readmissions over varying time frames, alongside the expedited detection of sepsis. The metrics are presented in percentages for the first three categories and hours for the last, underscoring the diverse yet profound impact of this technology in clinical settings. This visualization serves as a testament to the transformative potential of edge computing in optimizing healthcare delivery and patient outcomes.

16.6.3 Global adoption and risk assessment of edge computing in healthcare

The global adoption of Edge Computing in healthcare, coupled with the heightened focus on cybersecurity, illustrates the sector's commitment to embracing innovative technologies while acknowledging and addressing the associated risks. As Edge Computing continues to evolve, it is poised to play an increasingly vital role in shaping the future of healthcare, driving efficiencies, enhancing patient care, and fortifying data security.

- Widespread adoption of edge computing [29]. The adoption of Edge Computing in healthcare has been gaining significant momentum globally. According to recent statistics, 74% of healthcare organizations worldwide are either planning, partially, or have fully implemented Edge Computing use cases. This widespread adoption underscores the growing recognition of Edge Computing's potential to revolutionize healthcare delivery and data management. Among these organizations, those at a mature stage of Edge Computing implementation have identified consumer virtual care as the leading use case, accounting for 43% of the applications. This trend reflects the shifting focus toward patient-centric care models, where technology like

Edge Computing plays a crucial role in facilitating remote monitoring and telehealth services.

- Healthcare risk assessment [8,29,30]. With the increasing reliance on Edge Computing, cybersecurity has become a paramount concern for healthcare organizations. A significant 63.8% of these organizations perceive attacks on edge servers/data as the most significant cybersecurity threats. This concern is closely followed by the fear of attacks against connected cloud workloads, cited by 63.4% of organizations as one of the riskiest future attacks. These statistics highlight the critical need for robust cybersecurity measures in Edge Computing environments, especially considering the sensitive nature of healthcare data and the potential impact of data breaches on patient privacy and care.
- Cybersecurity investments [29,31,32]. In response to these cybersecurity challenges, healthcare organizations are significantly ramping up their investments in cybersecurity measures within Edge Computing projects. Currently, 44% of these organizations plan to allocate between 11% and 20% of their total Edge Computing use case expenditures directly to cybersecurity. This allocation marks a substantial increase compared to previous years, where only 1% of the total project budget was planned for cybersecurity at the planning stage. This shift in investment priorities indicates a growing awareness of the importance of cybersecurity in the successful implementation of Edge Computing in healthcare. It reflects an understanding that safeguarding data and systems is not just a technical necessity but a fundamental aspect of ensuring patient safety and trust in healthcare services.

Figure 16.11 presents a comprehensive overview of the current state of Edge Computing in healthcare. It highlights the widespread adoption and implementation stages of Edge Computing. This data underscores the critical role of Edge

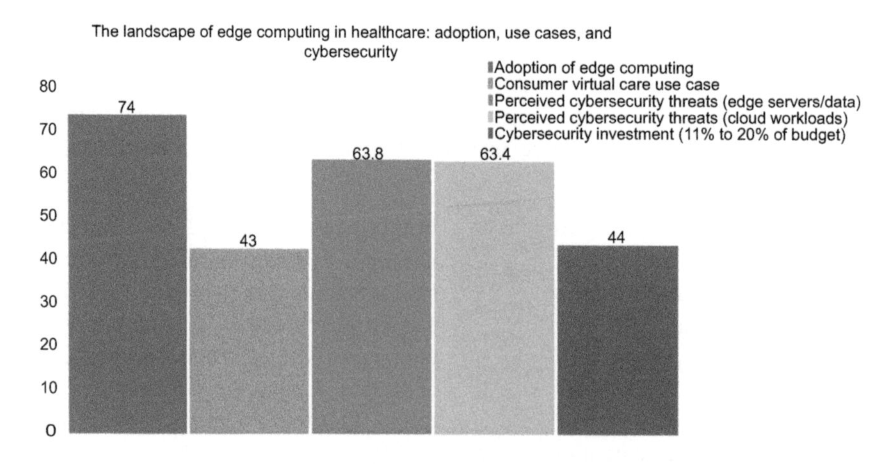

Figure 16.11 The landscape of edge computing in healthcare: adoption, use cases, and cybersecurity

Computing in modern healthcare, while also emphasizing the need for robust cybersecurity measures to protect sensitive healthcare data and maintain patient trust.

16.7 The future of edge computing and cybersecurity in healthcare

As we stand on the cusp of a new era in healthcare technology, Edge Computing and cybersecurity are poised to play increasingly pivotal roles. The integration of these technologies into healthcare systems is not just a trend but a paradigm shift, shaping the future of healthcare delivery and data security. This section explores the emerging trends and predictions in the realm of Edge Computing and cybersecurity within healthcare, offering insights into what the future may hold.

16.7.1 Trends and predictions

1. Increased integration of AI and ML:
   - Future Edge Computing systems in healthcare are expected to extensively integrate AI and ML. These technologies will enhance the capability of Edge Computing to analyze vast amounts of data in real-time, leading to more accurate and timely clinical decisions.
   - AI and ML will also play a crucial role in predictive analytics, enabling healthcare providers to anticipate and mitigate potential cybersecurity threats before they materialize.
2. Expansion of IoMT devices:
   - The IoMT is set to expand significantly, with a broader range of devices becoming interconnected. This expansion will necessitate more robust and scalable Edge Computing infrastructures to manage the increased data flow and ensure real-time data processing.
   - With more devices comes a greater surface area for cyber threats, thus driving advancements in cybersecurity measures tailored specifically for IoMT environments.
3. Enhanced focus on data privacy and compliance:
   - As Edge Computing becomes more prevalent, there will be an enhanced focus on data privacy and compliance with healthcare regulations such as HIPAA and GDPR. Edge Computing architectures will be designed with privacy-by-design principles, ensuring that patient data is protected at every stage of processing.
   - Compliance will also extend to the development of Edge Computing hardware and software, with stringent standards being applied to ensure data security and patient confidentiality.
4. Adoption of blockchain for data security:
   - Blockchain technology is predicted to be increasingly adopted in Edge Computing environments for its ability to provide secure, tamper-proof

data management. This will be particularly beneficial in managing patient records and ensuring the integrity of medical data.
- Blockchain, combined with Edge Computing, can create a decentralized and secure framework for data exchange in healthcare, enhancing trust and transparency in the system.

5. Development of edge-as-a-service (EaaS):
    - The concept of Edge-as-a-Service (EaaS) is expected to gain traction, offering healthcare organizations scalable and customizable Edge Computing solutions. EaaS will enable healthcare providers to deploy Edge Computing capabilities without the need for extensive in-house infrastructure, reducing costs, and enhancing flexibility.
    - EaaS providers will also offer integrated cybersecurity services, ensuring that healthcare organizations have access to the latest security technologies and expertise.

The future of Edge Computing and cybersecurity in healthcare is marked by rapid technological advancements and a shift toward more integrated, secure, and patient-centric systems. The trends and predictions outlined in this section highlight the potential of these technologies to revolutionize healthcare, offering improved patient care, enhanced data security, and more efficient healthcare delivery. As we move forward, it is clear that Edge Computing and cybersecurity will be at the forefront of healthcare innovation, shaping the landscape of medical technology for years to come.

16.7.2 The necessity of adapting healthcare infrastructure

The rapid evolution of Edge Computing and cybersecurity in healthcare necessitates a corresponding transformation in healthcare infrastructure. This adaptation is not merely a response to technological advancements but a proactive approach to meet the changing landscape of healthcare needs and challenges.

1. Upgrading network capabilities:
    - To accommodate the increased data flow from IoMT devices and Edge Computing systems, healthcare facilities must upgrade their network infrastructure. This includes enhancing bandwidth, improving network speed, and ensuring reliable connectivity to support real-time data processing and analysis.
    - Network security must also be bolstered to protect against potential cyber threats, which become more sophisticated with the advancement of technology.

2. Investing in advanced hardware and software:
    - Healthcare institutions need to invest in advanced hardware capable of supporting Edge Computing functionalities. This includes more powerful servers, dedicated Edge nodes, and secure storage solutions.
    - Software infrastructure also requires an upgrade, with a focus on integrating AI and ML capabilities for advanced data analytics and cybersecurity threat detection.

3. Training and development of IT staff:
   - As Edge Computing and cybersecurity technologies become more complex, the need for skilled IT professionals in healthcare becomes more critical. Healthcare organizations must invest in training and developing their IT staff to manage and maintain these advanced systems.
   - Continuous education and training programs will be essential to keep healthcare IT personnel abreast of the latest developments in Edge Computing and cybersecurity.
4. Implementing robust data management policies:
   - With the influx of patient data through IoMT devices, healthcare providers must establish robust data management policies. These policies should address data collection, storage, processing, and sharing while ensuring compliance with privacy regulations.
   - Data management policies must also include protocols for data backup, recovery, and secure disposal to maintain data integrity and patient confidentiality.
5. Collaboration with technology providers:
   - Healthcare institutions should collaborate with technology providers and industry experts to design and implement Edge Computing solutions tailored to their specific needs.
   - These collaborations can provide access to the latest technologies, expert insights, and support in developing a healthcare infrastructure that is both advanced and secure.

The necessity of adapting healthcare infrastructure to the evolving landscape of Edge Computing and cybersecurity is clear. This adaptation involves not only technological upgrades but also strategic planning, staff development, policy formulation, and collaborative efforts with technology experts. By embracing these changes, healthcare providers can ensure that their infrastructure is equipped to handle the demands of modern healthcare delivery, offering improved patient care, enhanced data security, and operational efficiency.

16.8 Lessons learned from the study

As we approach the conclusion of this comprehensive study on the integration of Edge Computing and cybersecurity within healthcare systems, it is imperative to reflect on the key lessons learned. These insights not only encapsulate the essence of our research but also provide valuable guidance for future endeavors in this rapidly evolving field.

1. The critical role of real-time data processing: One of the primary lessons is the undeniable importance of real-time data processing in healthcare. Edge Computing emerges as a pivotal solution, offering reduced latency and enhanced efficiency in handling vast amounts of medical data generated by IoMT devices.

2. Cybersecurity as a foundational element: The study underscores that cybersecurity is not an afterthought but a foundational element in the design and implementation of healthcare technologies. As healthcare systems become increasingly reliant on digital technologies, the integration of robust cybersecurity measures is essential for protecting sensitive patient data and ensuring system integrity.
3. Adaptability of healthcare infrastructure: The necessity for healthcare infrastructure to adapt and evolve in response to technological advancements is a key lesson. This includes upgrading network capabilities, investing in advanced hardware and software, and ensuring that healthcare professionals are adequately trained to manage these new technologies.
4. Interdisciplinary collaboration is key: The study highlights the importance of interdisciplinary collaboration between healthcare professionals, technology experts, and policymakers. Such collaborations are crucial for developing effective Edge Computing solutions that are secure, efficient, and tailored to the specific needs of the healthcare sector.
5. Balancing innovation with ethical considerations: As technological innovations like Edge Computing and AI continue to advance, it is crucial to balance these developments with ethical considerations, particularly regarding patient privacy and data security. Ethical guidelines and regulations must evolve alongside technological advancements to ensure responsible and secure use of technology in healthcare.
6. Preparedness for emerging threats: The dynamic nature of cybersecurity threats necessitates continuous vigilance and preparedness. The healthcare sector must stay abreast of emerging threats and continuously update its cybersecurity strategies to protect against evolving risks.
7. Importance of tailored cybersecurity frameworks: The study reinforces the need for cybersecurity frameworks that are specifically tailored to the unique challenges of healthcare Edge Computing environments. Generic solutions may not adequately address the specific security needs of healthcare systems.
8. Future-proofing healthcare technology: Finally, the study emphasizes the need for future-proofing healthcare technology. This involves not only anticipating future technological trends but also preparing for the potential challenges and opportunities these advancements may bring.

These lessons learned serve as guiding principles for future research and implementation in the field of Edge Computing and cybersecurity in healthcare. They underscore the complexity and multidimensionality of integrating advanced technologies in healthcare systems, highlighting the need for continuous innovation, collaboration, and ethical consideration.

16.9 Conclusion

As we conclude this comprehensive exploration of Edge Computing and cybersecurity in healthcare, it is evident that we are witnessing a paradigm shift in how healthcare data is managed, processed, and protected. The integration of Edge

Computing into healthcare systems represents not just a technological advancement but a fundamental rethinking of data handling and security strategies in response to the burgeoning demands of modern healthcare.

1. Transformative impact of edge computing: The adoption of Edge Computing has shown immense potential in enhancing the efficiency and effectiveness of healthcare services. By bringing data processing closer to the source, Edge Computing has enabled real-time analytics, faster decision-making, and improved patient outcomes. The integration with IoMT devices has further augmented the capabilities of healthcare systems, allowing for more comprehensive and continuous patient monitoring.
2. Evolving landscape of cybersecurity: Alongside the benefits, the increased reliance on digital technologies has underscored the critical importance of robust cybersecurity measures. The healthcare sector, being a repository of sensitive patient data, has become a prime target for cyber threats. The evolution of cybersecurity strategies, in tandem with Edge Computing, is crucial in safeguarding patient data against increasingly sophisticated cyberattacks.
3. The need for adaptive infrastructure: The shift toward Edge Computing and enhanced cybersecurity necessitates a corresponding evolution in healthcare infrastructure. This involves not only technological upgrades but also a strategic approach to network management, data policies, and staff training. The future of healthcare will depend significantly on the ability of healthcare providers to adapt their infrastructure to these emerging technologies.
4. Collaboration and continuous learning: The journey toward a fully integrated Edge Computing and cybersecurity ecosystem in healthcare is an ongoing process. It requires collaboration between healthcare providers, technology experts, policymakers, and researchers. Continuous learning and adaptation to new technologies and threats will be essential in navigating this evolving landscape.
5. Looking ahead: As we look to the future, it is clear that Edge Computing and cybersecurity will continue to play pivotal roles in shaping the healthcare sector. The potential for further innovations, such as the integration of AI and blockchain technologies, promises to further enhance the capabilities and security of healthcare systems.

In summary, the integration of Edge Computing and cybersecurity in healthcare is a critical step toward a more efficient, secure, and patient-centric healthcare system. As these technologies continue to evolve, they will undoubtedly bring new challenges, but also new opportunities to improve the quality and delivery of healthcare services. The proactive adaptation of healthcare infrastructure and the continuous evolution of cybersecurity strategies will be key in harnessing the full potential of these technological advancements.

Acknowledgment

- This project has received funding from the European Union's Horizon 2020 research and innovation program under the Marie Skłodowska-Curie grant agreement No. 101007820 – TRUST.

- This publication reflects only the author's view and the REA is not responsible for any use that may be made of the information it contains.

References

[1] M. Laroui, B. Nour, H. Moungla, M. A. Cherif, H. Afifi, and M. Guizani, "Edge and Fog Computing for IoT: A Survey on Current Research Activities and Future Directions," *Computer Communications*, vol. 180, pp. 210–231, 2021, doi:10.1016/j.comcom.2021.09.003.

[2] Y. Winnie, E. Umamaheswari, and D. M. Ajay, "Enhancing Data Security in IoT Healthcare Services Using Fog Computing," in *2018 International Conference on Recent Trends in Advance Computing (ICRTAC)*, 2018, pp. 200–205. IEEE. doi:10.1109/ICRTAC.2018.8679404.

[3] M. L. Hernandez-Jaimes, A. Martinez-Cruz, K. A. Ramírez-Gutiérrez, and C. Feregrino-Uribe, "Artificial Intelligence for IoMT Security: A Review of Intrusion Detection Systems, Attacks, Datasets and Cloud–Fog–Edge Architectures," *Internet of Things*, vol. 23, p. 100887, 2023, doi:10.1016/j.iot.2023.100887.

[4] P. Sarkhel and J. Chanda, "SecureHome: A Privacy Preserving Health Care Smart Home Systems," in *2021 8th International Conference on Internet of Things: Systems, Management and Security (IOTSMS)*, 2021, pp. 1–5. doi:10.1109/IOTSMS53705.2021.9704945.

[5] M. Paul, L. Maglaras, M. A. Ferrag, and I. Almomani, "Digitization of Healthcare Sector: A Study on Privacy and Security Concerns," *ICT Express*, vol. 9, no. 4, pp. 571–588, 2023, doi:10.1016/j.icte.2023.02.007.

[6] G. Aceto, V. Persico, and A. Pescapé, "Industry 4.0 and Health: Internet of Things, Big Data, and Cloud Computing for Healthcare 4.0," *Journal of Industrial Information Integration*, vol. 18, p. 100129, 2020, doi:10.1016/j.jii.2020.100129.

[7] R. Akkaoui, X. Hei, and W. Cheng, "EdgeMediChain: A Hybrid Edge Blockchain-Based Framework for Health Data Exchange," *IEEE Access*, vol. 8, pp. 113467–113486, 2020, doi:10.1109/ACCESS.2020.3003575.

[8] G. Pascarella, M. Rossi, E. Montella, *et al.*, "Risk Analysis in Healthcare Organizations: Methodological Framework and Critical Variables," *Risk Manag Healthc Policy*, vol. 14, pp. 2897–2911, 2021, doi:10.2147/RMHP.S309098.

[9] L. Tawalbeh, F. Muheidat, M. Tawalbeh, M. Quwaider, and A. A. Abd El-Latif, "Edge Enabled IoT System Model for Secure Healthcare," *Measurement*, vol. 191, p. 110792, 2022, doi:10.1016/j.measurement.2022.110792.

[10] D. Unal, S. Bennbaia, and F. O. Catak, "Chapter 12 – Machine Learning for the Security of Healthcare Systems Based on Internet of Things and Edge Computing – Qatar National Research Fund," in *Cybersecurity and Cognitive Science*, A. A. Moustafa, Ed., Academic Press, 2022, pp. 299–320. doi:10.1016/B978-0-323-90570-1.00007-3.

[11] L. Liu and Z. Li, "Permissioned Blockchain and Deep Reinforcement Learning Enabled Security and Energy Efficient Healthcare Internet of Things," *IEEE Access*, vol. 10, pp. 53640–53651, 2022, doi:10.1109/ACCESS.2022.3176444.

[12] M. Mahbub and R. M. Shubair, "Contemporary Advances in Multi-Access Edge Computing: A Survey of Fundamentals, Architecture, Technologies, Deployment Cases, Security, Challenges, and Directions," *Journal of Network and Computer Applications*, vol. 219, p. 103726, 2023, doi:10.1016/j.jnca.2023.103726.

[13] A. Yao, G. Li, X. Li, F. Jiang, J. Xu, and X. Liu, "Differential Privacy in Edge Computing-Based Smart City Applications: Security Issues, Solutions and Future Directions," *Array*, vol. 19, p. 100293, 2023, doi:10.1016/j.array.2023.100293.

[14] A. Hazra, A. Alkhayyat, and M. Adhikari, "Blockchain for Cybersecurity in Edge Networks," *IEEE Consumer Electronics Magazine*, vol. 13, no. 1, pp. 97–102, 2024, doi:10.1109/MCE.2022.3141068.

[15] R. Uddin, S. A. P. Kumar, and V. Chamola, "Denial of Service Attacks in Edge Computing Layers: Taxonomy, Vulnerabilities, Threats and Solutions," *Ad Hoc Networks*, vol. 152, p. 103322, 2024, doi:10.1016/j.adhoc.2023.103322.

[16] S. Ahmad, I. Shakeel, S. Mehfuz, and J. Ahmad, "Deep Learning Models for Cloud, Edge, Fog, and IoT Computing Paradigms: Survey, Recent Advances, and Future Directions," *Computer Science Review*, vol. 49, p. 100568, 2023, doi:10.1016/j.cosrev.2023.100568.

[17] C. Feng, Y. Wang, Q. Chen, Y. Ding, G. Strbac, and C. Kang, "Smart Grid Encounters Edge Computing: Opportunities and Applications," *Advances in Applied Energy*, vol. 1, p. 100006, 2021, doi:10.1016/j.adapen.2020.100006.

[18] M. Pawlicki, A. Pawlicka, R. Kozik, and M. Choraś, "The Survey and Meta-Analysis of the Attacks, Transgressions, Countermeasures and Security Aspects Common to the Cloud, Edge and IoT," *Neurocomputing*, vol. 551, p. 126533, 2023, doi:10.1016/j.neucom.2023.126533.

[19] "Secure Edge of Things for Smart Healthcare Surveillance Framework | IEEE Journals & Magazine | IEEE Xplore." Accessed: Dec. 23, 2023. [Online]. Available: https://ieeexplore.ieee.org/document/8654187

[20] S. E. Hassanin, "How Edge Computing Systems Lower Cybersecurity Risk in Healthcare while Enhancing Data Access," *Schneider Electric Blog*. Accessed: Dec. 22, 2023. [Online]. Available: https://blog.se.com/buildings/healthcare/2022/09/14/how-edge-computing-lower-cybersecurity-risk-healthcare-data-access/

[21] "EcoStruxure Asset Advisor | Schneider Electric | EcoStruxure IT." Accessed: Dec. 22, 2023. [Online]. Available: https://ecostruxureit.com/ecostruxure-asset-advisor/

[22] "Healthcare Managed Services Program (MSP) | AMN Healthcare." Accessed: Dec. 22, 2023. [Online]. Available: https://www.amnhealthcare.com/talent-planning/management/managed-services-programs/

[23] "Secure SDLC | Secure Software Development Life Cycle," Snyk. Accessed: Dec. 22, 2023. [Online]. Available: https://snyk.io/learn/secure-sdlc/
[24] C. Romeo, "Secure Development Lifecycle: The essential guide to safe software pipelines," TechBeacon. Accessed: Dec. 22, 2023. [Online]. Available: https://techbeacon.com/security/secure-development-lifecycle-essential-guide-safe-software-pipelines
[25] gluckd, "Microsoft Security Development Lifecycle (SDL) - Microsoft Service Assurance." Accessed: Dec. 22, 2023. [Online]. Available: https://learn.microsoft.com/it-it/compliance/assurance/assurance-microsoft-security-development-lifecycle
[26] HealthITSecurity, "As Adoption of Edge Computing in Healthcare Grows, So Do Security Needs," HealthITSecurity. Accessed: Dec. 22, 2023. [Online]. Available: https://healthitsecurity.com/news/as-adoption-of-edge-computing-in-healthcare-grows-so-do-security-needs
[27] W. the help of I. technologies, H. P. C. U. E. Computing, A. to C. D. into N. I. to H. I. P. O. W. D. Financial, and O. Value, "How Edge Computing Is Driving Advancements in Healthcare," Intel. Accessed: Dec. 23, 2023. [Online]. Available: https://www.intel.com/content/www/us/en/healthcare-it/edge-analytics.html
[28] "Edge computing in action: Healthcare." Accessed: Dec. 23, 2023. [Online]. Available: https://www.redhat.com/en/resources/edge-computing-health-care-brief
[29] T. Lanowitz, "AT&T Cybersecurity Insights Report: A Focus on Healthcare." Accessed: Dec. 23, 2023. [Online]. Available: https://cybersecurity.att.com/blogs/security-essentials/att-cybersecurity-insights-report-a-focus-on-healthcare
[30] O. US EPA, "Human Health Risk Assessment." Accessed: Dec. 23, 2023. [Online]. Available: https://www.epa.gov/risk/human-health-risk-assessment
[31] "European Cybersecurity Investment Platform," ECSO. Accessed: Dec. 23, 2023. [Online]. Available: https://ecs-org.eu/activities/european-cybersecurity-investment-platform/
[32] "Cybersecurity Investment: Spotlight on Vulnerability Management," ENISA. Accessed: Dec. 23, 2023. [Online]. Available: https://www.enisa.europa.eu/news/cybersecurity-investment-spotlight-on-vulnerability-management

Chapter 17

Enhancing healthcare data security: an intrusion detection system for web applications with SVM and decision tree algorithms

Micheal Olaolu Arowolo[1], Ominini Adango Jaja[2], Oluwatosin Faith Adeniyi[2], Prisca Olawoye[2], Oluwatomilola Babajide[3], Happiness Eric Aigbogun[4] and Mukhtar Damola Salawu[5]

Improving machine learning techniques for identifying attacks on healthcare web services is the focus of this study. Reliable intrusion detection systems are essential for the protection of sensitive medical data. This research introduces a new approach to K-means clustering by fusing the strengths of the Support Vector Machine (SVM) and the Decision Tree (DT) classifiers. Tests were successful using the "Friday-Working-Hours-Afternoon-DDos. pcap ISCX" scenario from the CIC-IDS2017 dataset. While both SVM and DT classifiers did well, Decision Tree's 99.96% accuracy was particularly outstanding. This state-of-the-art K-Means clustering method has become the de facto standard, with an associated accuracy of 99.96%. The need to keep medical records safe extends far beyond the obvious technology advantages. Intrusion detection systems must be adaptable since cyber threats are constantly evolving. This study examines the potential of cutting-edge intrusion detection systems for protecting electronic health records, as well as its limitations. In the midst of the ongoing digital revolutions in healthcare, this research charts a course toward a safer future for healthcare data.

Keywords: Artificial intelligence; medical information; Internet of Medical Things; AIoMT; COVID-19 pandemic data management; energy-efficient devices; wireless sensor nodes; security and privacy schemes

[1]Department of Electrical Engineering and Computer Science, University of Missouri, USA
[2]Department of Computer Science, Landmark University, Nigeria
[3]Department of Public Health, Western Illinois University, USA
[4]Stowers Institute for Medical Research, Kansas City, Missouri, USA
[5]Department of Computer Science, Kwara State University, Nigeria

17.1 Introduction

The security of sensitive data and digital infrastructure is of paramount importance in today's interconnected society. The widespread adoption of digital technologies has resulted in many positive outcomes, but it has also exposed consumers to unanticipated risks. The Intrusion Detection System (IDS) is a crucial part of today's security infrastructure. These devices (which can be hardware or software) act as watchful gatekeepers by monitoring network channels for any signs of trouble to stop malicious conduct or unauthorized access from disrupting software operations or leading to policy breaches [1].

To protect against both external and internal threats, intrusion detection was created. Scanning data from the network, the users, and the system logs, an IDS operates as a sentry, keeping a watchful eye out for any unusual behavior. When an intrusion attempt or other form of suspicious behavior is detected by the IDS, it immediately notifies the appropriate parties or takes the designated course of action [2]. It is impossible to exaggerate the value of IDS in today's linked society. Due to the increasing sophistication and frequency of cyberattacks, IDS functions have changed. Organizations and people require a security system that can detect not just the most prevalent but also the most unusual forms of cyberattack to stay ahead of the curve [3].

Different IDS are aimed at different types of threats, those utilized by signature-based intrusion prevention systems Similarities between a threat and previously recorded attacks are used by these systems to identify it. When new data arrives that fits the description of one of these patterns, an alert is generated [4]. They hold up well against well-known threats but may falter against more novel dangers. Anomaly-based IDS keep a watch out for anything out of the ordinary, while signature-based systems look for known malicious code. They can spot out-of-the-ordinary behavior that may indicate impending danger and act accordingly. Hybrid IDS combine signature-based and anomaly-based techniques to detect malicious activity. Hybrid IDS takes the best features of both approaches to guarantee that threats are identified as effectively as possible [5].

Cybersecurity is an ever-changing field since hackers are always improving their methods. Since then, IDS have come a long way, particularly thanks to developments in machine learning and Artificial Intelligence. As a result of these advancements, threat detection may become more complex and responsive to changing conditions [6]. In recent years, machine learning techniques have been applied to intrusion detection, considerably improving the capability to identify security breaches. Researchers have examined intercepted network packets using methods including Linear Discriminant Analysis (LDA), Classification and Regression Trees (CART), and Random Forest to better manage IP traffic for the sake of network security. Machine learning-based IDS are superior to their traditional counterparts because of their ability to spot novel threats [7].

IDS is also significantly more effective than other methods of network protection. IDS based on machine learning algorithms are crucial for safeguarding many applications in the modern era of IoT, big data, smart cities, and 5G network rollout. The demand for IDS has increased alongside the requirement for safeguarding vital infrastructure and IoT devices [8].

While there has been substantial development in the field of intrusion detection, there is still a way to go before it is completely problem-free. False alarms are one difficulty that must be overcome. A huge number of false warnings may be produced if it is unable to differentiate between harmless transients (which are common in complex systems), slowly accumulating faults, and actual cyber incursions. The security of IDS is compromised, and operational efficiency drops as a result [9].

Since cyber threats are always developing, it's important to take preventative measures to keep data safe. One of the newest methods fraudsters are using to get sensitive data is social engineering. Complex threats, such as ransomware, are becoming more sophisticated at an alarming rate, heightening the need for intrusion detection solutions that can keep up [10].

To improve the security of websites and web applications, this research proposes an intrusion detection method based on machine learning. The fundamental objective of this study is to classify and analyze data items for the purpose of analyzing and evaluating machine learning-based approaches to cybersecurity. The growing importance of digital healthcare data raises concerns about data security. It is crucial to safeguard hospital networks and patient data from hackers. As a result, this research will also investigate how intrusion detection relates to protecting sensitive healthcare information. Recent developments in machine learning, along with the ongoing importance of effective cybersecurity measures, are driving a paradigm shift in the IDS industry. By analyzing the efficacy of machine learning in intrusion detection, this study hopes to contribute to this rapidly expanding field by providing insight into the critically important topic of healthcare data security in today's increasingly digitalized world.

17.1.1 Chapter organization

Section 17.2 presents the related works on enhancing healthcare data security. Section 17.3 gives the methodologies used in enhancing healthcare data security. Section 17.4 presents the results and discussions of the proposed model. Section 17.5 concludes the chapter with future directions.

17.2 Related work

When comparing IDS for healthcare networks, it is best to take a comprehensive look at both the network infrastructure and the associated patient data [11]. As a result of the Internet of Things (IoT), doctors may remotely monitor their patients' vital signs and make an accurate diagnosis from any location. However, strict security standards are necessary to protect the privacy of patients' information. Vital patient records being hacked in an emergency could have devastating consequences. Due to the high dimensionality and extraordinary dynamism of the data involved, machine learning has the potential to become a useful intrusion detection technology. While there are still some outliers, most modern healthcare IDSs compile their databases using either network traffic metrics or patient biometric information. This research aimed to prove that by combining network and biometric measures, performance may be enhanced overusing method separately.

EHMS testbed can track network activity and gather data in real time from connected medical devices. The information is transmitted to a centralized computer for analysis to arrive at a diagnosis and plan of action. Over 16,000 healthcare records have been collected and analyzed by researchers, including both untouched and tampered with examples. To turn the dataset into usable training material, the system first secures it from further attack and then applies several machine learning algorithms. The results show that the proposed approach successfully detects intrusions, improving performance by as much as 25%.

Researchers developed a hybrid architecture based on deep learning to identify intrusions in healthcare IT systems [12]. Network IDS are under growing strain as both network traffic and user data expand at exponential rates. The healthcare business places a premium on reliable intrusion systems to ensure the security, confidentiality, and veracity of patients' electronic medical records. If the patient's actual statistics are different from the ones they provided, it could lead to diagnostic and therapeutic errors. Because they were trained on antiquated intrusion detection databases, many existing AI-based solutions necessitate starting from scratch when confronted with novel threats. The current intrusion detection methods used to protect healthcare institution computer networks may become obsolete sooner if these changes are implemented.

In this research, the authors introduce a hybrid system they call "ImmuneNet" that uses Deep Learning to defend modern healthcare databases from intrusion attempts. To achieve such high accuracy and performance, the proposed system uses a variety of feature engineering techniques, oversampling algorithms for improving class balance, and hyper-parameter optimization strategies. The design is suitable for installing the IDS on medical equipment and healthcare systems since it is lightweight, quick, and compatible with the IoT.

ImmuneNet's performance was measured against that of other machine learning algorithms using data from the Canadian Institute for Cybersecurity's Intrusion Detection System 2017 and 2018 and Bell DNS 2021 databases, which contain extensive real-time and most recent cyber assault data. Using the CIC Bell DNS 2021 dataset, ImmuneNet outperformed all other studies with an accuracy of 99.19%, precision of 99.22%, recall of 99.19%, and ROC-AUC of 99.2% when distinguishing between regular requests and intrusion attempts and other cyber threats.

Reliable intrusion detection was proposed [13] for application in e-healthcare systems. In IoT-network systems, IDS play a critical role in safeguarding electronic health records (EHR). The IoT network has significant security issues at its network layer because it is the most used infrastructure for both data transport and storage.

The security of data servers across all sectors, but especially in healthcare, is one of the most serious issues facing academics today. This study proposes an approach for efficient intrusion detection in the e-healthcare scenario using an ANFIS, with the end objective of maintaining PHR within a safe IoT-net. The results of the testing show that the proposed security paradigm can be employed with a security tool to recognize malicious network traffic. Results from testing and training the ANFIS model on the MATLAB® platform are compared with the accuracy rate from the original security research.

A novel method for intrusion detection in IoMT is the Mutual Information Feature Selection Method [14]. The Internet of Medical Things (IoMT) uses the IoT to enable remote patient monitoring and real-time diagnosis. If this connection is compromised, hackers could gain access to sensitive patient information and potentially compromise their health. Data manipulation from biosensors and hacking that disrupts IoMT are also major issues. Some have suggested bolstering IDS with deep learning algorithms to better spot intrusions.

It is difficult to build IDS for IoMT because of the high dimensionality of the data, which might induce model overfitting and reduce detection accuracy. Existing techniques mistakenly assume that feature redundancy rises linearly with feature size, even though feature selection has the potential to aid in avoiding overfitting. Insufficient data prevents us from drawing the conclusion that all characteristics transmit the same quantity of assault-related information. This is especially true of primitive designs. Because of this, the MIFS goal function overestimates the redundancy coefficient. Logistic Redundancy Coefficient Gradual Upweighting MIFS (LRGU-MIFS) is a new feature selection method proposed in this study that eliminates the necessity to find overlapping features.

Instead of using more traditional methods, LRGU employs the redundancy score computed by the logistic function to pick features. The logistic curve is utilized for this purpose of simplification. It shows how the mutual knowledge of the attributes in the given set is not linear. The MIFS criterion was modified to include the LRGU's computed redundancy coefficient. According to the results of the experiments, the suggested LRGU can choose a smaller but no less important set of features than the state-of-the-art methods. The proposed method is superior to existing strategies for detecting essential components, thus it can differentiate between identical traits even when there aren't enough assault patterns to go around.

The necessity to enhance intrusion detection without compromising users' personal information drove the creation of federated learning [15]. Network (including IoT) traffic anomalies, breaches, and security risks need the examination of massive amounts of sensitive data, which raises privacy and security problems. Federated learning allows for the collaborative training of a shared model while protecting the privacy and decentralization of the underlying data. Instead of training and evaluating the model on a single computer, clients in a federated learning environment each learn a local model with the same structure but are trained on distinct local datasets. These localized models are sent to an aggregate server, where they are averaged using a federated approach to get a more precise global prediction.

There are many benefits to using this strategy while developing innovative IDS. To evaluate federated learning, traditional deep learning models for IDSs were used for comparison. Our findings demonstrate that in settings where data privacy and security are of paramount importance, federated learning, which employs randomly selected clients, outperforms deep learning in terms of accuracy and loss. Our findings demonstrate that federated learning may be used to construct global models without revealing sensitive data, making them more secure against accidental disclosures. The results indicate that federated averaging in federated learning may have far-reaching consequences for the future development of IDS systems, leading to improved safety, efficiency, and efficacy.

A review of artificial intelligence-powered IDS, threats, datasets, and Cloud-Fog-Edge architectures for IoT protection was carried out [16]. Recent advancements in IoMT and its implications for conventional medical care are explored, as well as the evolution of data transmission in the Smart Healthcare setting. As a result, the neighborhood is now more welcoming to attackers. This has led to the incorporation of both tried-and-true intrusion detection models and novel detection algorithms tailored to the needs of IoMT in practical settings. Meanwhile, several AI algorithms have been implemented to enhance the ability of medical systems to identify attacks via their communication infrastructures.

A new classification of current datasets for insights into detection performance is introduced in this paper, along with a new taxonomy of intrusion detection methods for IoMT. We also assess potential cyber threats to IoMT's design and highlight the procedures needed to assure its safety. Additionally, we classify recent work based on AI approaches and analyze the duties performed by Cloud-Fog-Edge systems. The moral and legal ramifications of the security measures used by IoMT are also discussed. We wrap up by identifying some remaining puzzles and promising avenues of inquiry.

Investigation into the use of blockchain technology in the healthcare IoT to improve data security was undertaken [17]. Increased focus on IoT in recent years can be traced back to the integration of IoT devices with cloud storage for data management. Improving healthcare delivery through data sharing through the IoT, there is still the problem of keeping data secure and private when it is being uploaded and downloaded from the cloud. The limited storage space of IoT devices creates special difficulties for enforcing safety measures.

Sensitive data in the healthcare industry can be better protected by establishing a centrally located protected node. Blockchain has been widely used for various data management and security applications, but its potential has not yet been completely realized in the healthcare sector. To find the fastest way to transport the data, they perform some preliminary processing on the data and then use the Ant colony optimization technique. The use of blockchain technology for the safekeeping of medical records is also presented as part of a healthcare data management system. The major goal is to prevent malicious assaults on vulnerable medical records by enhancing safety measures. An immutable distributed ledger database protected by elliptic curve encryption and digital signatures is made available at the fog layer of the IoT. Time to generate a certificate, amount of data retrieved, and other metrics are used to confirm the effectiveness of the proposed approach.

For the sake of patient privacy, it was suggested that optimal deep learning be used for threat detection in the medical IoT [18]. In this research, they lay out the procedures necessary to put into effect deep learning architectural improvements for threat detection in BYOD medical IoT devices. Create a simulated medical facility complete with a variety of interconnected instruments and medical supplies. By compiling data on the characteristics of an attack, it is possible to identify the node or hardware component that was the subject of the assault. To detect attacks in a medical IoT network, information must be gathered from each connected device.

The information is subsequently fed into a deep belief network (DBN), an implementation of deep learning. Although DBN already exists, its detection accuracy could be improved using a meta-heuristic method, specifically, the combination of the grasshopper optimization algorithm (GOA) and the spider monkey optimization (SMO). The acronym "local leader phase-based GOA" (LLP-GOA) describes this method of fusion. To guarantee precise detection, nodes are trained using the DBN, and the attack data library is checked throughout testing. This research introduces a new way to ensure the security of medical IoT devices by employing a tailored deep learning architecture as BYOD. The research aims to prove that high-performance and high-convergence improved approaches for attack detection in hospital networks are feasible.

Particle swarm optimization (PSO)-DBN, grey wolf algorithm (GWO)-DBN, simulated annealing (SMO)-DBN, and GOA-DBN were all shown to be less accurate than the LLP-GOA-based DBN. The suggested LLP-GOA-DBN model improved accuracy by 13% when compared to SVM, 5.4% when compared to KNN, 8.7% when compared to NN, and 3.5% when compared to DBN. To identify unauthorized access in the medical IoT, this research makes use of LLP-GOA, a hybrid technique founded on optimum deep learning. They propose the first known implementation of the LLP-GOA algorithm, which improves DBN performance and, in turn, the security of healthcare data.

A quantum-trust and consultation-based transactional cybersecurity paradigm was developed for application in healthcare blockchains [19]. Academics have been interested in healthcare cybersecurity for some time now, understanding the critical nature of safeguarding personal health information. As a result, there have been major advancements in cybersecurity aimed at protecting the confidentiality of patients' medical records while they are being transmitted.

Persistent issues such as high computational complexity, rising time and resource requirements, and complex cost structures undermine the security system.

In this research, we offer a new technique called consultative transaction key generation and management (CTKGM) to increase the security of data transmission between healthcare networks. It generates a one-of-a-kind key pair using random integers, multiplication, and timestamps. Then, utilizing blockchain technology, the encrypted patient data is stored in blocks of hash values. By calculating a trust score from collected feedback data, the Quantum Trust Reconciliation Agreement Model (QTRAM) ensures secure data transfer.

The proposed architecture uses novel methods like feedback analysis and trust value to provide confidential two-way communication between patients and the healthcare system. The Tuna Swarm Optimization (TSO) method is used to check the legitimacy of nonce verification messages during phone calls. Message verification is a beneficial authentication feature that is built into QTRAM. It has been shown that the proposed approach is effective in testing the security model at hand by comparing it to other state-of-the-art models.

Researchers have found conflicting findings when looking at intrusion detection and network security in healthcare systems. The ubiquitous use of synthetic or small real-world datasets necessitates validation using larger, more diverse datasets. The reliability of hospital network traffic may have been overstated in several previous studies. It may also be difficult to apply deep learning and other resource-intensive models on low-computing-power healthcare equipment. While federated learning has many advantages, protecting patient information is a priority because of issues like rising communication costs and the potential for privacy breaches. The rising demand for IoT medical devices may outstrip network capacity, underlining the need for scalable solutions. Lack of standardized intrusion detection technologies may cause incompatibilities and adoption delays in healthcare networks.

Considering this, future research should prioritize fostering agreement. There is continuous investigation into IDS as a means of protecting networks from modern, complex attacks. When new IDS are not implemented correctly, it can cause major disruptions in healthcare operations. Ethical and legal considerations in the healthcare industry include things like obtaining patients' informed consent, safeguarding data ownership, and enforcing healthcare standards. Smaller healthcare facilities cannot afford expensive IDS and are thus looking into more cost-effective security options. Research has shown that healthcare networks are safer, more efficient, scalable, standardized, and able to detect advanced threats; they are also simple to incorporate, ethical, and affordable. Despite the evident limitations of these studies, they do provide a foundation for future research and progress in this crucial area.

Table 17.1 summarizes the critical literature and highlights the pros and cons while showcasing how the current work addresses the identified gaps in the field of healthcare network intrusion detection:

This table provides a concise summary of key contributions, advantages, disadvantages, and how the current work contributes to filling the gaps in the field of healthcare network intrusion detection.

Table 17.1 Summary of reviews

Reference	Key contributions	Pros	Cons	Current work's Contributions
[11]	Combined network and biometric data for IDS	Comprehensive approach	High dimensionality of data	Demonstrates improved performance using combined data sources
[12]	Introduced "ImmuneNet" for healthcare IDS	High accuracy, lightweight design	Limited to certain databases	Proposed an innovative system for intrusion detection using deep learning and hybrid techniques
[13]	Proposed ANFIS for efficient intrusion detection	Use of ANFIS model	Requires data from connected devices	Presented a new approach to intrusion detection using ANFIS model and tested its efficiency
[14]	Introduced Mutual Information Feature Selection	Efficient feature selection	Assumption of linear feature redundancy	Proposed a new feature selection method, LRGU, to address feature selection challenges in IoMT intrusion detection
[15]	Examined federated learning for intrusion detection	Privacy preservation, decentralized learning	Limited dataset privacy	Showed that federated learning outperforms traditional deep learning models in healthcare IDS
[16]	Reviewed AI-powered IDS and Cloud-Fog-Edge architectures	Detailed classification of IDS datasets	No new empirical findings	Provided a comprehensive review and classification of current research in IoT intrusion detection
[17]	Investigated blockchain for IoT data security	Improved data security, blockchain usage	Limited to cloud and fog architectures	Proposed a secure approach for using blockchain in healthcare data management
[18]	Explored deep learning for threat detection in BYOD medical IoT	Improved detection accuracy	Specific to the BYOD setting	Introduced a new deep learning architecture for healthcare network attack detection
[19]	Developed Quantum Trust and Consultative Transaction Key Generation	Enhanced security in data transmission	Limited practical implementation	Proposed a novel security paradigm and evaluated its effectiveness using consultative transaction key generation

17.3 Materials and methods

In healthcare, privacy and secrecy need even the most basic data processing and categorization. During this step, improved k-means clustering is used to find patterns in the raw data and extract useful information. The collected information is then classified using not one but two different decision tree classification techniques (DT, SVM) for further safety. The essential problem of healthcare data security is addressed in the study's comparison of results (Figure 17.1).

17.3.1 Experimental procedure

The "Friday-WorkingHours-Afternoon-DDos.pcap ISCX" subset of the CIC-IDS2017 dataset is processed for the purpose of executing the proposed approach. Since it includes both benign network activity and the more malicious intrusions that have become more common in PCAPs in recent years, this dataset provides a decent representation of real-world occurrences. CICFlowMeter's analysis of network traffic is also included in the bundle. The time-stamped, annotated CSV files include data such as IP addresses, protocol types, input/output ports, interfaces, and potential attack indicators. The system's ability to identify and remedy security flaws and to vigilantly guard the privacy of personal medical information relies on this extensive dataset.

17.3.2 Enhanced K-means clustering

K-means clustering, as an unsupervised learning technique, is crucial to many data analysis and machine learning applications. Its primary function is to group data elements into clusters based on their shared characteristics, making it an effective method for exploring unstructured datasets. To determine whether K-means clustering is useful, we will examine its strengths and drawbacks and suggest ways in which it could be enhanced [20]. K-means clustering is a technique for categorizing data into groups of a certain size ("K"). Data points are moved into the center cluster of the algorithm in an iterative process using a similarity measure, often Euclidean distance. Clusters are produced by redistributing data points to new centers and repeating the procedure until convergence is achieved [21].

The computational efficiency and scalability of K-means make it well-suited for real-world applications involving large data volumes. Its excellent efficiency and low learning curve have made it a popular tool for basic data segmentation and exploratory analysis. K-means can be utilized for a wide range of purposes, such as picture segmentation, customer segmentation, and anomaly detection [22].

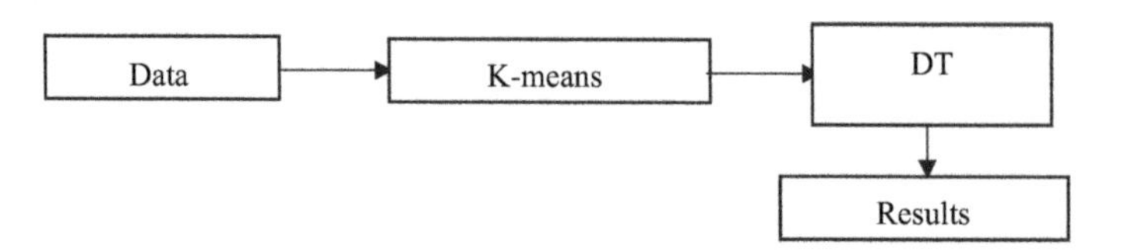

Figure 17.1 Proposed workflow

Due to the classical k-means clustering dependence on the positions of the initial cluster centers, K-means often generates poor results. Depending on the starting conditions, the results could be very different.

The method assumes implausibly that clusters are round of equal size and distributed randomly over the data [23]. This study recognizes the limitations of traditional K-means and tries to address them by exploring new avenues of inquiry. The study recommends more robust initialization techniques, such as K-means++, which provide stronger beginning cluster centers and are less vulnerable to initializations. To better capture complex cluster geometries, this work explores the use of alternative distance metrics or kernel-based K-means for dealing with non-spherical clusters. Real-world applications necessitate a level of robustness against outliers, thus understanding how to deal with them is crucial [24]. The reliability of clustering is improved by including strategies for locating and removing outliers. Here is the pseudocode of the enhanced K-means algorithm proposed in this chapter (see Algorithm 17.1).

Algorithm 17.1 Enhanced K-means algorithm approach

Input:
Data points: X
Number of clusters: K
Initialization:
1. Initialize cluster centers using K-means++ initialization (to ensure better starting points).
2. Create an empty array to store cluster assignments: cluster_assignments
3. Define a convergence threshold: convergence_threshold
4. Set an iteration counter: iteration = 0
Main Loop:
5. Repeat until convergence:
a. For each data point x in X:
i. Calculate the Euclidean distance between x and all cluster centers.
ii. Assign x to the cluster with the nearest center.
iii. Update cluster_assignments with the assigned cluster for x.
b. For each cluster k from 1 to K:
i. Calculate the new cluster center as the mean of all data points assigned to cluster k.
c. Check for convergence:
i. Calculate the change in cluster centers from the previous iteration.
ii. If the change is below the convergence_threshold, exit the loop.
d. Increment the iteration counter.
Output:
6. Return the final cluster assignments: cluster_assignments
7. Return the final cluster centers.
End of Algorithm.

This enhanced K-means method assigns data points to clusters iteratively based on the nearest cluster center, updates the cluster centers, and checks for convergence based on a predefined threshold. Until the algorithm converges, or a limit is reached, these steps will be repeated. The associated pseudocode has been updated to include improvements, such as more secure initialization and support for non-spherical clusters. The method ensures superior accuracy and efficiency in clustering by repeatedly iterating until convergence is obtained. K-means clustering is a powerful technique for grouping similar datasets into meaningful categories. Its utility, however, may be diminished by the method typically used to implement it. Because proper clustering of potentially sensitive data is so crucial to healthcare data security, this study acknowledges its limits and suggests new ways to overcome them.

17.3.3 Classification using decision tree and SVM

17.3.3.1 Support vector machines used in machine learning

Support Vector Machines (SVMs) have many practical uses since they are an effective supervised machine learning tool. To classify data most accurately, SVMs seek out the hyperplane in a high-dimensional space [25]. Dissimilarity maximization between classes is the hallmark of SVMs. Margin refers to the average distance of the hyperplane from the closest data point in each class while solving a problem requiring binary classification. The most accurate and generalizable result is produced by the hyperplane with the highest margin; hence this is the one that is favored by SVMs [26].

When describing a set of data points that are close to the hyperplane that delineates the decision boundary, the phrase "support vector" is often employed. You can't decide in the absence of these cornerstones. SVMs are beneficial even when the training dataset is limited since they can work with a low number of support vectors. When there is a lack of training data, SVMs can help SVMs generalize better than they would be able to on their own [27]. Because of its structure, SVMs excel at solving linear classification issues. SVMs do exceptionally well in hyperplane (or straight-line) methods of data separation. Text classification and image recognition are just two examples of applications where linear discrimination is enough [28].

Due to the nonlinear nature of most real-world data, a hyperplane split along a straight line is impractical. The usage of kernel functions allows SVMs to work past this restriction. Transforming the original feature space with kernel functions makes the data linearly separable in higher-dimensional spaces. This adjustment allows SVMs to perform exceptionally well with nonlinear data [29].

SVMs may be trusted to generate accurate results, but they are not immune to the effects of data noise. Noise occurs when individual data points do not conform to expectations or are wrongly classified. The predictive ability of the model will decrease if the noise is concentrated around the hyperplane. It is possible to improve SVMs' robustness against noise by careful data preprocessing and feature engineering.

SVMs can be used for more than just classifying data. Support Vector Regression is a powerful tool for both regression and anomaly detection. SVMs attempt to fit a hyperplane in regression that minimizes the gap between the datasets as much as possible. Due of their exceptional capacity to single out outliers, SVMs are well-suited for this task [30]. SVMs are a flexible machine learning tool for determining optimal decision criteria. They do quite well with linear data, and with the help of kernel functions, they can also deal with nonlinear data. Though reliable, SVMs can be affected by data noise, underscoring the importance of thorough preprocessing. Since SVMs are also effective at regression and anomaly detection, they can be used in fields as diverse as finance, health, and image analysis in addition to classification [31]. Algorithm 17.2 shows the SVM approach.

Algorithm 17.2 Support vector machine algorithm approach

Define SVM function

```
def svm(X, y, learning_rate=0.01, num_epochs=1000):
# Initialize weights and bias
w = np.zeros(X.shape[1])
b = 0
# Training loop
for epoch in range(num_epochs):
for i, x in enumerate(X):
# Calculate the decision boundary
decision = np.dot(w, x) + b
# Check if the data point is misclassified
if y[i] * decision <= 1:
# Update weights and bias
        w = w - learning_rate * (2 * (1/epoch) * w - np.dot(x, y[i]))
b = b + learning_rate * y[i]
return w, b
if __name__ == "__main__":
# Generate sample data
np.random.seed(0)
X = np.random.randn(100, 2)
y = np.where(X[:, 0] + X[:, 1] > 1, 1, -1)
# Train SVM
weights, bias = svm(X, y)
# Print the learned weights and bias
print("Learned Weights:", weights)
print("Learned Bias:", bias)
```

End of Algorithm.

17.3.3.2 Decision tree

A Decision Tree's fundamental purpose is to classify data sets by their most salient features. Each branch in the decision tree represents a different course of action taken once the first, top-level decision has been made. At each node, we look at a subset of the dataset determined by the feature and its associated values. Classification or regression findings are iterated upon until they are produced at the leaf nodes [32]. In the realm of intrusion detection, decision trees have proven indispensable when the goal is to identify harmful behaviors or trends in network traffic or system logs [33]. Decision trees can be used to prioritize features to classify network activity as either benign or malicious. The characteristic at the tree's root node is often indicative of the optimal initial split [34].

The characteristics' values determine the paths taken by the data using the Decision Tree classifier. The data is labeled as normal or cancerous based on a preset decision tree and feature values. These categorization concepts are built using the training data [35]. Decision trees excel at conducting assessments of data in real time. They can quickly sift through network data for indicators of intrusion. This kind of in-the-moment analysis is crucial for detecting intrusions in a timely manner and mitigating their effects [36]. Due to their useful features, decision trees are commonly utilized in intrusion detection. Since the rules are presented in a clear, chronological format in a decision tree, they are simple to grasp. Due to the ease with which security analysts can follow the algorithm's decision process, Decision Trees find a home in real-time security solutions. Since decision trees can detect even the most minor but relevant trends and patterns in network traffic, they are a powerful tool for pattern identification. Ability to discover and contribute new attack techniques to the attack signature library is invaluable [37].

Decision Trees are well-suited for use in IDS due to their ability to easily handle massive volumes of data. Security systems can keep up with the constant influx of network traffic because of their ability to handle data in real time [38,39]. Decision trees can use historical data to understand patterns that lead to low false positive rates (FPRs). As a result, security personnel will be less likely to be distracted by false alarms and more able to focus on actual threats. Decision Trees prove indispensable in the field of intrusion detection because they provide a rational and simply understood structure for evaluating network data. Because of their superior pattern recognition and trend detection in real-time data, they are a potent weapon in the fight against cyber threats. Decision trees are a great foundation on which to create trustworthy IDS that can adapt to new types of attack and boost network security in general [40]. Decision Trees are the preferred machine learning algorithm for tasks like classification and regression. The name stems from the fact that a diagram of the structure resembles the bare bones of a tree, including a trunk, branches, and nodes but no leaves. Branches represent rules or decisions, and leaf nodes represent class labels or output values in a decision tree. Decision trees are commonly used in cybersecurity for intrusion detection [41]. Algorithm 17.3 is for the Decision Tree Algorithm approach.

Algorithm 17.3 Decision tree algorithm approach

Procedure decision tree inducer (S,A,y)

Initialization:

1. Initialize cluster centers using K-means++ initialization (to ensure better starting points).
2. Create an empty array to store cluster assignments: cluster_assignments
3. Define a convergence threshold: convergence_threshold
4. Set an iteration counter: iteration = 0

Main Loop:

5. Repeat until convergence:

a. For each data point x in X:

   i. Calculate the Euclidean distance between x and all cluster centers.
   ii. Assign x to the cluster with the nearest center.
   iii. Update cluster_assignments with the assigned cluster for x.

b. For each cluster k from 1 to K:

   i. Calculate the new cluster center as the mean of all data points assigned to cluster k.

c. Check for convergence:

   i. Calculate the change in cluster centers from the previous iteration.
   ii. If the change is below the convergence_threshold, exit the loop.d. Increment the iteration counter.

Output:

6. Return the final cluster assignments: cluster_assignments
7. Return the final cluster centers.

End of Algorithm.

17.4 Results and discussions

The SVM and the Decision Tree are the main classifiers we employ at the commencement of our research. Second, the raw data is given a first round of processing by k-means clustering. The data is being processed on a fundamental level to make it more accessible and trustworthy.

In machine learning, data preparation is essential for improved model performance. For efficient data classification and organization prior to analysis, K-means clustering is used. Classifiers like SVM and Decision Trees are fed the collected data.

As a reflection of the complexity of healthcare data, the huge dataset used in our study has an impressive 225,711 features and 78 attributes. To guarantee reliable and accurate discoveries, we painstakingly compare the results and insights obtained from different classifiers.

Our investigation relies heavily on k-means clustering for data cleansing. This method not only improves the data's quality but also makes it easier to access and analyze. Separating a dataset into subsets for training, testing, and validation is also simplified. This partitioning approach is commonly used by machine learning experts to guarantee exhaustive testing and evaluation of their models.

Seventy-five percent of the data is contained in the training set, which is where the model is fitted, and its effectiveness is measured. The remaining 25% is used to do extensive testing to ensure the models' performance when making predictions based on completely new data.

The main classifiers in this research are the SVM and the Decision Tree. These classifiers are crucial for locating and resolving vulnerabilities in the security of healthcare data. These classifiers are applied to both the raw data and the k-means clustered data, as shown in Figures 17.2–17.5.

We employ several different metrics, including sensitivity, specificity, precision, negative predictive value, FPR, false discovery rate, false negative rate, accuracy, F1 score, and Matthew's correlation coefficient, to evaluate our models' performance. To better assess the efficacy of our IDS, we may use these measurements to build informative confusion matrices.

Table 17.2 gives a thorough picture of our system's capabilities and its potential influence on enhancing healthcare data security based on the substantial evaluation metrics we acquired from our trials.

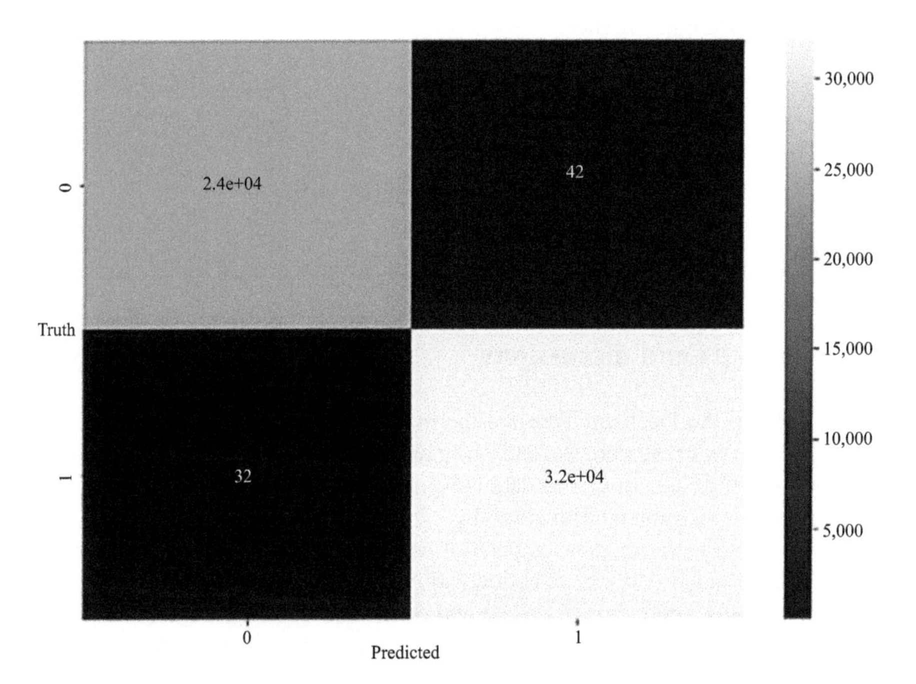

Figure 17.2 Confusion matrix for intrusion detection using SVM (TP=24245; TN=42; FP=32; FN=32109)

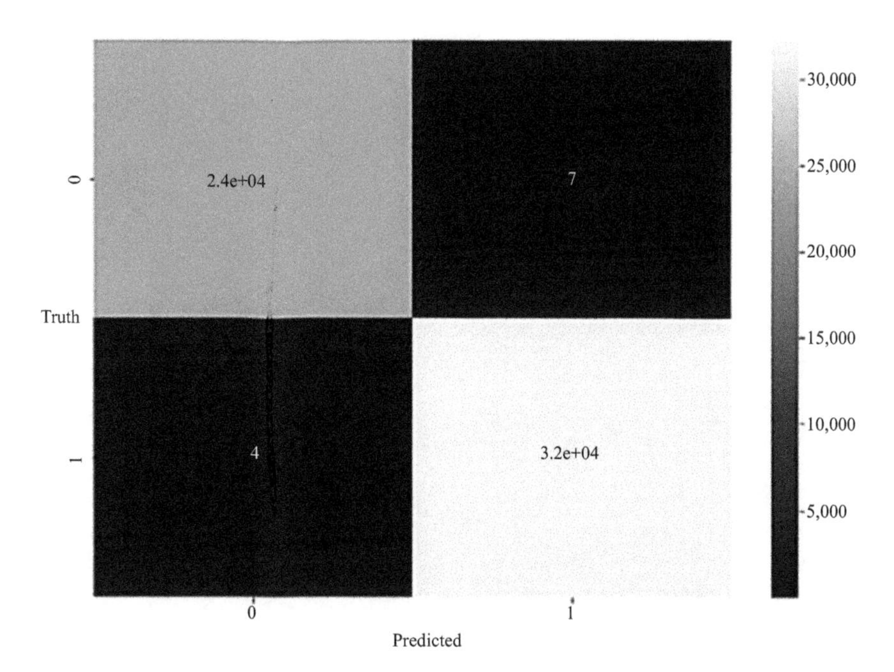

Figure 17.3 Confusion matrix for Intrusion Detection using Decision tree (TP=24280; TN=7; FP=4; FN=32137)

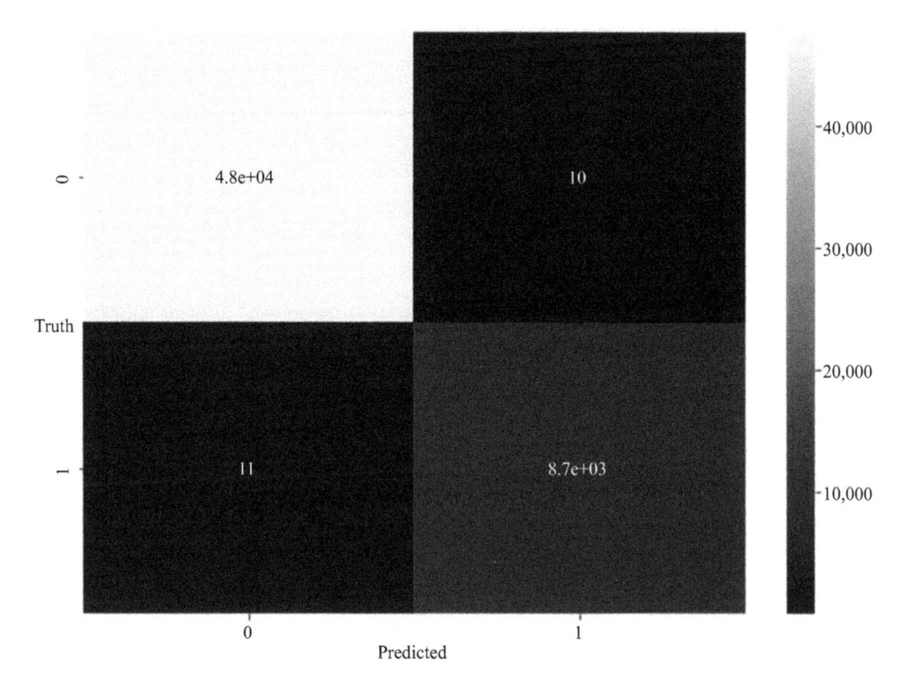

Figure 17.4 Confusion matrix for Intrusion Detection using SVM with k-means clustering technique (TP=47667; TN=10; FP=11; FN=8740)

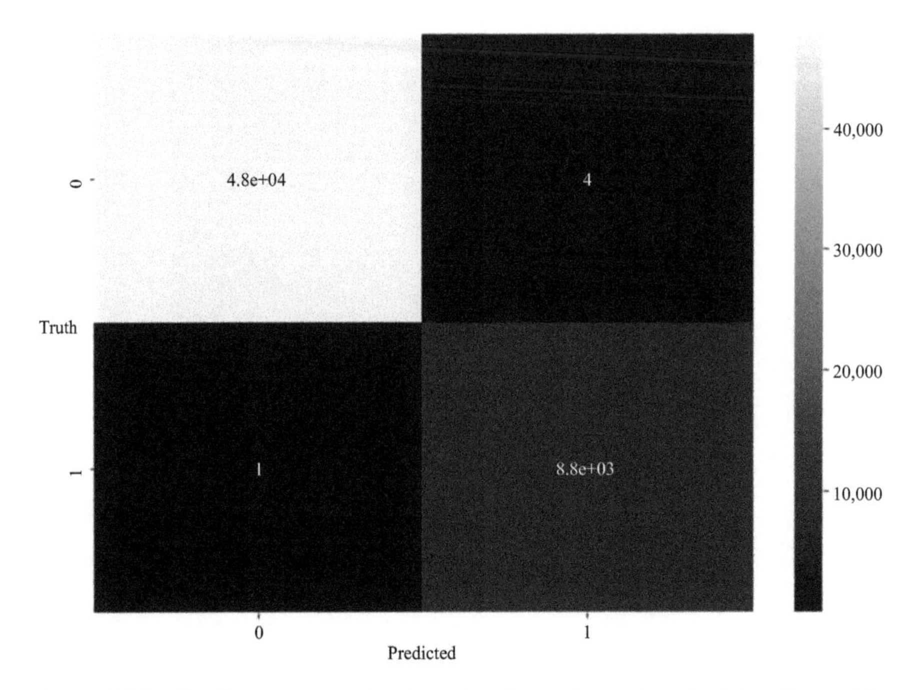

Figure 17.5 Confusion matrix for Intrusion Detection using Decision Tree with k-means clustering technique (TP=47673; TN=4; FP=1; FN=8750)

Table 17.2 Evaluation metrics

Performance measures (%)	Data + SVM	Data + decision tree	Data + k-means + SVM	Data + k-means + decision tree	Formulae
Accuracy	99.87	99.98	99.96	99.99	(TP+TN)/(P+N)
Specificity	99.87	99.98	99.89	99.95	TN/(FP+TN)
Precision	99.83	99.97	99.98	99.99	TP/(TP+FP)
Negative predictive value	99.90	99.99	99.87	99.99	TN/(TN+FN)
False positive rate	0.13	0.02	0.11	0.05	FP/(FP+TN)
False discovery rate	0.17	0.03	0.02	0.01	FP/(FP+TP)
False negative rate	0.13	0.02	0.02	0	FN/(FN+TP)
Sensitivity	99.87	99.98	99.98	100	TP/(TP+FN)
F1-score	99.85	99.98	99.98	99.99	2TP/(2TP+ FP+FN)

Table 17.2 summarizes the many criteria we employed to evaluate the efficacy of our IDS. The results of several scenarios are analyzed, including those that use SVM, Decision Tree, k-means preprocessing followed by SVM, and k-means preprocessing followed by Decision Tree. The results of these tests provide

important insight into the success of our approach. All scenarios are covered by the models with an accuracy of 99.87% to 99.99%. This demonstrates the consistency of our IDS across all preprocessing steps and classification strategies. In Table 17.3, we compare our results to those of similar studies. When compared to the state of the art, our results employing k-means preprocessing followed by Decision Tree (99.99% accuracy) greatly outperform the competition, proof positive that our approach can improve healthcare data security.

We conducted extensive testing and analysis of an IDS's behavior under different scenarios as part of our study. The combination of k-means preprocessing, and Decision Tree significantly increases the accuracy, precision, and dependability of our method, which could have a significant impact on healthcare data security. These results pave the path for taking our intrusion detection technique further and even using it in real healthcare settings, where safety is of the utmost importance.

For the sake of web-based system security and risk assessment, infiltration detection is crucial. Some of the difficulties it faces include false positives, low detection rates, skewed data, and delayed response times. Improving the safety of patient data is central to our research, hence we propose an IDS for web apps that uses machine learning.

We used machine learning methods like K-means clustering, Decision Tree, and SVM models to build a robust IDS. To simulate the complexity of real-world web traffic, we used the CIC-IDS2017 intrusion dataset (Friday-WorkingHours-Afternoon-DDos.pcap ISCX) to create a scenario with benign and frequent incursions. Time-stamped labeled flows, protocol categories, IP addresses, I/O ports, interfaces, and potential risks were all included in the dataset.

We gave the dataset a thorough cleaning before digging into the specifics of our methodology. The data was then divided into two groups: one for training, and another for evaluation. Seventy-five percent of the data was used as a training set to

Table 17.3 Comparison with the existing works in literature

Authors	Methods	Result
[42]	Decision trees	80.77 %
[43]	Decision trees and random forests	88.89%
[44]	LDA algorithm, CART algorithm, and Random Forest	98.1%, 98%, 99.81%, respectively
[45]	LTSM and CNN	97.60%
[12]	Hybrid Architecture based on Deep Learning	Outperformed other studies with 99.19% accuracy, 99.22% precision, 99.19% recall, and 99.2% ROC-AUC
[18]	Optimal Deep Learning for Threat Detection in Medical IoT	LLP-GOA-DBN model, improved accuracy by 13% compared to SVM, 5.4% to KNN, 8.7% to NN, and 3.5% to DBN

find out which variables worked best together. The final model's accuracy was checked by contrasting it with an external benchmark (the testing set, which was made up of 25% of the data).

It's possible that our experiments can be divided into three parts. We first used the raw data to train Decision Tree and SVM classifiers, both of which performed exceptionally well with an accuracy of 99.98% and 99.87%, respectively. Then, we applied the K-means clustering method to the raw data and achieved a 99.99% and 99.96% success rate. This clustering strategy greatly enhanced the system's accuracy.

Accuracy, sensitivity, precision, specificity, F1-score, and Matthew's correlation coefficient were only some of the performance indicators we used to evaluate our findings. These statistics offer a full picture of our system's capability to detect intrusion attempts.

In addition, we compared the learned precision to that of cutting-edge IDS to show how reliable and applicable our method is.

Protecting sensitive patient information is a top priority in the healthcare industry, making our intrusion detection technology essential. We have shown that web applications, and notably those dealing with medical records, can be made safer by combining machine learning approaches with advanced clustering methodologies. Our method provides an extra layer of protection for healthcare data management in the face of growing cyber threats.

17.5 Conclusions and future scope

This study provides network engineers with a valuable tool for identifying and avoiding harmful attacks. To help network engineers reduce the time it takes to detect and respond to threats, we set out to develop a straightforward, practical method for enhancing IDS. This method involves overcoming the challenge of gathering a large, targeted data collection. As cyber threats evolve over time, it will be increasingly important to learn more about IDS, and this work paves the way for that. Implementing the procedures outlined below is crucial for protecting websites and digital assets from the ever-present threats posed by hackers and cybercriminals.

The most effective methods of incorporating real-world data into the model are currently the subject of continuing study. IDS will benefit from this since they can better adjust to the specifics of real-world networks. Learning to handle larger datasets has the potential to significantly improve the performance of IDS. With more reliable data, we can have a deeper understanding of the risks. Adjusting to Specific Circumstances Extending the model's usefulness to include more network and business scenarios is crucial. IDS can be optimized for specific scenarios to increase their effectiveness. Exploring how methods like Random Forest, X-means, and fuzzy logic may be used to build more resilient and flexible IDS is a valuable endeavor.

The proposed idea is not without some important caveats that must be considered. The fact that we rely solely on one approach to our inquiries is problematic. Although this technique works well, it may not be able to fix all of the problems that companies have with intrusion detection. Researchers in all fields should never stop exploring new approaches and tools for the sake of maximum security. In conclusion, our study improves online safety by addressing longstanding issues with intrusion detection. No matter what the future of the internet holds, it will remain crucial to invest heavily in safeguarding websites, online apps, and anti-malware defenses in order to effectively combat cybercrime.

References

[1] J. Jang-Jaccard and S. Nepal, "A Survey of Emerging Threats in Cybersecurity," *J Comput Syst Sci*, vol. 80, no. 5, pp. 973–993, 2014, doi:10.1016/j.jcss.2014.02.005.

[2] J. Kizza and F. Migga Kizza, "Intrusion Detection and Prevention Systems," in *Securing the Information Infrastructure*, IGI Global, 2008, pp. 239–258. doi:10.4018/978-1-59904-379-1.ch012.

[3] T. Krause, R. Ernst, B. Klaer, I. Hacker, and M. Henze, "Cybersecurity in Power Grids: Challenges and Opportunities," *Sensors*, vol. 21, no. 18, p. 6225, 2021, doi:10.3390/s21186225.

[4] A. Khraisat, I. Gondal, P. Vamplew, and J. Kamruzzaman, "Survey of Intrusion Detection Systems: Techniques, Datasets and Challenges," *Cybersecurity*, vol. 2, no. 1, p. 20, 2019, doi:10.1186/s42400-019-0038-7.

[5] V. Jyothsna, V. V. Rama Prasad, and K. Munivara Prasad, "A Review of Anomaly based Intrusion Detection Systems," *Int J Comput Appl*, vol. 28, no. 7, pp. 26–35, 2011, doi:10.5120/3399-4730.

[6] J. M. Borky and T. H. Bradley, "Protecting Information with Cybersecurity," in *Effective Model-Based Systems Engineering*, Cham: Springer International Publishing, 2019, pp. 345–404. doi:10.1007/978-3-319-95669-5_10.

[7] P. Dini, A. Elhanashi, A. Begni, S. Saponara, Q. Zheng, and K. Gasmi, "Overview on Intrusion Detection Systems Design Exploiting Machine Learning for Networking Cybersecurity," *Applied Sciences*, vol. 13, no. 13, p. 7507, 2023, doi:10.3390/app13137507.

[8] N. Prazeres, R. L. de C. Costa, L. Santos, and C. Rabadão, "Engineering the Application of Machine Learning in an IDS Based on IoT Traffic Flow," *Intelligent Systems with Applications*, vol. 17, p. 200189, 2023, doi:10.1016/j.iswa.2023.200189.

[9] M. Ozkan-Okay, R. Samet, O. Aslan, and D. Gupta, "A Comprehensive Systematic Literature Review on Intrusion Detection Systems," *IEEE Access*, vol. 9, pp. 157727–157760, 2021, doi:10.1109/ACCESS.2021.3129336.

[10] H. Saleous, M. Ismail, S. H. AlDaajeh, *et al.*, "COVID-19 Pandemic and the Cyberthreat Landscape: Research Challenges and Opportunities," *Digital Communications and Networks*, vol. 9, no. 1, pp. 211–222, 2023, doi:10.1016/j.dcan.2022.06.005.

[11] A. A. Hady, A. Ghubaish, T. Salman, D. Unal, and R. Jain, "Intrusion Detection System for Healthcare Systems Using Medical and Network Data: A Comparison Study," *IEEE Access*, vol. 8, pp. 106576–106584, 2020, doi:10.1109/ACCESS.2020.3000421.

[12] M. Akshay Kumaar, D. Samiayya, P. M. D. R. Vincent, K. Srinivasan, C.-Y. Chang, and H. Ganesh, "A Hybrid Framework for Intrusion Detection in Healthcare Systems Using Deep Learning," *Front Public Health*, vol. 9, 2022, doi:10.3389/fpubh.2021.824898.

[13] F. Akram, D. Liu, P. Zhao, N. Kryvinska, S. Abbas, and M. Rizwan, "Trustworthy Intrusion Detection in E-Healthcare Systems," *Front Public Health*, vol. 9, 2021, doi:10.3389/fpubh.2021.788347.

[14] M. Alalhareth and S.-C. Hong, "An Improved Mutual Information Feature Selection Technique for Intrusion Detection Systems in the Internet of Medical Things," *Sensors*, vol. 23, no. 10, p. 4971, 2023, doi:10.3390/s23104971.

[15] A. Alazab, A. Khraisat, S. Singh, and T. Jan, "Enhancing Privacy-Preserving Intrusion Detection through Federated Learning," *Electronics (Basel)*, vol. 12, no. 16, p. 3382, 2023, doi:10.3390/electronics12163382.

[16] M. L. Hernandez-Jaimes, A. Martinez-Cruz, K. A. Ramírez-Gutiérrez, and C. Feregrino-Uribe, "Artificial Intelligence for IoMT Security: A Review of Intrusion Detection Systems, Attacks, Datasets and Cloud–Fog–Edge Architectures," *Internet of Things*, vol. 23, p. 100887, 2023, doi:10.1016/j.iot.2023.100887.

[17] J. Poongodi, K. Kavitha, and S. Sathish, "Healthcare Internet of Things (HIoT) Data Security Enhancement Using Blockchain Technology," *Journal of Intelligent & Fuzzy Systems*, vol. 43, no. 4, pp. 5063–5073, 2022, doi:10.3233/JIFS-220797.

[18] J. Aruna Santhi and T. Vijaya Saradhi, "Attack Detection in Medical Internet of Things Using Optimized Deep Learning: Enhanced Security in Healthcare Sector," *Data Technologies and Applications*, vol. 55, no. 5, pp. 682–714, 2021, doi:10.1108/DTA-10-2020-0239.

[19] S. Selvarajan and H. Mouratidis, "A Quantum Trust and Consultative Transaction-based Blockchain Cybersecurity Model for Healthcare Systems," *Sci Rep*, vol. 13, no. 1, p. 7107, 2023, doi:10.1038/s41598-023-34354-x.

[20] M. R. Karim, O. Beyan, A. Zappa, *et al*., "Deep Learning-based Clustering Approaches for Bioinformatics," *Brief Bioinform*, vol. 22, no. 1, pp. 393–415, 2021, doi:10.1093/bib/bbz170.

[21] R. Suwanda, Z. Syahputra, and E. M. Zamzami, "Analysis of Euclidean Distance and Manhattan Distance in the K-Means Algorithm for Variations Number of Centroid K," *J Phys Conf Ser*, vol. 1566, no. 1, p. 012058, 2020, doi:10.1088/1742-6596/1566/1/012058.

[22] Md. Zubair, MD. A. Iqbal, A. Shil, M. J. M. Chowdhury, M. A. Moni, and I. H. Sarker, "An Improved K-means Clustering Algorithm Towards an Efficient Data-Driven Modeling," *Annals of Data Science*, 2022, doi:10.1007/s40745-022-00428-2.

[23] R. Suryawanshi and S. Puthran, "A Novel Approach for Data Clustering using Improved K-means Algorithm," *Int J Comput Appl*, vol. 142, no. 12, pp. 13–18, 2016, doi:10.5120/ijca2016909949.

[24] A. M. Ikotun, A. E. Ezugwu, L. Abualigah, B. Abuhaija, and J. Heming, "K-means Clustering Algorithms: A Comprehensive Review, Variants Analysis, and Advances in the Era of Big Data," *Inf Sci (N Y)*, vol. 622, pp. 178–210, 2023, doi:10.1016/j.ins.2022.11.139.

[25] D. A. Pisner and D. M. Schnyer, "Support Vector Machine," in *Machine Learning*, Elsevier, 2020, pp. 101–121. doi:10.1016/B978-0-12-815739-8.00006-7.

[26] S. Upadhyaya and R. A. A. J. Ramsankaran, "Support Vector Machine (SVM) based Rain Area Detection from Kalpana-1 Satellite Data," *ISPRS Annals of the Photogrammetry, Remote Sensing and Spatial Information Sciences*, vol. II–8, pp. 21–27, 2014, doi:10.5194/isprsannals-II-8-21-2014.

[27] D. Nagaraj, M. Mutz, N. George, P. Bansal, and D. Werth, "A Semantic Segmentation Approach for Road Defect Detection and Quantification," in *2022 the 5th International Conference on Machine Vision and Applications (ICMVA)*, New York, NY: ACM, 2022, pp. 8–15. doi:10.1145/3523111.3523113.

[28] J. Shawe-Taylor and S. Sun, "Kernel Methods and Support Vector Machines," 2014, pp. 857–881. doi:10.1016/B978-0-12-396502-8.00016-4.

[29] H.-G. Yeom, S.-M. Park, J. Park, and K.-B. Sim, "Superiority Demonstration of Variance-considered Machines by Comparing Error Rate with Support Vector Machines," *Int J Control Autom Syst*, vol. 9, no. 3, pp. 595–600, 2011, doi:10.1007/s12555-011-0321-1.

[30] B. Frenay and M. Verleysen, "Classification in the Presence of Label Noise: A Survey," *IEEE Trans Neural Netw Learn Syst*, vol. 25, no. 5, pp. 845–869, 2014, doi:10.1109/TNNLS.2013.2292894.

[31] C. Campbell and Y. Ying, "Learning with Support Vector Machines," *Synthesis Lectures on Artificial Intelligence and Machine Learning*, vol. 5, no. 1, pp. 1–95, 2011, doi:10.2200/S00324ED1V01Y201102AIM010.

[32] B. N. Patel, "Efficient Classification of Data Using Decision Tree," *Bonfring International Journal of Data Mining*, vol. 2, no. 1, pp. 6–12, 2012, doi:10.9756/BIJDM.1098.

[33] S. Naeem, Aqib Ali, Sania Anam, and Muhammad Munawar Ahmed, "Machine Learning for Intrusion Detection in Cyber Security: Applications, Challenges, and Recommendations," *Innovative Computing Review*, vol. 2, no. 2, pp. 1126–1130, 2022, doi:10.32350/icr.0202.03.

[34] Y. Zhang and Z. Wang, "Feature Engineering and Model Optimization Based Classification Method for Network Intrusion Detection," *Applied Sciences*, vol. 13, no. 16, p. 9363, 2023, doi:10.3390/app13169363.

[35] N. Kh. Al-Salihy and T. Ibrikci, "Classifying Breast Cancer by Using Decision Tree Algorithms," in *Proceedings of the 6th International Conference on Software and Computer Applications*, New York, NY: ACM, 2017, pp. 144–148. doi:10.1145/3056662.3056716.

[36] A. Al-Saleh, "A Balanced Communication-avoiding Support Vector Machine Decision Tree Method for Smart Intrusion Detection Systems," *Sci Rep*, vol. 13, no. 1, p. 9083, 2023, doi:10.1038/s41598-023-36304-z.

[37] A. Guezzaz, S. Benkirane, M. Azrour, and S. Khurram, "A Reliable Network Intrusion Detection Approach Using Decision Tree with Enhanced Data Quality," *Security and Communication Networks*, vol. 2021, pp. 1–8, 2021, doi:10.1155/2021/1230593.

[38] O. Ayoade, T. Oladele, A. Imoize, J. Awotunde, A, Adeloye, S. Olorunyomi and A. Idowu, "Explainable Artificial Intelligence (XAI) in Medical Decision Systems (MDSSs): Healthcare Systems Perspective," *Explainable Artificial Intelligence in Medical Decision Support Systems*, 2022, doi:10.1049/pbhe050e_ch1

[39] Y. Hao, B. Qin, and Y. Sun, "Privacy-Preserving Decision-Tree Evaluation with Low Complexity for Communication," *Sensors*, vol. 23, no. 5, p. 2624, 2023, doi:10.3390/s23052624.

[40] A. Fernández, R. Usamentiaga, J. Carús, and R. Casado, "Driver Distraction Using Visual-Based Sensors and Algorithms," *Sensors*, vol. 16, no. 11, p. 1805, 2016, doi:10.3390/s16111805.

[41] K. Rai, M. S. Devi, and A. Guleria, "Decision Tree Based Algorithm for Intrusion Detection," *International Journal of Advanced Networking and Applications*, vol. 7, no. 4, pp. 2828–2834, 2016.

[42] M. Fratello and R. Tagliaferri, "Decision Trees and Random Forests," *Encyclopedia of Bioinformatics and Computational Biology: ABC of Bioinformatics*, vol. 1–3, pp. 374–383, 2018, doi:10.1016/B978-0-12-809633-8.20337-3.

[43] T. Saranya, S. Sridevi, C. Deisy, T. D. Chung, and M. K. A. A. Khan, "Performance Analysis of Machine Learning Algorithms in Intrusion Detection System: A Review," *Procedia Comput Sci*, vol. 171, pp. 1251–1260, 2020, doi:10.1016/j.procs.2020.04.133.

[44] H. Liu and B. Lang, "Machine Learning and Deep Learning Methods for Intrusion Detection Systems: A Survey," *Applied Sciences*, vol. 9, no. 20, p. 4396, 2019, doi:10.3390/app9204396.

Chapter 18

Legal and regulatory policies for cybersecurity and information assurance in emerging healthcare systems

Abdulwaheed Musa[1,2] and Segun Ezekiel Jacob[1]

Protecting data and information systems from unwanted access, use, change, or destruction is known as cybersecurity. The healthcare sector is among the most critical and challenging domains for cybersecurity. Healthcare systems comprise numerous entities and stakeholders, such as clinics, hospitals, laboratories, pharmacies, insurance companies, patients, and medical personnel. For these institutions to deliver efficient and superior healthcare services, including diagnosis, treatment, prevention, and research, they rely on information technology and data. However, these systems and data are also vulnerable to cyberattacks, which can endanger the security and well-being of patients and healthcare providers as well as the privacy, accuracy, and accessibility of medical records. Cyberattacks against healthcare systems can lead to several dangerous consequences, including ransomware, malware, sabotage, espionage, data breaches, identity theft, and fraud. These attacks may affect a country's general health and national security in addition to the targeted victims. As a result, it is imperative to ensure the information assurance and cybersecurity of developing healthcare systems using legislative and regulatory frameworks that take risk management, actual situations, and emerging trends into account.

Keywords: Cybersecurity; information assurance; healthcare systems; legal insight; risk management; real-world cases; future trends

18.1 Introduction

Protecting data and information systems against unauthorized access, use, change, or destruction is known as cybersecurity, and it is an essential field in today's world [1]. As the use of information technology permeates many industries, including

[1]Department of Electrical and Computer Engineering, Kwara State University, Nigeria
[2]Centre for Artificial Intelligence and Machine Learning Systems, Kwara State University, Nigeria

business, education, communication, and entertainment, cybersecurity becomes increasingly important in maintaining the security and integrity of digital environments. Because cybersecurity is dynamic and multifaceted, it calls for constant adaptation and increased awareness, especially in vital industries like healthcare.

The healthcare sector stands out as one of the most important and difficult sectors in the diverse field of cybersecurity [2]. Healthcare systems, which are made up of a wide range of stakeholders, mainly include patients, insurance companies, hospitals, clinics, labs, pharmacies, and healthcare professionals, mostly depend on information systems and data. These systems play a crucial role in providing efficient and superior healthcare services that include prevention, treatment, diagnosis, and research. But the very systems that enable these essential operations are vulnerable to a wide range of cyberattacks, which might endanger patient safety, the health of healthcare providers, and the privacy, accuracy, and accessibility of medical data [3].

Cyberattacks on healthcare systems come in many forms, from ransomware, malware, and sabotage to fraud, espionage, data breaches, and identity theft [2]. Beyond the immediate victims, there are wider implications for public health and national security. As such, it is critical to guarantee the cybersecurity and information assurance of healthcare systems. This entails making sure healthcare data is dependable, high-quality, and readily available in addition to guarding against unauthorized access, use, change, and destruction [4].

However, ensuring the information assurance and cybersecurity of healthcare systems is a difficult undertaking. It necessitates an all-encompassing, multidisciplinary strategy that considers a range of elements, such as organizational, legal, ethical, and technical issues. Furthermore, as healthcare systems are integrated beyond national boundaries, international cooperation is required. A thorough examination of the rules and regulations regulating cybersecurity and information assurance is necessary to comprehend their current position as well as to anticipate future developments in rapidly expanding healthcare systems. Therefore, in order to give important insights into preserving the digital foundation of healthcare globally, this chapter explores the complex web of legal and regulatory rules for cybersecurity and information assurance in developing healthcare systems.

18.1.1 Key contributions of the chapter

The following are the significant contributions of this chapter:

(i) In-depth legal insight: This chapter offers a deep dive into healthcare cybersecurity's legal and regulatory aspects.
(ii) Cybersecurity integration: It highlights the crucial role of cybersecurity in healthcare, connecting these critical domains.
(iii) Risk management guidance: Readers gain insights into risk assessment and proactive mitigation strategies.
(iv) Real-world cases: The chapter uses practical cases to illustrate cybersecurity challenges in healthcare.

(v) Future trends preview: It anticipates emerging trends, helping readers prepare for the future of healthcare cybersecurity.
(vi) Comprehensive resource: This chapter consolidates essential information, serving as a valuable reference for healthcare and cybersecurity professionals.

18.1.2 Chapter organization

In this chapter, Section 18.1 comprises an introduction and the key contributions. Section 18.2 discusses the basics of cyber security to lay the groundwork for understanding the rules in the emerging healthcare system. Section 18.3 then discusses the healthcare system and data, giving the context needed for putting these policies into action. In Section 18.4, cybersecurity frameworks as a guide for crafting policies are introduced. Section 18.5 is an in-depth analysis of legal and regulatory regulations, guaranteeing compliance with changing legal requirements. In Section 18.6, risk assessment and management, aligning strategies with what is required by the law, are tackled. Real-world stories are highlighted in Section 18.7 through case studies, offering practical lessons. Section 18.8 gives a summary and the key takeaways for the future of legal and regulatory policies in healthcare cybersecurity.

18.2 Cybersecurity fundamentals

The objective of this section is to establish a foundational understanding of key principles and concepts crucial for navigating the intricate landscape of cybersecurity in healthcare. It begins by explaining basic ideas that are necessary to understand the wide range of cyber threats and countermeasures. After that, it explores the fundamental ideas behind successful cybersecurity tactics, focusing on risk reduction and preventative actions. It also examines the cybersecurity triangle, emphasizing the complex interrelationships between availability, confidentiality, and integrity in safeguarding critical healthcare systems and data. Finally, the conversation moves on to new developments in cybersecurity, illuminating changing risks and creative methods for boosting cyber resilience in healthcare environments. With the help of this thorough review, readers will be better equipped to handle the complexity of cybersecurity in the ever-changing world of healthcare systems.

18.2.1 Key concepts of cybersecurity

Cybersecurity is the practice of protecting information systems and data from unauthorized access, use, modification, or destruction [1]. Cybersecurity is essential for ensuring the confidentiality, integrity, and availability of information in the digital world. Cybersecurity faces various threats from different sources, such as hackers, cybercriminals, nation-states, or even insiders within an organization [5]. These threats can exploit vulnerabilities in the information systems or use social engineering techniques to trick users into revealing sensitive information or installing malicious software. Some common types of threats are:

1. **Malware:** Malicious software that can infect, damage, or control a computer system or network. Examples of malware include viruses, worms, ransomware, spyware, and Trojans.
2. **Phishing:** A fraudulent attempt to obtain sensitive information or credentials by impersonating a legitimate entity or person via email or other online communication channels.
3. **Insider threats:** A threat that originates from within an organization, such as a disgruntled employee, a contractor, or a business partner who has access to the information systems or data and abuses their privileges for malicious purposes.

To protect against these threats, cybersecurity relies on various mechanisms that can prevent, detect, and respond to attacks. Some of these mechanisms are:

1. **Encryption:** A process of transforming information into an unreadable form that can only be decrypted by authorized parties who have the key. Encryption can protect the confidentiality and integrity of data in transit (such as over the internet) or at rest (such as on a hard drive).
2. **Access controls:** A set of rules and policies that define who can access what information and under what conditions. Access controls can limit the exposure of sensitive data to unauthorized parties and reduce the risk of insider threats.
3. **Authentication:** A process of verifying the identity of a user or a device before granting access to the information systems or data. Authentication can use various factors, such as passwords, biometrics, tokens, or certificates.

18.2.2 Principles of cybersecurity

Cybersecurity is the comprehensive practice of protecting information and systems from cyber threats, with a focus on ensuring the security, privacy, and reliability of data and services. Employing various principles, it encompasses defense-in-depth, risk management, confidentiality, integrity, availability, and non-repudiation, each playing a crucial role in maintaining a robust security posture. Defense-in-depth involves leveraging multiple security measures to safeguard organizational assets, while risk management is the process of identifying, assessing, and mitigating security risks. Confidentiality ensures sensitive information remains private, integrity guarantees data accuracy and trustworthiness, availability ensures accessibility and reliability of information and services, and non-repudiation verifies and proves the origin and destination of information. For a more detailed explanation of each principle, refer to Table 18.1.

In summary, cybersecurity principles play a vital role in safeguarding against cyber threats, with each principle addressing specific aspects of security. The detailed breakdown in Table 18.1 provides a comprehensive understanding of these principles and their practical applications in ensuring the resilience and protection of information and systems.

Table 18.1 Principles of cybersecurity

Principle	Description	Example
Defense-in-depth	Strategy leveraging multiple security measures to protect organizational assets [6].	Utilizing firewalls, antivirus software, web application firewalls, and intrusion detection systems for network security
Risk assessment	Process of identifying, assessing, and mitigating security risks [7].	Conducting regular security audits, implementing security policies, and allocating resources for security improvement
Confidentiality	Property ensuring sensitive information remains private and protected from unauthorized access [8].	Encrypting data at rest and in transit, using strong passwords, and applying access control mechanisms
Integrity	Property ensuring information accuracy and trustworthiness [9].	Employing digital signatures, checksums, and hashing algorithms to verify authenticity and integrity of data
Availability	Property ensuring accessibility and reliability of information and services [10].	Utilizing load balancing, redundancy, backup, and recovery strategies to prevent or minimize downtime and data loss
Non-repudiation	Property ensuring verification and proof of information origin and destination [11].	Employing certificates, timestamps, and audit logs to record and validate the identity and actions of users

18.2.3 The cybersecurity triad

In the realm of cybersecurity, understanding the fundamental principles is crucial. One key model that aids in comprehending the core objectives of cybersecurity is the Cybersecurity Triad, as illustrated in Figure 18.1.

The cybersecurity triad is a model that outlines the three primary objectives of cybersecurity: prevention, detection, and response [12]. These objectives are intricately interrelated and complementary, collectively working toward safeguarding the confidentiality, integrity, and availability of the system.

This model serves as a reference point throughout the discussion on cybersecurity fundamentals, providing a visual guide to the interconnected nature of prevention, detection, and response in ensuring robust cybersecurity.

1. **Prevention:** This objective refers to the actions taken to avoid or stop potential attacks before they happen. Prevention can be achieved by using security controls such as encryption, authentication, authorization, firewalls, antivirus software, etc.
2. **Detection:** This objective refers to the actions taken to identify and monitor possible attacks as they occur. Detection can be achieved by using security controls such as intrusion detection systems (IDS), log analysis, network traffic analysis, etc.
3. **Response:** This objective refers to the actions taken to contain and recover from an attack after it happens. Response can be achieved by using security

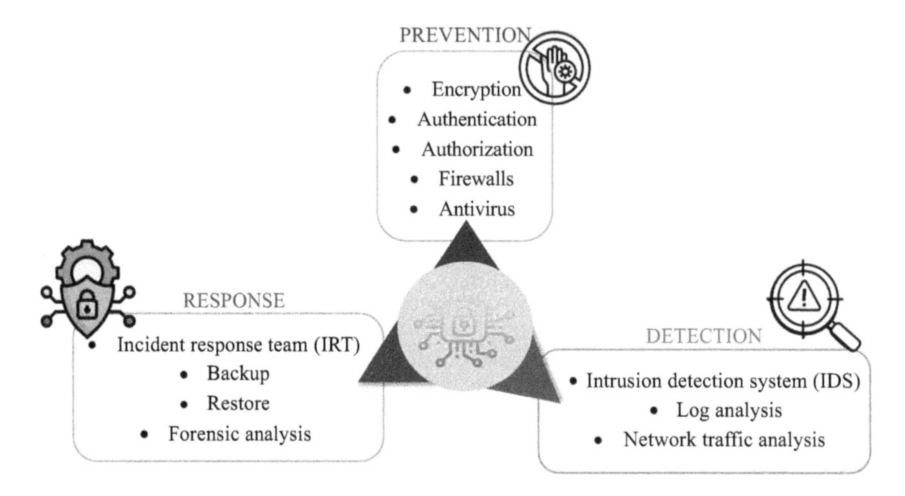

Figure 18.1 The cybersecurity triad

controls such as incident response teams (IRT), backup and restore procedures, forensic analysis, etc.

Security best practices are the recommended methods and standards that help to achieve effective and efficient cybersecurity [13]. Some of them include patch management and incident response planning. The patch management practice refers to the process of updating the software and firmware of the system with the latest security fixes and enhancements. Patch management can help to prevent or mitigate known vulnerabilities and improve the performance and functionality of the system. Incident response planning refers to the process of preparing for and handling security incidents in a systematic and coordinated manner. Incident response planning can help to minimize the impact and duration of an attack, preserve the evidence and information, and restore normal operations as soon as possible.

18.2.4 Emerging trends in cybersecurity

Cybersecurity is a dynamic and evolving field that constantly faces new challenges and opportunities. Healthcare systems are one of the most critical and sensitive sectors that require effective and efficient cybersecurity solutions [14]. In this subsection, certain current and emerging trends in cybersecurity that are pertinent to healthcare systems are emphasized. Additionally, their implications for applying cybersecurity fundamentals in healthcare contexts are explored. Table 18.2 depicts the emerging trends, which include AI-driven security, Internet of Things (IoT) device protection, and cloud computing security, with a description and the impacts on healthcare systems.

One of the current trends in cybersecurity is the use of artificial intelligence (AI) to enhance security capabilities and performance [26]. AI-driven security can

Table 18.2 Emerging trends in healthcare cybersecurity

Trend	Description	Impact on the health system	Examples
AI-Driven Security	Utilizes artificial intelligence (AI) for automating and enhancing security tasks, including threat detection, analysis, response, and prevention. Incorporates machine learning, natural language processing, and computer vision [15].	• Protects healthcare data's confidentiality, integrity, and availability. • Reduces the complexity and cost of security operations. • Enhances security awareness and education.	• IBM Watson Health: Uses AI for healthcare data analysis, diagnosis, and cybersecurity [15]. • Fortinet: Offers AI-driven security for healthcare IoT and OT devices [16]. • AltexSoft: Develops AI-based applications for healthcare cybersecurity, including anomaly detection and risk assessment [17].
IoT Device Protection	Addresses security risks associated with IoT devices in healthcare systems, covering issues like weak passwords and outdated software [18].	• Ensures the safety and quality of healthcare services. • Prevents harm from malicious attacks on IoT devices. • Preserves trust and reputation of healthcare providers.	• MedCrypt: Provides security solutions for medical devices, encrypting data and verifying device identity [19]. • Armis: Delivers agentless security for IoT and OT devices, monitoring behavior and responding to threats [20]. • Zingbox: Offers IoT security and analytics for healthcare, using machine learning to identify and protect devices [21].
Cloud Computing Security	Involves on-demand access to shared computing resources over the internet, introducing security challenges [22].	• Enhances performance and functionality of healthcare services. • Improves accessibility and availability of healthcare data. • Increases reliability and resilience of healthcare systems.	• AWS: Provides cloud computing services for healthcare, offering security features like encryption and identity management [23]. • Microsoft Azure: Delivers cloud solutions for healthcare, with security capabilities including threat protection and compliance [24]. • Google Cloud: Enables cloud applications for healthcare, supporting security functions such as access control and encryption [25].

leverage machine learning, natural language processing, computer vision, and other techniques to automate and improve various security tasks, such as threat detection, analysis, response, and prevention [27]. For example, AI can help to identify and classify malicious activities, anomalies, and patterns in large and complex data sets, such as network traffic, logs, or medical records [28]. AI can also help to generate and update security policies, rules, and configurations based on the changing environment and user behavior [29]. Moreover, AI can assist human security experts in decision-making, investigation, and remediation by providing insights, recommendations, and feedback.

AI-driven security can benefit healthcare systems in several ways. First, it can help to protect the confidentiality, integrity, and availability of healthcare data and services, which are essential for patient care, diagnosis, treatment, and research. Second, it can help to reduce the cost and complexity of security operations by automating and optimizing the security processes and resources. Third, it can help to enhance the security awareness and education of the healthcare staff and patients by providing interactive and personalized guidance and training.

Another current trend in cybersecurity is the protection of Internet of Things (IoT) devices. IoT devices are smart devices that can connect to the internet and communicate with other devices or systems. IoT devices are widely used in healthcare systems to provide various functions and benefits, such as remote monitoring, telemedicine, wearable sensors, smart implants, etc. However, IoT devices also pose significant security risks due to their heterogeneity, diversity, mobility, scalability, and resource constraints. For example, IoT devices may have weak or default passwords, outdated or unpatched software, insecure communication protocols or channels, or a lack of encryption or authentication mechanisms [30]. These vulnerabilities can expose IoT devices to various attacks, such as denial-of-service (DoS), ransomware, data theft or manipulation, device hijacking, or sabotage.

IoT device protection requires a holistic and multi-layered approach that involves both technical and non-technical measures. Some of the technical measures include device hardening (e.g., changing default passwords) [31], firmware updating (e.g., applying patches), encryption (e.g., using secure protocols), authentication (e.g., using biometrics), isolation (e.g., using separate networks), monitoring (e.g., using IDS), etc. Some of the non-technical measures include policy development (e.g., defining roles and responsibilities), regulation compliance (e.g., following standards and guidelines), user education (e.g., raising awareness and best practices), etc.

IoT device protection is crucial for healthcare systems because it can help to ensure the safety and quality of healthcare services and outcomes. For instance, it can help to prevent or mitigate the potential harm or damage caused by malicious attacks on IoT devices that may affect the health or life of the patients or staff. It can also help to preserve the trust and reputation of healthcare providers and organizations by safeguarding their data and assets.

The third emerging trend in cybersecurity is the role of cloud computing in healthcare cybersecurity. Cloud computing is a model that enables on-demand access to a shared pool of computing resources (such as servers, storage, applications, etc.) over the internet [32]. Cloud computing can offer various advantages for healthcare systems, such as scalability (e.g., adjusting resources according to demand), flexibility (e.g., accessing resources from anywhere), efficiency (e.g., reducing operational costs), innovation (e.g., enabling new services or features), etc. However, cloud computing also introduces new security challenges due to its characteristics, such as multi-tenancy (e.g., sharing resources with other users), dependency (e.g., relying on third-party providers), complexity (e.g., managing multiple components or layers), etc. These challenges can result in various threats, such as data breaches (e.g., unauthorized access or disclosure of data), data loss (e.g., accidental deletion or corruption of data), service disruption (e.g., unavailability or degradation of service), etc.

Cloud computing security requires a shared responsibility model that involves both the cloud service providers (CSPs) and the cloud service users (CSUs) [33]. The CSPs are responsible for securing the cloud infrastructure and platform, such as physical security (e.g., locking doors or cabinets), network security (e.g., using firewalls or VPNs), system security (e.g., using antivirus software or encryption), etc. The CSUs are responsible for securing the cloud data and applications, such as data security (e.g., using backup or recovery procedures), application security (e.g., using secure coding or testing practices), user security (e.g., using strong passwords or multifactor authentication), etc.

Cloud computing security is important for healthcare systems because it can help to enhance the performance and functionality of healthcare services and operations [34]. For example, it can help to improve the accessibility and availability of healthcare data and applications, which can facilitate collaboration and communication among healthcare stakeholders. It can also help to increase the reliability and resilience of the healthcare systems, which can cope with the increasing demand and complexity of healthcare needs.

The current and emerging trends in cybersecurity, such as AI-driven security, IoT device protection, and the role of cloud computing in healthcare cybersecurity, have significant implications for the application of cybersecurity fundamentals in healthcare contexts. These trends can help to protect the confidentiality, integrity, and availability of healthcare data and services, as well as to improve the efficiency and effectiveness of healthcare operations and outcomes. However, these trends also pose new challenges and risks that require continuous monitoring, evaluation, and adaptation of security measures and practices.

18.3 Healthcare system and data

An overview of the revolutionary effects on care delivery and quality that new healthcare systems and data management techniques are having is provided in this section. It begins by describing how the value-based care model evolved from the conventional fee-for-service approach, emphasizing patient pleasure, efficiency, and results. Health data kinds, sources, standards, purposes, and advantages and disadvantages of health data interchange are all covered in this talk about possibilities and problems in healthcare data management. Finally, it explores the importance of integration and interoperability, which enable safe health data exchange across various platforms, devices, and apps and promote cooperation and coordination amongst stakeholders.

18.3.1 Evolution of healthcare system

Healthcare systems are the organized networks of institutions, professionals, and resources that provide health services to populations [35,36]. The historical context of healthcare systems can be traced back to ancient civilizations, where medicine was often based on religious beliefs, natural remedies, and empirical observations. Some of the earliest examples of healthcare systems include the Ayurvedic system in India, the Traditional Chinese Medicine system in China, and the Hippocratic system in Greece [37,38].

Over time, healthcare systems evolved with the development of science, technology, and society. The modern era of healthcare systems began in the 19th and 20th centuries when advances in microbiology, immunology, surgery, anesthesia, and public health led to improved diagnosis, treatment, and prevention of diseases [39]. Healthcare systems also became more organized and regulated, with the establishment of professional associations, standards, and laws. Some of the key milestones in the modern history of healthcare systems include the creation of the National Health Service (NHS) in the United Kingdom in 1948, the adoption of the Alma-Ata Declaration by the World Health Organization (WHO) in 1978, and the launch of the Universal Health Coverage (UHC) initiative by the WHO in 2005.

In recent decades, healthcare systems have transformed into emerging healthcare systems, which are characterized by the integration of information and communication technologies (ICTs), such as telemedicine, IoT, and digital health records. Telemedicine is the delivery of health services and information via electronic means, such as phone, video, or online platforms. IoT is the network of physical devices, sensors, and software that collect and exchange data. Digital health records are electronic storage and management of health information. These technologies enable healthcare systems to provide more accessible, efficient, personalized, and coordinated care to patients.

The benefits of these advancements include improved access to health services for remote and underserved populations, reduced costs and errors in health delivery and administration, enhanced quality, and safety of care through data-driven decision-making and monitoring, increased patient empowerment and engagement through self-care and feedback mechanisms, and better health outcomes and equity through tailored and preventive interventions [40,41]. However, these advancements also pose some challenges for healthcare systems, such as ethical issues related to privacy, consent, and accountability of data use and sharing; technical issues related to interoperability, security, and reliability of ICTs; social issues related to digital literacy, trust, and human interaction; and economic issues related to affordability, sustainability, and impact of ICTs on health workforce and markets.

The healthcare systems have evolved from ancient to modern to emerging forms over time. The historical context of healthcare systems reflects the influence of various factors such as culture, science, technology, and society on health practices and policies. The transformation into emerging healthcare systems involves the adoption of ICTs such as telemedicine, IoT, and digital health records that offer both opportunities and challenges for improving health services and outcomes. Healthcare systems need to adapt to these changes by addressing the ethical, technical, social, and economic implications of ICTs for health.

18.3.2 Data management in healthcare

Data serves as the lifeblood of contemporary healthcare, facilitating the provision of high-quality, efficient, and personalized care to patients [42]. Data management encompasses the secure and ethical collection, storage, processing, analysis, and sharing of data [43]. Within healthcare, the critical role of data is undeniable. A myriad of data sources exists in this domain, ranging from patient records and diagnostic tools to wearables and IoT devices. Essential components of data management in healthcare include data governance, security, and privacy, as depicted in Figure 18.2. The subsequent list offers a more detailed exploration of each fundamental element of data management:

1. **Patient records:** Patient records are electronic or paper-based documentation of health information, such as medical history, medications, allergies, diagnoses, treatments, and outcomes.
2. **Diagnostic:** These tools are devices or software that measure or test various aspects of health, such as blood pressure, glucose level, heart rate, or genetic profile.

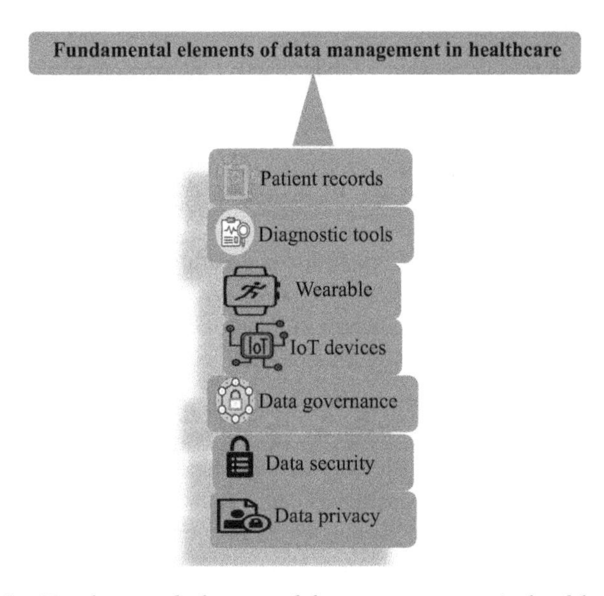

Figure 18.2 Fundamental element of data management in healthcare system

3. **Wearables:** These are the devices or accessories that monitor health or fitness data, such as activity level, sleep quality, or calories burned.
4. **IoT devices**: These are smart objects or systems that connect and communicate data via the internet, such as sensors, cameras, or robots.
5. **Data governance:** A set of policies and procedures that define roles, responsibilities, and rules for data collection, storage, processing, analysis, and sharing [44]. It ensures that data is accurate, consistent, complete, and compliant with legal and ethical standards.
6. **Data security:** involves the use of encryption, authentication, authorization, and auditing techniques to safeguard data from cyberattacks or breaches.
7. **Data privacy:** involves the use of consent, anonymization, de-identification, and minimization techniques to ensure that data is collected and used only for legitimate and agreed purposes.

In summary, effective data management is crucial within the healthcare domain, where data acts as the foundation for delivering high-quality, efficient, and personalized patient care. The comprehensive process of secure and ethical data collection, storage, processing, analysis, and sharing underscores the undeniable significance of data in modern healthcare. With a diverse array of data sources, spanning patient records, diagnostic tools, wearables, and IoT devices, the landscape demands meticulous attention to fundamental elements such as data governance, security, and privacy, as illustrated in Figure 18.2. The subsequent detailed exploration of each essential component aims to further underscore the critical role that these aspects play in shaping the landscape of data management within the healthcare sector.

18.3.3 Interoperability and integration

Interoperability refers to the seamless exchange of data among various healthcare systems and sources, ensuring standardized and meaningful communication. Integration, on the other hand, involves amalgamating disparate healthcare data into a cohesive and consistent format. Both interoperability and integration play pivotal roles in enhancing healthcare quality, efficiency, and innovation.

In this section, we explore the fundamental aspects of healthcare data interoperability and integration. For a comprehensive overview and detailed insights, refer to Table 18.3. This table presents a structured breakdown of challenges, solutions, and potential benefits, serving as a valuable resource for understanding the intricacies and advantages inherent in this critical domain.

The challenges for integrating diverse healthcare data include the following:

1. **Data heterogeneity:** Healthcare data can vary in terms of structure, format, semantics, and quality. For example, patient records can be stored in different electronic health record (EHR) systems that use different data models, terminologies, and coding schemes (Gamal *et al.*, 2021). Diagnostic tools can produce different types of data, such as images, signals, or texts. Wearables and IoT devices can generate large volumes of unstructured and streaming data that require real-time processing and analysis.

Table 18.3 Overview of healthcare data interoperability and integration

Aspect	Description
Definition	Interoperability: The ability of different healthcare systems and data sources to communicate and exchange data in a standardized way. Integration: Combining diverse healthcare data into a unified format.
Importance	Enhances healthcare quality, efficiency, and innovation by facilitating communication and harmonizing data.
Challenges	1. Data Heterogeneity: Variability in structure, format, semantics, and quality. 2. Data Fragmentation: Distribution across multiple locations, organizations, and domains. 3. Data Governance: Subject to regulations, policies, and standards.
Challenges Details	1. Patient records stored in different EHR systems with varying models, terminologies, and coding schemes. Diagnostic tools generate diverse data types. Wearables produce unstructured, streaming data. 2. Patient data scattered across healthcare providers, research repositories, and decision-making departments. 3. Healthcare data subject to privacy laws, ethical guidelines, and performance indicators.
Solutions	1. Data Standardization: Convert healthcare data into a common format (e.g., SNOMED CT, ICD). 2. Data Federation: Access data from multiple sources without consolidation (e.g., SHRINE, REDCap). 3. Data Stewardship: Manage data responsibly (e.g., PASOA, FAIR principles).
Solutions Details	1. Standardize patient records using SNOMED CT or ICD. Use common exchange protocols for diagnostic tools and wearables. 2. Query patient data through federated systems (e.g., SHRINE). Link research data with identifiers (e.g., REDCap). Aggregate decision-making data through federated dashboards (e.g., NHS Digital Dashboard). 3. Audit patient data using provenance systems (e.g., PASOA). Curate research data through the FAIR principles. Evaluate decision-making data with quality frameworks (e.g., DQAF).
Potential Benefits	1. Improved Patient Care: Access to comprehensive patient information enhances diagnosis, treatment, coordination, and patient participation. 2. Improved Research: Access to diverse datasets improves hypothesis generation, testing, and collaboration. 3. Improved Decision-Making: Timely access to relevant information supports evidence-based policy-making and management, enhancing healthcare services and transparency.
Benefits Details	1. Comprehensive patient information improves diagnosis, treatment, coordination, and patient engagement. 2. Access to diverse datasets enhances research processes and collaboration. 3. Timely information supports evidence-based decision-making, planning, evaluation, and transparency in healthcare services.

2. **Data fragmentation:** Healthcare data can be distributed across multiple locations, organizations, and domains. For example, patient data can be scattered among different healthcare providers, such as primary care physicians, specialists, hospitals, pharmacies, and laboratories. Research data can be isolated in different repositories, such as clinical trials, biobanks, or registries. Decision-making data can be siloed in different departments, such as administration, finance, or quality improvement.
3. **Data governance:** Healthcare data can be subject to various regulations, policies, and standards that govern the collection, storage, processing, analysis, and sharing of data. For example, patient data can be protected by privacy laws, such as the Health Insurance Portability and Accountability Act (HIPAA) in the United States or the General Data Protection Regulation (GDPR) in the European Union. Research data can be regulated by ethical guidelines, such as the Declaration of Helsinki or the Common Rule. Decision-making data can be influenced by performance indicators, such as the Healthcare Effectiveness Data and Information Set (HEDIS) or the National Quality Forum (NQF).

The solutions for integrating diverse healthcare data include the following:

1. **Data standardization**: Healthcare data can be converted into a common format that facilitates interoperability and integration. For example, patient records can be mapped to a standardized terminology system, such as the Systematized Nomenclature of Medicine—Clinical Terms (SNOMED CT) or the International Classification of Diseases (ICD). Diagnostic tools can use a common exchange protocol, such as Digital Imaging and Communications in Medicine (DICOM) or Health Level Seven (HL7). Wearables and IoT devices can adopt a universal platform, such as the Continua Health Alliance or Open mHealth.
2. **Data federation:** Healthcare data can be accessed from multiple sources without requiring physical consolidation or duplication. For example, patient data can be queried through a federated query system, such as the Shared Health Research Information Network (SHRINE) or the Informatics for Integrating Biology and the Bedside (i2b2). Research data can be linked through a federated identifier system, such as the Research Electronic Data Capture (REDCap) or the Global Unique Identifier (GUID). Decision-making data can be aggregated through a federated dashboard system, such as the NHS Digital Dashboard or the Health Catalyst Analytics Platform.
3. **Data stewardship:** Healthcare data can be managed in a responsible and accountable manner that ensures data quality, security, and privacy. For example, patient data can be audited through a data provenance system, such as the Provenance Aware Service Oriented Architecture (PASOA) or the Blockchain Health Information Exchange (B-HIE). Research data can be curated through a data lifecycle system, such as the FAIR principles (Findable, Accessible, Interoperable, Reusable) or the Data Documentation Initiative (DDI). Decision-making data can be evaluated through a data quality system,

such as the Data Quality Assessment Framework (DQAF) or the Data Quality Model (DQM).

The potential for improved patient care, research, and decision-making through data integration includes the following:

1. **Improved patient care:** Data integration can enable healthcare providers to access comprehensive and accurate information about patients' health status, history, preferences, and outcomes. This can improve diagnosis, treatment, coordination, and follow-up of care. Data integration can also empower patients to participate in their care through self-monitoring, feedback, and education.
2. **Improved research:** Data integration can enable researchers to access large and diverse datasets that span across multiple domains and disciplines. This can improve hypothesis generation, testing, validation, and dissemination of research findings. Data integration can also facilitate collaboration among researchers from different institutions and countries.
3. **Improved decision-making:** Data integration can enable decision-makers to access timely and relevant information that supports evidence-based policy-making and management. This can improve planning, evaluation, and improvement of healthcare services and systems. Data integration can also enhance transparency and accountability of healthcare performance and outcomes.

In conclusion, the pursuit of interoperability and integration in healthcare data management emerges as a paramount endeavor for advancing quality, efficiency, and innovation within the healthcare sector. By enabling seamless communication and harmonization of diverse data sources, interoperability and integration lay the foundation for improved patient care, enhanced research capabilities, and informed decision-making processes. While challenges such as data heterogeneity, fragmentation, and governance persist, the adoption of standardized practices, federated systems, and responsible data stewardship offers promising solutions. Through a concerted effort to address these challenges and leverage the potential benefits, healthcare systems can embrace a future where data interoperability and integration serve as catalysts for transformative change and sustained improvement.

18.4 Cybersecurity frameworks

Cybersecurity frameworks are sets of standards, guidelines, and best practices that help organizations manage their cybersecurity risks and improve their security posture. They provide a common language and a structured approach for identifying, assessing, and addressing cybersecurity challenges in various domains and sectors. While [45] discussed the legal frameworks for AI and blockchain technology in telehealth systems, [46] explored the legal frameworks for security schemes in wireless communication systems.

One of the sectors that can greatly benefit from cybersecurity frameworks is healthcare. Healthcare organizations deal with sensitive and personal data of patients, such as medical records, diagnoses, treatments, prescriptions, and insurance information [2]. These data are valuable for cybercriminals who can use them for identity theft, fraud, blackmail, or ransomware attacks. Moreover, healthcare organizations rely on various devices and systems that are connected to the internet, such as medical equipment, electronic health records, telemedicine platforms, and mobile applications. These devices and systems can be vulnerable to cyberattacks that can compromise their functionality, integrity, availability, and safety.

Therefore, cybersecurity frameworks are crucial in healthcare because they help healthcare organizations protect their data and systems from cyber threats. They also help them comply with relevant laws and regulations that govern the privacy and security of health information, such as the Health Insurance Portability and Accountability Act (HIPAA) in the United States or the General Data Protection Regulation (GDPR) in the European Union. By following a cybersecurity framework, healthcare organizations can establish a clear vision and strategy for their cybersecurity goals, identify their current strengths and weaknesses, prioritize their actions and investments, implement effective controls and measures, monitor, and evaluate their performance, and continuously improve their security culture and awareness [47].

Some of the key cybersecurity frameworks that apply to the healthcare sector are:

1. **NIST cybersecurity framework**: This is a voluntary framework developed by the National Institute of Standards and Technology (NIST) in collaboration with various stakeholders from the public and private sectors. It is based on existing standards, guidelines, and practices for improving critical infrastructure cybersecurity. It consists of five core functions: Identify, Protect, Detect, Respond, and Recover. Each function has a set of categories and subcategories that describe specific outcomes and activities for achieving cybersecurity objectives. The framework also provides informative references to various authoritative sources that can help implement the subcategories. The framework is flexible and adaptable to different types of organizations and risk profiles. It can be used to align security activities with business objectives, communicate risk management priorities to stakeholders, assess current security posture, identify gaps and opportunities for improvement, and measure progress over time.
2. **HITRUST CSF:** This is a certifiable framework developed by the Health Information Trust Alliance (HITRUST) in collaboration with data protection professionals from various industries. It rationalizes relevant regulations and standards into a single overarching security and privacy framework. It covers 19 domains of information security controls that address various aspects of people, processes, and technology. It also provides prescriptive and granular control requirements that can be customized through various factors such as organization type, size, systems, compliance requirements, risk appetite, etc.

The framework leverages a common assurance methodology across all HITRUST assessments and certifications. It helps organizations achieve compliance with multiple regulations and standards such as HIPAA, GDPR, PCI-DSS, NIST SP 800-53, ISO/IEC 27001/2/3/5/17/18/34, etc. [48].

3. **ISO/IEC 27001:** This is an international standard for information security management systems (ISMS) published jointly by the International Organization for Standardization (ISO) and the International Electro-Technical Commission (IEC). It defines requirements an ISMS must meet to ensure the confidentiality, integrity, and availability of information assets. It follows a Plan-Do-Check-Act (PDCA) cycle for establishing, implementing, maintaining, and continually improving an ISMS. It also specifies a set of 114 security controls that can be selected based on the results of a risk assessment. The standard is compatible with other management system standards such as ISO 9001 (quality management) or ISO 22301 (business continuity management) [48]. It enables organizations to demonstrate their compliance with various regulations and standards through an independent certification by an accredited certification body. These frameworks have different scopes, structures, contents, and levels of detail. However, they share some common principles and objectives such as:

(i) Adopting a risk-based approach to information security management.
(ii) Aligning security activities with business goals.
(iii) Implementing a comprehensive set of security controls.
(iv) Following a continuous improvement process.
(v) Engaging stakeholders and fostering a security culture.

Table 18.4 meticulously outlines key cybersecurity frameworks tailored to the healthcare sector, offering insights into their unique approaches for safeguarding sensitive medical information and ensuring regulatory compliance. This comprehensive resource serves as an invaluable reference for healthcare professionals and cybersecurity experts seeking to enhance the resilience of healthcare systems against evolving cyber threats.

Healthcare organizations can choose one or more of these frameworks to suit their specific needs and contexts. They can also use them as complementary or supplementary resources to enhance their security capabilities and performance. For example, they can use the NIST Cybersecurity Framework as a high-level guide to define their security objectives and outcomes, the HITRUST CSF as a detailed and tailored roadmap to achieve compliance with multiple regulations and standards, and the ISO/IEC 27001 as a globally recognized certification to demonstrate their security maturity and credibility.

18.4.1 Implementing and adapting frameworks for healthcare

Implementing cybersecurity frameworks in healthcare organizations is not a trivial task. It requires a clear vision, a strong commitment, a dedicated team, and a

Table 18.4 Key cybersecurity frameworks for healthcare

Framework	Developer/organization	Core functions	Applicability and flexibility
NIST Cybersecurity Framework	National Institute of Standards and Technology (NIST)	Identify, Protect, Detect, Respond, Recover	Voluntary, adaptable to various organizations, aligns security with business goals
HITRUST CSF	Health Information Trust Alliance (HITRUST)	Unified security and privacy framework	Certifiable, covers multiple domains, customizable based on various factors
ISO/IEC 27001	International Organization for Standardization (ISO) and International Electro Technical Commission (IEC)	Plan-Do-Check-Act (PDCA) cycle, 114 security controls	International standard, independent certification, compatible with other management system standards

systematic process. Some of the practical aspects of implementing cybersecurity frameworks in healthcare organizations are:

1. **Framework selection:** Selecting a suitable framework or a combination of frameworks that match the organization's goals, needs, and context. This may involve conducting a gap analysis, benchmarking with peers, consulting with experts, and evaluating the costs and benefits of different options.
2. **Scope definition:** Defining the scope and boundaries of the framework implementation, such as the organizational units, functions, processes, assets, and stakeholders that are involved or affected by the framework.
3. **Roles and responsibilities:** Establishing the roles and responsibilities of the framework implementation team, such as the project manager, the security officer, the risk manager, the compliance officer, the technical staff, and the business owners.
4. **Project planning**: Developing a project plan and a timeline for the framework implementation, including the tasks, milestones, deliverables, resources, dependencies, and risks.
5. **Risk assessment:** Conducting a risk assessment to identify and prioritize the cybersecurity threats and vulnerabilities that affect the organization's data and systems. This may involve using tools and methods such as threat modeling, vulnerability scanning, penetration testing, etc.
6. **Security controls implementation:** Implementing the security controls and measures that are recommended or required by the framework to mitigate the risks. This may involve using tools and methods such as policies, procedures, standards, guidelines, training, awareness, audits, monitoring, testing, etc.

7. **Progress measurement**: Measuring and reporting the progress and performance of the framework implementation, using metrics and indicators that are defined or suggested by the framework. This may involve using tools and methods such as dashboards, scorecards, reports, surveys, feedback, etc.
8. **Review and update:** Reviewing and updating the framework implementation regularly to ensure its effectiveness and alignment with changing requirements and conditions. This may involve using tools and methods such as audits, reviews, evaluations, feedback, lessons learned, etc.

Adapting cybersecurity frameworks to meet the unique needs and compliance requirements of healthcare cybersecurity is also a challenging task. It requires a deep understanding of the healthcare sector's characteristics, such as:

(i) The diversity and complexity of healthcare data and systems.
(ii) The high value and sensitivity of health information.
(iii) The dynamic and collaborative nature of healthcare processes.
(iv) The regulatory and ethical obligations of healthcare providers.
(v) The innovation and evolution of healthcare technologies.

Some of the challenges and best practices for adapting cybersecurity frameworks to meet the unique needs and compliance requirements of healthcare cybersecurity are:

1. **Balancing security and usability:** Healthcare organizations need to ensure that their security controls do not interfere with their core functions of providing quality care to patients. They need to consider factors such as user experience, workflow efficiency, accessibility, availability, and reliability when implementing security measures. They also need to involve users in designing, testing, and evaluating security solutions to ensure their acceptance and adoption.
2. **Integrating security into the lifecycle:** Healthcare organizations need to incorporate security into every stage of their data and system lifecycle, from planning, design, development, deployment, operation, and maintenance, to disposal. They need to apply security principles such as privacy by design, security by design, and secure development lifecycle (SDLC) to ensure that their data and systems are secure from inception to retirement.
3. **Aligning security with compliance:** Healthcare organizations need to comply with various laws and regulations that govern the privacy and security of health information, such as HIPAA in the United States or GDPR in the European Union. They need to map their security controls to their compliance requirements and demonstrate their adherence to them through documentation, evidence, and certification. They also need to monitor and update their security and compliance status regularly to cope with changing rules and expectations.
4. **Leveraging security standards and best practices:** Healthcare organizations need to adopt and adapt security standards and best practices that are relevant and applicable to their sector, such as the NIST Cybersecurity Framework, HITRUST CSF, or ISO/IEC 27001. They need to customize these frameworks

according to their specific needs and contexts, using factors such as organization type, size, systems, compliance requirements, risk appetite, etc. They also need to benchmark their security performance with their peers and learn from their experiences and challenges.

18.5 Legal and regulatory policies

In order to protect patients' rights and interests and make sure healthcare organizations are in accordance with all current laws and regulations, this section examines the important legal and ethical aspects of healthcare cybersecurity. It begins with a summary of the main cybersecurity frameworks and laws that are pertinent to the healthcare industry, such as the Health Information Technology for Economic and Clinical Health (HITECH) Act, the Health Insurance Portability and Accountability Act HIPAA Security Rule, Health and Human Services Section HHS 405(d) recommendations and others. In light of changing cyber threats and resource limitations, the conversation also covers best practices and obstacles for attaining cybersecurity compliance in the dynamic and diversified healthcare sector. It also explores the moral dimensions of cybersecurity in healthcare, covering ransomware attacks, the function of ethical hackers, the possible consequences of data breaches, and the moral standards that inform cybersecurity choices in the medical field.

18.5.1 Healthcare data privacy laws and regulations

Healthcare data privacy is the protection of personal health information (PHI) from unauthorized access, use, disclosure, or modification [49]. PHI includes any information that relates to the past, present, or future physical or mental health or condition of an individual, the provision of healthcare to an individual, or the payment for the provision of healthcare to an individual. Healthcare data privacy is important for ensuring patient trust, confidentiality, and quality of care, as well as for complying with legal and ethical obligations. Various healthcare data privacy regulations apply to different regions and jurisdictions.

1. **The Health Information Technology for Economic and Clinical Health (HITECH) Act**: A federal law included in the American Recovery and Reinvestment Act of 2009 is the Health Information Technology for Economic and Clinical Health (HITECH) Act [50]. The objective is to promote the use of electronic health records (EHRs) by consumers and healthcare providers while strengthening HIPAA's security and privacy safeguards. The Act contains provisions such as the Health Information Exchange (HIE) support, which encourages secure health information sharing, the Meaningful Use Programme, which offers financial incentives for the adoption of EHRs, and the Health Information Technology (HIT) Workforce Development, which addresses the shortage of qualified professionals. Furthermore, it expands HIPAA's privacy and security regulations to include business partners. The healthcare industry

has been greatly influenced by the HITECH Act, which has improved information sharing, encouraged the use of EHRs, and trained HIT workers. However, challenges include the complexity of meaningful use criteria, interoperability issues, cybersecurity risks, and ethical/legal considerations in health information technology. Despite challenges, the HITECH Act has transformed the US healthcare sector, advancing technology adoption, enhancing patient engagement, and improving overall healthcare quality and coordination.

2. **Health Insurance Portability and Accountability Act (HIPAA):** HIPAA was enacted in the United States in 1996 to improve the efficiency and effectiveness of the healthcare system by establishing national standards for the security and privacy of personal health information (PHI) [51,52]. HIPAA applies to covered entities, such as health plans, healthcare clearinghouses, and healthcare providers that transmit PHI electronically, and their business associates, such as vendors, contractors, and consultants, that access or handle PHI on their behalf. HIPAA requires covered entities and business associates to implement administrative, technical, and physical safeguards to protect PHI from unauthorized or accidental access, use, disclosure, or destruction. HIPAA also grants patients certain rights regarding their PHI, such as the right to access, amend, request an accounting of disclosures, and file complaints. HIPAA mandates that covered entities and business associates notify affected individuals and the Department of Health and Human Services in case of a breach of unsecured PHI.
3. **Health and Human Services Section HHS 405(d):** The HHS 405(d) Task Group was tasked under the Cybersecurity Act of 2015 to design a collaborative endeavor, and as a result, the suggestions it made are voluntary and industry-led [53]. By following these recommendations, the healthcare and public health (HPH) industry's cybersecurity will be better protected against online attacks. Based on tenets like considering cybersecurity as essential to patient safety, affordability, and usefulness, the suggestions may be customized for use in a variety of healthcare settings. They tackle prevalent risks like as ransomware and phishing, and they update often to keep up with the changing threat environment. The Health Industry Cybersecurity Practices (HICP) and the Health Industry Cybersecurity Tactical Crisis Response Guide (TCRG) are two publications that offer a crisis response guide and a risk management framework, respectively. While voluntary, the HHS 405(d) Task Group encourages HPH organizations to adopt a cybersecurity-aware culture and leverage these recommendations to enhance their cybersecurity posture and protect patients and services. This public-private partnership illustrates an effective strategy in tackling cybersecurity challenges in the HPH sector by providing a unified framework and tools for resilience.
4. **General Data Protection Regulation (GDPR):** GDPR was adopted in the European Union (EU) in 2016 and became effective in 2018 to harmonize and strengthen data protection laws across the EU member states [54,55]. GDPR applies to any organization that processes the personal data of individuals in

the EU, regardless of where the organization is located or where the data is processed. Personal data is any information that relates to an identified or identifiable natural person. GDPR requires organizations to process personal data lawfully, fairly, and transparently; collect personal data for specified, explicit, and legitimate purposes; limit personal data collection to what is necessary; keep personal data accurate and up to date; retain personal data for no longer than necessary; and ensure personal data security. GDPR also grants individuals certain rights regarding their data, such as the right to access, rectify, erase, restrict, port, object, and withdraw consent. GDPR obliges organizations to notify the relevant supervisory authority and the affected individuals in case of a personal data breach.

5. **The California Consumer Privacy Act (CCPA):** CCPA was enacted in 2018 and became effective in 2020 to grant California residents certain rights regarding their personal information, such as the right to know, access, delete, opt out of sale, and non-discrimination. CCPA applies to any business that collects, sells, or shares the personal information of California residents and meets certain thresholds [56]. Personal information is any information that identifies, relates to, describes, is reasonably capable of being associated with, or could reasonably be linked, directly or indirectly, with a particular consumer or household. CCPA requires businesses to provide notices to consumers at or before the point of collecting their personal information; respond to consumer requests within specified time frames; implement reasonable security measures to protect personal information; and comply with the California Attorney General's regulations.
6. **The Personal Health Information Protection Act (PHIPA):** PHIPA was enacted in 2004 in Ontario, Canada to govern the collection, use, disclosure, retention, and disposal of personal health information by health information custodians (HICs) [57], such as healthcare practitioners, hospitals, pharmacies, laboratories, and healthcare organizations. PHIPA requires HICs to obtain consent from individuals before collecting, using, or disclosing their personal health information; protect personal health information from theft, loss, unauthorized access, use, disclosure, copying, or modification; notify individuals at the first reasonable opportunity if their personal health information is stolen, lost or accessed by unauthorized persons; and comply with individuals' requests for access or correction of their personal health information.
7. **The Data Protection Act (DPA):** DPA was enacted in 2012 in Singapore to regulate the collection, use, disclosure, transfer, retention, disposal, protection, access, correction, accuracy, consent withdrawal, accountability, openness, complaints handling, enforcement, penalties, exemptions, appeals, codes of practice, guidelines, notices, orders, directions, decisions, rules, regulations, subsidiary legislation, and other matters relating to personal data in Singapore [58,59]. DPA requires organizations to obtain consent from individuals before collecting, using, or disclosing their data; notify individuals of the purposes of the collection, use, or disclosure; collect, use, or disclose personal data only for reasonable and appropriate purposes; make reasonable efforts to ensure that

personal data is accurate and complete; protect personal data from unauthorized access, modification, disclosure, copying, use, disposal, or similar risks; retain personal data only for as long as necessary; provide individuals with access to and correction of their personal data; designate a data protection officer to ensure compliance with DPA; develop and implement data protection policies and practices; and cooperate with the Personal Data Protection Commission (PDPC) in the performance of its functions.

Healthcare data privacy regulations are constantly evolving and adapting to the changing needs and challenges of the healthcare sector. Some of the recent updates, enforcement actions, and emerging trends in healthcare data privacy regulations are:

1. **HIPAA updates and enforcement**: In 2020, HHS issued a notice of enforcement discretion to allow covered entities and business associates to use certain video communication technologies to provide telehealth services during the COVID-19 public health emergency, without being subject to penalties for noncompliance with HIPAA rules. HHS also issued guidance on how HIPAA permits covered entities and business associates to disclose PHI to public health authorities, health oversight agencies, law enforcement, and first responders during the COVID-19 public health emergency. In 2021, HHS announced a proposed rule to modify the HIPAA Privacy Rule to enhance individuals' access to their PHI, improve information sharing for care coordination and case management, reduce administrative burdens on covered entities, and promote value-based healthcare [57]. HHS also announced a settlement of $200,000 with a healthcare provider for failing to respond timely to a patient's request for access to her medical records.
2. **GDPR updates and enforcement:** In 2020, the Court of Justice of the European Union (CJEU) invalidated the EU-US Privacy Shield framework, which was a mechanism for transferring personal data from the EU to the United States in compliance with GDPR, due to concerns about the adequacy of US data protection laws and the lack of effective remedies for EU individuals [60]. The CJEU also upheld the validity of another mechanism for transferring personal data from the EU to third countries, namely the standard contractual clauses (SCCs), subject to certain conditions and safeguards. The European Commission issued a draft decision on new SCCs for international transfers of personal data in 2020 and adopted it in 2021. The European Data Protection Board (EDPB) issued guidelines on various aspects of GDPR, such as consent, data protection by design and by default, data protection impact assessment, territorial scope, codes of conduct, certification, cooperation and consistency, accountability, transparency, right to be forgotten, profiling, breach notification, and international transfers. The EDPB also issued recommendations on measures that supplement transfer tools to ensure compliance with GDPR considering the CJEU ruling on the EU-US Privacy Shield. The EDPB also coordinated several joint enforcement actions by national supervisory authorities against organizations that violated GDPR, such as Google, Amazon, Twitter, Marriott, British Airways, H&M, Vodafone, and others.

18.5.2 Cybersecurity compliance challenges in healthcare

Cybersecurity compliance is the adherence to the rules and standards that govern the protection of information systems and data from cyber threats. It is especially important for healthcare organizations, as they handle sensitive and valuable personal health information (PHI) of patients, as well as critical medical devices and systems that affect patient safety and quality of care. However, achieving cybersecurity compliance in healthcare is not an easy task, as healthcare organizations face various challenges.

1. Complex and evolving regulations: Healthcare organizations must comply with multiple cybersecurity regulations that apply to different regions, jurisdictions, and sectors.
2. Third-party risk management: Healthcare organizations often rely on third parties, such as vendors, contractors, consultants, or affiliates, to provide them with products, services, or support that involve access to or handling of PHI or other sensitive data. However, these third parties may pose significant cybersecurity risks to healthcare organizations, as they may not have adequate security measures or controls in place to protect the data they receive or process.
3. Cloud computing security: Healthcare organizations are increasingly adopting cloud computing solutions to store, process, and access their data and applications. Cloud computing offers many benefits to healthcare organizations, such as scalability, flexibility, efficiency, cost-effectiveness, and innovation. However, cloud computing also introduces new cybersecurity challenges.
4. Data sovereignty: Healthcare organizations must ensure that they comply with the data protection laws and regulations of the countries or regions where their data is stored, processed, or transferred by their CSPs. This may involve verifying the location of the cloud servers and data centers, obtaining the consent of the data subjects, ensuring the adequacy of the data protection measures, and implementing appropriate safeguards for cross-border data transfers.
5. Data security: Healthcare organizations have to ensure that their data is protected from unauthorized or accidental access, use, disclosure, modification, or deletion by their CSPs or other parties. This may involve encrypting the data at rest and in transit, implementing strong authentication and authorization mechanisms, applying security patches and updates, monitoring and auditing the cloud activities and logs, and detecting and responding to any security incidents or breaches.
6. Medical device cybersecurity: Healthcare organizations use various medical devices, such as pacemakers, insulin pumps, infusion pumps, MRI machines, CT scanners, X-ray machines, ventilators, etc., to diagnose, treat, monitor, or support patients. These medical devices are often connected to the internet, networks, systems, or other devices, enabling remote access, control, update, or integration. However, these medical devices may also be vulnerable to cyberattacks that could compromise their functionality, integrity, or safety. For example, cyber attackers could hack into a medical device and alter its settings,

disable its features, inject malicious code, steal or corrupt its data, or cause physical harm to the patient or the device.

18.5.3 Legal and ethical implications of healthcare cybersecurity

The possible responsibility of healthcare organizations and technology vendors in the event of data breaches, cyberattacks, or regulatory noncompliance is one of the primary legal challenges in healthcare cybersecurity. Cyberattacks and data breaches may reveal patients' private health information (PHI), which may lead to identity theft, fraud, extortion, discrimination, or worsening of mental or physical health. Legal repercussions, including fines, lawsuits, or criminal charges, may result from breaking legislation like the General Data Protection Regulation (GDPR) in the EU or the Health Insurance Portability and Accountability Act (HIPAA) in the United States [61]. Consequently, it is legally required for healthcare institutions and technology suppliers to put in place sufficient cybersecurity safeguards to secure PHI and to abide by all relevant laws and regulations.

Dealing with cross-border data flows and intrusions presents a jurisdictional barrier, which is another legal concern in healthcare cybersecurity. Healthcare data may be subject to various legal regimes and enforcement methods depending on the location of the data or the attacker as it is increasingly processed and stored in cloud services or transferred through telemedicine platforms. For instance, a Chinese hacker could be able to access PHI that a US-based healthcare provider stores in an Irish cloud service [62]. It might be challenging to decide which laws apply in this situation, who has the authority to investigate and prosecute the occurrence, and how to work with foreign authorities to resolve the matter.

A related legal issue is the harmonization of cybersecurity laws and standards across different countries and regions. As healthcare data is becoming more globalized and interconnected, there is a need for consistent and interoperable cybersecurity frameworks that can facilitate data sharing and collaboration while ensuring data protection and security. However, there may be divergent or conflicting approaches to cybersecurity regulation among different jurisdictions, which can create barriers or uncertainties for healthcare organizations and technology vendors operating across borders. For example, the GDPR has stricter requirements for data protection and consent than some other countries, which may limit the ability of EU-based healthcare organizations to share data with non-EU partners or to use certain cloud services or AI applications that do not comply with the GDPR.

One of the main ethical issues in healthcare cybersecurity is the balance between data privacy and data utility. Data privacy refers to the right of individuals to control their own PHI and to decide who can access, use, or disclose it. Data utility refers to the value of PHI for improving healthcare quality, efficiency, and innovation. For example, PHI can be used for diagnosis, treatment, research, public health or policy-making purposes. However, there may be trade-offs or tensions between data privacy and data utility, as increasing one may decrease the other. For example, anonymizing PHI may enhance data privacy but reduce data utility, as some information may be lost or distorted in the process. Conversely, sharing PHI with third parties may increase data utility but compromise data privacy, as some information may be misused or leaked without consent or knowledge.

The role that cybersecurity plays in fostering patient trust and informed consent in the healthcare system raises additional ethical concerns. The confidence that people have in their healthcare professionals and technology suppliers to safeguard their personal health information and behave in their best interests is known as patient trust. The practice of getting patients' free and explicit approval before gathering, utilizing, or releasing their PHI for certain reasons is known as "informed consent." Ensuring ethical and respectful interactions between patients, healthcare practitioners, and technology suppliers requires both informed consent and patient trust [63]. However, by putting patients in danger or raising doubts about their PHI, cybersecurity concerns can erode patient confidence and informed consent. For example, patients may lose trust in their healthcare providers or technology vendors if they experience or hear about data breaches or cyberattacks that affect their PHI. Patients may also feel coerced or manipulated into giving consent for their PHI if they are not adequately informed or given meaningful choices about the potential benefits and risks of data sharing or use.

A third ethical issue in healthcare cybersecurity is the emerging debate on the ethical implications of AI-driven healthcare [64]. AI-driven healthcare refers to the use of AI techniques, such as machine learning or natural language processing, to analyze large amounts of PHI and to provide insights or recommendations for healthcare decision-making. AI-driven healthcare can offer many advantages for improving healthcare outcomes, such as enhancing diagnosis accuracy, optimizing treatment plans, discovering new drugs, or detecting disease outbreaks. However, AI-driven healthcare also poses many ethical challenges for ensuring cybersecurity and patient data protection. For example,

1. How can hacks that could jeopardize the integrity or dependability of AI-driven healthcare systems be prevented?
2. How can transparency and accountability about the sources, processes, and outcomes of data be ensured in AI-driven healthcare systems?
3. How can AI-powered healthcare systems be made to uphold justice, diversity, and human dignity while protecting patients from injury or discrimination because of their PHI?
4. How can AI-driven healthcare systems be made to conform to human values and preferences without compromising or erasing human agency or autonomy?

Healthcare cybersecurity faces some ethical and legal challenges in the present and the future. It has social and moral aspects in addition to technological ones, requiring cooperation and coordination across a variety of stakeholders, such as healthcare providers, technology suppliers, regulators, researchers, patients, and the public. To ensure that healthcare cybersecurity protects patient rights, interests, and PHI while improving healthcare quality, efficiency, and innovation, these challenges must be addressed.

18.6 Risk and assessment and management

The importance and difficulties of managing cybersecurity risks in the healthcare industry are discussed in this section. These risks include identifying, evaluating, and mitigating possible threats and vulnerabilities that might compromise the privacy, availability, and integrity of health data and systems. Along with tools and techniques for risk assessment and analysis, it starts by providing concepts and methods for identifying risks in healthcare cybersecurity. It covers the types, origins, and implications of cyber hazards. The topic of risk mitigation techniques for healthcare organizations is then discussed, with a focus on best practices and implementation frameworks. These strategies include risk acceptance, avoidance, reduction, and transfer. Finally, it underscores the necessity for continuous risk management and adaptation in healthcare cybersecurity, necessitating regular monitoring, evaluation, and improvement of risk management processes and outcomes, along with the capability to respond and recover from cyber incidents [65].

18.6.1 Risk identification in healthcare cybersecurity

Risk identification is the process of finding and analyzing the potential sources and types of cybersecurity threats that could affect a healthcare organization [66]. It is an essential step in developing a risk management plan and implementing effective security measures. Risk identification helps healthcare organizations to understand their risk exposure, prioritize their resources, and mitigate the impact of cyberattacks.

Cybersecurity hazards in the healthcare industry come from a variety of sources, including both internal and external attacks [67]. Internal risks are those that come from people who work for the company, such as partners, contractors, or employees who have access to systems or critical data. These dangers, which include malevolent insiders, carelessness, and human mistakes, might be deliberate or inadvertent. External risks are those that originate from outside the company, including rivals, state-sponsored actors, hackers, and cybercriminals that target the company's systems or data for a variety of reasons. These threats, which include ransomware, phishing, DoS assaults, and advanced persistent threats, can be targeted or opportunistic.

The healthcare sector faces a unique risk landscape due to its complex and interconnected nature. Healthcare organizations store and process large amounts of sensitive and valuable data, such as personal health information, medical records, research data, or financial data [68]. These data are often shared among multiple stakeholders, such as patients, providers, payers, researchers, or regulators. Healthcare organizations also rely on various devices and systems, such as medical devices, electronic health records, telemedicine platforms, or cloud services [69]. These devices and systems are often outdated, unpatched, or incompatible with each other. Moreover, healthcare organizations have to comply with various laws and regulations, such as the Health Insurance Portability and Accountability Act (HIPAA), the General Data Protection Regulation (GDPR), or the National Institute of Standards and Technology (NIST) frameworks [70]. These laws and regulations impose strict requirements and penalties for data protection and security.

Therefore, risk identification in healthcare cybersecurity is a challenging and ongoing task that requires a comprehensive and systematic approach. Healthcare organizations should adopt a risk-based mindset and use various methods and tools to identify their risks. Some of these methods and tools include:

1. **Risk assessment:** A process of evaluating the likelihood and impact of potential threats on the organization's assets, objectives, and operations.
2. **Risk matrix:** A tool that visualizes the risk level of each threat based on its likelihood and impact.
3. **Risk register:** A tool that documents the identified risks, their sources, types, causes, consequences, and mitigation strategies.
4. **Risk analysis:** A process of analyzing the root causes and contributing factors of each risk and estimating its probability and severity.
5. **Risk monitoring:** A process of tracking and reviewing the status and performance of each risk and its mitigation actions.
6. **Risk reporting:** A process of communicating risk information to relevant stakeholders and decision-makers.

By identifying their cybersecurity risks, healthcare organizations can enhance their security posture and resilience. They can also improve their quality of care, patient safety, operational efficiency, and regulatory compliance. Risk identification is not a one-time activity but a continuous process that requires regular updates and revisions. Healthcare organizations should always be aware of their changing environment and adapt accordingly.

18.6.2 Risk mitigation strategies for healthcare organizations

Cybersecurity risks are a major threat to the healthcare sector, as they can compromise the confidentiality, integrity, and availability of sensitive data and systems. Cyberattacks can also endanger patient safety, quality of care, operational efficiency, and regulatory compliance. Therefore, healthcare organizations need to adopt proactive measures and strategies to mitigate cybersecurity risks and protect their assets and stakeholders.

One of the key measures for risk mitigation is to establish and implement effective policies and procedures that define the roles, responsibilities, and expectations of all staff members regarding cybersecurity. Policies and procedures should cover topics such as data classification, access control, encryption, backup, incident response, disaster recovery, and security awareness. Policies and procedures should also be aligned with relevant laws and regulations, such as HIPAA, GDPR, or NIST frameworks. Policies and procedures should be regularly reviewed and updated to reflect the changing risk environment and best practices.

Another important measure for risk mitigation is to deploy and maintain security controls that can prevent, detect, and respond to cyberattacks. Security controls can be technical, such as firewalls, antivirus software, IDS, or multifactor authentication. Security controls can also be administrative, such as security audits, risk assessments, or security training [71]. Security controls should be based on a risk-based approach that identifies the most critical assets and threats and prioritizes the resources and actions accordingly.

Some examples of successful risk mitigation in healthcare are:

1. A Florida hospital launched a comprehensive cybersecurity program in 2019 that comprised incident response plans, security controls, security training, and rules and procedures. In only a single year, the program assisted the hospital in lowering its cyber risk score by 64% [72].
2. To detect and prioritize cybersecurity concerns in 2020, a hospital network in New York employed a cloud-based platform that combined data from several sources and used AI. In just six months, the network was able to minimize its vulnerability exposure by 75% thanks to the platform [73].
3. A zero-trust approach was used in 2021 by a medical facility in California. Before allowing access to data or systems, every user and device's identity and context were confirmed. By preventing unwanted access and data breaches, the model improved the center's security posture [74].
4. To detect and prioritize cybersecurity concerns in 2022, a hospital network in New York employed cloud-based technology that combined data from several sources and applied AI. In just six months, the network was able to minimize its vulnerability exposure by 75% thanks to the platform [73].
5. A complete cybersecurity program comprising policies and procedures, security controls, security training, and incident response plans was put into place by a Florida hospital in 2023. In only a single year, the program assisted the hospital in lowering its cyber risk score by 64% [75].

In conclusion, risk mitigation strategies for healthcare organizations are essential to safeguard their data and systems from cyberattacks. By implementing effective policies and procedures and security controls, healthcare organizations can reduce their risk exposure and improve their security resilience.

18.6.3 Continuous risk management and adaptation

Healthcare organizations need to adopt effective risk mitigation strategies and best practices tailored to the healthcare industry. Risk mitigation strategies for healthcare are essential to safeguard data and systems from cyberattacks. By implementing robust access controls, regular security training and awareness programs, encryption of sensitive data, network monitoring, and incident response planning, healthcare organizations can reduce risk exposure and improve their security resilience.

1. **Implementing robust access controls:** Access controls are security measures that regulate who can access what data or systems and under what conditions. Access controls can include various methods, such as passwords, biometrics,

tokens, or certificates. Access controls should be based on the principle of least privilege, which means granting the minimum level of access necessary for each user or role. Access controls should also be enforced by policies and procedures that define the rules and responsibilities for granting, revoking, or changing access rights.

2. **Conducting regular security training and awareness programs**: Security training and awareness programs are educational activities that aim to increase the knowledge and skills of staff members regarding cybersecurity. Security training and awareness programs should cover topics such as security policies and procedures, common threats and vulnerabilities, best practices, and tips, or incident reporting and response. Security training and awareness programs should also be tailored to the specific needs and roles of different staff members, such as clinicians, administrators, or IT personnel.
3. **Encrypting sensitive data:** Encryption is a process that transforms data into an unreadable form using a secret key. Encryption can protect data from unauthorized access or disclosure, both in transit and at rest. Encryption can be applied to various types of data, such as PHI, medical records, research data, or financial data. Encryption can also be implemented at different levels, such as file level, disk level, or network level.
4. **Monitoring network activity**: Network monitoring is a process that collects and analyzes data about the traffic and performance of a network. Network monitoring can help detect and prevent cyberattacks, such as malware infections, DoS attacks, or unauthorized access. Network monitoring can also help identify and resolve network issues, such as bottlenecks, errors, or failures. Network monitoring can use various tools and techniques, such as firewalls, IDS, or log analysis.
5. **Planning for incident response:** Incident response is a process that defines the actions and procedures to be taken in the event of a cybersecurity incident. Incident response can help minimize the impact and damage of cyberattacks, such as data loss, system downtime, or patient harm. Incident response can also help restore normal operations and prevent the recurrence of similar incidents. Incident response should include steps such as preparation, identification, containment, eradication, recovery, and lessons learned.

18.7 Case studies

Examples of cybersecurity problems in the healthcare industry are shown in this part. Three common types of incidents are covered: ransomware, malware, and data breaches; insider threats and staff carelessness are also included. In addition to highlighting the risks and vulnerabilities facing healthcare organizations in the digital age, it also describes the reasons, effects, and lessons learned from each occurrence. With the goal of improving the overall cybersecurity posture and resilience of healthcare organizations, the section also provides advice and best practices for preventing, identifying, and handling these occurrences.

18.7.1 Data breach incidents

Incidents involving data breaches entail the unapproved or illegal acquisition or revelation of private health information (PHI) or other confidential information. Such occurrences may result in severe repercussions for patients as well as healthcare institutions, such as monetary losses, harm to one's reputation, legal troubles, fines from authorities, identity theft, fraud, or extortion. The case studies of actual data breaches in the healthcare industry are examined below, with an emphasis on the methods used, the effects these breaches had on patients and organizations, and the lessons that could be drawn from them.

1. **Tricare data breach:** The September 2011 theft of backup tapes containing electronic health records resulted in a major data breach for Tricare, a healthcare program serving active-duty military personnel, their dependents, and retirees [76]. The backups were taken from the driver's automobile who oversaw moving the tapes from one location to another. Whether or not the thieves knew what they were taking is unknown, as is their level of expertise in deciphering the data on the tapes. The event was handled as a data breach because of necessity. Five million patients had their personal information compromised, including names, social security numbers, phone numbers, addresses, and medication information. A class-action lawsuit against Tricare and its contractor SAIC arose from the breach, and the case was resolved for $4.9 million in 2017 [77]. Tricare also reviewed and strengthened its security policies and procedures in response to the intrusion, limiting access to sensitive data and encrypting backup tapes following federal regulations [78].
2. **Community Health Systems data breach:** One of the biggest hospital chains in the United States, Community Health Systems (CHS), disclosed a data breach that happened in April and June of 2014 [79,80]. Cybercriminals thought to be based in China used highly sophisticated malware to take advantage of a software flaw, which allowed them to steal private patient information. Anyone who had treatment from a facility connected to the CHS network within the previous five years was affected by the event. 4.5 million patients' names, birth dates, Social Security numbers, phone numbers, and addresses were disclosed because of the hack [81]. CHS paid $100 million in legal fees and security measures because of the hack [82]. Federal authorities and state attorneys general launched many lawsuits and investigations. The hack also made CHS improve its security protocols, including network segmentation, software vulnerability patches, and security audits [83].
3. **Eskenazi Health data breach:** The Indiana-based public health institution, Eskenazi Health, revealed a data breach that happened between January and May of 2021 [84–86]. By taking advantage of a flaw in the system of a third-party software vendor, cybercriminals were able to access their network for over three months. Some files with patient and personnel data were accessible to and exfiltrated by the hackers. A total of 1.5 million people had their personal information compromised due to the breach, including names, dates of birth, Social Security numbers, driver's license numbers, patient account

numbers, numbers from medical records, information about treatments received, health insurance, and financial accounts [87]. A class-action lawsuit alleging negligence and privacy law violations was filed against Eskenazi Health because of the incident. Eskenazi Health also informed the impacted parties and provided free credit monitoring and identity protection services. Additionally, Eskenazi Health said that it was collaborating with its outside partners to guarantee the security of its systems.

18.7.2 Malware attacks and ransomware

Ransomware events and malware attacks are terms used to describe malicious software programs that harm or infect networks or machines. The regular operation of healthcare systems, such as electronic health records (EHRs), medical equipment, or telemedicine platforms, may be interfered with by these incidents. They could lead to ransom demands in exchange for decryption or restoration, jeopardize system security or performance, or result in data theft or destruction. The following discusses case studies of ransomware and malware occurrences in the healthcare industry.

1. **WannaCry ransomware attack:** A Windows operating system vulnerability was disclosed by a hacker collective known as the Shadow Brokers, and this vulnerability was leveraged by the worldwide ransomware assault known as WannaCry in May 2017 [88]. The files on compromised machines were encrypted by this attack and their decryption cost between $300 and $600 in Bitcoin. The NHS in the UK was one of the most badly impacted institutions, with over 200,000 computers across 150 nations being impacted. About 19,000 appointments had to be canceled, ambulances had to be rerouted, and some services had to be suspended by the NHS. The NHS spent an estimated £92 million on IT expenses and lost productivity because of the hack. As a result of the event, the NHS strengthened its cybersecurity protocols, which now include patching software vulnerabilities, upgrading operating systems, and funding security awareness and training programs.
2. **Universal Health Services ransomware attack:** In September 2020, a ransomware assault happened to Universal Health Services (UHS). One of the biggest hospital groups in the United States, UHS has more than 400 locations nationwide [89]. The attack was directed at its IT systems. On the compromised systems, the attack encrypts the files and presents a ransom notice on the screens. UHS was compelled by the attack to go into offline mode and shut down its IT systems. Due to the need for workers to use phones, fax machines, and paper records, the attack interfered with patient care and operations. Some patients had to wait longer for treatment or be sent to different clinics. UHS suffered an estimated $67 million in missed income and recovery costs because of the attack. The incident also prompted UHS to strengthen its security protocols, including network segmentation, backup restoration, and security assessments.

3. **Scripps Health ransomware attack:** In May 2021, a ransomware attack was launched on Scripps Health. The California-based nonprofit health organization Scripps Health, which operates four hospitals and numerous outpatient clinics, was impacted by the attack on its IT infrastructure [90]. The hack requested an undisclosed fee to unlock the encrypted contents on the infected PCs. Due to the attack, Scripps Health was obliged to halt some services and take down its IT systems. Due to the need for staff to utilize manual processes, reschedule appointments and procedures, and alert patients of potential data breaches, the attack had an impact on patient care and privacy. The attack resulted in undetermined revenue losses and recovery expenses for Scripps Health. Additionally, Scripps Health informed the impacted parties and provided them with free identity protection and credit monitoring services. Additionally, Scripps Health announced that it was collaborating with law enforcement and cybersecurity specialists to investigate and address the situation.

18.7.3 Insider threats and employee negligence

Insider threats and employee carelessness are two major cybersecurity concerns in the healthcare industry that could jeopardize the availability, confidentiality, and integrity of sensitive data and systems. These dangers could result from carelessness, incompetence, malevolent intent, or outside factors. The following case studies from healthcare organizations will be examined to shed light on situations in which workers violated cybersecurity whether intentionally or unintentionally resulting in breaches or vulnerabilities:

1. **Anthem data breach:** An important data breach occurred at Anthem, one of the biggest health insurance providers in the United States, between December 2014 and January 2015. A phishing campaign that targeted Anthem employees and persuaded them to download infected attachments or click on dangerous links was the first step in this attack. The attackers obtained the login credentials of a minimum of five Anthem staff members, including a system administrator, through the phishing campaign. With these credentials, the attackers gained access to Anthem's database and took out about 78.8 million people's data [91]. Due to the incident, Anthem improved its cybersecurity protocols, adding two-factor authentication, encrypting data while it was in transit and at rest, and putting security awareness training into place.
2. **Allina Health insider theft:** A Minnesota-based nonprofit health system called Allina Health has revealed that it was the victim of an insider theft that took place from February 2019 to June 2020 [92]. In the event, a worker gained unauthorized access to around 3,800 individuals' medical records without a legitimate business requirement. The staff member examined the names, birth dates, medical record numbers, insurance details, and clinical data of the patients. Additionally, the worker took roughly 160 patients' Social Security numbers and used them to file false tax forms. The internal audit staff at Allina Health found the occurrence and notified law enforcement. The worker was fired and taken into custody. Due to this occurrence, Allina Health was the

target of a class-action lawsuit alleging negligence and privacy law violations. Allina Health also informed the impacted patients and provided them with free credit monitoring and identity protection services because of the event. Additionally, Allina Health announced that it was improving its monitoring and security controls.

3. **University of Vermont Medical Center ransomware attack:** The University of Vermont Medical Center (UVMMC), a teaching hospital affiliated with the University of Vermont, was a victim of a ransomware attack that occurred in October 2020 [93]. The attack was caused by an employee who opened an email attachment that contained malicious code. The attachment launched a ransomware program that encrypted the files on the affected systems and demanded $5.5 million for their decryption. The attack affected more than 5,000 computers and disrupted patient care and operations for several weeks. Staff had to use paper records, fax machines, and phones. Some patients had to be diverted to other facilities or rescheduled for appointments and procedures. The attack cost UVMMC an estimated $63 million in lost revenue and recovery expenses. The attack also forced UVMMC to restore its systems from backups and enhance its security measures, such as updating antivirus software, blocking suspicious email domains, and conducting security awareness training [94].

These case studies illustrate the common causes and consequences of insider threats and employee negligence in healthcare. They also highlight the importance of implementing effective security measures and practices to prevent or mitigate such incidents. Some of these measures and practices include:

(i) Encrypting sensitive data both in transit and at rest.
(ii) Patching software vulnerabilities promptly.
(iii) Implementing robust access controls based on the principle of least privilege.
(iv) Conducting regular security training and awareness programs for staff members.
(v) Monitoring network activity for signs of intrusion or anomaly.
(vi) Planning for incident response and recovery.
(vii) Reviewing and updating security policies and procedures.
(viii) Evaluating and verifying the security of third-party vendors.

18.8 Future trends

The changing trends and difficulties in healthcare cybersecurity are covered in detail in this section. It starts by looking at recent and upcoming advancements in telemedicine, AI [95], digital transformation, and the Internet of Medical Things [96], and evaluating how this affects cybersecurity. The conversation then focuses on developments in threat prevention and response, including fresh approaches, frameworks, and instruments to improve the security and adaptability of healthcare institutions. Ultimately, it highlights the necessity of a comprehensive, cooperative, and proactive approach to healthcare cybersecurity and summarizes the main lessons learned, drawing the chapter to a close. Additionally, the section offers suggestions and best practices to improve the healthcare industry's cybersecurity preparedness and posture.

18.8.1 Emerging trends in healthcare

The increasing incidents of cyberattacks on healthcare systems in recent years underscore the importance of healthcare cybersecurity as a critical issue. Some of the latest and noteworthy developments in healthcare cybersecurity are explored here.

1. **AI and machine learning for threat detection:** Healthcare is using AI and machine learning more and more to identify and stop cyberattacks. These tools can examine vast volumes of data and spot trends that can point to a possible danger. They can also adjust to new threats and learn from previous attacks, which increases their efficacy in identifying and stopping intrusions.
2. **Impact of IoT devices in healthcare:** IoT device usage in the medical field has grown dramatically in the last several years. These gadgets can lower expenses, enhance patient outcomes, and enable remote patient monitoring for healthcare practitioners. They do, meanwhile, also present serious cybersecurity dangers. IoT devices are susceptible to hacks since security is frequently not considered in their design. To safeguard IoT devices from cyberattacks, strong security protocols must be developed as their use grows.
3. **Advancements in encryption and data protection**: Data security and encryption are essential elements of healthcare cybersecurity. Thanks to developments in encryption technology, private patient information may now be shielded from online attacks. Patient data may be kept private and safe by using encryption to help prevent unwanted access.
4. **Evolving regulations and compliance standards:** Healthcare cybersecurity laws and compliance requirements are always changing to stay up with the ever-evolving threat landscape. To guarantee that healthcare organizations are sufficiently safeguarding patient data from cyber risks, compliance with these criteria is necessary. A few of the most important laws and guidelines include HITECH, GDPR, and HIPAA.

The future of cybersecurity in healthcare is being shaped by these factors. To safeguard patient data from cyber-attacks, healthcare institutions must establish strong cybersecurity procedures as they become increasingly technologically integrated and interconnected. Healthcare organizations can guarantee that patient data is secure and private by utilizing AI and machine learning for threat detection, creating strong security protocols for IoT devices, improving encryption and data protection, and adhering to changing legal requirements and compliance standards.

18.8.2 Innovation in threat prevention and response

Novel techniques and cutting-edge tools are being created to stop and address cyberattacks in the healthcare industry. The following are a few recent developments:

1. **Threat intelligence:** This entails identifying and analyzing possible cyber threats using machine learning algorithms and sophisticated analytics. Healthcare companies can keep ahead of new risks and take proactive steps to stop them from harming by utilizing this technology.
2. **Proactive security measures:** These consist of a variety of tactics and equipment intended to stop cyberattacks before they start. Firewalls, IDS, and access controls are a few examples. Healthcare organizations may lower their chance of becoming a target for cybercriminals by putting these precautions into place.
3. **Automated incident response systems:** Real-time cyberattack detection and response is built into these systems. They can lessen the harm that a breach causes by assisting healthcare organizations in promptly identifying and containing risks.
4. **Cyber security awareness training:** This is a crucial part of any successful cybersecurity plan. Healthcare companies may foster a culture of security that helps ward off assaults by teaching staff members about the dangers of cyber threats and how to avoid them.

With these developments, healthcare organizations are proactively tackling cyber risks and safeguarding sensitive patient data. By utilizing cutting-edge technology and following the industry's best practices, healthcare providers can make sure they are ready to stop and respond to cyberattacks.

The key elements of innovation in danger prevention and response in the healthcare sector are shown in Figure 18.3. The arrows represent the information flow and mutual effect between these elements, which together improve healthcare organizations' overall cybersecurity posture. It is noteworthy that in real-world circumstances, the actual implementation and linkages could be more complex.

It is obvious that cybersecurity will be important in the healthcare sector going ahead. The sophistication of cyberattacks will increase in tandem with technological advancements. To safeguard patient data and guarantee the security of their systems, healthcare organizations need to continue being watchful and proactive. Healthcare organizations may assist with defending against cyber threats and protect the health and well-being of their patients by putting the best practices into practice and keeping up to speed with the newest security technology.

18.8.3 Lessons learned from the study

The legal and regulatory environment that affects cybersecurity and information assurance in developing healthcare systems is examined in depth in this chapter. Its main objectives are to analyze the current state of cybersecurity laws and regulations in the healthcare industry, identify any gaps or difficulties in the current legal frameworks, and provide best practices and recommendations for improving cybersecurity governance and compliance in the healthcare industry.

In order to gather and examine data from a variety of sources and viewpoints, the study employed a mixed-methods strategy that included surveys, case studies,

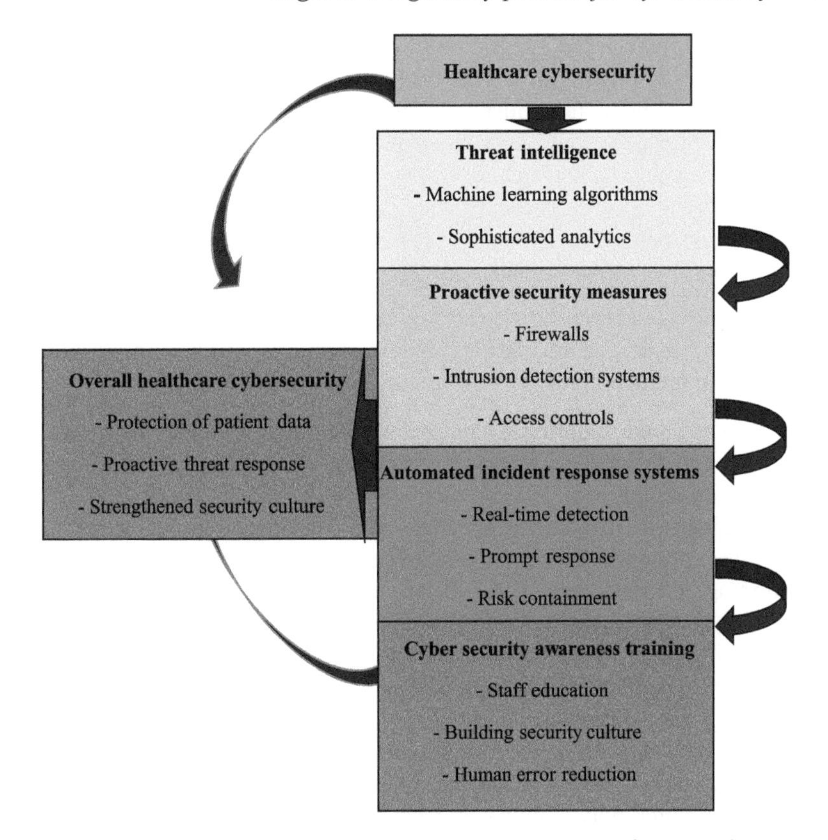

Figure 18.3 Integrated healthcare cybersecurity framework

interviews, and literature reviews. Aspects of cybersecurity and information assurance in the healthcare industry, including data protection, privacy, confidentiality, integrity, availability, accountability, and resilience, have all been covered in the research.

The results of the study show that the cybersecurity environment facing the healthcare industry is dynamic and complicated, with a wide range of threats and vulnerabilities that might seriously jeopardize the safety and quality of healthcare services. Additionally, the study has demonstrated that the legal and regulatory framework governing the healthcare industry is varied and dispersed, with several rules and regulations at various levels and jurisdictions that are applicable to various players and activities within the healthcare ecosystem. The research has shown several obstacles and deficiencies in the existing legal and regulatory structures, including:

1. Lack of harmonization and coordination among different laws and regulations.
2. Lack of clarity and consistency in the definitions and scope of cybersecurity and information assurance concepts and terms.

3. Lack of alignment and integration of cybersecurity and information assurance objectives and requirements with other healthcare goals and standards.
4. Lack of awareness and understanding of the legal and regulatory obligations and implications among the healthcare stakeholders.
5. Lack of capacity and resources to implement and enforce the legal and regulatory measures and mechanisms.
6. Lack of incentives and sanctions to motivate and deter the compliance and non-compliance behaviors of healthcare stakeholders.

Additionally, the report offers several best practices and recommendations for enhancing the legal and regulatory frameworks pertaining to cybersecurity and information assurance in the healthcare industry, including:

1. Developing and adopting a comprehensive and coherent cybersecurity and information assurance framework that covers all aspects and dimensions of the healthcare sector.
2. Enhancing and harmonizing the legal and regulatory definitions and scope of cybersecurity and information assurance concepts and terms.
3. Aligning and integrating the cybersecurity and information assurance objectives and requirements with other healthcare goals and standards.
4. Increasing the awareness and understanding of the legal and regulatory obligations and implications among the healthcare stakeholders.
5. Building and strengthening the capacity and resources to implement and enforce the legal and regulatory measures and mechanisms.
6. Creating and applying incentives and sanctions to motivate and deter the compliance and non-compliance behaviors of healthcare stakeholders.

By offering a thorough and methodical examination of the legal and regulatory laws and their effects on the security and caliber of healthcare services, the research has advanced our understanding of cybersecurity and information assurance in the industry. Additionally, the report has provided some useful recommendations and principles for improving cybersecurity governance and compliance in the healthcare industry. The study aims to stimulate and guide more investigation and action on this significant and relevant subject.

18.9 Conclusion

The legal and regulatory frameworks for information assurance and cybersecurity in developing healthcare systems have been covered in this chapter. The chapter emphasized the difficulties and shortcomings in the present legal and regulatory frameworks, as well as the significance and complexity of cybersecurity in the healthcare industry. Additionally, the chapter offers some best practices and suggestions for enhancing cybersecurity governance and compliance in the healthcare industry. These were developed using a mixed-methods study that included case studies, interviews, questionnaires, and literature analysis. By providing a thorough and methodical study of the legal and regulatory laws and their effects on the security and caliber of healthcare services, the chapter has advanced knowledge and practice in cybersecurity and information assurance in the healthcare industry. Additionally, the chapter offers several recommendations for future study and action on this subject, including:

1. Conducting more empirical studies to evaluate the effectiveness and efficiency of the legal and regulatory measures and mechanisms in the healthcare sector
2. Developing and testing new models and tools for cybersecurity and information assurance assessment and management in the healthcare sector
3. Exploring and addressing the ethical and social implications of cybersecurity and information assurance in the healthcare sector
4. Fostering and facilitating the collaboration and coordination among the healthcare stakeholders and other sectors on cybersecurity and information assurance issues and initiatives

Information assurance and cybersecurity are vital, ever-changing components of the healthcare industry that demand ongoing development and attention. The healthcare industry may improve its cybersecurity posture and performance by embracing and putting into practice the suggestions and best practices offered in this chapter. This will eventually allow it to provide the public and its clients with more secure, dependable, and trustworthy healthcare services.

References

[1] Y. Bk, "Overview of cyber security," *International Journal of Advanced Research in Science, Communication and Technology*, pp. 489–492, 22 2022.
[2] K. A. Ali and S. Alyounis, "Cybersecurity in healthcare industry," in *2021 International Conference on Information Technology (ICIT)*, Amman, Jordan, 2021.
[3] K. Saleem, Z. Tan and W. J. Buchanan, *Security for Cyber-Physical Systems in Healthcare*, Springer eBooks, pp. 233–251, 2017.
[4] M. I. Khan, M. Nadeem, M. Kaleem and S. Nazir, "Blockchain based secure data management for healthcare applications," in *2023 International Conference on Communication, Computing and Digital Systems (C-CODE)*, Islamabad, Pakistan, 2023.
[5] A. Pawlicka, M. Choraś and M. Pawlicki, "Cyberspace threats: not only hackers and criminals. Raising the awareness of selected unusual cyberspace actors – cybersecurity researchers' perspective," in *Proceedings of the 15th International Conference on Availability, Reliability and Security*, 2020.
[6] G. Béla, G. Flavius and H. Piroska, "Experimental assessment of network design approaches for protecting industrial control systems," *International Journal of Critical Infrastructure Protection*, vol. 11, pp. 24–38, 2015.
[7] P. A. S. Ralston, J. H. Graham and J. L. Hieb, "Cyber security risk assessment for SCADA and DCS networks," *ISA Transactions*, vol. 46, no. 4, pp. 583–594, 2007.
[8] J. David, "Confidentiality and security of information," *Anaesthesia & Intensive Care Medicine*, vol. 5, no. 12, pp. 404–406, 2004.

[9] H. Keysley and C. Rodney, "Information integrity: Are we there yet?," *ACM Computing Surveys*, vol. 54, no. 2, pp. 1–35, 2021.

[10] J. Pennekamp, R. Matzutt, C. Klinkmüller, *et al.*, "An Interdisciplinary survey on information flows in supply chains," *ACM Computing Surveys*, vol. 56, no. 2, pp. 1–38, 2023.

[11] J. L. Ferrer-Gomilla, J. A. Onieva, M. Payeras and J. López, "Certified electronic mail: Properties revisited," *Computers & Security*, vol. 29, no. 2, pp. 167–179, 2010.

[12] A. A. Garba, A. M. Bade, M. Yahuza and Y. Nuhu, "Cybersecurity capability maturity models review and application domain," *International Journal of Engineering & Technology*, vol. 9, no. 3, p. 779, 2020.

[13] R. Hill, *Best Practices in Cybersecurity from Intergovernmental Discussions and a Private Sector Proposal*, Springer eBooks, pp. 253–259, 2018.

[14] N. Shingari, S. Verma, B. Mago and M. S. Javeid, "A review of cybersecurity challenges and recommendations in the healthcare sector," *023 International Conference on Business Analytics for Technology and Security (ICBATS)*, pp. 1–8, 2023.

[15] I. H. Sarker, H. Furhad and R. Nowrozy, "AI-driven cybersecurity: An overview, security intelligence modeling and research directions," *SN Computer Science*, vol. 2, p. 3, 2021.

[16] "CSO – The Role of Artificial Intelligence in IoT and OT Security," [Online]. Available: https://www.csoonline.com/article/566503/the-role-of-artificial-intelligence-in-iot-and-ot-security.html.

[17] E. Segal, "AltexSoft – AI Applications in Cybersecurity with Real-Life Examples," *AltexSoft*, 2 June 2020. [Online]. Available: https://www.altexsoft.com/blog/ai-cybersecurity/.

[18] A.-A. O. Affia, H. Finch, W. Jung, I. A. Samori, L. Potter and X.-L. Palmer, "IoT health devices: Exploring security risks in the connected landscape," *IoT*, vol. 4, no. 2, pp. 150–182, 2023.

[19] "Medcrypt – The Future of Medical Devices Is Secure by Design," [Online]. Available: https://www.medcrypt.com.

[20] C. RAY, "ARMIS – Armis Wins 2024 Frost & Sullivan Customer Value Leadership Award for OT Cybersecurity Solutions," 2024. [Online]. Available: https://www.medcrypt.com.

[21] "ZingBox," [Online]. Available: https://theinternetofthings.report/Resources/Whitepapers/24333da0-6ee3-402c-993e-5503f09c05ec_ZingBox_WP_IoT-Guardian-for-the-Healthcare-Industry.pdf.

[22] M. Ali, S. U. Khan and A. V. Vasilakos, "Security in cloud computing: Opportunities and challenges," *Information Sciences*, vol. 305, pp. 357–283, 2015.

[23] "AWS – AWS for Healthcare & Life Sciences," [Online]. Available: https://aws.amazon.com/health/.

[24] "Microsoft – Microsoft Cloud for Healthcare," [Online]. Available: https://www.microsoft.com/en-us/industry/health/microsoft-cloud-for-healthcare?rtc=1.

[25] G. Cloud, "Google Cloud Whitepaper – Protecting Healthcare Data on Google Cloud," *Google*, 2023. [Online]. Available: https://services.google.com/fh/files/misc/protecting_healthcare_data_on_google_cloud_wp.pdf.

[26] B. S. Rawat, D. Gangodkar, V. Talukdar, K. Saxena, C. Kaur and S. P. Singh, "The Empirical Analysis of Artificial Intelligence Approaches for Enhancing the Cyber Security for Better Quality," *2022 5th International Conference on Contemporary Computing and Informatics (IC3I)*, pp. 247–250, 2022.

[27] D. D. D. Alionsi, "AI-driven cybersecurity: Utilizing machine learning and deep learning techniques for real-time threat detection, analysis, and mitigation in complex IT networks," *Advances in Engineering Innovation*, vol. 3, pp. 27–31, 2023.

[28] S. Andropov, A. Guirik, M. Budko and M. Budko, "Network anomaly detection using artificial neural networks," in *2017 20th Conference of Open Innovations Association (FRUCT)*, St. Petersburg, Russia, 2017.

[29] K. Ghazinour and M. Ghayoumi, "An autonomous model to enforce security policies based on user's behavior," in *2015 IEEE/ACIS 14th International Conference on Computer and Information Science (ICIS)*, Las Vegas, NV, USA, 2015.

[30] F. Meneghello, M. Calore, D. Zucchetto, M. Polese and A. Zanella, "IoT: Internet of Threats? A survey of practical security vulnerabilities in real IoT devices," *IEEE Internet of Things Journal*, vol. 6, no. 5, pp. 8182–8201, 2019.

[31] A. Echeverría, C. Cevallos, I. Ortiz-Garcés and R. Andrade, "Cybersecurity model based on hardening for secure internet of things implementation," *Applied Sciences*, vol. 11, no. 7, p. 3260, 2021.

[32] R. Sikka and M. K. Ojha, "An overview of cloud computing," *International Journal of Innovative Research in Computer Science & Technology*, vol. 9, no. 6, pp. 135–138, 2021.

[33] F. S. Al-Anzi, S. K. Yadav and J. Soni, "Cloud computing: Security model comprising governance, risk management and compliance," 2014.

[34] M. H. L. Louk, H. Lim and H. J. Lee, "Security system for healthcare data in cloud computing," *International Journal of Security and Its Applications*, vol. 8, no. 3, pp. 241–248, 2014.

[35] N. Wickramasinghe, S. Chalasani, R. V. Boppana and A. Madni, "Healthcare system of systems," in *2007 IEEE International Conference on System of Systems Engineering*, San Antonio, TX, USA, 2007.

[36] S. K. Rajamani and R. S. Iyer, "Networks in healthcare: A systematic review," *BioMedInformatics*, vol. 3, no. 2, pp. 391–404, 2023.

[37] S. B. "The roots of ancient medicine: an historical outline," *Journal of Biosciences*, vol. 26, no. 2, pp. 135–143, 2001.

[38] Y. Tountas, "The historical origins of the basic concepts of health promotion and education: the role of ancient Greek philosophy and medicine," *Health Promotion International*, vol. 24, no. 2, pp. 185–192, 2009.

[39] A. Polte, S. Haunss, A. Schmid, G. de Carvalho and H. Rothgang, "The emergence of healthcare systems," in M. Windzio, I. Mossig, F. Besche-Truthe, and H. Seitzer (eds.), *Networks and Geographies of Global Social Policy Diffusion*, Cham: Palgrave Macmillan, 2022.

[40] E. J. Pérez-Stable, B. Jean-Francois and C. F. Aklin, “Leveraging advances in technology to promote health equity,” *Medical Care*, vol. 57, no. Suppl 2, pp. S101–S103, 2019.
[41] M. LeBlanc, S. Petrie, S. Paskaran, D. B. Carson and P. A. Peters, “Patient and provider perspectives on eHealth interventions in Canada and Australia: A scoping review,” *Rural and Remote Health*, vol. 20, no. 3, p. 5754, 2020.
[42] M. &. L. M. Spruit, “Applied data science in patient-centric healthcare: Adaptive analytic systems for empowering physicians and patients,” *Telematics and Informatics*, vol. 35, no. 4, pp. 643–653, 2018.
[43] Z. Arnob, J. K. Poulsen, R. Sharma and S. C. Wingreen, “A systematic review of emerging information technologies for sustainable data-centric health-care,” *International Journal of Medical Informatics*, vol. 149, p. 104420, 2021.
[44] M. D. Bergren, “Data governance and stewardship,” *NASN School Nurse*, vol. 34, no. 3, pp. 149–151, 2019.
[45] A. Musa, A. Abdulfatai, D. Oluyemi, S. Jacob and A. L. Imoize, “Legal frameworks for artificial intelligence and blockchain technology in telehealth systems,” in *Artificial Intelligence and Blockchain Technology in Modern Telehealth Systems*, London, United Kingdom, The Institution of Engineering and Technology, pp. 441–470, 2023.
[46] A. Musa, “Legal frameworks for security schemes in wireless communication systems,” in *Security and Privacy Schemes for Dense 6G Wireless Communication Networks*, London, United Kingdom, The Institution of Engineering and Technology, pp. 423–444, 2023.
[47] N. Shingari, S. Verma, B. Mago and M. S. Javeid, “A review of cybersecurity challenges and recommendations in the healthcare sector,” in *2023 International Conference on Business Analytics for Technology and Security (ICBATS)*, pp. 1–8, 2023.
[48] D. Lindgren, “Framework for assessing compliance,” in *An Assessment Framework for Compliance with International Space Law and Norms, Southern Space Studies*. Cham: Springer, 2020.
[49] M. Puppala, T. He, X. Yu, S. Chen, R. Ogunti and S. T. C. Wong, “Data security and privacy management in healthcare applications and clinical data warehouse environment,” in *2016 IEEE-EMBS International Conference on Biomedical and Health Informatics (BHI)*, pp. 5–8, 2016.
[50] M. B. Buntin, S. H. Jain and D. Blumenthal, “Health information technology: laying the infrastructure for national health reform,” *Health Affairs*, vol. 29, no. 6, pp. 1214–1219, 2010.
[51] F. Akowuah, Y. Xioahong, J. Xu and W. Hong, “A survey of U.S. laws for health information security and privacy,” *International Journal of Information Security and Privacy*, vol. 6, no. 4, pp. 40–54, 2012.
[52] “Health Care Reform In the United States: HITECH Act and HIPAA Privacy, Security, and Enforcement Issues[dagger] – ProQuest,” [Online]. Available: https://www.proquest.com/openview/deb9bbf0d095e69b6927ef308271f0b9/1?pq-origsite=gscholar&cbl=8980.

[53] "An Official Website of the United States Government," HHS 405(d) – Aligning Health Care Industry Security Approaches, 2023. [Online]. Available: https://405d.hhs.gov/about.

[54] E. Salami, "An Analysis of the General Data Protection Regulation (EU) 2016/679," *Social Science Research Network*, 2017.

[55] C. Kuner, L. A. Bygrave and C. Docksey, *Background and Evolution of the EU General Data Protection Regulation (GDPR),* Oxford University Press eBooks, 2020.

[56] T. D. Nguyen, "An Empirical Evaluation of the Implementation of the California Consumer Privacy Act (CCPA)," *arXiv* (*Cornell University*), 19 May 2022.

[57] M. Bodie, "HIPPA," *Social Science Research Network*, 2021.

[58] Cookieyes, "Cookieyes – Singapore's Personal Data Protection Act (PDPA)," 2023. [Online]. Available: https://www.cookieyes.com/blog/singapore-pdpa/.

[59] O. D. Guidance, "Data Guidance," 2023. [Online]. Available: https://www.dataguidance.com/notes/singapore-data-protection-overview#:~:text=26%20of%202012)%20(%27PDPA,that%20a%20reasonable%20person%20 would.

[60] A. Hoxhaj, "The CJEU Validates in C-156/21 and C-157/21 the Rule of Law Conditionality Regulation Regime to Protect the EU Budget," *Nordic Journal of European Law*, vol. 5, no. 1, pp. 131–144, 2016.

[61] S. Blanke and E. McGrady, "When it comes to securing patient health information from breaches, your best medicine is a dose of prevention: A cybersecurity risk assessment checklist," *Journal of Healthcare Risk Management*, vol. 36, no. 1, pp. 14–24, 2016.

[62] M. Huo, M. Bland and K. Levchenko, "All eyes on me: inside third party trackers exfiltration of phi from healthcare providers online systems," in *WPES 2022 – Proceedings of the 21st Workshop on Privacy in the Electronic Society, co-located with CCS 2022*, pp. 197–211, 2022.

[63] P. Kalina, "Ethical and legal manifestations of informed consent," *Technium Social Sciences Journal*, vol. 8, pp. 753–758, 2020.

[64] M. Abdulraheem, E. A. Adeniyi, J. Awotunde, *et al.*, *Artificial Intelligence of Medical Things for Medical Information Systems Privacy and Security*, CRC Press, pp. 63–96, 2024.

[65] J. Awotunde, A. Imoize, R. Jimoh, *et al.*, "AIoMT enabling real-time monitoring of healthcare systems: Security and privacy considerations," *Handbook of Security and Privacy of AI-Enabled Healthcare Systems and Internet of Medical Things*, CRC Press, pp. 97–133, 2024.

[66] M. Van Devender and J. T. McDonald, "A quantitative risk assessment framework for the cybersecurity of networked medical devices," *Proceedings of the International Conference on Information Warfare and Security*, vol. 18, no. 1, pp. 402–411, 2023.

[67] R. Luna, E. Rhine, M. Myhra, R. Sullivan and C. S. Kruse, "Cyber threats to health information systems: A systematic review," *Technology and Health Care*, vol. 24, no. 1, pp. 1–9, 2016.

[68] A. G. Alzahrani, A. Ahmed and G. Wills, "A framework of the critical factors for healthcare providers to share data securely using blockchain," *IEEE Access*, vol. 10, pp. 41064–41077, 2022.

[69] S. Shenai and M. Aramudhan, "Cloud computing framework to securely share health and medical records among federations of healthcare information systems," *Biomedical Research-Tokyo*, vol. 29, pp. 133–136, 2018.

[70] M. T. Kwong, D. Stell and E. Akinluyi, "Medical device regulation from a health service provider's perspective," *Prosthesis*, vol. 3, no. 3, pp. 261–266, 2021.

[71] "Neumetric," 2 October 2023. [Online]. Available: https://www.neumetric.com/types-of-cybersecurity-measures/.

[72] S. J. Choi and M. E. Johnson, "The relationship between cybersecurity ratings and the risk of hospital data breaches," *Journal of the American Medical Informatics Association*, vol. 28, no. 10, pp. 2085–2092, 2021.

[73] S. S. Gopalan, A. Raza and W. Almobaideen, "IoT security in healthcare using AI: A survey," in *2020 International Conference on Communications, Signal Processing, and their Applications (ICCSPA)*, pp. 1–6, 2021.

[74] K. Abu Ali and S. Alyounis, "CyberSecurity in healthcare industry," in *2021 International Conference on Information Technology (ICIT)*, pp. 695–701, 2021.

[75] T. Fezzey, J. Batchelor, G. Burch and R. Reid, "Cybersecurity continuity risks: Lessons learned from the COVID-19 pandemic," *Journal of Cybersecurity Education Research and Practice*, vol. 2022, no. 2, 2023.

[76] J. Reddy, N. Elsayed, Z. ElSayed and M. Özer, "A review on data breaches in healthcare security systems," *International Journal of Computer Applications*, vol. 184, no. 45, pp. 1–7, 2023.

[77] O. Dyer, "Teva pays $54M to settle claims it paid doctors kickbacks to prescribe its drugs," *BMJ*, vol. 368, p. 53, 2020.

[78] K. Chatterjee, "A secure three factor-based authentication scheme for telecare medicine information systems with privacy preservation," *International Journal of Information Security and Privacy*, vol. 16, no. 1, pp. 1–24, 2022.

[79] M. Chernyshev, S. Zeadally and Z. A. Baig, "Healthcare data breaches: Implications for digital forensic readiness," *Journal of Medical Systems*, vol. 43, no. 1, 2018.

[80] J. Reddy, N. Elsayed, Z. ElSayed and M. Özer, "A review on data breaches in healthcare security systems," *International Journal of Computer Applications*, vol. 184, no. 45, 2023.

[81] W. W. Koczkodaj, J. Masiak, M. Mazurek, D. Strzałka and P. F. Zabrodskii, "Massive health record breaches evidenced by the Office for Civil Rights Data," *Iranian Journal of Public Health*, vol. 48, no. 2, pp. 278–288, 2019.

[82] J. Lenzer, "Hackers demand $10m for eight million medical records they are holding "hostage"," *The BMJ*, vol. 338, no. 1, p. b1917, 2009.

[83] C. Provost, E. Dishman and N. Paul, "Monitoring corporate compliance through cooperative federalism: Trends in multistate settlements by State Attorneys General," *Publius: The Journal of Federalism*, vol. 52, no. 3, pp. 497–522, 2022.

[84] S. J. C. a. A. M. M. Alkinoon, "Measuring healthcare data breaches," *Lecture Notes in Computer Science*, pp. 265–277, 2021.
[85] S. T. D. C. L. a. S. B. B. M. Gibson, "Vulnerability in massive API scraping: 2021 LinkedIn data breach," *2021 International Conference on Computational Science and Computational Intelligence (CSCI)*, 1 December 2021.
[86] "A systematic review of 2021 Microsoft Exchange data breach exploiting multiple vulnerabilities," *2022 7th International Conference on Smart and Sustainable Technologies (SpliTech)*, 5 July 2022.
[87] J. Jiang and G. Bai, "Types of information compromised in breaches of protected health information," *Annals of Internal Medicine*, vol. 172, no. 2, p. 159, 2019.
[88] S. Gaitond and R. Patil, "Leveraging machine learning algorithms for zero-day ransomware attack," *International Journal of Engineering and Advanced Technology*, vol. 8, no. 6, pp. 4104–4107, 2019.
[89] M. Abusaqer, M. B. Senouci and K. Magel, "Twitter user sentiments analysis: Health system cyberattacks case study," in *2023 International Conference on Artificial Intelligence in Information and Communication (ICAIIC)*, pp. 18–24, 2023.
[90] L. Van Boven, R. W. J. Kusters, D. Tin, *et al.*, "Hacking acute care: A qualitative study on the healthcare impacts of ransomware attacks against hospitals," *medRxiv (Cold Spring Harbor Laboratory)*, 2023.
[91] D. Kolevski, K. Michael, R. Abbas and M. Freeman, "Cloud computing data breaches: A review of U.S. regulation and data breach notification literature," in *2021 IEEE International Symposium on Technology and Society (ISTAS)*, pp. 1–7, 2021.
[92] A. S. Al-Harrasi, A. K. Shaikh and A. H. Al-Badi, "Towards protecting organisations' data by preventing data theft by malicious insiders," *The International Journal of Organizational Analysis*, vol. 31, no. 3, pp. 875–888, 2021.
[93] S. Ades, D. Herrera, T. Lahey, *et al.*, "Cancer care in the wake of a cyberattack: How to prepare and what to expect," *JCO Oncology Practice*, vol. 18, no. 1, pp. 23–34, 2022.
[94] R. S. Hallyburton, Q. Zhang, Z. M. Mao and M. Pajić, "Partial-information, longitudinal cyber attacks on LiDAR in autonomous vehicles," *arXiv (Cornell University)*, 2023.
[95] A. Edmund, C. Alabi, O. Tooki, A. Imoize and T. Salka, "Artificial intelligence-assisted Internet of Medical Things enabling medical image processing.," in *Handbook of Security and Privacy of AI-Enabled Healthcare Systems and Internet of Medical Things*, CRC Press, pp. 309–334, 2024.
[96] V. Iguoba and A. Imoize, "AIoMT training, testing, and validation.," in *Handbook of Security and Privacy of AI-Enabled Healthcare Systems and Internet of Medical Things*, CRC Press, pp. 394–410, 2024.

Chapter 19

Federated learning for enhanced cybersecurity in modern digital healthcare systems

Rufai Yusuf Zakari[1], Kassim Kalinaki[2,3], Zaharaddeen Karami Lawal[4,5] and Najib Abdulrazak[6]

Recent advancements in emerging technologies, like artificial intelligence (AI) and the Internet of Health Things (IoHT), have propelled a remarkable revolution in smart healthcare. However, traditional AI approaches that rely on centralized data collection and processing have proven impractical and unattainable in healthcare due to expanding network scale and escalating privacy concerns. Federated Learning (FL), an emerging distributed and collaborative technique, appears as a potential solution to address the security and privacy challenges associated with conventional AI. By enabling the training of machine learning (ML) models on decentralized data stored across diverse wearable devices, including fitness trackers, smartwatches, implantable devices, and other IoHT devices, FL facilitates the analysis and interpretation of data while upholding the security and privacy of the participating devices and raw data. Accordingly, this comprehensive study reviews the different FL techniques aimed at bolstering security and privacy in modern digital healthcare systems. Moreover, it highlights the benefits and challenges of FL in healthcare and presents future research trends aimed at enhancing the cybersecurity posture of FL in modern healthcare systems.

Keywords: Federated learning; artificial intelligence; electronic health records; digital healthcare systems; healthcare cybersecurity

[1]Department of Computer Science, School of Science, and Information Technology (SSIT), Skyline University, Nigeria
[2]Department of Computer Science, Islamic University in Uganda (IUIU), Uganda
[3]Department of Computer Science, Borderline Research Laboratory, Uganda
[4]Department of Computer Science, Federal University, Dutse, Nigeria
[5]Faculty of Integrated Technologies, Universiti Brunei Darussalam, Brunei
[6]Department of Computer Science, Bayero University, Kano, Nigeria

19.1 Introduction

Modern healthcare systems rely heavily on digital technologies and vast amounts of sensitive patient data. From electronic health records (EHRs) to connected healthcare devices through the IoHT and telemedicine platforms, healthcare organizations are generating and storing unprecedented amounts of health data. The IoHT encompasses a network of interconnected medical devices, software applications, and sensors, fostering seamless data exchanges and generating substantial EHR from diverse IoT devices [1,2]. This surge in data plays a pivotal role, enabling myriad analytical techniques to unveil valuable insights and enhance medical applications. Additionally, IoHT devices, including wearable gadgets, have evolved into indispensable health assistants, facilitating real-time health tracking, safety surveillance, rehabilitation monitoring, therapy outcome assessment, preemptive illness screening, and various other health metrics 3–5]. While this data enables innovations in preventive care and personalized medicine, healthcare systems stand as prime targets for cyber adversaries, who seek to steal patient data or disrupt vital care services via ransomware and comparable assaults. Recent years have seen major breaches at healthcare organizations, jeopardizing millions of patient records containing detailed medical histories, payment information, and more. As digital healthcare expands, so too do vulnerabilities that bad actors can exploit. This poses data privacy issues and significant patient safety threats if hackers can access connected medical devices and systems. Enhanced cybersecurity measures are essential.

Despite the promising advancements, the escalating data generation in IoHT raises concerns about data privacy and security [6–11]. Unauthorized access and manipulation of patient information pose significant threats to individual well-being. Compounding these challenges is the current reality of a data-driven world, where access to healthcare services often requires the voluntary surrender of personal information [12,13]. Traditional machine learning (ML) approaches to ensure healthcare data security and privacy have proven futile, mainly when valuable user data resides in a central server [14,15]. Centralized models pose challenges such as limited processing capacity, time constraints, and critical issues regarding the security and privacy of personal information [16,17]. As healthcare systems evolve toward decentralization, a collaborative and artificial intelligence (AI)-centered approach becomes imperative to address privacy concerns and ensure the scalability of intelligent healthcare systems.

Federated learning (FL) has emerged as a prominent solution, offering a decentralized data model to overcome these challenges and enhance ML model performance. Introduced in 2017, FL is a privacy-preserving and distributed ML approach that allows multiple stakeholders to train an ML model collaboratively without sharing raw data [18]. This innovative approach exchanges model parameters instead of raw data, fostering a client-server structure where the server coordinates the training process. This decentralized method has transformed ML in IoT systems, particularly healthcare, where data is generated from multiple devices with limited processing and storage capabilities [19]. FL's local training on individual devices significantly reduces the risks of data breaches, minimizes data transmission, and provides better control over data ownership [20]. It also enhances training efficiency by utilizing local IoHT devices' datasets and computational resources that may be inaccessible with a centralized approach.

FL has several potential applications in digital healthcare systems. One of the most promising applications is personalized medicine [21]. By leveraging data from various sources, including EHR and wearable devices, FL models can be trained to provide personalized patient treatment recommendations. This can help improve the effectiveness of treatments while minimizing side effects and reducing costs. Another application of FL in digital healthcare is clinical decision support [22]. FL models can be trained to analyze patient data and provide clinicians with insights and recommendations for treatment. This can help clinicians make more informed decisions and improve patient outcomes [23]. FL can also be used for disease detection and diagnosis [24]. By analyzing data from various sources, including medical imaging, clinical records, and genetic data, FL models can be trained to detect and diagnose diseases accurately. This can aid in enhancing the accuracy of diagnoses while minimizing the time and costs linked with conventional diagnostic methods [25]. Finally, by analyzing data from wearable devices and other remote monitoring technologies, FL models can be trained to detect early warning signs of potential health issues [26]. This can help improve patient outcomes and reduce the need for hospitalizations and other costly interventions.

While FL has many potential applications in digital healthcare, several challenges must be addressed. These include data heterogeneity, privacy concerns, and the need for standardized data formats [27]. Ongoing research in this area is focused on developing techniques to overcome these challenges and effectively implement FL in digital healthcare systems [28]. As this research progresses, we can expect to see new and innovative approaches to improving patient outcomes and transforming the delivery of healthcare services.

This study underscores the significance of FL in enhancing data privacy and security in modern healthcare systems. FL incorporates cryptographic and privacy-preserving techniques to protect sensitive data while enabling collaborative ML model training without sharing raw data. Various privacy-preserving methods based on FL, such as Differential Privacy (DP), Secure Multi-Party Computation (SMC), and Homomorphic Encryption (HE), have been proposed to safeguard patient data and ensure privacy [29–33]. The existing literature in this emerging domain is insufficient, and many proposed techniques have not been fully deployed. As health data generated by IoHT devices grows, developing efficient and effective FL techniques becomes crucial to protect patient data. A comprehensive review of FL techniques is essential to identify strengths and weaknesses, paving the way for more robust approaches to address current challenges.

19.1.1 Main chapter contributions

The following are the significant contributions of this chapter:

- Presentation of a comprehensive overview of FL in digital healthcare systems, highlighting the urgent need for patient data security and privacy.

- A highlight of different terminologies used in FL in modern digital healthcare systems.
- A comprehensive discussion of different FL techniques for Enhanced Cybersecurity in Modern Digital Healthcare Systems.
- A discussion of the different benefits and challenges associated with deploying FL approaches in modern digital healthcare systems.
- A Highlight of the future research trends of FL in modern healthcare systems.

19.1.2 Chapter organization

After the introduction in Section 19.1, the rest of this chapter is structured as follows: Section 19.2 details the different terminologies of FL in modern digital healthcare systems. Section 19.3 comprehensively discusses the various FL techniques for enhanced cybersecurity of modern digital healthcare systems. Section 19.4 presents the benefits of FL in modern digital healthcare systems. The challenges of FL in modern digital healthcare systems are depicted in Section 19.5. The lessons learned are highlighted in section 19.6. Future research trends are presented in Section 19.7, and the conclusion is provided in section 19.8.

19.2 Terminologies of FL in modern digital healthcare systems

This section endeavors to unravel the foundational terminologies intrinsic to FL, offering a comprehension of the principles and methodologies that underscore this innovative paradigm. We aim to cultivate a profound insight into the application and inherent potential of FL, particularly in bolstering the security framework within digital healthcare ecosystems.

19.2.1 Vertical FL

Vertical FL is a variant of FL where different entities possess heterogeneous data types like medical records, genomic data, and imaging data [34]. This allows collaborative modeling while preserving privacy across data silos. The key technical challenges involve handling varying feature spaces, developing privacy-preserving aggregation methods for diverse data types, and ensuring model robustness [35]. The application of advanced cryptography, like HE, offers promise in enabling secure computation across data partitions with different schemas.

19.2.2 Horizontal FL

Horizontal FL facilitates collaborative learning where different entities, like hospitals, have similar data types, such as EHRs [36]. This decentralizes model training while keeping sensitive patient data localized on institutional servers. Current research focuses on developing statistical methods for varying data distributions across hospitals. Robust aggregation mechanisms are also needed to prevent faults or biases from being introduced by outlier client models.

19.2.3 On-device FL

On-device FL refers to model training directly on user devices like wearables and smartphones without relying on a central server [37]. This provides enhanced privacy but poses computational challenges regarding communication overhead and platform heterogeneity across devices. Efficient model compression algorithms are being studied to reduce bandwidth usage. Personalized models can also be cultivated locally using on-device learning and later contributed to the global model.

19.2.4 Central server/aggregator

The central server or aggregator is the coordinating entity that manages the collaborative training process [38]. It orchestrates secure model aggregation from participating clients without directly accessing raw data [39]. Robust defense mechanisms are needed to prevent model poisoning or dimensionality attacks that can compromise server integrity. Trusted execution environments like Intel SGX offer hardware-based attestation to protect Aggregation.

19.2.5 Local model/client model

Local or client models are trained on individual data sources like hospitals or patient devices in an FL setup [38]. This decentralized approach ensures data privacy and sovereignty. However, statistical heterogeneity between clients can introduce bias during Aggregation. Robust federation methods and incentive mechanisms are being researched to promote quality local model development.

19.2.6 Secure aggregation

Secure Aggregation enables privacy-preserving consolidation of local model updates at the coordinating server without exposing raw data [35]. Advanced multi-party computation and HE provide the cryptographic building blocks. However, high computational complexity warrants efficiency enhancements through protocol optimization and hardware acceleration. Fully HE enabling arbitrary computation on encrypted data is also being investigated.

19.2.7 Decentralized data storage

Decentralized data storage retains information within respective source domains while only sharing model updates [40]. This mitigates privacy concerns and single points of failure in centralized training. Integration with blockchain further enhances tamper-proofing, transparency, and access control over sensitive records [41]. Ongoing research focuses on scalable architectures for decentralized learning suitable for healthcare workloads. Compute-efficient cryptographic methods also warrant further investigation.

19.2.8 Cross-validation

Cross-validation enables decentralized model performance evaluation by partitioning local datasets [42]. This prevents information leakage while allowing assessment of metrics like accuracy, providing insights into model generalizability. Privacy-preserving analytics methods like federated statistics can further derive global insights from local validations.

19.2.9 Federated transfer learning (FTL)

This combination of FL and transfer learning techniques addresses the challenge of training models on distributed data sources with non-overlapping features [43]. Traditional FL requires data sources to share the same feature space, which is impractical in industries including healthcare and finance [44]. FTL allows a global model trained on one dataset to be fine-tuned using data from different participants, even if their features do not overlap [45]. In the medical domain, FTL has been applied to tasks such as disease diagnosis and prediction, medical image analysis, and remote patient monitoring [46].

19.2.10 Federated reinforcement learning (FRL)

Reinforcement learning allows intelligent agents to optimize behaviors through environmental interaction [47]. Governing dynamics like delayed rewards and partial observability make it suitable for decentralized learning. FRL thus emerges as a natural extension to enable collaborative agent modeling while preserving privacy. Current research focuses on distributed reward modeling and policy aggregation mechanisms tailored for non-stationary healthcare environments. Table 19.1 summarizes the above terminologies.

Table 19.1 Summary of terminologies in FL

Terminology	Summary	References
Vertical FL	Allows different entities with different types of data (e.g., medical records, genomic data, imaging data) to collaborate on model training without sharing raw data. Preserves privacy.	[34]
Horizontal FL	Enables collaboration between entities with similar/related datasets (e.g., EHR across hospitals). Allows decentralized training and aggregation while keeping raw data decentralized and private.	[36]
On-Device FL	Enables model training directly on user devices like smartphones or wearables. Does not require the sharing of raw data with the central server. Offers enhanced privacy and reduced communication overhead. Allows personalized on-device models.	[37]
Central Server/ Aggregator	Acts as coordinating entity to manage the overall FL process. Receives model update summaries from clients, aggregates them, and sends updated global models back to clients. Has no direct access to raw data - only processes encrypted/summarized updates.	[38,39]

(Continues)

Table 19.1 (Continued)

Terminology	Summary	References
Local Model/ Client Model	Refers to models that are trained on individual participating devices/data sources in FL setup. Allows decentralized training to maintain the privacy/security of data. Local model updates are then sent to the aggregator to improve the global model.	[38]
Secure Aggregation	Privacy-preserving aggregation method that allows a central server to combine local model updates without direct access to the underlying raw private data. Typically uses encryption (e.g., MPC, homomorphic encryption) to enable secure Aggregation and preserve confidentiality.	[35]
Decentralized data storage	Allows data to remain stored within respective domains while only sharing model parameters for Aggregation. Provides data sovereignty and tackles issues like central points of failure and increased latency. Blockchain can be leveraged to make the system more robust, tamper-proof, and transparent through features like collective maintenance traceability.	[40,41]
Cross-Validation	Assesses model performance by partitioning local decentralized data into training and validation sets to get an unbiased evaluation. Allows validation of models in a privacy-preserving decentralized way during FL.	[42]
FTL	Enables transfer learning to adapt models trained on one dataset to other datasets with non-overlapping features/ sample spaces. Useful when decentralized datasets have heterogeneous features/sample spaces.	[43,45]
FRL	Merges FL and reinforcement learning. Allows decentralized agents/devices to collaboratively learn policies while keeping local data private. Enables knowledge sharing and policy aggregation in distributed environments like healthcare.	[47]

19.3 FL for enhanced cybersecurity in modern digital healthcare systems

As digital healthcare expands, so too do vulnerabilities that bad actors can exploit. This poses data privacy issues and significant patient safety threats if hackers can access connected medical devices and systems. Hence, enhanced cybersecurity measures are essential and are discussed in this section.

19.3.1 Differential privacy (DP) in modern digital healthcare systems

DP, first introduced by [48], is a framework for developing privacy-preserving data analysis algorithms and systems. By adding controlled random noise to computations and outputs, DP obscures the contribution of any single data point, making it challenging to trace outcomes back to specific inputs. This provides plausible

Table 19.2 Summary of DP techniques in healthcare systems

Technique	Summary	References
Novel DPFL framework with 3-D contract approach	Introduces artificial noise into local datasets to address task expenditure and privacy considerations. Uses a 3-D contract incentive mechanism to optimize the model owner's utility.	[50]
DP-based FL framework for decentralized health data	Refrains from sharing raw data between sites. Uses a DP scheme to protect patient privacy. Tested on large healthcare datasets while preserving utility.	[51]
BFG - Blockchain+DP +GAN framework	Combines blockchain, DP, and GANs. Withstands poisoning attacks and constraints storage problem. Optimizes between privacy budget and global model proficiency.	[52]
Edge computing DP framework	Fortifies privacy by mitigating vulnerabilities in data transfer and incorporating user anonymity and load reduction. Uses Laplacian noise for DP.	[39]
Differentially private FL for histopathology	Distributed training using DP performs similarly to conventional methods while ensuring strong privacy guarantees.	[33]

deniability for individuals' data [48]. DP was later adapted to FL settings by [49] to mitigate gradient leakage of sensitive information. Numerous studies have since explored differentially private FL (DPFL) for various applications. For instance, [50] proposed a DPFL approach that balances privacy risk and computation/communication costs using a 3D contract incentive mechanism. Simulations showed this optimizes model utility within an inherent information asymmetry between parties. Moreover, [51] developed a DPFL healthcare framework that combines not sharing raw data between sites with a DP scheme to protect patient privacy. Evaluations on large real-world medical datasets demonstrated this preserves utility while upholding privacy. Additionally, [52] combined blockchain, DP, and generative adversarial networks (GANs) into an IoHT privacy protection framework called BFG. BFG withstands various attacks, optimizes the privacy-utility tradeoff, and tackles blockchain storage limitations in decentralized learning. Experiments confirm BFG's precision, resilience, and privacy capabilities. Furthermore, [39] introduced an edge computing DPFL framework focused on strengthening privacy in IoHT via data transfer protections, user anonymity, and load reduction. Laplacian noise DP further fortifies data security. Finally, [33] proposed a DPFL approach for healthcare, using histopathology images as a case study. Despite distributed private training, results matched conventional methods while ensuring strong privacy guarantees. This helps overcome medical data limitations due to privacy concerns. Table 19.2 summarizes the different DP techniques in healthcare systems.

While the above studies depict the effectiveness of DP in preserving patient information security and privacy in the healthcare sector, one limitation of DP is its effectiveness dwindles when dealing with a small amount of data. This is because injecting noise into a diminutive data set while training the model can negatively impact the outcome [36]. Hence, with colossal datasets, DP is guaranteed to provide the necessary privacy in healthcare systems.

19.3.2 Homomorphic encryption (HE) for secure modern digital healthcare systems

Traditional encryption systems have drawbacks for sensitive data analysis, including the need to share keys and the inability to process encrypted data computationally [53]. HE methods address this by enabling computations on ciphertexts without decryption [54]. HE supports addition, multiplication, or both on encrypted data [55,56]. This suits secure offloading, ML, and sensitive data manipulation applications like IoHT. HE categories include partially homomorphic (limited operations), somewhat homomorphic (restricted computations within a robustness bound), and fully homomorphic encryption (FHE). FHE supports unlimited operations for any computable function, enhancing multi-party computation efficiency [57–59]. Figure 19.1 depicts the scheme of HE in healthcare systems.

As FL relies on multi-platform computation, HE improves security, as various studies demonstrate. For instance, [60] proposed an FL approach using homomorphic re-encryption between fog and server. This protects IoT data and resolves computational/storage issues while achieving resilience to node failures. To prevent model reconstruction privacy attacks in IoHT, [32] applied masks and HE, judging dataset impact by intrinsic attributes over quantity alone. Their scheme withstands participant dropouts. Finally, [61] developed a HE-based architecture

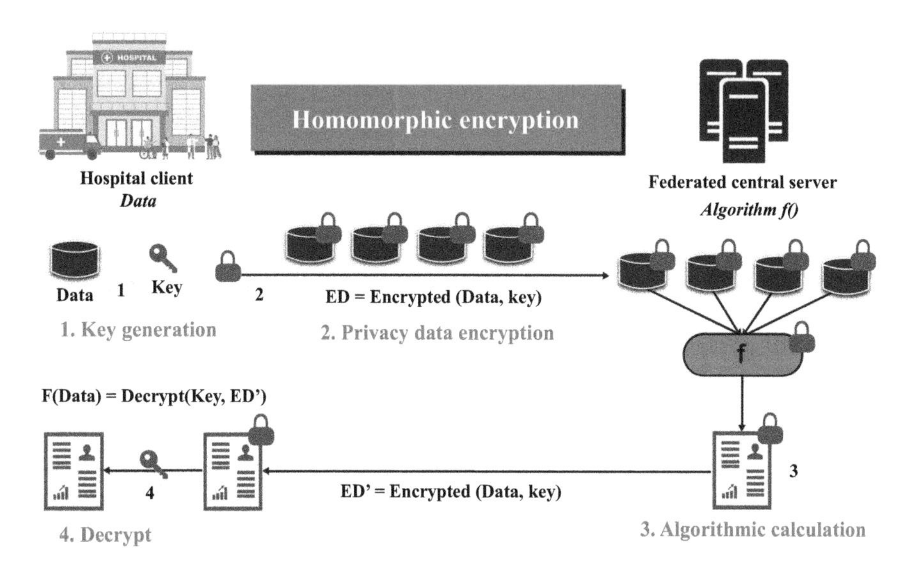

Figure 19.1 Homomorphic encryption scheme

Table 19.3 Summary of HE techniques in healthcare systems

Technique	Summary	References
FL using homomorphic re-encryption	Uses homomorphic re-encryption for model aggregation between fog nodes and server. Protects data from IoT devices and resolves computational/storage costs. Resilient to node failures.	[60]
Masks and homomorphic encryption	Uses masks and homomorphic encryption to protect local medical models from reconstruction attacks. Contribution rate based on intrinsic dataset attributes. Resilient to participant dropouts.	[32]
HE-based architecture with encrypted query	Implements homomorphic encryption and encrypted query technology for privacy-preserving FL. Enables data exploration and model training without compromising privacy.	[61]

for privacy-preserving FL in IoHT, implementing encrypted query technology so data providers can enable model training without exposing task requirements. Table 19.3 summarizes the studies on HE for bolstering cybersecurity in healthcare systems.

19.3.3 Secure multi-party computation (SMC) for secure modern digital healthcare systems

SMC, a sub-domain of cryptography, safeguards confidential data by enabling collaborative computing without any party having access to other participants' information. This technique facilitates the secure calculation of functions for multiple participants without relying on third-party trust or revealing inputs [62]. Nevertheless, SMC's computational overhead and high communication costs stem from the added encryption and decryption operations [63]. Several studies have been undertaken to address security and privacy concerns using SMC. For instance, a novel scheme based on SMC was proposed to mitigate the significant privacy challenges of handling patients' sensitive medical data during the diagnostic process [64]. The authors introduce a methodology that encrypts registered patients' healthcare data before transmitting it to the healthcare facility server to achieve their objectives.

Through the application of HE, a novel approach to FL in healthcare was introduced in this study, emphasizing privacy preservation [65]. To combat potential threats from malicious entities, a secure MPC protocol is utilized to protect the integrity of the DL model. In another study [66], authors proposed a novel FL framework for 6G and IoMT, based on a convolutional neural network (CNN) and incorporating both SMC and Encrypted Inference methods. Their framework addresses privacy and security challenges by enabling several healthcare facilities with clusters of varied IoMT and edge devices to train locally and encrypt their models before transmitting them for encryption and Aggregation in the cloud based on SMC. To optimize the model's efficacy, their innovative approach yields an

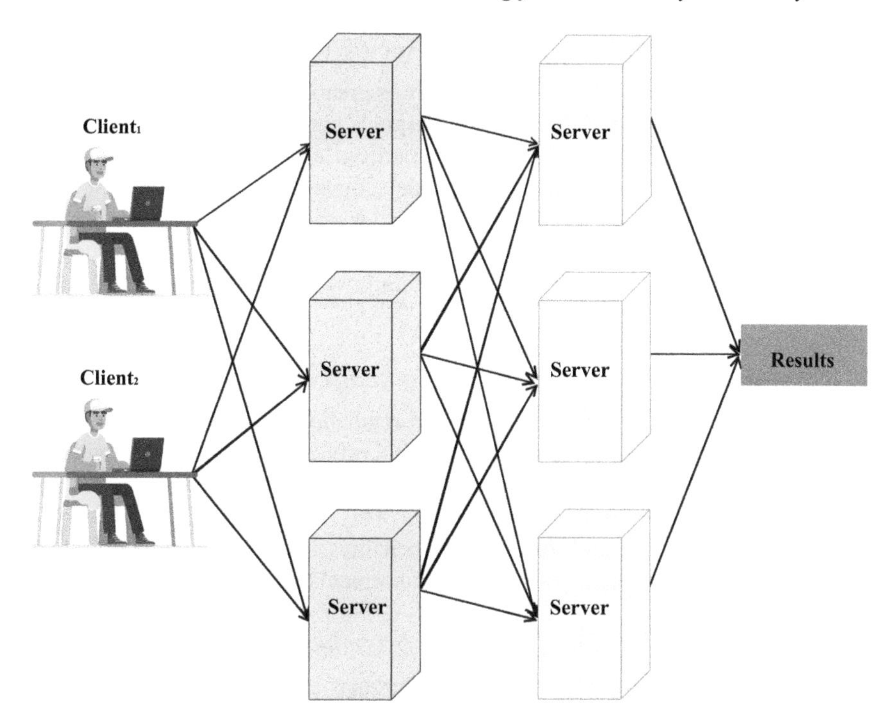

Figure 19.2 Secure multi-party computation scheme

encrypted global model distributed back to individual healthcare institutions for further refinement through localized training. Additionally, their method enables hospitals to execute encrypted inference seamlessly on their edge servers or within the cloud, ensuring the utmost confidentiality of both data and model throughout the entire procedure. Figure 19.2 depicts the SMC scheme.

Although these approaches provide an additional layer of data privacy and security, they do come at a cost to communication efficiency and model performance. For instance, DP incorporates random noise into client training data, enhancing privacy albeit at the potential cost of diminished model proficiency. On the other hand, HE encrypts model parameters exclusively, which safeguards data but also has performance implications. Lastly, SMC maintains client input privacy, which is computationally demanding and requires substantial communication among the involved parties [67].

19.4 Benefits of FL in modern digital healthcare systems

In healthcare, there are immense benefits to leveraging FL approaches due to stringent data privacy regulations and the sensitivity of health data. This section discusses the benefits of FL in healthcare.

19.4.1 Improved data privacy and security

One of the main appeals of FL for healthcare is greatly enhanced data privacy and security. Under traditional ML methods, hospitals and health systems would need to transfer real-world patient data to third parties, leading to risks of hacking or misuse. With federated approaches, model development can occur without exposing patient data [68]. Each hospital or clinic trains an algorithm on their local data silos, and only the models or updates need to be shared rather than raw patient information. This prevents single points of failure where entire healthcare datasets could be compromised.

19.4.2 Regulatory alignment for the healthcare industry

Healthcare organizations must comply with regulations like HIPAA that enforce strict safeguards around patient data sharing and privacy. FL is consistent with data minimization principles emphasized in these policies, only requiring model parameters rather than underlying data [69,70]. This helps healthcare stakeholders demonstrate compliance and avoid heavy penalties. FL will become even better aligned with healthcare data governance requirements as data regulations expand.

19.4.3 Reduced liability from data breaches

By training deep learning (DL) algorithms through federated approaches without central patient data repositories, healthcare groups can significantly limit their liability in the event of cyberattacks. Successful hacking attempts may steal model information without the underlying data samples. While disruptive, this prevents the compromise of patient records [71]. The reduced liability risk profile makes FL approaches more appealing for risk-averse hospital administrators and insurers.

19.4.4 Ability to utilize more real-world patient data

Federated architectures give hospitals and clinics the confidence to feed more real-world observational data into ML pipelines. Under traditional centralized methods, healthcare groups heavily filter their datasets before sharing due to justifiable privacy concerns or regulatory ambiguity. Federated techniques sidestep this issue. Each participant can use extensive sets of actual patient data for on-device model training without disclosure concerns, leading to algorithms better grounded in reality [72].

19.4.5 Fostering collaboration across healthcare institutions

While hospitals and health systems compete in many ways, improving patient outcomes is an area ripe for collaboration. FL enables healthcare institutions to jointly improve AI models on specific conditions without compromising patient data independence or competitive dynamics [73]. This allows tapping into collective intelligence and diverse population datasets that are not possible for single entities to achieve alone. Patient subgroups that may be underrepresented within one hospital can be supplemented by federated data contributions across many care sites.

19.4.6 Accelerating model development through large collective datasets

The federated approach of distributed on-device training followed by secure model aggregation provides a means of rapidly developing healthcare algorithms. Rather than rely solely on their patient dataset, which may lack cases for unusual presentations, each organization contributes patterns found across their local data silos into an anonymized modeling pool [74,75]. The collective model is thereby trained on what may amount to millions of diverse medical records across varied populations and geographies. Acceleration of algorithm performance is possible without ever combining raw data stores.

19.4.7 Rare disease advancement through increased data volumes

One major challenge in health AI is having adequate training data for rare diseases and conditions. By bringing federated updates across a global network of hospitals, even sparse illnesses have increased the potential for intelligent algorithm development. Whereas an individual academic medical center may see one or two dozen cases of a given condition per decade, collectively, this turns into thousands of cases. Rare disease profiling and discovery efforts can progress rapidly in the federated construct without requiring centralized warehousing of data [76,77].

19.4.8 Stronger generalizability to new healthcare settings

A perennial issue with many modern AI algorithms is the lack of transportability to new medical institutions with different equipment, workflows, or demographics. FL helps enable sophisticated models trained across myriad settings with diversity on multiple levels [78,79]. This allows healthcare AI development to be grounded on broader generalizability rather than overfitting a single population or care delivery paradigm. Simulation findings demonstrate superior portability for federated models into unseen data distributions relative to traditional approaches.

19.4.9 Reducing algorithmic bias through population diversity

It is widely recognized that bias can unintentionally be introduced into healthcare AI systems due to a lack of diversity in the underlying training data. FL has the potential to reduce this algorithmic bias by enabling secure contribution of data patterns across patient subgroups that may experience inequities in the traditional healthcare system [80–82]. Responsible data scientists can proactively utilize the federated approach to give equal representation where imbalance has historically occurred.

In summary, FL opens new possibilities in healthcare AI, leveraging DL techniques applied securely across decentralized datasets. Benefits span multiple dimensions, from privacy and compliance to model performance and algorithmic responsibility. Federated architectures help healthcare stakeholders tap into collective intelligence to develop robust algorithms even for rare conditions. By maintaining patient data control locally while allowing anonymous model sharing, health organizations can advance AI capabilities in a trusted fashion compliant with existing governance frameworks. Emerging privacy-enhanced methods like FL will enable healthcare players to confidently pursue AI progress grounded in real-world evidence without undue risks. Healthcare delivery stands to be transformed through this next evolution in distributed ML paradigms tailored for the modern medical ecosystem.

19.5 Challenges of FL in modern digital healthcare systems

While FL offers various benefits, it falls short of addressing all the challenges associated with medical data learning. Achieving an effective model still heavily relies on variables such as data quality, standardization, and avoiding biases. This section details the different challenges of FL in healthcare.

19.5.1 Heterogeneity of medical data

The intricate nature of medical data heterogeneity is a tapestry of diverse aspects, including but not limited to modality, dimensionality, and overarching traits. Moreover, this heterogeneity extends within a specific protocol, attributed to factors like dissimilarities in acquisition methods, the medical equipment brand, or localized demographics [9,83,84]. Although FL can potentially alleviate certain biases by enriching data diversity, non-uniform data distribution poses a formidable hurdle for FL algorithms and strategies, as they heavily rely on the assumption of independent and identically distributed (IID) data across participants [85]. Addressing the data diversity issue involves developing robust FL algorithms capable of handling data heterogeneity while preserving data privacy and security. Techniques like FedProx, part-sharing strategy, and domain adaptation have yielded promising results [86]. Moreover, data heterogeneity poses another challenge, as it may create a scenario where the perfect global solution is not necessarily the most optimal choice for a local participant. To avoid this, a consensus on model training optimality must be reached among all participants before commencing the training process.

19.5.2 Security and privacy

The sanctity of healthcare data cannot be overstated; it requires the utmost protection through strict adherence to confidentiality protocols. In this regard, crucial factors to be considered are the delicate balance between risks and benefits, the methodologies employed, and the remaining risks associated with safeguarding FL's privacy-preserving capabilities. Like ML algorithms, FL techniques provide security and privacy solutions, albeit with some risks. For instance, the privacy-preserving methodologies of FL provide unparalleled security, surpassing that of contemporary commercially accessible ML models. Nonetheless, this heightened protection comes at a cost—the compromise of model performance, potentially impacting the ultimate precision of the model [87]. Moreover, the advent of novel techniques and accompanying data may threaten the security of previously deemed low-risk models. Additionally, FL is susceptible to attacks such as membership attacks, GAN-based inference attacks, backdoor attacks, and free-riding attacks, along with unintentional information leakage as a result of shared information, which may indirectly expose private data of participating healthcare institutions [7,8,88–91].

19.5.3 Scalability issues

Effective management of inbound and outbound networks is critical in the healthcare industry, but this can be hindered by the significant scalability obstacle posed by FL. When numerous high-speed wireless systems are supported, system speed degradation [92] may occur, jeopardizing patient care. Maintaining high speed, quality, and low cost is becoming increasingly difficult [93]. As the array of interconnected gadgets expands and the torrent of data traffic relentlessly surges, the network's capacity constraints are provoked to their limits. Additionally, the network's hybrid architecture includes devices from multiple providers, further complicating scalability [94]. The daunting challenge of remotely managing numerous devices without any time or management losses must also be considered. A holistic approach is necessary to integrate the devices and their data and information from different sources while considering the unique needs of each device and the data it generates.

19.5.4 Data quality

In the healthcare domain, data is frequently marred by incompleteness, noise, and bias, which can significantly hinder the performance and generalization of models. FL emerges as a captivating tapestry that weaves together disparate healthcare institutions, hospitals, and cutting-edge gadgets, granting them the power to exchange invaluable experiences while safeguarding privacy. Yet, amidst this promising tapestry, many health systems are locked in a relentless dance with the intricacies of data chaos and the quest for optimal efficiency [95]. The heterogeneity of data obtained from diverse sources exhibits variances, and the absence of a standardized data protocol hinders uniformity. The interpretation of findings loses significance when samples are tainted by impure data [96]. The strategic leveraging of medical data is paramount; therefore, ensuring the cleanliness, accuracy, and completeness of data is key to improving ML models, whether they are being developed for an FL scenario or not [23]. Thus, to overcome these obstacles, FL must integrate data cleaning and quality control measures into the training process.

19.5.5 Infrastructure and computational challenges

Collaborative ML that relies on centralized data storage is further impeded by the significant expenses associated with establishing and sustaining the infrastructure needed for such storage [67]. Furthermore, the iterative training procedure necessitates recurrent exchanges between the central server and the collaborating clients, wherein each client actively imparts progressive enhancements to the model by leveraging its localized dataset [97]. The computational demands of this communication can prove unreasonable, particularly in scenarios entailing substantial data volumes or intricate models. Furthermore, implementing FL necessitates a bespoke infrastructure that facilitates expedient communication channels between the clients and the central server [19]. This infrastructure must ensure that patient data is protected and secured throughout training, from data collection to model updates. This can be challenging, as healthcare data is susceptible and subject to strict privacy regulations. Hence, healthcare systems must invest in the necessary infrastructure and resources to support large-scale FL.

19.5.6 Ethical and legal challenges

FL raises ethical and legal questions about ownership of data, informed consent, and patient privacy due to its dynamic, heterogeneous, distributed, and collaborative mechanisms [98]. Efficiently safeguarding and transferring healthcare data while ensuring anonymity and regulated access can be arduous and occasionally insurmountable. Despite the General Data Protection Regulation (GDPR) compliance in anonymized data sourced from EHR by healthcare providers, the mere presence of a few data elements can lead to identifying patients [99] a significant privacy concern for affected parties. Therefore, healthcare systems must ensure that they have appropriate policies and regulations in place to address these crucial concerns.

19.6 Lessons learned

The chapter provides an illuminating look into the promising yet complex intersection of FL and digital healthcare. Right from the outset, it emphasizes the urgent imperative to leverage FL specifically to amplify patient data privacy and security within an increasingly digitalized healthcare ecosystem. The chapter clearly explains a range of fundamental FL terminologies, including Vertical FL, Horizontal FL, and Secure Aggregation. Defining these key terms furnishes readers with the prerequisite context to strategize FL implementation. The chapter astutely examines how specific avant-garde FL approaches, chiefly DP, SMC, and HE, can concretely reinforce the cybersecurity posture of cutting-edge digital healthcare infrastructure.

Notably, the chapter sheds light on the wide-ranging benefits that FL adoption can unleash within healthcare, from strengthening data privacy protections and better regulatory alignment to opening the doors for increased collaboration between disparate healthcare stakeholders. However, rather than take an exclusively optimistic standpoint, the text maintains a balanced perspective by addressing the obstacles that FL deployment faces in domains like healthcare with unique challenges. The chapter provides a nuanced look, from grappling with heterogeneous medical data types to valid cybersecurity apprehensions, ethical dilemmas, and scaling hurdles.

Ultimately, the chapter empowers readers to walk away with an enlightened, balanced outlook by wielding both academic rigor and pragmatic lens regarding FL's promise and impediments influencing digital healthcare advancement. This sets the stage for stakeholders to strategize the prudent adoption or support for FL within the mission-critical healthcare realm with eyes fully open to this complex technological frontier.

19.7 Future research directions of FL in modern digital healthcare systems

FL has sparked tremendous interest in healthcare but remains an early-stage field requiring extensive research across multiple dimensions. This section highlights the future trends of FL in modern digital healthcare systems.

19.7.1 Enhancing algorithmic efficiency

While proof-of-concept healthcare studies demonstrate the feasibility of FL, model convergence times can be prolonged compared to centralized approaches since Aggregation occurs after limited local update steps. Further research on efficiency enhancements allowing more rapid model convergence even across thousands of remote participating devices will expand applicability. Areas like structured or sketched updates, pre-trained bootstrap models, and hierarchical aggregation present promising directions. Multi-task architectures that allow joint learning across related predictive problems may likewise improve efficiency [100–102].

19.7.2 Strengthening differential privacy implementations

A core motivation of federated healthcare analytics is maintaining patient data privacy. Mathematical guarantees to ensure no individual data characteristics can be inferred from shared model updates, even by a malicious actor, are provided in frameworks like DP [103]. However, strict privacy comes at the cost of degraded model utility. Advancing privacy-preserving techniques specialized to healthcare tasks with minimal accuracy loss is an open challenge. Trade-offs between privacy budgets across institutions and their impact on model performance also require further analysis.

19.7.3 Hybridizing FL with external knowledge

While FL pools knowledge across institutions through model parameter sharing, supplementing with medical ontology information in standardized formats holds further potential. More explainable and robust predictions become feasible by hybridizing learned distributed embeddings with formalized entity-relationship graphs of healthcare knowledge. Research on representational bridges between declarative expert systems and probabilistic deep models is still developing [104]. Projects at this intersection may uncover new techniques that merge FL with healthcare domain knowledge graphs.

19.7.4 Mitigating bias and ensuring fairness

While FL can provide more representative population coverage than single health systems, algorithmic bias remains a challenge if certain subgroups are under-represented across devices or generate limited prediction updates [80–82]. Developing bias detection and resolution techniques tailored to healthcare tasks on federated frameworks will be critical. This includes research on technical tools to mitigate unfairness and governance policies on participant inclusion rules and monitoring requirements.

19.7.5 Lightweight architectures for edge devices

While early federated healthcare demonstrations concentrated on server computing within hospitals, expanding to edge devices like wearables or IoT sensors was a strategic priority [102,105]. Many monitoring use cases rely on streaming data sources, requiring research innovations on lightweight federated implementations. Mini-batch model updates or decentralized knowledge distillation present possible directions well-matched to intermittent connectivity and inferencing on battery-powered devices.

19.7.6 Trustworthy and ethical FL

Trust in FL software and hardware stacks is imperative for broad healthcare adoption. Formal verification tooling and standards around secure multi-party analytics will play a key role. Additionally, upholding principles of transparency and algorithmic ethics around issues like bias testing or using restrictions on prediction insights will be crucial [106]. Developing governance frameworks on operationalizing and monitoring trustworthy FL across stakeholders is vital to scalable maturation.

19.7.7 Real-world validation and impact assessment

Technical experiments represent initial progress, but rigorous evidence proving the benefits and harms of FL in practice is limited. Methodical production rollouts with clinical integration and outcomes measurement through pragmatic trials or living laboratories could strengthen the evidence. Economic analyses clarifying ROI would likewise spur adoption. Priorities include cheaper and faster trials, safer interventions, genomic advances, and tailored population health. Creating model risk management guidelines and software tooling to validate impact will accelerate learning [107].

In summary, FL for modern digital healthcare ecosystems remains an emergent scientific field with abundant open frontiers requiring interdisciplinary perspectives spanning ML, security engineering, behavioral economics, and regulatory policy. While promising in concept, realizing benefits while guaranteeing privacy with demonstrable clinical utility at scale is non-trivial, necessitating extensive research along multiple dimensions, from efficient algorithms to trustworthy system design. If technical and adoption obstacles are overcome, federated architectures may transform how predictive healthcare AI is developed and responsibly deployed across decentralized networks. The extent and timing of paradigm shifts toward this future remain active research questions warranting ongoing investigation over the next decade across both academia and industry.

19.8 Conclusion

In conclusion, the chapter underscores the importance of integrating FL into the digital healthcare landscape to address pressing patient data security and privacy challenges. The comprehensive overview of FL terminologies, ranging from Vertical and Horizontal FL to Secure Aggregation, establishes a solid foundation for understanding the nuances of this technology in healthcare settings. The detailed exploration of FL techniques, including DP, SMC, and HE, highlights their pivotal role in fortifying cybersecurity. The myriad benefits of FL in modern digital healthcare, such as improved data privacy, regulatory alignment, and collaborative potential, showcase its transformative potential. However, the chapter also acknowledges the inherent challenges, including the heterogeneity of medical data, security and privacy concerns, scalability issues, and ethical and legal considerations. Recognizing these challenges is crucial for fostering responsible implementation. The chapter further highlights the future trends of FL in modern digital healthcare systems for bolstering the cybersecurity posture. Overall, this chapter serves as a comprehensive guide, providing valuable insights into leveraging FL for enhanced cybersecurity while navigating the complexities of the digital healthcare landscape.

References

[1] K. E. Fahim, K. Kalinaki, and W. Shafik, 'Electronic Devices in the Artificial Intelligence of the Internet of Medical Things (AIoMT)', in *Handbook of Security and Privacy of AI-Enabled Healthcare Systems and Internet of Medical Things*, 1st ed., CRC Press, 2023, pp. 41–62. doi: 10.1201/9781003370321-3.

[2] J. B. Awotunde, A. L. Imoize, R. G. Jimoh, *et al.*, 'AIoMT Enabling Real-Time Monitoring of Healthcare Systems Security and Privacy Considerations', in *Handbook of Security and Privacy of AI-Enabled Healthcare Systems and Internet of Medical Things*. Boca Raton, FL: CRC Press, pp. 97–133, 2023, doi: 10.1201/9781003370321-5.

[3] J. Srivastava, S. Routray, S. Ahmad, and M. M. Waris, 'Internet of Medical Things (IoMT)-Based Smart Healthcare System: Trends and Progress', *Comput Intell Neurosci*, vol. 2022, pp. 1–17, 2022, doi:10.1155/2022/7218113.

[4] K. Kalinaki, M. Fahadi, A. A. Alli, W. Shafik, M. Yasin, and N. Mutwalibi, 'Artificial Intelligence of Internet of Medical Things (AIoMT) in Smart Cities: A Review of Cybersecurity for Smart Healthcare', in *Handbook of*

Security and Privacy of AI-Enabled Healthcare Systems and Internet of Medical Things, 1st ed., CRC Press, 2023, pp. 271–292. doi: 10.1201/9781003370321-11.

[5] A. U. Rufai, E. P. Fasina, C. O. Uwadia, A. T. Rufai, and A. L. Imoize, 'Cyberattacks against Artificial Intelligence- Enabled Internet of Medical Things', *Handbook of Security and Privacy of AI-Enabled Healthcare Systems and Internet of Medical Things*, pp. 191–216, 2023, doi: 10.1201/9781003370321-8.

[6] M. Ali, F. Naeem, M. Tariq, and G. Kaddoum, 'Federated Learning for Privacy Preservation in Smart Healthcare Systems: A Comprehensive Survey', *IEEE J Biomed Health Inform*, vol. 27, no. 2, pp. 778–789, 2023, doi:10.1109/JBHI.2022.3181823.

[7] A. A. Alli, K. Kassim, N. Mutwalibi, H. Hamid, and L. Ibrahim, 'Secure Fog-Cloud of Things: Architectures, Opportunities and Challenges', in *Secure Edge Computing*, 1st ed., M. Ahmed and P. Haskell-Dowland, Eds., CRC Press, 2021, pp. 3–20. doi:10.1201/9781003028635-2.

[8] K. Kalinaki, N. N. Thilakarathne, H. R. Mubarak, O. A. Malik, and M. Abdullatif, 'Cybersafe Capabilities and Utilities for Smart Cities', in *Cybersecurity for Smart Cities*, Springer, Cham, 2023, pp. 71–86. doi:10.1007/978-3-031-24946-4_6.

[9] A. Alabdulatif, N. N. Thilakarathne, and K. Kalinaki, 'A Novel Cloud Enabled Access Control Model for Preserving the Security and Privacy of Medical Big Data', *Electronics (Basel)*, vol. 12, no. 12, p. 2646, 2023, doi:10.3390/electronics12122646.

[10] A. L. Imoize, V. E. Balas, V. K. Solanki, C.-C. Lee, and M. S. Obaidat, *Handbook of Security and Privacy of AI-Enabled Healthcare Systems and Internet of Medical Things*. Boca Raton, FL: CRC Press, 2023.

[11] W. Shafik and K. Kalinaki, 'Smart City Ecosystem: An Exploration of Requirements, Architecture, Applications, Security, and Emerging Motivations', in *Handbook of Research on Network-Enabled IoT Applications for Smart City Services*, IGI Global, 2023, pp. 75–98. doi:10.4018/979-8-3693-0744-1.CH005.

[12] B. Pfitzner, N. Steckhan, and B. Arnrich, 'Federated Learning in a Medical Context: A Systematic Literature Review', *ACM Transactions on Internet Technology (TOIT)*, vol. 21, no. 2, 2021, doi:10.1145/3412357.

[13] A. N. Edmund, C. A. Alabi, O. O. Tooki, A. L. Imoize, and T. D. Salka, 'Artificial Intelligence-Assisted Internet of Medical Things Enabling Medical Image Processing', *Handbook of Security and Privacy of AI-Enabled Healthcare Systems and Internet of Medical Things*, pp. 309–334, 2023, doi: 10.1201/9781003370321-13.

[14] X. Yin, Y. Zhu, and J. Hu, 'A Comprehensive Survey of Privacy-preserving Federated Learning', *ACM Computing Surveys (CSUR)*, vol. 54, no. 6, 2021, doi:10.1145/3460427.

[15] M. Abdulraheem, E. A. Adeniyi, J. B. Awotunde, *et al.*, 'Artificial Intelligence of Medical Things for Medical Information Systems Privacy and

Security', *Handbook of Security and Privacy of AI-Enabled Healthcare Systems and Internet of Medical Things*. Boca Raton, FL: CRC Press, pp. 63–96, 2023, doi: 10.1201/9781003370321-4.

[16] V. Mothukuri, R. M. Parizi, S. Pouriyeh, Y. Huang, A. Dehghantanha, and G. Srivastava, 'A survey on security and privacy of federated learning', *Future Generation Computer Systems*, vol. 115, pp. 619–640, 2021, doi:10.1016/J.FUTURE.2020.10.007.

[17] M. Chemisto, T. J. Gutu, K. Kalinaki, *et al.*, 'Artificial Intelligence for Improved Maternal Healthcare: A Systematic Literature Review', *2023 IEEE AFRICON*, pp. 1–6, 2023, doi:10.1109/AFRICON55910.2023.10293674.

[18] B. McMahan, E. Moore, D. Ramage, S. Hampson, and B. A. y. Arcas, 'Communication-Efficient Learning of Deep Networks from Decentralized Data'. *PMLR*, pp. 1273–1282, Apr. 10, 2017. Accessed: May 08, 2023. [Online]. Available: https://proceedings.mlr.press/v54/mcmahan17a.html

[19] S. Gaba, I. Buddhiraja, V. Kumar, and A. Makkar, 'Federated Learning Based Secured Computational Offloading in Cyber-Physical IoST Systems', *Communications in Computer and Information Science*, vol. 1704 CCIS, pp. 344–355, 2023, doi:10.1007/978-3-031-23599-3_26.

[20] D. C. Nguyen, P. Quoc-Viet, P. N. Pathirana, *et al.*, 'Federated Learning for Smart Healthcare: A Survey', *ACM Computing Surveys (CSUR)*, vol. 55, no. 3, 2022, doi:10.1145/3501296.

[21] K. Zhang, X. Song, C. Zhang, and S. Yu, 'Challenges and future directions of secure federated learning: a survey', *Frontiers of Computer Science*, vol. 16, no. 5. 2022. doi:10.1007/s11704-021-0598-z.

[22] A. Ghosh, J. Chung, D. Yin, and K. Ramchandran, 'An Efficient Framework for Clustered Federated Learning', *IEEE Trans Inf Theory*, vol. 68, no. 12, 2022, doi:10.1109/TIT.2022.3192506.

[23] J. Xu, B. S. Glicksberg, C. Su, P. Walker, J. Bian, and F. Wang, 'Federated Learning for Healthcare Informatics', *J Healthc Inform Res*, vol. 5, no. 1, pp. 1–19, 2021, doi:10.1007/s41666-020-00082-4.

[24] V. Rey, P. M. Sánchez Sánchez, A. Huertas Celdrán, and G. Bovet, 'Federated Learning for Malware Detection in IoT Devices', *Computer Networks*, vol. 204, 2022, doi:10.1016/j.comnet.2021.108693.

[25] E. Darzidehkalani, M. Ghasemi-rad, and P. M. A. van Ooijen, 'Federated Learning in Medical Imaging: Part I: Toward Multicentral Health Care Ecosystems', *Journal of the American College of Radiology*, vol. 19, no. 8, 2022, doi:10.1016/j.jacr.2022.03.015.

[26] A. Bogdanova, N. Attoh-Okine, and T. Sakurai, 'Risk and Advantages of Federated Learning for Health Care Data Collaboration', *ASCE ASME J Risk Uncertain Eng Syst A Civ Eng*, vol. 6, no. 3, 2020, doi:10.1061/ajrua6.0001078.

[27] W. Oh and G. N. Nadkarni, 'Federated Learning in Health Care Using Structured Medical Data', *Advances in Kidney Disease and Health*, vol. 30, no. 1, 2023, doi:10.1053/j.akdh.2022.11.007.

[28] F. Zerka, S. Barakat, S. Walsh, *et al.*, 'Systematic Review of Privacy-Preserving Distributed Machine Learning from Federated Databases in Health Care', *JCO Clin Cancer Inform*, no. 4, 2020, doi:10.1200/cci.19.00047.

[29] R. S. Antunes, C. A. Da Costa, A. Küderle, I. A. Yari, and B. Eskofier, 'Federated Learning for Healthcare: Systematic Review and Architecture Proposal', *ACM Transactions on Intelligent Systems and Technology (TIST)*, vol. 13, no. 4, 2022, doi:10.1145/3501813.

[30] S. M. Hosseini, M. Sikaroudi, M. Babaei, and H. R. Tizhoosh, 'Cluster Based Secure Multi-party Computation in Federated Learning for Histopathology Images', *Lecture Notes in Computer Science (including subseries Lecture Notes in Artificial Intelligence and Lecture Notes in Bioinformatics)*, vol. 13573 LNCS, pp. 110–118, 2022, doi:10.1007/978-3-031-18523-6_11.

[31] T. U. Islam, R. Ghasemi, and N. Mohammed, 'Privacy-Preserving Federated Learning Model for Healthcare Data', 2022 *IEEE 12th Annual Computing and Communication Workshop and Conference, CCWC 2022*, pp. 281–287, 2022, doi:10.1109/CCWC54503.2022.9720752.

[32] L. Zhang, J. Xu, P. Vijayakumar, P. K. Sharma, and U. Ghosh, 'Homomorphic Encryption-based Privacy-preserving Federated Learning in IoT-enabled Healthcare System', *IEEE Trans Netw Sci Eng*, vol. 10, no. 5, pp. 2864–2880, 2022, doi:10.1109/TNSE.2022.3185327.

[33] M. Adnan, S. Kalra, J. C. Cresswell, G. W. Taylor, and H. R. Tizhoosh, 'Federated Learning and Differential Privacy for Medical Image Analysis', *Scientific Reports*, vol. 12, no. 1, pp. 1–10, 2022, doi:10.1038/s41598-022-05539-7.

[34] K. K. Coelho, M. Nogueira, A. B. Vieira, E. F. Silva, and J. A. M. Nacif, 'A Survey on Federated Learning for Security and Privacy in Healthcare Applications', *Comput Commun*, vol. 207, pp. 113–127, 2023, doi:10.1016/J.COMCOM.2023.05.012.

[35] G. A. Kaissis, M. R. Makowski, D. Rückert, and R. F. Braren, 'Secure, Privacy-preserving and Federated Machine Learning in Medical Imaging', *Nat Mach Intell*, vol. 2, no. 6, 2020, doi:10.1038/s42256-020-0186-1.

[36] H. Li, C. Li, J. Wang, *et al.*, 'Review on Security of Federated Learning and Its Application in Healthcare', *Future Generation Computer Systems*, vol. 144, pp. 271–290, 2023, doi:10.1016/J.FUTURE.2023.02.021.

[37] R. Myrzashova, S. H. Alsamhi, A. V. Shvetsov, A. Hawbani, and X. Wei, 'Blockchain Meets Federated Learning in Healthcare: A Systematic Review with Challenges and Opportunities', *IEEE Internet Things J*, vol. 10, no. 16, pp. 14418–14437, 2023, doi:10.1109/JIOT.2023.3263598.

[38] D. Sirohi, N. Kumar, P. S. Rana, S. Tanwar, R. Iqbal, and M. Hijjii, 'Federated Learning for 6G-enabled Secure Communication Systems: A Comprehensive Survey', *Artificial Intelligence Review*, vol. 56, pp. 1–93, 2023, doi:10.1007/S10462-023-10417-3.

[39] A. K. Nair, J. Sahoo, and E. D. Raj, 'Privacy Preserving Federated Learning Framework for IoMT Based Big Data Analysis Using Edge Computing',

Comput Stand Interfaces, vol. 86, p. 103720, 2023, doi:10.1016/J.CSI.2023.103720.

[40] Y. Chang, C. Fang, and W. Sun, 'A Blockchain-Based Federated Learning Method for Smart Healthcare', *Comput Intell Neurosci*, vol. 2021, 2021, doi:10.1155/2021/4376418.

[41] S. Ji, T. Saravirta, S. Pan, G. Long, and A. Walid, 'Emerging Trends in Federated Learning: From Model Fusion to Federated X Learning', 2021, Accessed: Jun. 25, 2023. [Online]. Available: https://arxiv.org/abs/2102.12920v2

[42] A. Linardos, K. Kushibar, S. Walsh, P. Gkontra, and K. Lekadir, 'Federated Learning for Multi-center Imaging Diagnostics: A Simulation Study in Cardiovascular Disease', *Scientific Reports*, vol. 12, no. 1, pp. 1–12, 2022, doi:10.1038/s41598-022-07186-4.

[43] S. Saha and T. Ahmad, 'Federated Transfer Learning: Concept and Applications', *Intelligenza Artificiale*, vol. 15, no. 1, 2021, doi:10.3233/IA-200075.

[44] R. Ramadoss, 'Blockchain Technology: An Overview', *IEEE Potentials*, vol. 41, no. 6, 2022, doi:10.1109/MPOT.2022.3208395.

[45] Y. Chen, X. Qin, J. Wang, C. Yu, and W. Gao, 'FedHealth: A Federated Transfer Learning Framework for Wearable Healthcare', *IEEE Intell Syst*, vol. 35, no. 4, pp. 83–93, 2020, doi:10.1109/MIS.2020.2988604.

[46] A. S. Zhang and N. F. Li, 'A Two-Stage Federated Transfer Learning Framework in Medical Images Classification on Limited Data: A COVID-19 Case Study', *in Lecture Notes in Networks and Systems*, 2023. doi:10.1007/978-3-031-18461-1_13.

[47] J. Qi, Q. Zhou, L. Lei, and K. Zheng, 'Federated Reinforcement Learning: Techniques, Applications, and Open Challenges', *Intelligence & Robotics*, 2021, doi:10.20517/ir.2021.02.

[48] M. Abadi, A. Chu, I. Goodfellow, *et al.*, 'Deep Learning with Differential Privacy', *Proceedings of the ACM Conference on Computer and Communications Security*, vol. 24, pp. 308–318, Oct. 2016, doi:10.1145/2976749.2978318.

[49] R. C. Geyer, T. Klein, M. Nabi, S. Se, and E. Zurich, 'Differentially Private Federated Learning: A Client Level *Perspective*', Dec. 2017, Accessed: May 17, 2023. [Online]. Available: https://arxiv.org/abs/1712.07557v2

[50] M. Wu, D. Ye, J. Ding, Y. Guo, R. Yu, and M. Pan, 'Incentivizing Differentially Private Federated Learning: A Multidimensional Contract Approach', *IEEE Internet Things J*, vol. 8, no. 13, pp. 10639–10651, 2021, doi:10.1109/JIOT.2021.3050163.

[51] O. Choudhury, A. Gkoulalas-Divanis, T. Salonidis, *et al.*, 'Differential Privacy-enabled Federated Learning for Sensitive Health Data', 2019, Accessed: May 17, 2023. [Online]. Available: https://arxiv.org/abs/1910.02578v3

[52] W. Liu, Y. He, X. Wang, Z. Duan, W. Liang, and Y. Liu, 'BFG: Privacy Protection Framework for Internet of Medical Things Based on Blockchain and Federated Learning', *Conn Sci*, vol. 35, no. 1, p. 2199951, 2023, doi:10.1080/09540091.2023.2199951.

[53] M. Singh and A. K. Singh, 'A Comprehensive Survey on Encryption Techniques for Digital Images', *Multimed Tools Appl*, vol. 82, no. 8, pp. 11155–11187, 2023, doi:10.1007/S11042-022-12791-6.

[54] M. Ogburn, C. Turner, and P. Dahal, 'Homomorphic Encryption', *Procedia Comput Sci*, vol. 20, pp. 502–509, 2013, doi:10.1016/J.PROCS.2013.09.310.

[55] A. Acar, H. Aksu, A. S. Uluagac, and M. Conti, 'A Survey on Homomorphic Encryption Schemes: Theory and Implementation', *ACM Comput Surv*, vol. 51, no. 4, 2018, doi:10.1145/3214303.

[56] W. Yang, S. Wang, H. Cui, Z. Tang, and Y. Li, 'A Review of Homomorphic Encryption for Privacy-Preserving Biometrics', *Sensors*, vol. 23, no. 7, p. 3566, 2023, doi:10.3390/S23073566.

[57] T. Wu, C. Zhao, and Y. J. A. Zhang, 'Privacy-Preserving Distributed Optimal Power Flow with Partially Homomorphic Encryption', *IEEE Trans Smart Grid*, vol. 12, no. 5, pp. 4506–4521, 2021, doi:10.1109/TSG.2021.3084934.

[58] H. Chen, I. Iliashenko, and K. Laine, 'When HEAAN Meets FV: A New Somewhat Homomorphic Encryption with Reduced Memory Overhead', *Lecture Notes in Computer Science (including subseries Lecture Notes in Artificial Intelligence and Lecture Notes in Bioinformatics)*, vol. 13129 LNCS, pp. 265–285, 2021, doi:10.1007/978-3-030-92641-0_13.

[59] S. Meftah, B. H. M. Tan, C. F. Mun, K. M. M. Aung, B. Veeravalli, and V. Chandrasekhar, 'DOReN: Toward Efficient Deep Convolutional Neural Networks with Fully Homomorphic Encryption', *IEEE Transactions on Information Forensics and Security*, vol. 16, pp. 3740–3752, 2021, doi:10.1109/TIFS.2021.3090959.

[60] H. Ku, W. Susilo, Y. Zhang, W. Liu, and M. Zhang, 'Privacy-Preserving Federated Learning in Medical Diagnosis with Homomorphic Re-Encryption', *Comput Stand Interfaces*, vol. 80, p. 103583, 2022, doi:10.1016/J.CSI.2021.103583.

[61] R. H. Hsu and T. Y. Huang, 'Private Data Preprocessing for Privacy-preserving Federated Learning', *Proceedings of the 2022 5th IEEE International Conference on Knowledge Innovation and Invention, ICKII 2022*, pp. 173–178, 2022, doi:10.1109/ICKII55100.2022.9983518.

[62] N. Khalid, A. Qayyum, M. Bilal, A. Al-Fuqaha, and J. Qadir, 'Privacy-preserving Artificial Intelligence in Healthcare: Techniques and Applications', *Comput Biol Med*, vol. 158, p. 106848, 2023, doi:10.1016/J.COMPBIOMED.2023.106848.

[63] X. Ma, L. Liao, Z. Li, R. X. Lai, and M. Zhang, 'Applying Federated Learning in Software-Defined Networks: A Survey', *Symmetry 2022, Vol. 14, Page 195*, vol. 14, no. 2, p. 195, 2022, doi:10.3390/SYM14020195.

[64] D. Li, X. Liao, T. Xiang, J. Wu, and J. Le, 'Privacy-preserving Self-serviced Medical Diagnosis Scheme Based on Secure Multi-party Computation', *Comput Secur*, vol. 90, p. 101701, 2020, doi:10.1016/J.COSE.2019.101701.

[65] F. Wibawa, F. O. Catak, S. Sarp, and M. Kuzlu, 'BFV-Based Homomorphic Encryption for Privacy-Preserving CNN Models', *Cryptography 2022, Vol. 6, Page 34*, vol. 6, no. 3, p. 34, 2022, doi:10.3390/CRYPTOGRAPHY6030034.

[66] A. P. Kalapaaking, V. Stephanie, I. Khalil, M. Atiquzzaman, X. Yi, and M. Almashor, 'SMPC-Based Federated Learning for 6G-Enabled Internet of Medical Things', *IEEE Netw*, vol. 36, no. 4, pp. 182–189, 2022, doi:10.1109/MNET.007.2100717.

[67] T. K. Dang, X. Lan, J. Weng, and M. Feng, 'Federated Learning for Electronic Health Records', *ACM Trans Intell Syst Technol*, vol. 13, no. 5, p. 72, 2022, doi:10.1145/3514500.

[68] A. Lakhan, M. A. Mohammed, J. Nedoma, *et al.*, 'Federated-Learning Based Privacy Preservation and Fraud-Enabled Blockchain IoMT System for Healthcare', *IEEE J Biomed Health Inform*, vol. 27, no. 2, pp. 664–672, 2023, doi:10.1109/JBHI.2022.3165945.

[69] A. Rahman, M. S. Hossain, G. Muhammad, *et al.*, 'Federated Learning-based AI Approaches in Smart Healthcare: Concepts, Taxonomies, Challenges and Open Issues', *Cluster Computing*, vol. 26, pp. 1–41, 2022, doi:10.1007/S10586-022-03658-4.

[70] S. R. Chalamala, N. K. Kummari, A. K. Singh, A. Saibewar, and K. M. Chalavadi, 'Federated Learning to Comply with Data Protection Regulations', *CSI Transactions on ICT*, vol. 10, no. 1, pp. 47–60, 2022, doi:10.1007/S40012-022-00351-0.

[71] F. Cremonesi, V. Planat, V. Kalokyri, *et al.*, 'The Need for Multimodal Health Data Modeling: A Practical Approach for a Federated-learning Healthcare Platform', *J Biomed Inform*, vol. 141, p. 104338, 2023, doi:10.1016/J.JBI.2023.104338.

[72] C. Thapa, M. A. P. Chamikara, and S. A. Camtepe, 'Advancements of Federated Learning Towards Privacy Preservation: From Federated Learning to Split Learning', *Studies in Computational Intelligence*, vol. 965, pp. 79–109, 2021, doi:10.1007/978-3-030-70604-3_4.

[73] M. M. Salim and J. H. Park, 'Federated Learning-Based Secure Electronic Health Record Sharing Scheme in Medical Informatics', *IEEE J Biomed Health Inform*, vol. 27, no. 2, pp. 617–624, 2023, doi:10.1109/JBHI.2022.3174823.

[74] P. Qi, D. Chiaro, A. Guzzo, M. Ianni, G. Fortino, and F. Piccialli, 'Model Aggregation Techniques in Federated Learning: A Comprehensive Survey', *Future Generation Computer Systems*, vol. 150, pp. 272–293, 2024, doi:10.1016/J.FUTURE.2023.09.008.

[75] E. T. Martínez Beltrán, Á. L. P. Gómez, C. Feng, *et al.*, 'Fedstellar: A Platform for Decentralized Federated Learning', *Expert Syst Appl*, vol. 242, p. 122861, 2024, doi:10.1016/J.ESWA.2023.122861.

[76] J. Lekstrom-Himes, E. F. Augustine, A. Brower, *et al.*, 'Data Sharing to Advance Gene-targeted Therapies in Rare Diseases', *Am J Med Genet C Semin Med Genet*, vol. 193, no. 1, pp. 87–98, 2023, doi:10.1002/AJMG.C.32028.

[77] B. Chen, T. Chen, X. Zeng, *et al.*, 'DFML: Dynamic Federated Meta-Learning for Rare Disease Prediction', *IEEE/ACM Trans Comput Biol Bioinform,* pp. 1–11, 2023, doi:10.1109/TCBB.2023.3239848.

[78] A. Rauniyar, D. H. Hagos, D. Jha, *et al.*, 'Federated Learning for Medical Applications: A Taxonomy, Current Trends, Challenges, and Future Research Directions', *IEEE Internet Things J*, vol. 11, no. 5, pp. 7374–7398, 2023, doi:10.1109/JIOT.2023.3329061.

[79] W. Ding, M. Abdel-Basset, H. Hawash, M. Pratama, and W. Pedrycz, 'Generalizable Segmentation of COVID-19 Infection From Multi-Site Tomography Scans: A Federated Learning Framework', *IEEE Trans Emerg Top Comput Intell*, vol. 8, no. 1, 2023, doi:10.1109/TETCI.2023.3245103.

[80] R. J. Chen, J. J. Wang, D. F. K. Williamson, *et al.*, 'Algorithmic Fairness in Artificial Intelligence for Medicine and Healthcare', *Nature Biomedical Engineering*, vol. 7, no. 6, pp. 719–742, 2023, doi:10.1038/s41551-023-01056-8.

[81] T. Salazar, M. Fernandes, H. Araújo, and P. H. Abreu, 'FAIR-FATE: Fair Federated Learning with Momentum', *Lecture Notes in Computer Science (including subseries Lecture Notes in Artificial Intelligence and Lecture Notes in Bioinformatics)*, vol. 14073 LNCS, pp. 524–538, 2023, doi: 10.1007/978-3-031-35995-8_37/COVER.

[82] Y. H. Ezzeldin, S. Yan, C. He, E. Ferrara, and S. Avestimehr, 'FairFed: Enabling Group Fairness in Federated Learning', *Proceedings of the AAAI Conference on Artificial Intelligence*, vol. 37, no. 6, pp. 7494–7502, 2023, doi:10.1609/AAAI.V37I6.25911.

[83] A. L. Imoize, P. A. Gbadega, H. I. Obakhena, D. O. Irabor, K. V. N. Kavitha, and C. Chakraborty, 'Artificial Intelligence-enabled Internet of Medical Things for COVID-19 Pandemic Data Management', *in Explainable Artificial Intelligence in Medical Decision Support Systems*, Institution of Engineering and Technology, 2022, pp. 357–380. doi:10.1049/PBHE050E_ch13.

[84] K. Kalinaki, U. Yahya, O. A. Malik, and D. T. C. Lai, 'A Review of Big Data Analytics and Artificial Intelligence in Industry 5.0 for Smart Decision-Making', in *Human-Centered Approaches in Industry 5.0: Human-Machine Interaction, Virtual Reality Training, and Customer Sentiment Analysis*, 2023, pp. 24–47. doi:10.4018/979-8-3693-2647-3.ch002.

[85] Prayitno, C.-R. Shyu, K. T. Putra, *et al.*, 'A Systematic Review of Federated Learning in the Healthcare Area: From the Perspective of Data Properties and Applications', *Applied Sciences (Switzerland)*, vol. 11, no. 23, 2021. doi:10.3390/app112311191.

[86] N. Rieke, J. Hancox, W. Li, *et al.*, 'The Future of Digital Health with Federated Learning', *NPJ Digit Med*, vol. 3, no. 1, 2020, doi:10.1038/s41746-020-00323-1.

[87] T. Li, A. K. Sahu, A. Talwalkar, and V. Smith, 'Federated Learning: Challenges, Methods, and Future Directions', *IEEE Signal Process Mag*, vol. 37, no. 3, 2020, doi:10.1109/MSP.2020.2975749.

[88] S. Singh, S. Rathore, O. Alfarraj, A. Tolba, and B. Yoon, 'A Framework for Privacy-preservation of IoT Healthcare Data Using Federated Learning and Blockchain Technology', *Future Generation Computer Systems*, vol. 129, 2022, doi:10.1016/j.future.2021.11.028.

[89] D. Yang, Z. Xu, W. Li, *et al.*, 'Federated Semi-supervised Learning for COVID Region Segmentation in Chest CT Using Multi-national Data from China, Italy, Japan', *Med Image Anal*, vol. 70, 2021, doi:10.1016/j.media.2021.101992.

[90] M. Ahmed and P. Haskell-Dowland, *Cybersecurity for Smart Cities*. Cham: *Springer International Publishing*, 2023. doi: 10.1007/978-3-031-24946-4.

[91] M. Ahmed and P. Haskell-Dowland, *Secure Edge Computing: Applications, Techniques and Challenges*. 2021. Accessed: Jan. 18, 2024. [Online]. Available: https://www.routledge.com/Secure-Edge-Computing-Applications-Techniques-and-Challenges/Ahmed-Haskell-Dowland/p/book/9780367464141

[92] G. Muhammad, M. S. Hossain, and N. Kumar, 'EEG-Based Pathology Detection for Home Health Monitoring', *IEEE Journal on Selected Areas in Communications*, vol. 39, no. 2, 2021, doi:10.1109/JSAC.2020.3020654.

[93] F. Hussain, S. G. Abbas, G. A. Shah, *et al.*, 'A Framework for Malicious Traffic Detection in IoT Healthcare Environment', *Sensors*, vol. 21, no. 9, 2021, doi:10.3390/s21093025.

[94] A. Ullah, M. Azeem, H. Ashraf, A. A. Alaboudi, M. Humayun, and N. Z. Jhanjhi, 'Secure Healthcare Data Aggregation and Transmission in IoT - A Survey', *IEEE Access*, vol. 9. 2021. doi:10.1109/ACCESS.2021.3052850.

[95] X. Ma, J. Zhu, Z. Lin, S. Chen, and Y. Qin, 'A State-of-the-art Survey on Solving Non-IID Data in Federated Learning', *Future Generation Computer Systems*, vol. 135, 2022, doi:10.1016/j.future.2022.05.003.

[96] R. S. Antunes, C. A. Da Costa, A. Küderle, I. A. Yari, and B. Eskofier, 'Federated Learning for Healthcare: Systematic Review and Architecture Proposal', *ACM Trans Intell Syst Technol*, vol. 13, no. 4, 2022, doi:10.1145/3501813.

[97] P. Treleaven, M. Smietanka, and H. Pithadia, 'Federated Learning: The Pioneering Distributed Machine Learning and Privacy-Preserving Data Technology', *Computer (Long Beach Calif)*, vol. 55, no. 4, 2022, doi:10.1109/MC.2021.3052390.

[98] N. Truong, K. Sun, S. Wang, F. Guitton, and Y. K. Guo, 'Privacy Preservation in Federated Learning: An Insightful Survey from the GDPR Perspective', *Comput Secur*, vol. 110, 2021, doi:10.1016/j.cose.2021.102402.

[99] L. Rocher, J. M. Hendrickx, and Y. A. de Montjoye, 'Estimating the Success of Re-identifications in Incomplete Datasets Using Generative Models', *Nat Commun*, vol. 10, no. 1, 2019, doi:10.1038/s41467-019-10933-3.

[100] Z. Li, J. Chen, P. Zhang, H. Huang, and G. Li, 'DSFedCon: Dynamic Sparse Federated Contrastive Learning for Data-Driven Intelligent Systems', *IEEE Trans Neural Netw Learn Syst*, pp. 1–13, 2024, doi:10.1109/TNNLS.2024.3349400.

[101] Y. Li, Z. He, X. Gu, H. Xu, and S. Ren, 'AFedAvg: Communication-efficient Federated Learning Aggregation with Adaptive Communication Frequency and Gradient Sparse', *Journal of Experimental & Theoretical*

Artificial Intelligence, vol. 36, no. 1, pp. 47–69, 2024, doi:10.1080/0952813X.2022.2079730.

[102] M. Ficco, A. Guerriero, E. Milite, F. Palmieri, R. Pietrantuono, and S. Russo, 'Federated Learning for IoT Devices: Enhancing TinyML with On-board Training', *Information Fusion*, vol. 104, p. 102189, 2024, doi:10.1016/J.INFFUS.2023.102189.

[103] F. Elhattab, S. Bouchenak, and C. Boscher, 'PASTEL', *Proc ACM Interact Mob Wearable Ubiquitous Technol*, vol. 7, no. 4, pp. 1–29, 2023, doi:10.1145/3633808.

[104] S. Kumbhare, A. B.Kathole, and S. Shinde, 'Federated Learning Aided Breast Cancer Detection with Intelligent Heuristic-based Deep Learning Framework', *Biomed Signal Process Control*, vol. 86, p. 105080, 2023, doi:10.1016/J.BSPC.2023.105080.

[105] K. Kalinaki, M. Abdullatif, S. A.-K. Nasser, R. Nsubuga, and J. Kugonza, 'Paving the Path to a Sustainable Digital Future with Green Cloud Computing', *Emerging Trends in Cloud Computing Analytics, Scalability, and Service Models*, pp. 44–66, 2024, doi:10.4018/979-8-3693-0900-1.CH002.

[106] P. M. Sánchez Sánchez, A. Huertas Celdrán, N. Xie, G. Bovet, G. Martínez Pérez, and B. Stiller, 'FederatedTrust: A Solution for Trustworthy Federated Learning', *Future Generation Computer Systems*, vol. 152, pp. 83–98, 2024, doi:10.1016/J.FUTURE.2023.10.013.

[107] Z. Zhang, G. Chen, Y. Xu, L. Huang, C. Zhang, and S. Xiao, 'FedDQA: A Novel Regularization-based Deep Learning Method for Data Quality Assessment in Federated Learning', *Decis Support Syst*, vol. 180, p. 114183, 2024, doi:10.1016/J.DSS.2024.114183.

Chapter 20

Directed acyclic graph-based blockchains for enhanced cybersecurity in the Internet of Medical Things

Abubakar Aliyu[1], Abubakar Aminu Mu'azu[1] and Aminu Adamu[1]

To strengthen cybersecurity in the Internet of Medical Things (IoMT), this chapter examines the use of blockchains based on Directed Acyclic Graphs (DAGs). Securing private medical data and guaranteeing the integrity of networked medical devices become critical challenges as the IoMT scenario changes. The chapter leverages the efficiency and resilience of DAG-based blockchains against certain attacks. The proposed access control approach is built on the decentralised and impenetrable structure of Tangle, a DAG-based consensus technique. A novel framework for access control is presented, which represents IoMT entities with DAG structures. Directed edges encode dynamic relationships and permissions, whereas nodes represent medical equipment, healthcare providers, and patients. Blockchain-integrated smart contracts automate access decisions, guaranteeing adherence to healthcare laws and enabling real-time modifications to access rights. Security considerations encompass encryption protocols for secure communication, decentralised identity solutions for authentication, and immutable audit trails to meet regulatory requirements. To facilitate interoperability and smooth data sharing, the chapter puts a strong emphasis on integrating the access control mechanism with the current healthcare systems. The proposed solution aims to revolutionise IoMT cybersecurity by addressing the particular difficulties faced by the healthcare industry, namely security, and scalability. Furthermore, metrics like Elapsed Time *vs.* Number of Nodes, Access Rate *vs.* Number of Nodes, and Throughput *vs.* Number of Nodes are used to evaluate the implementation of the suggested access control, demonstrating observable improvements. The chapter emphasises how DAG-based blockchains might improve IoMT cybersecurity in a revolutionary way. This study enhances the security of developing healthcare systems amid the growth of

[1]Department of Computer Science, Umaru Musa Yar'adua University, Nigeria

linked medical devices and digital health technologies by providing a clear and flexible access control mechanism.

Keywords: Blockchains; cyber security; medical data; IoMT; DAG; security and scalability

20.1 Introduction

The Internet of Medical Things (IoMT), is a game-changer for the healthcare industry [1]. It integrates cutting-edge technologies and networked devices to improve patient care, optimise healthcare operations, and eventually improve health results all around [2]. The Internet of Medical Things (IoMT) is a broad network of linked wearables, sensors, medical equipment, and healthcare systems that exchange data in real time and communicate with one another to enable remote monitoring, diagnosis, and customised treatment [3]. Wearables, implanted devices, remote monitoring equipment, and other medical devices and sensors are all part of the IoMT [4]. Blood pressure and blood glucose levels are just two examples of the physiological data that these devices record and provide [5]. Furthermore, hospital information systems and Electronic Health Records (EHRs) are two examples of healthcare information systems that are essential to managing the massive amounts of data produced by IoMT devices [6]. The Internet and other communication networks serve as the backbone of safe and effective data interchange between healthcare systems and equipment [7]. IoMT is extremely important to the healthcare industry [8]. It allows for remote patient monitoring, which benefits older people and those with chronic illnesses in particular by providing ongoing supervision of their condition and health problems outside of typical healthcare settings [9]. Healthcare personnel are better equipped to respond quickly and wisely when using real-time data collecting, particularly in emergencies [5]. IoMT supports data-driven diagnostics, which makes it possible to create individualised treatment programmes based on information about each patient [10]. By automating procedures and allocating resources optimally, it increases total efficiency [11].

IoMT is also essential to preventative healthcare because it uses continuous monitoring to spot possible health problems early on [12]. In the long term, this proactive strategy helps to avoid issues and lower healthcare expenses [13]. IoMT has many advantages, but it also has drawbacks. These include issues with data security, patient privacy, interoperability across different devices, and regulatory compliance [14]. IoMT represents a paradigm shift in the medical field, presenting hitherto unheard-of chances to boost diagnostics, optimise patient care, and improve workflows [15]. The ongoing development and integration of IoMT technologies have enormous potential to revolutionise the provision of healthcare services in a connected and data-driven society, despite certain obstacles [16]. Robust cybersecurity protections are becoming increasingly important as the IoMT becomes more integrated into healthcare [17]. Sensitive patient data is being transferred and analysed in real time in greater quantities as the healthcare industry evolves to include wearables, smart sensors, and interconnected medical devices [18]. This increase raises serious cybersecurity concerns that require quick attention in addition to chances for improving patient care [19]. The large amount of health data that IoMT devices create is one of the main issues. Sensitive data, such as treatment plans, medical histories, and patient vitals, is continuously gathered and transmitted by these devices [20]. Due to the large attack surface, this data inflow creates, bad actors looking to gain unauthorised access, compromise data, or interfere with healthcare operations are drawn to it [21].

Furthermore, the interconnectedness of IoMT makes it more difficult to secure the lines of communication between healthcare systems and devices [22]. Safeguards against potential vulnerabilities, strict authentication procedures, and encryption protocols are necessary for the seamless transfer of data between various platforms [16]. These communication routes become vulnerable to data modification, eavesdropping, and unauthorised access in the absence of strong cybersecurity safeguards, posing major hazards to patient privacy and the accuracy of healthcare data [23]. Moreover, the widespread use of IoMT devices in diverse healthcare environments presents difficulties with device upkeep and upgrades [24]. Retaining a robust cybersecurity posture requires that every device is compliant with the most recent security patches, standards, and compliance requirements [25]. Inadequate attention to these elements may reveal weaknesses that cybercriminals could take advantage of, jeopardising the privacy, availability, and integrity of medical records [26]. IoMT is becoming more and more important to patient care, thus lawmakers, device makers, and healthcare providers need to work together to prioritise and put strong cybersecurity safeguards in place [6]. This entails anticipating and proactively minimising potential hazards in addition to tackling current ones. Establishing a reliable and secure IoMT ecosystem is the aim of preserving patient confidence, regulatory compliance, and the general integrity of healthcare services [21].

The healthcare industry faces numerous cybersecurity concerns as a result of the IoMT integration. These challenges must be addressed. With the constant flow of health data from IoMT devices, data integrity is a key concern because any compromise in quality could result in inaccurate diagnosis and treatment decisions [17]. To prevent unauthorised changes to patient records or treatment plans, tamper resistance must be guaranteed [5]. Due to the interconnectedness of IoMT, secure communication becomes crucial, necessitating strong encryption techniques to protect against data interception, eavesdropping, and unauthorised access during data transmission [14]. The problem of safeguarding the variegated environment of IoMT is made more difficult by the lack of standardised communication protocols and interoperability issues [11]. There are serious hazards associated with unauthorised access that result from compromised authentication systems or device vulnerabilities [5]. If these vulnerabilities are taken advantage of, they could result in medical record modification, unauthorised access to private health information, or disruption of device functionality [2]. Furthermore, the inherent remote monitoring and control capabilities of IoMT devices pose problems to cloud-based infrastructure security and remote device management, requiring strict procedures to prevent unauthorised access and manipulation [26]. To tackle these obstacles, a holistic strategy is needed, which includes strong encryption procedures, continual surveillance, standardised security guidelines, and continuing instruction to promote a cybersecurity-aware culture in the quickly changing IoMT environment.

Cyber threats have the potential to have a wide range of negative effects on healthcare settings, including patient safety, data privacy, and the general operation of healthcare systems [27]. Cyberattacks that manipulate or interfere with medical devices directly endanger patient safety, especially in situations involving critical care [28]. Unauthorised access to patient records can result in data breaches and privacy violations, which can compromise patient confidence in healthcare providers to protect their private information and cause fraud and identity theft [29]. Cyber threats, such as ransomware attacks, have the potential to interfere with vital healthcare functions, making it more difficult for medical personnel to access patient records and to provide timely care [27].

The financial ramifications are significant and include possible legal and regulatory fines as well as the expenses of defending against attacks, recovering systems, and putting stronger cybersecurity measures in place [30]. Attacks on the infrastructure supporting healthcare can jeopardise public health as well as patient care, particularly in an emergency [28]. Theft of intellectual property, including patented designs or medical research obtained without authorisation, reduces competition and might have wider social repercussions [20]. Most importantly, people may be deterred from seeking medical attention and from providing correct information to healthcare providers as a result of the confidence that is being destroyed by cybersecurity breaches, which might affect public health [21]. A thorough and proactive cybersecurity approach, including risk assessments, cutting-edge cybersecurity solutions, continuing education for medical professionals, and constant monitoring to identify and address emerging cyber threats, is needed to address these possible outcomes.

Blockchains based on Directed Acyclic Graphs (DAGs) are a novel and exciting advancement in the field of distributed ledger technology [31]. The DAG blockchain design presents a non-linear, acyclic structure that has distinct benefits in comparison to conventional blockchain systems that depend on a linear structure [32]. We explore the fundamental ideas of DAG-based blockchains, emphasising their potential to address some of the issues that traditional blockchain systems encounter. The conventional blockchain employs a sequential sequence of blocks, every one of which has a collection of transactions, as demonstrated by digital currencies such as Ethereum and Bitcoin [33]. This linear structure limits scalability and transaction speed even if it is good at ensuring security and transparency. By adopting a decentralised and non-sequential structure, DAG overcomes these drawbacks and promotes a more effective and scalable method of reaching consensus [34].

The lack of a single, linear chain is fundamental to DAG-based blockchains. Alternatively, each transaction validates and approves two preceding transactions in a directed acyclic network [35]. Because of this structure, transactions can happen concurrently and miners are not required, increasing its throughput in general [36]. The Tangle, which is employed by IOTA, a cryptocurrency created especially for the Internet of Things (IoT), is one of the noteworthy applications of DAG [37]. By involving users in the validation process, the Tangle develops a decentralised, self-sustaining ecosystem [38]. In contrast to conventional proof-of-work or proof-of-stake systems, this one lessens the need for devoted miners and might allay worries about centralisation [39].

DAG-based blockchains have several benefits, such as better confirmation speeds, lower transaction costs, and more scalability. Their characteristics render them especially appropriate for usage in nascent technologies such as real-time transaction processing and the IoT. The inventive and decentralised characteristics of DAG-based blockchains come to light as a viable way to meet the changing needs of diverse industries and applications as we investigate the landscape of blockchain technologies. As the IoMT continues to revolutionise healthcare, the increasing interconnectivity of medical devices poses significant cybersecurity challenges. Existing security measures often struggle to adapt to the dynamic nature of IoMT, leading to vulnerabilities in data integrity, secure communication, and access control. Traditional blockchain architectures face scalability issues in handling the growing volume of health data generated by IoMT devices. This problem statement highlights the need for a tailored cybersecurity solution. DAG-based blockchains show promise in addressing these challenges by offering scalability, efficient access control, and dynamic adaptability. However, a comprehensive understanding of how to harness the full potential of DAG-based blockchains for enhanced cybersecurity in IoMT is lacking. This research aims to bridge this gap by investigating and developing robust, secured, scalable, and efficient cybersecurity mechanisms leveraging DAG-based blockchains to secure the IoMT.

20.1.1 Key contributions of the chapter

The key contribution of this chapter is the development of an access control mechanism, which is a ground-breaking development in the security and scalability of the IoMT. This novel contribution marks a significant advancement in addressing the complex challenges related to securing medical data and guaranteeing the smooth expansion of IoMT networks. By introducing an inventive access control mechanism, the chapter not only improves the overall cybersecurity posture of IoMT but also establishes a scalable and resilient ecosystem. This significant development is to have a broad impact and establish an innovative standard for protecting private health data in the dynamic rapidly evolving IoMT ecosystem.

20.1.2 Chapter organisation

The chapter begins with a thorough introduction to the IoMT in Section 20.1, emphasising the critical need for comprehensive cybersecurity measures in this constantly changing and dynamic environment. To properly solve the severe security concerns that IoMT systems face, this section proposes DAG-based blockchains as a novel and promising solution. This introduction carefully defines the research challenge and highlights how crucial the proposed study is to achieving the overall goals of protecting sensitive medical data in a healthcare setting that is becoming more linked. The introduction provides a foundational framework, laying the groundwork for further sections that explore the nuances of DAG-based blockchains, methods, results, and discussions. These sections come to a thorough conclusion that enumerates the main findings and implications of the research. A thorough examination of pertinent works is offered in Section 20.2, which thoroughly examines the body of research on DAG-based blockchains and cybersecurity in IoMT. This important section provides a comprehensive knowledge of the state of research currently and highlights gaps that the current study aims to fill by critically analysing important papers, techniques, and conclusions. The foundations of DAG-Based blockchains are explained in Section 20.3, which provides a thorough examination of their architectures, consensus processes, and incorporation of quantum-resistant cryptographic techniques. The study approach, experimental design, and application of the suggested access control mechanism are all described in great depth in the methodology section of Section 20.4, which offers an open and honest description of the procedures used. Elapsed Time *vs.* Number of Nodes, Access Rate *vs.* Number of Nodes, and Throughput *vs.* Number of Nodes are just a few of the important performance metrics that are evaluated as the implementation results are presented and analysed in Section 20.5 with ease. Section 20.6 summarises the discoveries and modifications made while reflecting on the study process and the lessons learned. Based on research findings, strategic recommendations are presented in Section 20.7 to assist IoMT stakeholders in deploying DAG-based blockchains for improved cybersecurity and to identify possible directions for future investigation. Section 20.8 concludes the chapter by highlighting major contributions, conclusions, and wider ramifications. This section serves as a coherent conclusion to the investigation of improved cybersecurity in IoMT.

20.2 Review of related works

A promising approach to improving cybersecurity in healthcare settings is the use of DAG-based blockchains in the context of the IoMT. To handle the particular difficulties brought about by the growing integration of linked medical devices, several academics and business professionals have investigated the junction of DAG-based blockchains with IoMT. Here, we offer a concise synopsis of relevant research in this area, emphasising investigations and advancements that advance knowledge and the application of DAG-based blockchains for IoMT cybersecurity. Table 20.1 gives a summary review of related works.

20.2.1 Gap analysis

Healthcare cybersecurity has advanced significantly with the incorporation of DAG-based blockchains into the IoMT framework. As IoMT develops as a crucial

Table 20.1 Review of related works

Reference	Description of work done	Limitations of the work
[40]	They examined the application of Tangle in IoMT security and how its functionalities improve data integrity and safe protocols for medical device connection.	Inadequate empirical support; issues with scalability in large networks.
[41]	Studied the use of smart contracts in DAG-based blockchains to provide sophisticated access control for the medical field. Smart contract-encoded permissions and access controls.	Lack of standardised frameworks for smart contracts; possible intricacy.
[42]	Investigated decentralised identity solutions for better user identification and authorisation in IoMT within DAG-based blockchains. Examined models of self-sovereign identity.	Inadequate investigation of scalability issues; obstacles related to regulations.
[43]	Investigated DAG consensus techniques, such as asynchronous Byzantine fault tolerance (aBFT), to address issues with scalability in the IoMT networks.	Dependency on theoretical frameworks; possible implementation challenges.
[44]	Explored dynamic permissioning frameworks that enable real-time modifications to access permissions on DAG-based blockchains for IoMT. Adjusted to modifications in user responsibilities or device features.	Restricted use in the actual world and possible resistance to dynamic modifications.
[45]	Presented example studies and implementations demonstrating the viability of DAG-based blockchains in actual Internet of Medical Things situations. Highlighted advancements in access control, secure communication, and data integrity.	Variable results in various healthcare environments; standardisation is necessary.
[46]	Investigated the use of Tangle in IoMT to provide safe, instantaneous data exchange. Examined the effects on the accessibility and integrity of healthcare data.	Restricted scalability testing with a focus on particular use cases in large-scale IoMT deployments.
[47]	Looked into the security of medical IoT devices using DAG-based blockchains. Suggested an innovative consensus technique to improve security and shorten the time it takes for transactions to be confirmed.	Limited empirical backing and possible difficulties in implementing new consensus-building techniques.
[48]	Investigated the use of DAG smart contracts to create granular access control for IoMT devices.	Complex logic execution difficulties on devices with limited resources and possible latency.

(Continues)

Table 20.1 Review of related works (Continued)

Reference	Description of work done	Limitations of the work
[49]	Developed a lightweight and scalable mechanism, to maintain the identity of IoT devices and access control of large-scale IoT data, the author proposes a distributed ledger technology (IOTA) with low energy consumption. This will help to assure source dependability and sharing security of IoT data.	Limited investigation of practical implementation issues.
[50]	A blockchain-based architectural solution for scalable reconfiguration of huge IoT devices is proposed in this article. To reduce resource utilisation, the IoT devices are decoupled from the blockchain processes via an event-based publish/subscribe method via a REST API.	Limited assessment in IoT environments that are dynamic and change quickly; possible latency problems.
[51]	Proposes a blockchain-based device registration algorithm to improve transaction security and scalability.	Heavyweight, inadequate mitigation and detection mechanism.
[52]	Presented a thorough analysis of case studies using DAG-based blockchains in IoMT. Examined the advantages and difficulties in practice, focusing on data security and integrity results.	Variable outcomes in various healthcare environments; possible problems with interoperability.
[53]	Examined the security ramifications of blockchains based on DAG in the context of IoT in healthcare. Investigated possible weaknesses and suggested fixes to improve overall cybersecurity.	Limited coverage of real-world attack scenarios; possible bias in favour of particular security features.
[44]	Investigated using DAG consensus techniques in IoMT to overcome issues with scalability. Assessed the efficiency and performance improvements in the processing of healthcare data in real-time.	Insufficient attention to energy consumption in IoMT devices with limited resources; possible network overhead.
[54]	Examined the use of DAG for transparent and safe exchange of health data. Suggested a DAG-based system for safe interoperability between various healthcare providers.	Insufficient investigation of difficulties related to regulatory compliance; and possible discrepancies in data types.
[2]	Investigated how to secure supply chains for medical devices using DAG-based blockchains. Looked into how DAG can improve medical device integrity, lower counterfeiting, and improve traceability.	Inadequate focus on the real-time components of IoMT; possible obstacles in supplier adoption.

(Continues)

Table 20.1 Review of related works (Continued)

Reference	Description of work done	Limitations of the work
[55]	Examined how secure patient-centric healthcare records might be created using DAG. Suggested a decentralised, unchangeable method for handling patient data, and resolving issues with data ownership.	Inadequate investigation of user-centred design; possible opposition from conventional healthcare systems.
[56]	Investigated how to improve the security and privacy of health data stored in IoMT using DAG. Looked at consensus processes and cryptographic solutions to guarantee private and unchangeable data.	Cryptographic processes pay little attention to computational cost, which could harm device performance.
[57]	Explored integrating DAG with secure, auditable medical billing systems. Examined how DAG might help provide tamper-proof, transparent records for financial activities related to healthcare.	Inadequate investigation of billing systems' conformity with regulations; possible opposition from well-established financial systems.

component of healthcare ecosystems, improved cybersecurity protocols are essential. This section evaluates the current IoMT cybersecurity situation and points out gaps that can be filled by utilising DAG-based blockchains, highlighting how crucial these blockchains are to reducing current issues. There are many obstacles in the way of IoMT cybersecurity right now. The fast growth of connected medical equipment frequently outpaces traditional security safeguards, creating gaps that bad actors might take advantage of. Data integrity issues, problems with secure transmission, and the possibility of unauthorised access to private health information are significant challenges. Innovative solutions that can adjust to the dynamic and linked nature of IoMT are required to meet these problems.

When utilised with IoMT, traditional blockchain architectures—like those seen in well-known cryptocurrencies—have scalability problems. The transaction constraints caused by the linear structure and reliance on miners impede the real-time processing requirements of IoMT. DAG-based blockchains are a gap-filling option because of their built-in scalability and efficiency gains. By enabling parallel transaction processing, they reduce latency and can handle the growing amount of data produced by IoMT devices. This is enlightening to examine DAG consensus algorithms for IoMT scalability. However, there is a gap in the scant attention paid to energy usage, particularly in IoMT devices with low resources. To ensure sustainable and useful implementations, future research should examine how DAG-based consensus processes affect the energy efficiency of IoMT devices. Safeguarding patient data and preserving privacy in IoMT requires strong access control methods. The dynamic nature of healthcare environments, where responsibilities and permissions can change quickly, is a challenge for existing solutions.

Access control on DAG-based blockchains, especially those with smart contracts integrated, can be programmed and decentralised.

Automating authorisation procedures closes the gap and guarantees that only legitimate organisations have access to and the ability to alter sensitive health data. Rapid changes are possible in the IoMT environment, including the addition of new devices, updates for already-existing ones, and changes in security risks. It might be difficult for conventional security measures to quickly adjust to these changes. DAG-based blockchains can close this gap by offering a flexible and adaptable cybersecurity framework thanks to their decentralised consensus methods and dynamic authorisation systems. This guarantees that defences against new attacks and modifications to the IoMT environment can adapt in real-time. The suggestion of decentralised identity solutions within DAG for enhanced user authentication in IoMT highlights a vacuum in the scant investigation of practical implementation issues, such as user acceptability and regulatory compliance. To guarantee that decentralised identification systems comply with legal standards and win the confidence of users in healthcare contexts, future research should fill in these areas.

Blockchains based on DAGs are emerging as a critical way to close the holes in IoMT cybersecurity that currently exist. DAG is positioned as an effective and customised cybersecurity solution for the changing difficulties in healthcare due to its intrinsic qualities, which include scalability, efficiency, programmable access control, and dynamic flexibility. In addition to filling in the gaps, integrating DAG-based blockchains into IoMT lays the groundwork for a safe, open, and robust healthcare ecosystem. DAG-based blockchains must be incorporated as IoMT develops to guarantee the availability, confidentiality, and integrity of sensitive health data. The gap analysis highlights the necessity of focused research initiatives to overcome certain constraints noted in Table 20.1. By addressing these shortcomings, the IoMT integration of DAG-based blockchains can be optimised to offer scalable, standardised, and energy-efficient cybersecurity solutions, supporting the IoMT' safe and robust expansion.

20.3 Fundamentals of DAG-based blockchains

The DAG is a data structure made up of nodes connected by edges. As shown in Figure 20.1, each edge has a direction and is not a cycle. The structure of a distributed ledger is represented by a DAG in the context of blockchain technology. DAG adds an acyclic, non-linear structure to typical blockchains, which are linear and made up of blocks connected in a chain [45].

Each transaction is represented as a node in a DAG-based blockchain, and instead of having a predetermined order of blocks, transactions are connected directly [49]. Put more simply, as shown in Figure 20.1, every transaction approves two preceding ones, resulting in a branching and connected structure that does not require a central chain. Transactions can be handled concurrently rather than sequentially with this structure.

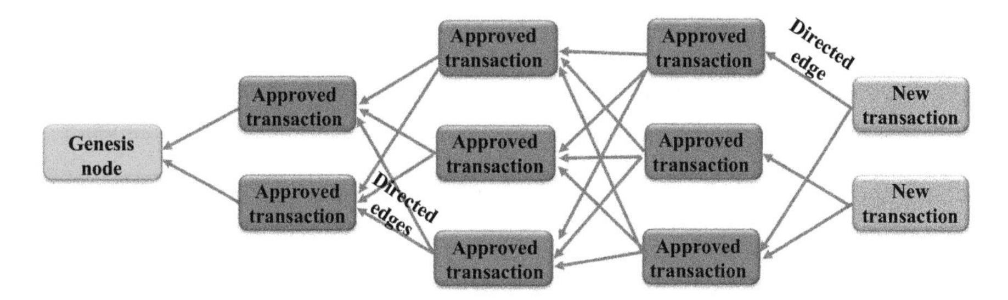

Figure 20.1 DAG network

An important property of a DAG is that it is a finite directed graph structure with nodes connected by directed edges but no cycles. Because of its acyclic structure, the network lacks any closed loops or circular node sequences [58]. The elements of a DAG are specified in formal terms as follows:

(a) Nodes (Vertices)
A DAG is made up of several nodes, also known as vertices. In the graph, every node denotes a distinct element or item.

(b) Edges
In a graph, edges are connections that are directed between nodes. Each edge indicates how information flows from one node to another. The directionality guarantees that a closed loop or cycle cannot form inside the graph.

(c) Directedness
A DAG has directed edges, which have a head as the terminal node and a tail as the starting node. Directionality denotes a connection or interdependence among nodes.

(d) Acyclic nature
The acyclic structure of a DAG is one of its distinguishing features. This indicates that no closed loops are formed by node sequences connected by directed edges. There is a distinct directionality, and following the boundaries of a cycle will not allow one to complete it.

A DAG can be formally expressed mathematically as a pair (V, E), where:

V is the set of nodes or vertices.
E is the set of directed edges, each defined as an ordered pair (u, v), where u is the tail node, and v is the head node.

In a DAG, the absence of cycles introduces specific features and ramifications:

(a) Topological ordering
A topological ordering of a DAG allows the nodes to be organised in a linear sequence so that, for each directed edge, (u, v), in the ordering, node u is ahead of node v. For a DAG, this topological ordering is distinct.

(b) Dependency representation
Dependencies and relationships between various elements are often represented using DAGs. A DAG, for instance, can be used to describe jobs and

their dependencies in project management, guaranteeing that no task is dependent on another in a cyclic fashion.

(c) Efficient data structures
Because DAGs are acyclic, efficient data structures and processing techniques can be used to navigate and manipulate the graph. Topological ordering is one algorithm that may be used to analyse and work with the graph quickly.

A finite collection of nodes (vertices) and a set of directed edges linking these nodes constitute the formal representation of a DAG. The graph is guaranteed to include no closed loops or circular dependencies if there are no cycles.

(a) Mathematical representation
A DAG is mathematically represented as a pair (V, E), where:
V is the set of nodes or vertices.
E is the set of directed edges, each defined as an ordered pair *(u, v), where:*
u is the tail node, and
v is the head node.

Mathematically

$$DAG = (V, E)$$
$$V = \{v_1, v_2, \ldots, v_n\}$$
$$E = \{(u_1, v_1), (u_2, v_2), \ldots, (u_m, v_m)\}$$

(b) Directedness
Each directed edge *(u, v)* signifies a directed connection from node *u* to node *v*. The directionality of edges establishes a clear order and dependency relationship between nodes.

(c) Acyclic property
The absence of closed loops or cycles in the graph is guaranteed by the acyclic property. Formally, if there may not be a directed path that begins and ends at the same node, a DAG is acyclic.

Mathematically
$\nexists$ the directed path from *vi* to v_j such that $v_i = v_j$

(d) Topological ordering
The topological ordering of a DAG yields a linear sequence of nodes such that node *u* appears before node *v* in the ordering for each directed edge (u, v). For a DAG, topological ordering is distinct.

Mathematically:
$\forall$ *(u,v)*$\in$ *E*, Node *u* comes before node *v*.

20.3.1 Advantages of DAG structures over traditional blockchains

A structured overview in Table 20.2 outlines and briefly explains these benefits, showcasing how DAG introduces novel solutions to common challenges in

Table 20.2 Advantages of DAG structures over traditional blockchains

Benefit	**Explanation**
Scalability [49]	Scalability issues are a common problem for traditional blockchains, particularly as the network expands. Consensus regarding the transaction order is necessary for the linear structure, which could result in bottlenecks. By enabling concurrent and independent transactions, DAG improves scalability by doing away with the requirement for a single chain and the related consensus constraints.
Efficiency and Throughput [49]	Traditional blockchains frequently experience scalability problems, especially as the network grows. The linear structure requires agreement on the transaction order, which could lead to bottlenecks. By eliminating the need for a single chain and the associated consensus limitations, DAG increases scalability by permitting concurrent and independent transactions.
Decentralisation [39]	A more decentralised consensus process is frequently encouraged by DAG structures. Concerns with centralisation may arise from the fact that traditional blockchains could depend on miners or validators to validate transactions. The approval-based paradigm of DAG encourages a more dispersed and cooperative method of reaching an agreement because transactions verify earlier transactions.
Reduced Transaction Fees [57]	Transaction costs are lowered in DAG because there is less competition for block space due to the concurrent nature of transactions. Users on traditional blockchains can bid more to get their transactions added to the next block as soon as possible. Naturally, this competitive fee environment is mitigated by the structure of DAG.
Dynamic Consensus Mechanism [43]	A more adaptable and dynamic consensus process is made possible by DAG. The consensus algorithms used by traditional blockchains such as Proof of Work or Proof of Stake are frequently inflexible. Different techniques can be used in DAG to reach an agreement, and the structure allows for future enhancements and adjustments to account for shifting network conditions.
Resistance to Centralization [39]	Because DAG does not have a single chain, there is less possibility of centralisation, which occurs when strong mining companies control the order in which transactions are completed. The decentralised philosophy of blockchain technology is supported by this feature.

(Continues)

Table 20.2 Advantages of DAG structures over traditional blockchains (Continued)

Benefit	Explanation
Adaptability to the Internet of Things (IoT) and Real-time Systems [49]	Because of its scalability and efficiency, DAG is particularly well-suited for real-time systems and the Internet of Things (IoT), where processing transactions quickly and concurrently is essential.
Energy Efficiency [59]	In general, DAG topologies use less energy than conventional Proof of Work (PoW) blockchain consensus techniques. Energy-intensive mining operations are a feature of traditional Proof of Work (PoW) blockchains; however, DAG-based systems frequently use more energy-efficient consensus algorithms, making them more environmentally friendly.
Resistance to 51% Attacks [44]	Conventional blockchains are susceptible to 51% attacks, in which the ledger is manipulated by a malevolent party possessing more than half of the network's processing power. Because DAG does not utilise a single point of control and instead uses distributed consensus, it is more resistant to these kinds of assaults.
Asynchronous Validation [49]	Transactions can be validated asynchronously (i.e., without requiring confirmation from the entire network) thanks to DAG. This is in contrast to traditional blockchains, where synchronisation is frequently necessary for the consensus, potentially delaying the validation of transactions.
Adaptive Block Sizes [60]	The block size in DAG-based systems is not fixed. Because of its flexibility, the network may grow more naturally in response to demand. During times of high activity, traditional blockchains may find it difficult to alter block sizes, which could affect transaction throughput.
No Mining Competition [57]	In traditional blockchains, transactions are validated and new blocks are added by miners competing to solve challenging mathematical puzzles. The approval-based paradigm in DAG reduces the resource-intensiveness of traditional blockchain mining by doing away with the requirement for competitive mining.
Reduced Latency [49]	The structure of DAG minimises latency and reduces transaction confirmation times because of its parallel processing capability. Applications that need responses in real-time, such as those in the Internet of Things (IoT) and healthcare systems, would especially benefit from this.
Tamper Resistance [44]	Due to its interconnectedness, DAG is less susceptible to manipulation or backward modifications. Every transaction builds a visible and tamper-evident record of the transaction history by explicitly referencing and validating earlier transactions.

distributed ledger systems. In this section, we explore and highlight the key advantages of DAG structures over traditional blockchains. DAG structures have emerged as a compelling alternative to traditional blockchain architectures, offering a range of advantages that address some of the inherent limitations in linear blockchain designs.

With a wide range of benefits, DAG architectures are a strong contender to replace conventional blockchains. Because of these characteristics, DAG is ideally suited to meet the changing requirements of a wide range of applications, including those that call for improved cybersecurity safeguards in dynamic, networked systems like the IoMT.

20.3.2 Consensus algorithms in DAG-based blockchains, with a focus on tangle

Revolutionary consensus techniques, distinct from the conventional Proof of Work (PoW) or Proof of Stake (PoS) algorithms typically observed in blockchain systems, are introduced by DAG architectures. In particular, Tangle the consensus mechanism connected to IOTA. An asynchronous approval mechanism powers the Tangle consensus mechanism [49]. The DAG structure is a dynamic web of approvals, with each transaction approving two before it. Tangle lacks miners and set blocks, in contrast to conventional blockchains [61]. The Tangle receives transactions asynchronously, and the consensus is reached when the transactions confirm one another. Revolutionary consensus techniques, distinct from the conventional PoW or PoS algorithms typically observed in blockchain systems, are introduced by DAG architectures. In particular, Tangle the consensus mechanism connected to IOTA, is highlighted as we delve into the consensus algorithms found in DAG-based blockchains [60]. An asynchronous approval mechanism powers the Tangle consensus mechanism. The DAG structure is a dynamic web of approvals, with each transaction approving two before it [37]. Tangle lacks miners and set blocks, in contrast to conventional blockchains. The Tangle receives transactions asynchronously, and the consensus is reached when the transactions confirm one another [49].

Tangle stands out for its ability to enable parallel transaction validation. The network can validate more transactions at once with greater capacity as more transactions take place. Tangle is different from other blockchain models in that it sequentially processes data. This is due to its inherent scalability [57]. By doing away with the requirement for miners, the consensus mechanism of Tangle significantly deviates from conventional blockchain conventions. Rather, through the approval of earlier transactions, users take an active part in the validation process [43]. In addition to improving security, this decentralised validation removes transaction fees, creating a more affordable environment [39].

Tangle includes quantum-resistant cryptographic techniques, including the Winternitz one-time signature scheme, to counter growing risks from quantum computing. This calculated action protects the network from future quantum assaults by guaranteeing the strength of the cryptographic layer that underpins the consensus process. Tangle uses an adaptive PoW technique for every transaction to prevent spam transactions [60]. By prioritising genuine transactions and discouraging hostile actors, this lightweight PoW requirement enhances the network's overall security and dependability. One important accomplishment of the consensus method Tangle is decentralisation, which is achieved by active user involvement. By approving transactions, each user becomes a crucial component of ensuring network safety and consensus, supporting the idea of a decentralised and cooperative ecosystem [43]. Tangle offers novel approaches, but there are drawbacks as well, like the existence of a security "Coordinator" and the possibility of network segmentation. The objective of ongoing research and development endeavours is to tackle these obstacles and augment the general resilience of Tangle as a consensus mechanism.

In DAG-based blockchains, the Tangle consensus algorithm offers a decentralised, scalable, and feeless method of reaching a consensus on transaction validity. In the rapidly changing field of distributed ledger technologies, Tangle is positioned as a novel and exciting consensus mechanism thanks to its removal of miners, parallel validation, and quantum-resistant security characteristics. Tangle is being improved and optimised for a wider range of uses, including possible consequences for cybersecurity in the IoMT, thanks to ongoing research and community contributions.

20.3.3 Evaluation of how DAG characteristics align with the requirements of IoMT

Evaluating the degree to which the properties of DAGs correspond with the needs of the IoMT is essential to comprehending the possible advantages that DAG-based frameworks provide for healthcare systems. We provide a thorough analysis of the compliance of DAG in particular concerning IoMT standards as outlined and explained in Table 20.3. This review focuses on the distinctive qualities of DAG,

Table 20.3 An assessment of the alignment between DAG characteristics and IoMT requirements

IoMT requirement	Alignment with DAG characteristics
Scalability	The parallel processing of DAG satisfies the scalability requirements of IoMT, effectively managing the increasing amount of health data.
Efficiency and Throughput	The parallel processing of DAG increases productivity and efficiency, satisfying the real-time or near-real-time data processing requirements of IoMT.

(Continues)

Table 20.3 An assessment of the alignment between DAG characteristics and IoMT requirements (Continued)

IoMT requirement	Alignment with DAG characteristics
Decentralisation	The consensus processes of DAG encourage decentralisation, which lessens dependency on centralised entities and increases system resilience as a whole.
Security and Resistance to Attacks	Strong security is facilitated by cryptographic methods used by DAG and resilience to 51% of attacks, which is consistent with concern for data security in IoMT.
Adaptive Consensus Mechanism	Because DAG has a flexible consensus algorithm selection process, it can adapt to changing network conditions in the heterogeneous IoMT ecosystem.
Low Transaction Fees	DAG is more cost-effective since it does away with miners and related costs, which is in line with the requirement of IoMT for affordable data exchange.
Quantum-Resistant Security	The integration of quantum-resistant cryptographic algorithms by DAG tackles upcoming security issues in IoMT and is consistent with the proactive stance.
Adaptive Proof of Work for Spam Prevention	By preventing spam and ensuring the integrity of IoMT transactions, DAG satisfies quality and reliability standards through the use of lightweight Proof of Work.
Data Integrity and Tamper Resistance	Data integrity is required by IoMT, and the interconnected structure of DAG and cryptographic methods provide tamper-resistant data.
Interoperability and Device Heterogeneity	Since DAG is flexible and decentralised, it makes it easier for different devices in the IoMT ecosystem to work together.

including security, decentralisation, efficiency, and scalability, and it investigates how these traits directly meet the complex requirements of IoMT. Table 20.3 provides insightful information about the possible uses and benefits of DAG in the rapidly changing medical technology landscape.

Table 20.3 presents a concise synopsis of how the features of DAG correspond with the particular needs of the IoMT.

20.4 Methodology

The IoMT access control mechanism is the main focus of this approach. It is more precisely related to the execution of an IoMT Directed Acyclic Graph-Based Access Control Mechanism. In the context of the IoMT deployments, this approach aims to mitigate the security and scalability issues related to conventional, heavy-weight blockchain-based access control systems by utilising the lightweight characteristics of DAG.

20.4.1 The proposed system

The three key components of the proposed IoMT access control mechanism are device registration, device configuration, and the DAG network (tangle) are covered in this section.

20.4.1.1 Access control mechanism

The IoMT device logs, generates, and updates an access control policy as transactions take place in the tangle ledger, allowing it to uniquely identify each piece of data it receives. The access policy entries in the tangle ledger provide fine-grained access control for device resources. An access request is transmitted by the IoMT device that wishes to use a resource to the node that manages itself. The node finds the resource covered by the access policy and the attribute set of the requester and then verifies that the attribute set conforms to the policy. Following successful verification, the requester receives an authorisation certificate, which is then entered into the tangle ledger. Access to the relevant resources is restricted to the device that possesses the authorisation certificate. Each device will be assigned an authentic identification based on its unique make/brand *ID (D_ID)* and cluster *id (C_ID)* by the Access Control Server (AC). The identity number will be used to provide access, authenticate, register, and configure each device. The IOTA Tangle Network will retain the identity, verification, and transaction data of each device. Any device from any cluster that wishes to send or receive a transaction to or from the DAG Network must first have its registration and configuration details carefully checked to gain or lose access to the system. The entire procedure is illustrated in Figure 20.1.

The proposed system is composed of five different components: IoMT device pool, Gateway (device management hub), device registration unit, device configuration unit, and the DAG network. The device management hub is a unit where device-related operations are handled, which guarantees a secure scalable, and well-organised setting for the wide range of devices linked together in the IoMT ecosystem. Its function is essential to achieving the proposed DAG-Based Access Control's capability in handling the intricacies of access control in a dynamic, networked IoMT ecosystem, while the IoMT Device Pool, as used in the proposed system, is a dynamic, well-organised group of IoMT devices that are controlled and supervised by the access control system. The proposed system infrastructure manages and orchestrates this pool to guarantee safe, effective, and scalable interactions throughout the IoT ecosystem. Device registration and Configuration units are explained in more detail in the following sections.

Device registration

The structure of registering a device is illustrated in Figure 20.2. Creating and maintaining nodes within a DAG structure is the main step in the registration process of a DAG-based device registration system for the IoMT ecosystem, these steps are depicted in Figure 20.3. The graph represents every device in the IoMT network as a node, along with attributes like *device ID*, *type, owner*, and other relevant data. The structure of the graph is acyclic, meaning there are no loops in the relationships. A new node is added to the DAG whenever an IoMT device has

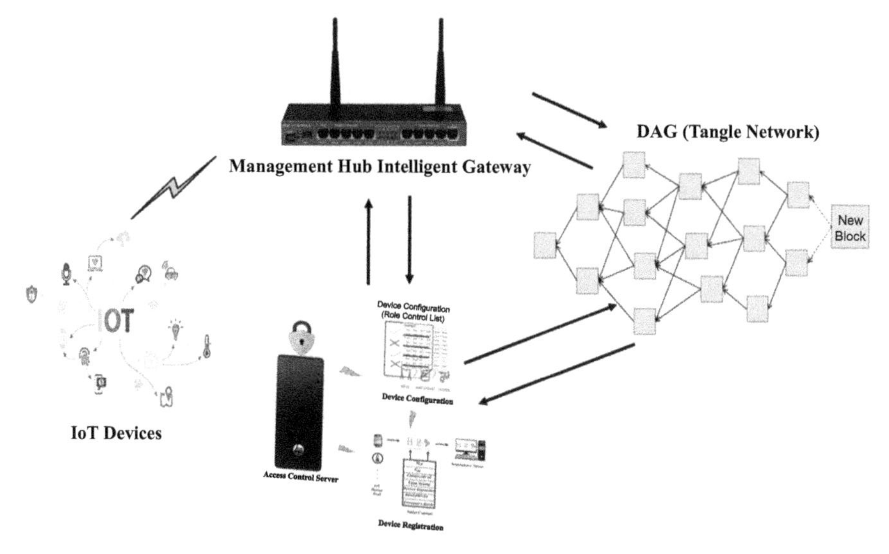

Figure 20.2 Access control mechanism

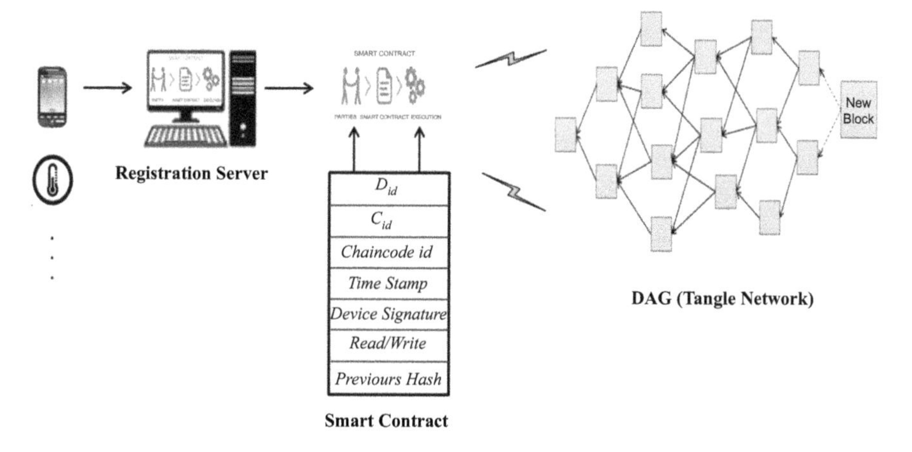

Figure 20.3 Device registration

to be registered. The relationships between this new device node and other pertinent nodes in the graph are then indicated. These connections could be related to ownership, communication channels, or anything else that is thought to be important to the IoMT ecosystem. Information about the device that the node represents is one of its properties. An important factor is the directed relationships in the graph. They stand for communication or control flow. For example, data may be sent from a device to a gateway, but data may not be returned to the device from the gateway. Since different nodes may have varying levels of access, this directed structure naturally accommodates access control. A gateway node may have more control than a user node about the devices that are connected to it.

The system searches the graph during the device registration process to determine where the new device should fit. Finding an appropriate parent node for the new device and verifying access rights are the two tasks involved in this traversal. Before registering the device, the system frequently confirms and validates the accuracy of its information. This could entail verifying ownership information, digital signatures, or other security protocols. Every registration event is recorded in the graph, allowing for the tracking of changes over time and offering an audit trail. By its very nature, the DAG structure facilitates the efficient and logical modelling of links between devices in the IoT ecosystem. It provides a clear hierarchy and supports complicated network topologies. Scalability is incorporated into the architecture of the system so that it can grow with the number of devices in the IoT ecosystem. Moreover, security protocols must be put in place at every stage to guarantee the confidentiality and integrity of the data in the graph.

The IoMT device logs identity information as a transaction into the IOTA network to guarantee the validity of devices engaging in network operations. The transaction record is immutable and the identification cannot be disputed thanks to the curl hash algorithm, which takes an arbitrary ternary value as input and outputs a 243-trit hash. To tie the identity and public key and enable security services like identity authentication and non-repudiation, the node issues a public key certificate to the device upon successful registration. Algorithm 20.1 outlines the basic registration process. If a device consistently engages in harmful activity, the management IoMT device node will send a revocation transaction to the network to remove it from its eligibility to participate in network activities.

Algorithm 20.1 **Name:** DAG-Based Device Registration in IoT Ecosystem

---

Input

(a) *Graph G represents the current state of the IoMT ecosystem.*
(b) *DeviceID, ClusterID, Timestamp, ChaincodeID, DeviceSignature, and DeviceHash are the registration details.*

Output

(a) *Updated graph G with the new device added.*

Steps

1. *Create a new node for the NewDevice in the DAG*
   CreateNode(DeviceID, ClusterID, Timestamp, ChaincodeID, DeviceSignature, DeviceHash)
2. *Perform Validation*
   If IsValid (DeviceID, ClusterID, Timestamp, ChaincodeID, DeviceSignature, DeviceHash)

Proceed to Step 3
- Else
Display Error Message
Exit Registration Process

3. *Traverse the Graph to Find a Suitable Location:*
   parent = TraverseGraph(G, DeviceID)
4. *Update the Graph*
   AddNodeToGraph (G, DeviceID, ClusterID, Timestamp, ChaincodeID, DeviceSignature, DeviceHash, parent)
5. *Log the Registration Event*
   LogEvent ("Device Registered", DeviceID, ClusterID, Timestamp, ChaincodeID, DeviceSignature, DeviceHash)
6. *Return Updated Graph*

Return G

A new node is created in the DAG to represent the device to be registered, which is one of the few crucial processes in the pseudocode for device registration. Important details like *DeviceID*, *ClusterID*, *Timestamp*, *ChaincodeID*, *DeviceSignature*, and DeviceHash are all included in the node. The *CreateNode* method helps do this. The *IsValid* method is used to validate the registration details. If the information is correct, the process of registration continues; if not, an error message appears and the process is terminated. The graph is traversed to locate the new device in an appropriate location. The parent node that the new device ought to be linked to is provided by the *TraverseGraph function*. Based on the traversal result, the new device node is added to the graph and relationships are made with existing nodes. For this, the *AddNodeToGraph* method is used. The device registration event is recorded in an event log along with information about the device, including its ID, *cluster ID*, *timestamp*, *chaincode ID*, device signature, and device hash. This is made possible using the *LogEvent* function. The final step involves returning the updated graph, denoted as G, with the newly registered device. The systematic process for adding a new device to the DAG is described in the pseudocode. It involves node creation, registration detail validation, and graph traversal for an appropriate position, graph updating, registration event logging, and graph return. Together, these actions provide a strong and organised method for registering devices with the DAG-based access control system.

Device configuration

After a successful registration, configuration will take place. The goal is to have the DAG Network act as a root trust for all communications between the administrator and the IoMT devices. The system will scale extremely well with this design as well. *Cluster-ID*, *Device ID*, *Configuration Status (Submit, Commit, and Error)*, Configuration Update, Module Configuration, and Module Configuration Status (*indicating the status of the update on the module*) are the details that need to be configured. These setup parameters will be kept in the DAG network. Allowing devices to complete the task allocated to them is the heart of device setup. Algorithm 20.2 outlines the fundamental step of configuring any IoT device, and Figure 20.4 is the sequence flow which illustrates how those steps are carried out. The device configuration is described in Figure 20.5, and the device configuration sequence flow is given in Figure 20.6.

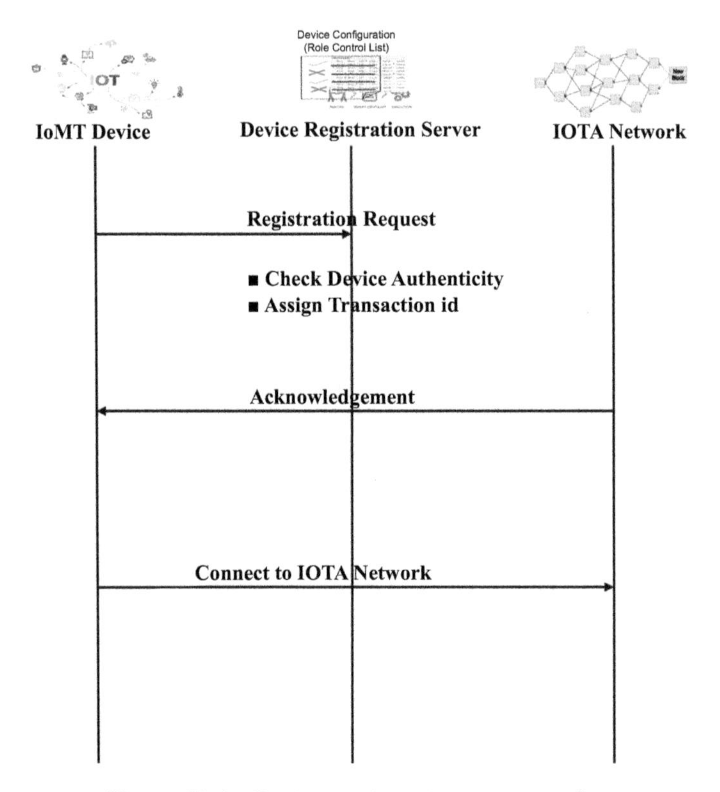

Figure 20.4 Device registration sequence flow

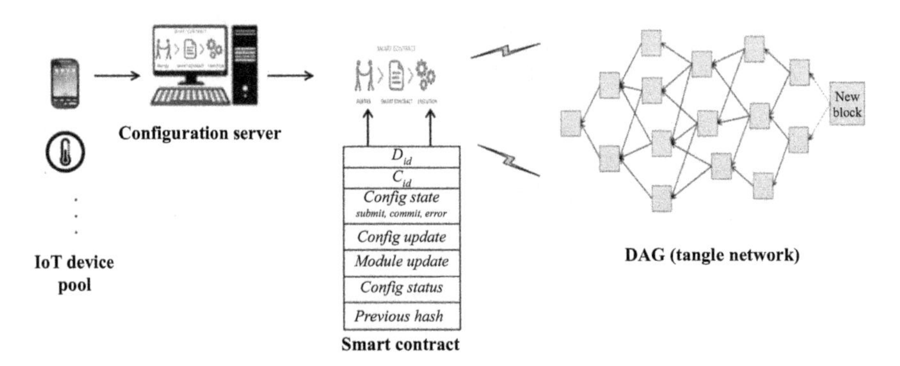

Figure 20.5 Device configuration

Algorithm 20.2 **Name:** *DAG-Based Device Configuration in IoT Ecosystem*

Inputs

(a) *Graph G represents the current state of the IoT ecosystem.*
(b) *DeviceID specifies the device to be configured.*
(c) *ClusterID, ConfigStatus, ConfigUpdate, ModuleConfig, and ModuleConfigStatus provide configuration details.*

Outputs

(a) *Updated graph G with the updated device configuration.*

Steps

1. *Find the Device Node in the DAG*
   deviceNode = FindDeviceNode(G, DeviceID)
2. *Update Configuration Details*
   SetNodeAttributes(deviceNode, ClusterID, ConfigStatus, ConfigUpdate, ModuleConfig, ModuleConfigStatus)
3. *Log the Configuration Event*
   LogEvent("Device Configuration Updated", DeviceID, ClusterID, ConfigStatus, ConfigUpdate, ModuleConfig, ModuleConfigStatus, CurrentTime())
4. *Return Updated Graph*

Return G

In an IoMT ecosystem DAG-based device configuration system, the procedure entails creating a graph structure in which nodes stand for individual devices. Configuration settings, status data, and other facts are contained in each node. The DAG format allows for dynamic configuration modifications, and relationships between nodes show dependencies and linkages between devices. Access control techniques within the DAG determine authorisation for device configuration. To ensure that only allowed modifications are done, configuration changes are validated. System responsiveness and scalability are enhanced by the DAG structure, which makes configuration information retrieval and querying more efficient. The entire functionality and integrity of the IoMT ecosystem are improved by fault tolerance, security measures, and the smooth integration of device registration and setup.

The DAG node that represents the device to be configured must be located to begin the device setup pseudocode. The FindDeviceNode function accomplishes this by iterating across the graph and returning the node that corresponds to the given device. The configuration details, such as *ClusterID*, *ConfigStatus*, *ConfigUpdate*, *ModuleConfig*, and *ModuleConfigStatus*, are updated after the device node has been found. For this, the *SetNodeAttributes* method is used. After the configuration details are updated, an event log is made to document the

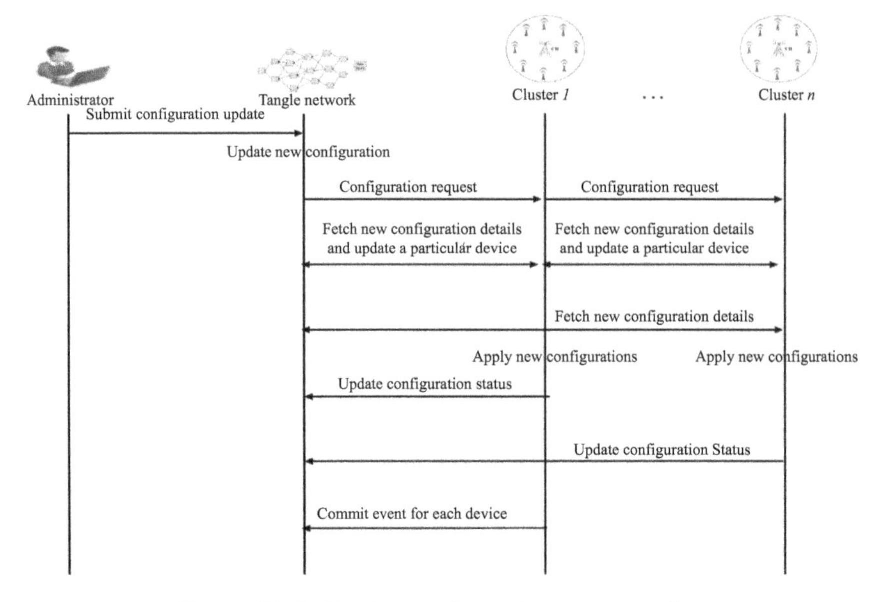

Figure 20.6 Device configuration sequence flow

modifications. *EventType* ("Device Configuration Updated"), DeviceID, *ClusterID*, *ConfigStatus*, *ConfigUpdate*, *ModuleConfig*, *ModuleConfigStatus*, and the current Timestamp are among the details included in this work. Returning the adjusted configuration along with the updated graph, G is the last step. A systematic approach to device configuration within the DAG-based access control mechanism is described in the pseudocode. Finding the device node, modifying configuration information, recording the configuration event, and then providing the revised graph are all included. Together, these actions create a methodical and thorough procedure for setting devices inside the DAG framework.

20.5 Results and discussion

This section is crucial for outlining and illustrating the outcomes of the access control system implementation within the IoMT ecosystem. Table 20.4 summarises the empirical results, discusses their consequences, and offers a thorough understanding of how the proposed access control overcomes the difficulties and achieves the desired goals.

The number of nodes in the system, which reflects the size of the IoMT network, is indicated by the number of nodes. The effectiveness of the system is demonstrated by the Elapsed Time, the access and the throughput, which is a measure of the overall efficiency of the system. Figure 20.7 shows a graph of the elapsed time vs. number of nodes. Figure 20.8 gives the access rate vs. number of nodes, and Figure 20.9 presents the throughput vs. number of nodes.

Table 20.4 Performance metrics of access control mechanism with varying number of nodes

Number of nodes	Elapsed time (s)	Access rate (accesses per second)	Throughput (iterations per second)
100	0.0014	697307.3982	697307.3982
200	0.0014	735197.8966	735197.8966
300	0.0019	519675.8766	519675.8766
400	0.0015	670123.6619	670123.6619
500	0.0015	681114.6476	681114.6476

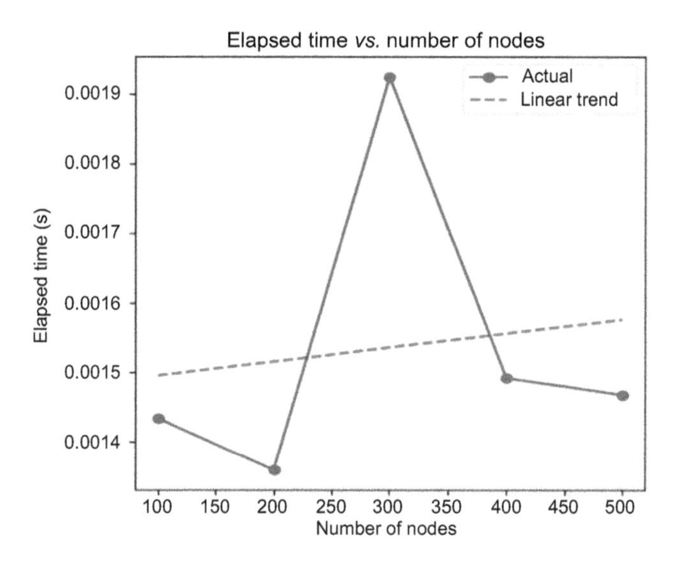

Figure 20.7 Elapsed time vs. number of nodes

20.5.1 Elapsed time vs. number of nodes

Figure 20.7 shows how the number of nodes (devices) and the elapsed time are related. Elapsed time is the amount of time that passes between when an access request is made and when it is either granted or denied. It shows how long it takes the access control system to handle and react to an access request from a device or user. For varying numbers of nodes, the blue markers show the actual data points of elapsed time. The linear trend line fitted to the data points using linear regression is shown by the red dashed line. The y-axis displays the elapsed time in seconds, and the x-axis displays the number of nodes.

20.5.2 Access rate vs. number of nodes

Figure 20.8 illustrates how the number of nodes and the access rate are related. The pace at which access requests are sent to the access control system over a given

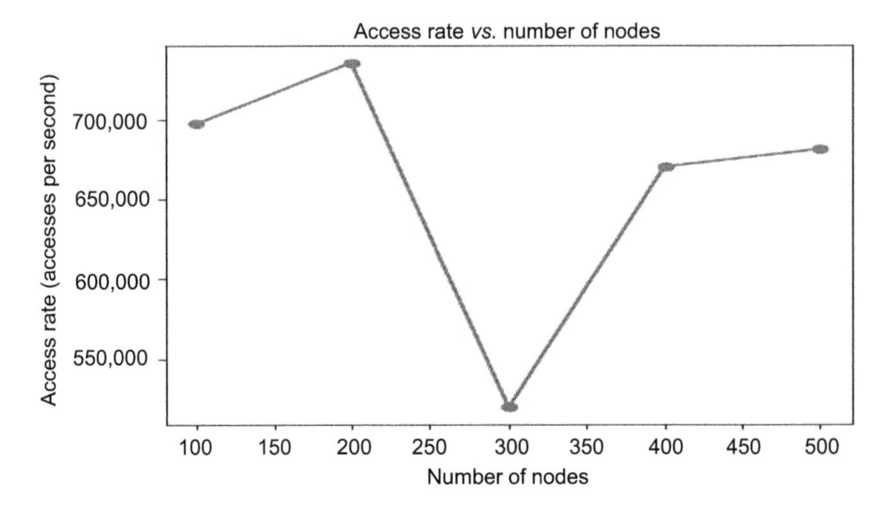

Figure 20.8 Access rate vs. number of nodes

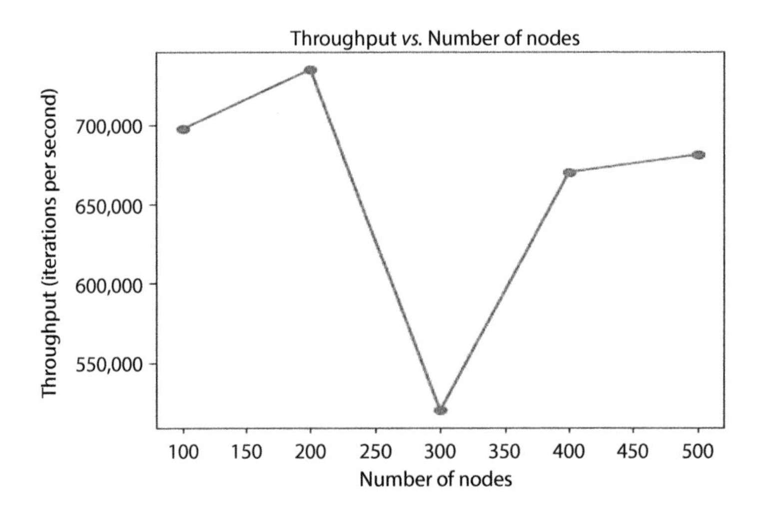

Figure 20.9 Throughput vs. number of nodes

time frame is known as the access rate. Access rate is an important indicator of how frequently users or devices ask for permission to access system resources. The red markers show the access rates for various node counts. The y-axis displays the access rate in accesses per second, while the x-axis displays the number of nodes.

20.5.3 Throughput vs. number of nodes

Figure 20.9 depicts how the number of nodes and the throughput are related. The amount of successful access requests or transactions that the access control system can process in a predetermined amount of time is referred to as throughput. It is a

Table 20.5 Performance comparison with the existing works

Metric number of nodes	Proposed system	Reference [49]	Reference [51]	Reference [52]
100	Efficient processing with low elapsed time, high access rate, and throughput.	Access Rate: HighThroughput: High	Throughput: High	Throughput: High.
200	Consistent performance with minimal elapsed time, high access rate, and throughput.	Access Rate: HighThroughput: High	Throughput: Low	Throughput: High
300	Robust performance with slightly increased elapsed time, maintaining high access rate and throughput.	Access Rate: LowThroughput: Low	Throughput: Low.	Throughput: High
400	Consistent and efficient processing with low elapsed time, maintaining high access rate and throughput.	Access Rate: LowThroughput: Low	Throughput: Low	Throughput: High.
500	Optimal performance with minimal elapsed time, high access rate, and throughput.	Access Rate: LowThroughput: Low	Throughput: Low	Throughput: Low

crucial performance indicator that measures how effectively the system handles and grants access rights. For varying numbers of nodes, the throughput is indicated by the green markers. The number of nodes is displayed on the x-axis and throughput, measured in iterations per second, is displayed on the y-axis.

Table 20.5 presents the performance analysis of the proposed Access control with the existing literature. The analysis shows that the proposed system performs efficiently with varying workloads.

The performance metric that is being compared is indicated by the metric. The measured performance of the proposed access control system for each metric and number of nodes is highlighted in the proposed system. A comprehension of the efficiency and efficacy of the proposed access control system about referenced works is made easier by comparing its performance with current literature across a range of node counts.

The Directed Acyclic Graph-Based Access Control Mechanism performance test results show promising features. The system maintains efficiency regardless of scale, as evidenced by the amazingly consistent elapsed time for access request processing across a range of node numbers. Furthermore, the proposed system can process a significant number of access requests per second because the access rate consistently increases as the number of nodes grows. The high throughput of the proposed system further indicates its ability to manage a substantial volume of access requests. Interestingly, the system maintains high-performance metrics as the number of nodes rises, indicating that the proposed system may grow successfully without seeing a noticeable drop in performance.

The Directed Acyclic Graph-Based Access Control Mechanism system is stable in the IoMT ecosystem. This entails assessing the security of smart contracts, securing

Table 20.6 Security analysis of the proposed access control

Metric	Proposed system	Reference [49]	Reference [50]	Reference [51]
Malicious Node Attack	Robust defence against malicious nodes, efficient detection, and mitigation.	Robust, Efficient detection and Mitigation	Robust,Weak detection and Mitigation	Robust, Weak detection and Mitigation
Spam Attacks	Effective measures to resist and mitigate spam attacks, maintaining network integrity.	Resilience: Strong	Resilience: Weak	Resilience: Weak
Double Spend Attack	Strong defences against double-spend attacks, ensuring secure IoMT transactions.	Double spending attack prevention, system: Strong	Double spending attack prevention, system: Weak	Double spending attack prevention, system: Weak

authentication and authorisation mechanisms for nodes, putting cryptographic safeguards in place to protect medical data integrity and confidentiality, looking into granular access control policies with dynamic updates, assessing resilience against Sybil and denial-of-service attacks, and securely managing user and device identities.

The security analysis of the proposed access control mechanism assesses its robustness against various types of attacks, specifically focusing on malicious node attacks, spam attacks, and double-spend attacks. Comparisons are drawn in Table 20.6 with the findings from reference works [49–51] to highlight the strengths of the proposed system.

20.5.3.1 Malicious node attack

The proposed access control mechanism undergoes a thorough evaluation regarding its resilience to malicious node attacks. This involves scrutinising the system's ability to detect and mitigate attempts by nodes with malicious intent to compromise the integrity of the IoMT network. Comparative analysis with reference [49–51] reveals the effectiveness of the proposed system in thwarting malicious node attacks, showcasing its superior security measures.

20.5.3.2 Spam attacks

The security analysis includes an examination of the proposed access control mechanism's capability to resist spam attacks, where malicious entities flood the network with a large volume of illegitimate transactions. By comparing the system's performance against references [49–51], the analysis highlights the proposed system's robust defences against spam attacks, demonstrating its efficiency in maintaining the integrity and functionality of the IoMT network.

20.5.3.3 Double spend attack

The proposed access control mechanism is scrutinised for its ability to prevent double-spend attacks, a critical consideration in ensuring the integrity of financial transactions within the IoMT ecosystem. The analysis compares the system's resilience to double-spend attacks with the findings from references [49–51], showcasing the proposed system's effectiveness in mitigating this type of attack and providing a secure foundation for IoMT transactions.

The security analysis of the proposed access control mechanism demonstrates its strength in safeguarding against malicious node attacks, spam attacks, and double-spend attacks. Comparative assessments with reference works [49], [50], and [51] underscore the superior security features of the proposed system, positioning it as a robust and reliable solution for ensuring the security and integrity of IoMT transactions in the face of various potential threats.

Metric identifies the particular security metric under comparison. The suggested system emphasises how well the suggested access control system has been observed to function in each relevant parameter. Understanding the strengths of the proposed solution in comparison to the existing works is made easier by comparing it with the existing research on various security metrics.

20.6 Lessons learned

This chapter provides a wealth of information about several facets of cybersecurity in the context of the IoMT. A few of the most important teachings include:

(a) The significance of developing tailored security solutions, especially for the IoMT environment is one of the main lessons learned. The chapter highlights the shortcomings of general cybersecurity measures and the necessity for solutions that take into consideration the particular difficulties and needs of healthcare systems.
(b) To improve cybersecurity in IoMT, the chapter emphasises the significance of investigating cutting-edge technologies like DAG-based blockchains. Examining alternative consensus methods such as Tangle provides important insights into how these technologies can handle issues related to scalability and security.
(c) Efficiency and scalability turn out to be important factors in IoMT cybersecurity. Among the lessons learned is the need to put in place solutions that can handle the increasing amount of medical data while guaranteeing prompt access and processing to properly support healthcare operations.
(d) One important takeaway is how crucial it is for IoMT systems to balance security and usability. Strong security protocols are necessary to protect patient data, but this is also critical to make sure that these protocols avoid making healthcare technologies harder for patients and clinicians to use and access.
(e) The chapter emphasises how cybersecurity risks in IoMT require a proactive response. The necessity of consistently identifying and evaluating such vulnerabilities as well as putting policies in place to reduce risks before bad actors may take advantage of them are among the lessons that have been learned.

(f) IoMT cybersecurity tactics need to be flexible enough to counter new threats as they arise, such as those brought on by cutting-edge technologies like quantum computing. Among the lessons gained is the need to future-proof security systems so that, in the face of changing cyber threats, they continue to be effective.
(g) The chapter concludes by highlighting the significance of legal and ethical issues for IoMT cybersecurity. Among the lessons learned is the necessity of protecting patient privacy and confidentiality while adhering to the laws and guidelines that are pertinent to the security of healthcare data.

Stakeholders interested in IoMT system security can benefit greatly from the lessons learned in this chapter. Through comprehension of the distinct obstacles and possibilities posed by IoMT cybersecurity, institutions can formulate more resilient and efficient security approaches to safeguard patient information and guarantee the integrity of healthcare functions.

20.7 Recommendations

The chapter offers both practical measures and strategic advice for improving cybersecurity in the IoMT. Among the crucial recommendations are:

(a) Embrace DAG-based blockchains to get beyond the drawbacks of conventional blockchain techniques, especially those that use the Tangle consensus mechanism. For increased security and scalability in IoMT, the chapter suggests investigating the advantages of using Tangle as parallel validation, asynchronous approval process, and decentralised user involvement.
(b) Design and implement access control systems designed especially for IoMT environments. The chapter recommends developing access control methods that address the particular needs and difficulties presented by medical data within IoMT systems rather than relying on universal security solutions.
(c) When developing and implementing security solutions for IoMT, give scalability priority. Acknowledge that the amount of medical data produced by linked devices is growing exponentially, and make sure that security measures can adapt to the volume of data without sacrificing effectiveness.
(d) Integrate cryptographic techniques that are resistant to quantum computing in IoMT security protocols. To ensure the long-term robustness of IoMT security, the chapter suggests implementing cryptographic algorithms that can withstand quantum assaults, given the future developments in quantum computing.
(e) Engage users in the validation process to promote decentralisation inside IoMT systems. The chapter suggests creating a cooperative atmosphere where users actively take part in network security, strengthening the distributed nature of the network and its resilience to cybersecurity infrastructure.
(f) Establish an equilibrium between IoMT system usability and strong security measures. The chapter suggests creating security measures that protect patient

information while allowing healthcare technologies to be used and accessed by both patients and physicians.

(g) Encourage interdisciplinary collaboration by bringing together technology developers, cybersecurity specialists, and healthcare practitioners. The chapter suggests interdisciplinary cooperation to create thorough and efficient security plans that comply with cybersecurity best practices and healthcare regulations.

(h) Keep up with the regulations controlling healthcare data security compliance needs. The chapter suggests that to protect patient privacy and preserve the integrity of IoMT activities, ongoing adherence to ethical principles and compliance with pertinent regulations is advised.

(i) To continuously improve and optimise IoMT cybersecurity safeguards, and allocate resources to continuous research and development initiatives. The chapter emphasises how crucial it is to remain ahead of new dangers by doing ongoing research and innovation.

Collectively, these suggestions give stakeholders tasked with protecting IoMT systems a road map that includes concrete actions to strengthen cybersecurity defences, adjust to changing risks, and guarantee the accuracy of medical data in the ever-changing context of the IoMT.

20.8 Conclusions

This chapter has explored the complex world of cybersecurity in the context of the IoMT, offering a progressive solution to the ever-changing problems associated with healthcare data security. Investigating blockchains based on DAGs and concentrating on the Tangle consensus mechanism has revealed novel ideas that have the potential to completely alter the cybersecurity landscape in the medical field. One key development that offers a major improvement in IoMT security and scalability is the development of a tailored access control mechanism. This chapter promotes a decentralised and cooperative approach to medical data security by utilising the special qualities of DAG structures, especially the parallel validation and asynchronous approval mechanism. By incorporating quantum-resistant encryption, future threats are anticipated and a strong defence against developing technologies is ensured. The suggestions made offer useful information that promotes the uptake of DAG-based blockchains, proactive threat detection, and cross-disciplinary cooperation. Maintaining an accurate equilibrium between usability and security, the chapter emphasises how crucial user involvement is in strengthening the IoMT cybersecurity ecosystem. As we head towards a future where healthcare technology becomes more and more important, stakeholders can refer to the lessons gained and suggestions presented in this chapter for guidance. The IoMT community can steer towards a future that is secure and robust, where patient data is protected and healthcare operations flourish in a setting of efficiency and trust, by embracing innovation, scalability, and adaptation.

References

[1] M. Zhao, C. Shi, and Y. Yuan, "Blockchain-Based Lightweight Authentication Mechanisms for Industrial Internet of Things and Information Systems," *International Journal on Semantic Web and Information Systems (IJSWIS)*, vol. 20, no. 1, pp. 1–30, 2024.

[2] J. Tan, J. Shi, J. Wan, H. N. Dai, J. Jin, and R. Zhang, "Blockchain-Based Data Security and Sharing for Resource-Constrained Devices in Manufacturing IoT," *IEEE Internet of Things Journal*, 2024.

[3] D. M. Mathkor, N. Mathkor, Z. Bassfar, *et al.*, "Multirole of the Internet of Medical Things (IoMT) in Biomedical Systems for Managing Smart Healthcare Systems: An Overview of Current and Future Innovative Trends," *Journal of Infection and Public Health*, vol. 17, no. 4, pp. 559–572, 2024.

[4] K. T. Putra, A. Z. Arrayyan, N. Hayati, C. Damarjati, A. Bakar, and H. C. Chen, "A Review on the Application of Internet of Medical Things in Wearable Personal Health Monitoring: A Cloud-Edge Artificial Intelligence Approach," *IEEE Access*, vol. 12, pp. 21437–21452, 2024.

[5] J. B. Awotunde, A. L. Imoize, R. G. Jimoh, *et al.*, "AIoMT Enabling Real-Time Monitoring of Healthcare Systems: Security and Privacy Considerations," *in Handbook of Security and Privacy of AI-Enabled Healthcare Systems and Internet of Medical Things*. London: CRC Press, Taylor & Francis Group, pp. 97–133, 2024.

[6] K. K. Baseer, K. Sivakumar, D. Veeraiah, *et al.*, "Healthcare Diagnostics with an Adaptive Deep Learning Model Integrated with the Internet of medical Things (IoMT) for Predicting Heart Disease," *Biomedical Signal Processing and Control*, vol. 92, p. 105988, 2024.

[7] Y. A. Qadri, H. Jung, and D. Niyato, "Towards the Internet of Medical Things for Real-Time Health Monitoring over Wi-Fi," *IEEE Network*, 2024.

[8] M. Nalluri, C. Babu Mupparaju, R. Pulimamidi, and A. S. Rongali, "Integration Of AI, ML, and IoT in Healthcare Data Fusion: Integrating Data from Various Sources, Including IoT Devices and Electronic Health Records, Provides a More Comprehensive View of Patient Health," *Pakistan Heart Journal*, vol. 57, no. 1, pp. 34–42, 2024.

[9] A. T. Rufai, A. U. Rufai, and A. L. Imoize, "Application of AIoMT in Medical Robotics," in *Handbook of Security and Privacy of AI-Enabled Healthcare Systems and Internet of Medical Things*. London: CRC Press, Taylor & Francis Group, pp. 335–364, 2024.

[10] S. Ramakrishnan, S. Jijitha, and T. Amudha, "Roadmap of AI and IoMT in Smart Healthcare: Current Applications and Future Perspectives," in *Internet of Medical Things in Smart Healthcare*. London: Apple Academic Press, Taylor & Francis Group, pp. 137–161, 2024.

[11] P. Y. Chen, Y. C. Cheng, Z. H. Zhong, *et al.*, "Information Security and Artificial Intelligence–Assisted Diagnosis in an Internet of Medical Thing System (IoMTS)," *IEEE Access*, vol. 12, pp. 9757–9775, 2024.

[12] K. Sharma, "Personalized Telemedicine Utilizing Artificial Intelligence, Robotics, and Internet of Medical Things (IOMT)," in *Handbook of Research on Artificial Intelligence and Soft Computing Techniques in Personalized Healthcare Services*. London: Apple Academic Press, Taylor & Francis Group, pp. 301–323, 2024.

[13] T. Kesavan, E. Kaliappan, S. Sivaranjani, K. Rameshkumar, and P. Kathirvel, "IoMT-Based Telemedicine Monitoring Machine for COVID Patients," in *Internet of Medical Things in Smart Healthcare*. London: Apple Academic Press, Taylor & Francis Group, pp. 1–10, 2024.

[14] S. F. Ahmed, M. S. B. Alam, S. Afrin, S. J. Rafa, N. Rafa, and A. H. Gandomi, "Insights into Internet of Medical Things (IoMT): Data Fusion, Security Issues and Potential Solutions," *Information Fusion*, vol. 102, p. 102060, 2024.

[15] A. Husnain, S. Rasool, A. Saeed, A. Y. Gill, and H. K. Hussain, "AI's Healing Touch: Examining Machine Learning's Transformative Effects on Healthcare," *Journal of World Science*, vol. 2, no. 10, pp. 1681–1695, 2023.

[16] S. Messinis, N. Temenos, N. E. Protonotarios, I. Rallis, D. Kalogeras, and N. Doulamis, "Enhancing Internet of Medical Things Security with Artificial Intelligence: A Comprehensive Review," *Computers in Biology and Medicine*, vol. 108036, 2024.

[17] A. U. Rufai, E. P. Fasina, C. O. Uwadia, A. T. Rufai, and A. L. Imoize, "Cyberattacks against Artificial Intelligence-Enabled Internet of Medical Things," in *Handbook of Security and Privacy of AI-Enabled Healthcare Systems and Internet of Medical Things*. London: CRC Press, Taylor & Francis Group, pp. 191–216, 2024.

[18] Y. Sei, A. Ohsuga, J. A. Onesimu, and A. L. Imoize, "Local Differential Privacy for Artificial Intelligence of Medical Things," in *Handbook of Security and Privacy of AI-Enabled Healthcare Systems and Internet of Medical Things*. London: CRC Press, Taylor & Francis Group, pp. 241–270, 2024.

[19] M. Abdulraheem, E. A. Adeniyi, J. B. Awotunde, *et al.*, "Artificial Intelligence of Medical Things for Medical Information Systems Privacy and Security," in *Handbook of Security and Privacy of AI-Enabled Healthcare Systems and Internet of Medical Things*. London: CRC Press, Taylor & Francis Group, pp. 63–96, 2024.

[20] V. A. Iguoba and A. L. Imoize, "AIoMT Training, Testing, and Validation," in *Handbook of Security and Privacy of AI-Enabled Healthcare Systems and Internet of Medical Things*. London: CRC Press, Taylor & Francis Group, pp. 394–410.

[21] S. I. Popoola, A. L. Imoize, M. Hammoudeh, B. Adebisi, O. Jogunola, and A. M. Aibinu, "Federated Deep Learning for Intrusion Detection in Consumer-Centric Internet of Things," in *IEEE Transactions on Consumer Electronics*, vol. 70, no. 1, pp. 1610–1622, doi:10.1109/TCE.2023.3347170.

[22] M. Z. Nezhad, A. J. J. Bojnordi, M. Mehraeen, R. Bagheri, and J. Rezazadeh, "Securing the Future of IoT-Healthcare Systems: A Meta-Synthesis of Mandatory Security Requirements," *International Journal of Medical Informatics*, vol. 185, p. 105379, 2024.

[23] A. Samadhiya, A. Kumar, J. A. Garza-Reyes, S. Luthra, and F. del Olmo García, "Unlock the potential: Unveiling the Untapped Possibilities of Blockchain Technology in Revolutionizing Internet of Medical Things-based Environments through Systematic Review and Future Research Propositions," *Information Sciences*, vol. 170, p. 120140, 2024.

[24] A. S. Nadhan and I. J. Jacob, "Enhancing Healthcare Security in the Digital Era: Safeguarding Medical Images with Lightweight Cryptographic Techniques in IoT Healthcare Applications," *Biomedical Signal Processing and Control*, vol. 88, p. 105511, 2024.

[25] A. M. A. Modarres, N. S. Anzabi-Nezhad, and M. Zare, "A New PUF-Based Protocol for Mutual Authentication and Key Agreement Between Three Layers of Entities in Cloud-Based IoMT Networks," *IEEE Access*, vol. 12, pp. 21807–21824, 2024.

[26] S. Dadkhah, E. Carlos Pinto Neto, R. Ferreira, R. Chukwuka Molokwu, S. Sadeghi, and A. Ghorbani, "CICIoMT2024: Attack Vectors in Healthcare devices-A Multi-Protocol Dataset for Assessing IoMT Device Security," *CiCIoMT2024: Attack Vectors in Healthcare Devices-A Multi-Protocol Dataset for Assessing IoMT Device Security*, 2024.

[27] L. Coventry, D. Branley-Bell, E. Sillence, *et al.*, "Cyber-risk in Healthcare: Exploring Facilitators and Barriers to Secure Behaviour," in *International Conference on Human–Computer Interaction*, pp. 105–122, Cham: Springer International Publishing, 2020.

[28] S. Aminabee, "The Future of Healthcare and Patient-Centric Care: Digital Innovations, Trends, and Predictions," in *Emerging Technologies for Health Literacy and Medical Practice*, pp. 240–262, IGI Global, 2024.

[29] M. U. Tariq, "Revolutionizing Health Data Management with Blockchain Technology: Enhancing Security and Efficiency in a Digital Era," in *Emerging Technologies for Health Literacy and Medical Practice*, pp. 153–175, IGI Global, 2024.

[30] S. Konar, G. Mukherjee, and G. Dutta, "Understanding the Relationship Between Trust and Faith in Micro-Enterprises to Cyber Hygiene: An Empirical Review," in *Strengthening Industrial Cybersecurity to Protect Business Intelligence*, pp. 125–148, 2024.

[31] J. D. Preece and J. M. Easton, "To Blockchain or Not to Blockchain, These Are the Questions: A Structured Analysis of Blockchain Decision Schemes," *Telematics and Informatics Reports*, p. 100115, 2024.

[32] A. Ferenczi and C. Bădică, "Optimization of IOTA Tangle Cumulative Weight Calculation Using Depth-First and Iterative Deepening Search Algorithms," *Vietnam Journal of Computer Science*, pp. 1–21, 2024.

[33] A. Mehrban and P. Ahadian, "An Adaptive Network-based Approach for Advanced Forecasting of Cryptocurrency Values," *arXiv preprint arXiv:2401.05441*, 2024.

[34] I. S. Rao, M. L. Kiah, M. M. Hameed, and Z. A. Memon, "Scalability of Blockchain: A Comprehensive Review and Future Research Direction," *Cluster Computing*, vol. 11, no. 2, pp. 1–24, 2024.

[35] A. Aliyu, H. Abdu, A. Suleiman, M. M. Yakubu, and M. Abubakar, "Blockchain Technology: An Overview," in *2nd International Conference on Applied ICT (ICAICT): Theme – ICT for All*, pp. 1–1, Lead City University, Ibadan, 2019.
[36] R. Sharad Mangrulkar and P. Vijay Chavan, "Introduction to Blockchain," in *Blockchain Essentials: Core Concepts and Implementations*, pp. 1–46, Berkeley, CA: Apress, 2024.
[37] N. Gligoric, D. Escuín, L. Polo, A. Amditis, T. Georgakopoulos, and A. Fraile, "IOTA-Based Distributed Ledger in the Mining Industry: Efficiency, Sustainability and Transparency," *Sensors*, vol. 24, no. 3, p. 923, 2024.
[38] C. Mazzocca, N. Romandini, R. Montanari, and P. Bellavista, "Enabling Federated Learning at the Edge through the IOTA Tangle," *Future Generation Computer Systems*, vol. 152, pp. 17–29, 2024.
[39] L. Jiang, Y. Liu, H. Tian, L. Tang, and S. Xie, "Resource Efficient Federated Learning and DAG Blockchain with Sharding in Digital Twin Driven Industrial IoT," *IEEE Internet of Things Journal*, 2024.
[40] D. Dione, I. Diop, I. Gueye, and S. M. Farssi, "Survey on Internet of Things Security and Medical Data Protection: Challenges and Perspectives," in *AIP Conference Proceedings (Vol. 2814, No. 1)*, 2023.
[41] A. Deep, A. Perrusquía, L. Aljaburi, S. Al-Rubaye, and W. Guo, "A Novel Distributed Authentication of Blockchain Technology Integration in IoT Services," *IEEE Access*, vol. 12, pp. 9550–9562, 2024.
[42] B. Bhushan, A. Kumar, A. K. Agarwal, A. Kumar, P. Bhattacharya, and A. Kumar, "Towards a Secure and Sustainable Internet of Medical Things (IoMT): Requirements, Design Challenges, Security Techniques, and Future Trends," *Sustainability*, vol. 15, no. 7, pp. 6177, 2023.
[43] A. J. Alkhodair, S. P. Mohanty, and E. Kougianos, "Consensus Algorithms of Distributed Ledger Technology–A Comprehensive Analysis," *arXiv preprint arXiv:2309.13498*, 2023.
[44] K. Venkatesan and S. B. Rahayu, "Blockchain Security Enhancement: An Approach Towards Hybrid Consensus Algorithms and Machine Learning Techniques," *Scientific Reports*, vol. 14, no. 1, p. 1149, 2024.
[45] D. M. Reoukadji, P. L. Bokonda, A. A. Madi, and I. Alihamidi, "Protecting Patient Privacy and Data Integrity With DAG Technology for IoMT and EHR: A Systematic Review," in *4th International Conference on Innovative Research in Applied Science, Engineering and Technology (IRASET)*, pp. 1–7, May 2024, IEEE.
[46] A. A. Jolfaei, S. F. Aghili, and D. Singelee, "A Survey on Blockchain-based IoMT Systems: Towards Scalability," *IEEE Access*, vol. 9, pp. 148948–148975, 2021.
[47] X. Lai, Y. Zhang, and H. Luo, "A Low-cost Blockchain Node Deployment Algorithm for the Internet of Things," *Peer-to-Peer Networking and Applications*, vol. 17, pp. 756–766, 2024.
[48] C. Mazzocca, A. Acar, S. Uluagac, R. Montanari, P. Bellavista, and M. Conti, "A Survey on Decentralized Identifiers and Verifiable Credentials," *arXiv preprint arXiv:2402.02455*, 2024.

[49] S. Wang, H. Li, J. Chen, J. Wang, and Y. Deng, "DAG Blockchain-based Lightweight Authentication and Authorization Scheme for IoT Devices," *Journal of Information Security and Applications*, vol. 66, p. 103134, 2022.

[50] S. R. Mallick, R. K. Lenka, P. K. Tripathy, D. C. Rao, S. Sharma, and N. K. Ray, "A Lightweight, Secure, and Scalable Blockchain-Fog-IoMT Healthcare Framework with IPFS Data Storage for Healthcare 4.0," *SN Computer Science*, vol. 5, no. 1, p. 198, 2024.

[51] Q. Le-Dang and T. Le-Ngoc, "Scalable Blockchain-based Architecture for Massive IoT Reconfiguration," in *2019 IEEE Canadian Conference of Electrical and Computer Engineering (CCECE)*, May 2019, pp. 1–4.

[52] S. Biswas, K. Sharif, F. Li, B. Nour, and Y. Wang, "A Scalable Blockchain Framework for Secure Transactions in IoT," *IEEE Internet of Things Journal*, vol. 6, no. 3, pp. 4650–4659, 2018.

[53] H. Purnama and M. Mambo, "IHIBE: A Hierarchical and Delegated Access Control Mechanism for IoT Environments," *Sensors*, vol. 24, no. 3, p. 979, 2024.

[54] J. A. Bartell, S. B. Valentin, A. Krogh, H. Langberg, and M. Bøgsted, "A Primer on Synthetic Health Data," *arXiv preprint arXiv:2401.17653*, 2024.

[55] R. Shinde, S. Patil, K. Kotecha, V. Potdar, G. Selvachandran, and A. Abraham, "Securing AI-based Healthcare Systems Using Blockchain Technology: A State-of-the-art Systematic Literature Review and Future Research Directions," *Transactions on Emerging Telecommunications Technologies*, vol. 35, no. 1, p. e4884, 2024.

[56] I. C. Lin, P. C. Tseng, P. H. Chen, and S. J. Chiou, "Securing Industrial Control Systems: Enhancing Data Preservation in IoT with Streamlined IOTA Integration," *Automation, Robotics & Communications for Industry 4. 0/5.0*, p. 332, 2024.

[57] Y. Chen, Y. Zhang, Y. Zhuang, K. Miao, S. Pouriyeh, and M. Han, "Efficient and Secure Blockchain Consensus Algorithm for Heterogeneous Industrial Internet of Things Nodes Based on Double-DAG," *IEEE Transactions on Industrial Informatics*, vol. 20, no. 4, pp. 6300–6312, 2024.

[58] V. Gandarillas, A. J. Joshy, M. Z. Sperry, A. K. Ivanov, and J. T. Hwang, "A graph-based methodology for constructing computational models that automates adjoint-based sensitivity analysis," *Structural and Multidisciplinary Optimization*, vol. 67, no. 5, p. 76, 2024.

[59] Z. Gao, G. Luo, S. Zhan, B. Liu, L. Huang, and H. C. Chao, "ST-HO: Symmetry-Enhanced Energy-Efficient DAG Task Offloading Algorithm in Intelligent Transport System," *Symmetry*, vol. 16, no. 2, p. 164, 2024.

[60] X. Xiao, "Accelerating Tip Selection in Burst Message Arrivals for DAG-based Blockchain Systems," *IEEE Transactions on Services Computing*, vol. 17, no. 2, pp. 392–405, 2024.

[61] S. Li, H. Xu, Q. Li, and Q. Han, "Simulation Study on the Security of Consensus Algorithms in DAG-based Distributed Ledger," *Frontiers of Computer Science*, vol. 18, no. 3, p. 183704, 2024.

Chapter 21
Detection and mitigation of cyber attacks in healthcare systems

Adeyemo Adetoye[1], Abiodun Adeyinka[2], Abidemi Emmanuel Adeniyi[3], Ozichi Nweke Emuoyibofarhe[3], Olanloye Odunayo[3] and Chinecherem Umezuruike[4]

In the era of digital transformation, the healthcare sector has been exposed to a new set of challenges, chief among them being the security of delicate patient data and the potential consequences of cyberattacks on healthcare systems. Healthcare organizations are often the main target because of the value of the patient data they own, making it critical for them to invest in robust cybersecurity measures to defend against these threats. This chapter focuses on healthcare cybersecurity and ways to detect ransomware, malware, denial of service attacks, and insider threats using security information and event management (SIEM), User and entity behavior analytic (UEBA), and security onion. The aim of this study is to look into the different methods of detecting healthcare threat techniques. In addition, we will provide insights into mitigation strategies.

Keywords: Healthcare; deepfake; security information and event management (SIEM); user and entity behavior analytic (UEBA); electronic healthcare records; telemedicine; netflow; NBAR

21.1 Introduction

Given the rise in dependence on technology in healthcare, the research of lethal cybersecurity risks in developing healthcare systems is a vital field. It emphasizes on understanding and addressing the risks linked with AI-driven assaults, deepfake technologies, and sensitive data breaches [1,2]. This field of study is vital because

[1]Cybersecurity Programme, Bowen University, Nigeria
[2]Africa Centre of Excellence on Technology Enhanced Learning, National Open University of Nigeria, Nigeria
[3]Computer Science Programme, Bowen University, Nigeria
[4]Software Engineering Programme, Bowen University, Nigeria

it tries to protect patient information, preserve confidence in healthcare systems, and assure continuity of service in the face of dynamic cybersecurity breaches. In the rapidly evolving landscape of modern healthcare, the integration of information technology has ushered in an era of unprecedented progress and innovation. The digital transformation has enabled remote consultations, improved patient monitoring, and streamlined healthcare operations [3]. Electronic health records (EHRs), telemedicine, wearable health devices, and interconnected medical devices have revolutionized patient care, enabling better diagnosis, treatment, and monitoring [4–8]. However, this digital transformation has also exposed the healthcare sector to a new set of challenges—chief among them being the security of delicate patient data and the potential consequences of cyberattacks on healthcare systems.

The importance of cybersecurity in healthcare is underscored not only by technological advancements but also by the collective opinions of experts in the field. In an age where patient data is a precious commodity, and the consequences of security breaches can be life-threatening and altering, healthcare organizations face an existential imperative to safeguard their digital assets. While the promise of interconnected healthcare systems is immense, the vulnerabilities that accompany this digital revolution are equally profound. It is within this delicate balance between technological advancement and security vulnerability that the true importance of robust cybersecurity measures in healthcare becomes evident.

21.1.1 Key contributions of the chapter

Listed below are the significant contributions of this chapter:

(i) The chapter critically examines ransomware and malware threats in the context of healthcare with prominent examples of attacks and consequences.
(ii) In addition, the chapter explores and discusses the number of incidence malware and ransomware incidents in the healthcare sector.
(iii) Discusses insider threats in healthcare cybersecurity and ways to detect insider threats using security information and event management (SIEM) and User and entity behavior analytic (UEBA).
(iv) The last section attempts to proffer ways to mitigate malware, ransomware, and insider attacks in healthcare organizations.

21.1.2 Chapter organization

Section 21.2 examines the related works and expert opinions on healthcare cybersecurity. The section also covers ransomware and malware threats in the context of healthcare, prominent healthcare-related malware, and ransomware incidents. Section 21.3 discusses life-threatening consequences of malware and ransomware attacks in healthcare systems. Section 21.4 presents evidence of the deadly impacts of cybersecurity threats in healthcare. Section 21.5 discusses the methodology and experimental design for the detection of insider threats in healthcare cybersecurity. Section 21.6 sheds light on the detection of Denial of Service attacks. Section 21.7

presents the results and discussions. Finally, Section 21.8 presents the concluding part and highlights the way forward.

21.2 Related works

Leading voices in healthcare and cybersecurity have emphasized the critical importance of robust cybersecurity measures in the healthcare sector. Dr. Brett Sacks, a renowned Plastic Surgery Registrar, asserts, "Data security is paramount in healthcare, given the sensitivity of medical information and the focus of malicious actors on the global industry" [9]. In this data-driven age, healthcare organizations handle vast volumes of patient data. Certifying the confidentiality, integrity, and availability of this data is of utmost importance, as breaches can have serious implications for patient safety and trust.

Furthermore, in the healthcare sector the most predominant and major hazard is healthcare cybersecurity. Information technology (IT) must constantly provide a shock absorber for healthcare data security issues due to the requirements to help patients and the harm that healthcare security breaches may do to their lives [10,11].

21.2.1 The increasing frequency of attacks

The urgency of the matter is further underscored by the growing frequency and complexity of cyber-attacks directed at healthcare organizations. Ransomware attacks, in particular, have become alarmingly prevalent, with criminal actors holding healthcare systems hostage in exchange for hefty ransoms. These attacks not only disrupt critical healthcare services but also expose patient data to potential compromise. In conclusion, the significance of cybersecurity in healthcare is not merely a technical concern but a multifaceted issue that impacts patients, policy-makers, healthcare providers, and society as a whole. It is a subject that resonates with experts, patients, and ethical principles, emphasizing its paramount importance in an increasingly digital healthcare landscape.

In the following segments of this chapter, we will examine specific deadly cybersecurity threats that have plagued emerging healthcare systems, shedding light on their consequences and providing insights into mitigation strategies. Understanding these threats is essential for healthcare professionals, administrators, and policymakers alike, as they collectively strive to fortify the healthcare sector against a growing and ever-evolving digital threat landscape.

21.2.2 Ransomware and malware threats in the context of healthcare

Defining malware and ransomware threats in the context of healthcare, they are specific types of malicious software and attacks respectively that target and exploit healthcare systems, networks, devices, and data. These threats pose enormous risks to patient privacy, the integrity of medical records, and the availability of critical healthcare services. Below is a breakdown of these threats:

21.2.3 Malware in healthcare

Malware is a wide term that includes any form of software purposefully designed to compromise, exploit, or damage computer infrastructures, data, or networks. In healthcare, malware can take innumerable forms, including adware, viruses, spyware worms, Trojans, and many more.

Impact in healthcare

(i) **Data theft:** Malicious software can be deployed to steal delicate patient information or data, such as medical, personal identification, and financial records.
(ii) **Manipulation of data:** Malware can manipulate or modify patient records, treatment schedules, or medication doses, which consequently lead to improper medical decisions.
(iii) **Services disruption:** Malware can disrupt healthcare operations by infecting systems, leading to system crash, and making data unreachable.

Examples

(i) **Botnets:** can generate networks of compromised devices that launch synchronized attacks on healthcare facilities, overwhelming them with traffic thereby causing denial of service (DoS) [12].
(ii) **Spyware:** can be used to spy on healthcare providers' activities, including keystroke logging to capture passwords and other sensitive information.

21.2.4 Ransomware in healthcare

Ransomwares are types of malware that encode a victim's data or lock the victim out of their system. Attackers request for ransom from the victim in exchange for the key to decryption the encrypted files or to recover access to their data or systems.

Impact in healthcare

(i) **Data encryption:** Ransomware encrypts patient data, making it unreachable to healthcare workers. This can interrupt patient care and treatment.
(ii) **Payment of ransom:** Attacker demands for ransom payment, often in cryptocurrency, in return for the decryption key. Paying ransom is not the best option owing to ethical, legal, and security concerns.
(iii) **Data loss:** In some cases, after a ransom is paid, there is no assurance that the attacker will make available the decryption key, resulting in permanent loss of data [9].

Examples

(i) **WannaCry:** WannaCry otherwise known as WannaCrypt ransomware was introduced in May 2017. In 2017, the WannaCry ransomware attack affected several healthcare organizations worldwide, barring them from gaining access to their systems and demanding ransom payments [13,14].

(ii) **Ryuk:** Ryuk is another deadly ransomware variant that has targeted healthcare organizations, causing significant disruptions of service.

In healthcare sector, the effect of malware and ransomware attacks can be predominantly severe because patient care, privacy, and safety are a stack. Healthcare organizations are often the main target because of the value of the patient data they own, making it critical for them to invest in robust cybersecurity measures to defend against these threats. Prevention, regular backups, employee training, and incident response plans are indispensable components of healthcare cybersecurity tactics to lessen the risks posed by malware and ransomware attacks.

21.2.5 Prominent healthcare-related malware and ransomware incidents

Certainly, there have been several prominent healthcare-related malware and ransomware incidents in recent years, and have posed significant threats to patient safety, data security, and healthcare organizations' operations, highlighting the vulnerability of the healthcare sector to cyberattacks. From the prevalent disruption triggered by WannaCry to the targeted attacks of Ryuk ransomware, healthcare organizations have become primary targets for cybercriminals in quest of exploiting vulnerabilities and collecting ransoms. In this section of the chapter, landscape of prominent healthcare-related malware and ransomware incidents will be discussed, examining the impact on healthcare organizations, patient care, and organizational stability.

21.2.5.1 WannaCry ransomware attack (2017)

The WannaCry ransomware exploits the vulnerability in the Microsoft Windows operating system to spread quickly across the internet and encrypt data to hold its victim hostage and promise to return the data after the payment of ransom. It encrypts files using cryptographically secure algorithms so that targeted victims are required to pay ransom in cryptocurrency like Bitcoin to acquire the private key to decrypt the encrypted data or file [15,16]. The WannaCry ransomware attack affected numerous computers globally. Telefónica, a Spanish mobile company, was the first company to be attacked by WannaCry ransomware, and in a short time, it spread across the United Kingdom thousands of NHS hospitals and surgeries were affected [17].

The attack affected several hospitals, clinics, and healthcare facilities, leading to patient appointment cancellations, delayed medical surgeries, and loss of access to patient records and critical systems, ambulances were allegedly diverted and redirected, leaving people in need of critical care stranded. It was estimated to cost the NHS a whopping £92 million after thousands of appointments were annulled because of the attack [18]. The WannaCry incident underscored the importance of promptly patching and updating systems to protect against known vulnerabilities. It also highlighted the need for robust cybersecurity practices in healthcare [18].

21.2.5.2 NotPetya (Petya) ransomware attack (2017)

The NotPetya ransomware attack, also known as Petya or ExPetr, occurred in June 2017. In order to gain administrative access, NotPetya injects malicious codes in the computer using EternalBlue Server Message Block (SMB) exploit to conduct the attacks thereby encrypting the hard drive, when the computer is booted, the ransom note is displayed [19,20]. It initially targeted organizations in Ukraine but quickly spread globally. It used a modified version of the Petya ransomware. Hospitals in Ukraine were severely impacted, with disruptions in patient care and administrative functions. However, the attack also affected multinational healthcare companies, causing significant financial losses. The incident emphasized the need for robust backup and disaster recovery plans to restore operations quickly. It also emphasized the importance of employee training to recognize phishing attempts.

21.2.5.3 Ryuk ransomware attacks

Ryuk is a notorious ransomware strain known for targeting healthcare organizations. It usually sneaks into their systems through tricky emails and, once it's in, it locks up all the important files and asks for money to unlock them. Several healthcare establishments, including hospitals and clinics, have fallen prey to Ryuk attacks. These occurrences have given rise to disruptions to patient care and data breaches. Defending against Ryuk and similar ransomware threats encompasses strong email security procedures, consistent backups, network segmentation, and robust cybersecurity training for staff.

21.2.5.4 Clop ransomware attacks

Another ransomware variant that has targeted healthcare organizations is clop. It not only encrypts data but also steals sensitive information, threatening to release it after the ransom is paid. Over the years, clop attacks have compromised patient data and interrupted healthcare operations. The combination of data encryption and data theft makes these attacks predominantly destructive. Healthcare establishments must prioritize not only data recovery plans but also defending against data theft. This undermines the significance of comprehensive security controls and incident response plans. These incidents highlighted and explained in the previous section explain the serious need for healthcare establishments to invest in cybersecurity measures and infrastructures, including intrusion detection systems, intrusion prevention systems, systematic and regular updates, employee training, and incident response plans. Healthcare information is highly delicate and sensitive, and patient care can be brutally impacted by cyberattacks, making cybersecurity an utmost priority in the healthcare industry. Furthermore, sharing information about threats and best practices among healthcare professionals and the community is critical for building collective resilience against cyber threats and attacks.

21.2.6 Insider threats in healthcare cybersecurity

Insider threats in healthcare cybersecurity refer to security risks posed by individuals within healthcare organizations who have legal or authorized permission to access healthcare information, systems, networks, data, facilities, and patient records. These individuals may be third-party vendors, contractors, part-time or full-time staff. Insider threats can be deliberate or planned or accidental and involve a range of activities that threaten the confidentiality, integrity, or availability of healthcare data and facilities. Insider threats can come in different forms. It can be:

21.2.6.1 Malicious insider threats

Malicious insider threats are a major cybersecurity risk for organizations across different industries, including healthcare. These threats happen when individuals within an organization misuse their access privileges to cause harm, steal sensitive information, or disrupt operations. In the healthcare sector, malicious insider threats can have severe consequences for patient safety, data integrity, and the organization's reputation.

Examples

(i) An employee maliciously stealing patient data with the intention of exchanging it with financial gain.
(ii) A disgruntled staff looking for a way to take revenge against the organization by deleting critical patient records.
(iii) An IT administrator installing malware to compromise the security of healthcare systems.

21.2.6.2 Unintentional insider threats

Unintentional insider threats, also known as negligent or accidental insider threats, represent a significant cybersecurity risk for organizations, including those in the healthcare sector. This involves when individuals often well-meaning employees or vendors carelessly compromise cybersecurity as a result of disregard, negligence, errors, or lack of awareness. These threats can occur when employees become targets of phishing attacks, unintentionally click on harmful links, or misplace work devices that contain sensitive data. While these individuals involved may not have malicious intent, their actions can still have serious consequences for patient safety, data security, and organizational resilience.

Examples

(i) Accidentally distributing sensitive patient information to unintended recipients through email.
(ii) Installation of malware on a healthcare system through phishing.
(iii) Misconfiguring security settings on a healthcare devices and applications, thereby exposing devices or applications vulnerable to attacks.

21.3 Life-threatening consequences of malware and ransomware attacks in healthcare

The incidence of malware and ransomware attacks in healthcare can be life-threatening because of the serious nature of healthcare services and the delicate nature of patient data involved. Listed below are several ways these attacks can directly or indirectly affect patient data, safety, and well-being:

(i) **Medical services disruption**: Malware and ransomware attacks can disrupt the operation of healthcare systems, hospitals, and clinics. This disruption can cause delayed or cancellation of surgeries, postponed medical treatments, and complications in accessing and providing timely care to patients with life-threatening conditions. Patients may experience protracted suffering or worsening of their health because of these prolonged delays.

(ii) **Medical records inaccessibility**: To be precise, ransomware attacks encode medical records and files and make them inaccessible or unreadable to healthcare providers and professionals. This can result in professionals lacking vital patient information required to make well-versed medical verdicts. Without access to previous medical records, medication lists, allergies, and test results of patients, healthcare providers may run into blunders in diagnosis and treatment and possibly harming patients.

(iii) **Medication errors:** Malware attacks can compromise EHRs and those systems that help in the management of medications. When that happens, it can cause some major problems with giving the right dosages or medicines to patients. It can lead to some serious consequences like adverse drug reactions or even life-threatening complications.

(iv) **Patient misidentification:** If patient identification systems get messed up by some malware or ransomware, things can go totally haywire. There might be cases where patients get mixed up and identified all wrong. And guess what? That means the wrong person could end up getting treatment or procedures meant for someone else. And it could totally mess things up and even cause harm.

(v) **Medical device vulnerabilities**: Malware can actually go after medical gadgets and infrastructures like infusion pumps, ventilators, and pacemakers. If these devices get attacked, they might start malfunctioning or even be controlled remotely the hackers thereby putting the lives of patients in danger.

(vi) **Delayed emergency response**: In cases where malware or ransomware attacks distort communication facilities or interrupt the accessibility of critical patient data, emergency response times can be seriously affected. Patients in life-threatening conditions may not receive the instantaneous care they need, leading to worsened consequences.

(vii) **Data privacy breaches**: In the event of a data compromise as a result of a cyberattack, patient records, as well as medical history and personal information, can be exposed consequently leading to fraud, identity theft, and financial harm to patients, furthermore compromising their medical privacy.

(viii) **Psychological stress**: Due to ransomware and malware attacks, patients may be subjected to significant psychological, and emotional stress and anxiety knowing fully well that their personal health information has been tampered with. This stress can adversely affect their general well-being and recovery.

(ix) **Legal and ethical issues**: Malware and ransomware attacks can lead to legal and ethical problems for healthcare providers. Verdicts concerning how to respond to ransom demands and payments and whether to divulge incidents to patients can be multifaceted and may have life-altering consequences for all parties involved.

21.4 Evidence of the deadly impacts of cybersecurity threats in healthcare

In today's healthcare landscape, digital technologies are playing an increasingly important role. However, this also means that the threat of cybersecurity attacks is a major concern. These attacks can have serious consequences on patient safety, data integrity, and the overall healthcare infrastructure. The impact of these threats is evident in various ways, such as ransomware attacks that paralyze hospital operations or data breaches that compromise sensitive patient information. This section aims to shed light on the alarming reality of cyber attacks on healthcare organizations by providing real-world examples of incidents that have resulted in patient harm, disrupted medical services and eroded public trust. The deadly impacts of cybersecurity threats in healthcare are well-documented and include the following (see Table 21.1).

By highlighting the weighty consequences of cybersecurity vulnerabilities in healthcare, there is the need to emphasize the urgent necessity for strong cybersecurity measures, proactive risk management strategies, and collaborative efforts to protect patient well-being and maintain the integrity of healthcare systems.

Table 21.1 Lists of facilities that have recorded a form of cyberattack in the past

Year	Health facility/ attack	Description	Impact	Reference
2023	UK's National Health Service. Ransomware Attack	May 12, 2017, the UK's National Health Service was targeted by WannaCry ransomware, exploiting a vulnerability in outdated Windows computers. The malware encrypted host files and requested for payment in Bitcoin.	The attack disrupted health services in hospitals across Britain, canceling approximately 19,000 appointments and diverting emergency ambulances to unaffected facilities. The WannaCry attack is the most widespread and expensive in NHS history, resulting in a loss of £20M and a £72M investment in technology.	[21]

(Continues)

Table 21.1 (Continued)

Year	Health facility/ attack	Description	Impact	Reference
2020	Lukaskrankenhaus Neuss (Germany). Ransomware attack	Lukaskrankenhaus Neuss, a German public hospital, experienced a ransomware attack in February 2016, causing staff to take their computers offline to assess and clean infected systems. Despite not receiving a direct demand for money, staff were given an email address for further instructions. The hospital reported keeping its backup system and EHR, but a backlog of handwritten records needs to be integrated with the system.		[22]
2020	South-eastern Norway regional health authority (Norway)	The South-Eastern Norway Regional Health Authority (South-East RHF) reported that nearly 2.9 million people's personal health information (PHI) and records were compromised in January 2018. The attack was believed to have been led by a foreign spy or state agency, targeting patient health data and the health service's interaction with Norway's armed forces. The vulnerability was believed to have come from the legacy system, Windows XP for GDPR.	Although the attack did not pose risks to patient safety or delays in hospital operations, it raised concerns about future health data attacks for political gain and served as a wake-up call.	[22]
2020	Hancock regional hospital (United States)	Hancock Regional Hospital in Greenfield, Indiana, faced a ransomware attack by SamSam in January	The hackers corrupted backup files, except for electronic medical record backup files. The hospital shut down all	[22]

(Continues)

Table 21.1 (*Continued*)

Year	Health facility/ attack	Description	Impact	Reference
		2018. The attacker directed the attack to a server in their emergency IT backup system and spread through the electronic connection between the backup site and the server farm. The CEO reported that the attack was deliberate and was carried out by a sophisticated criminal group.	systems, but operations continued.	
2021, 2023	Hammersmith Medicines Study (HMR). Maze Ransomware.	According to the HMR, their IT department discovered the attack on the 14th of March 2020 but was able to restore both services effectively before the day runs out. On the 21st of March 2020, the attackers reported tens of thousands of patients' information from 8 years to 20. There were medical records compromised, including copies of passports, driving licenses, details on insurance, and more.	Managing Director and clinical manager of HMR, the doctor clarified that they don't want to charge a ransom for compensation: "I would rather quit company instead of charging ransom to these men."	[23,24]
2023	Hancock regional hospital (United States). Malware SamSam	On January 11, 2018, a ransomware attack by malware SamSam was conducted against Hancock Regional [14]. The attack focused on a backup server that is located in their IT emergency-standby environment and propagated via the electronic link from the standby site, situated miles away from the main campus to the server farm at the hospital.	It was found that parts of the backup files from all systems were irreversibly damaged by the hackers, except for the electronic medical record backup files. It used an entry point into the server, Microsoft's Remote Desktop Protocol, and the first step made by the hackers was taking control over the administrative account of a hardware vendor in order to initiate the attack.	[21,25,26]

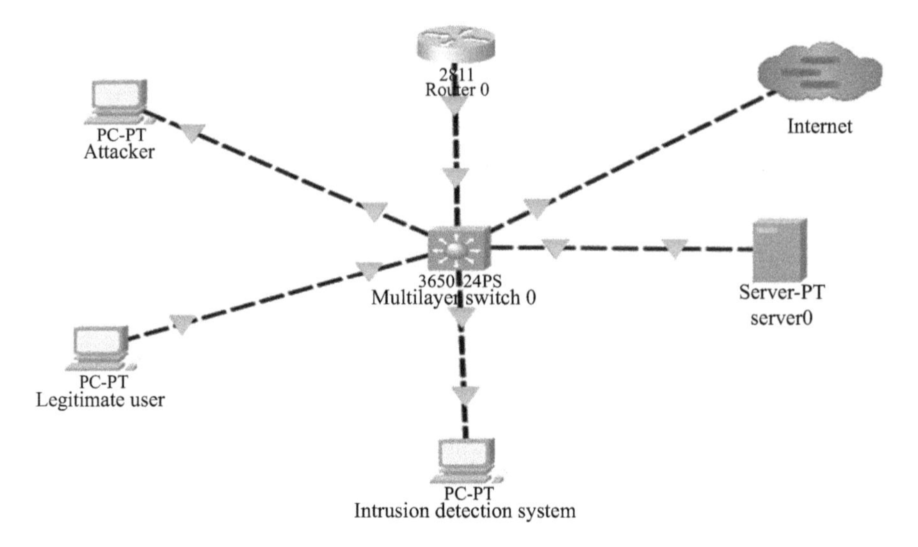

Figure 21.1 Network connection and configuration

21.5 Experimental design

The LAN setup as shown in Figure 21.1 is connected to the Internet through the switch for the purpose of accessing the Internet. The aim of this study is to look into the different methods of detecting healthcare threats and mitigation techniques. The experiment setup consists of a Cisco layer 3 Switch (Catalyst 3550 series) and three PCs.

For this experiment to run easily and successfully, the experiment has been divided into different stages. Stage 1: Connecting and Configuring the Network. Stage 2: Testing connections and installing data collection software installation. Stage 3: Performing the DoS attacks detection and mitigation.

21.6 Detection of denial of service attack

Detecting and mitigating DoS attacks is a critical aspect of maintaining cybersecurity and protecting sensitive information in organizations. The following gives insights into both detecting and mitigating DoS attacks, along with proper references to reputable sources for further information:

21.6.1 Security information and event management (SIEM) systems

Employing network traffic analysis tools to monitor network communications for unusual patterns or data exfiltration attempts will go a long way to safeguard healthcare facilities. Looking for anomalies in traffic volume, destinations, or protocol usage. Also, use SIEM solutions to aggregate and analyze security event

```
Router(config)#int fa0/0
Router(config-if)#ip flow ingress
Router(config-if)#ip flow egress
Router(config-if)#exit
Router(config)#ip flow-export version 9
Router(config)#ip flow-cache timeout active 1
Router(config)#ip flow-cache timeout inactive 15
Router(config)#ip flow-export destination 192.168.2.6 9996
Router(config)#ip flow-export source fa0/0
```

Figure 21.2 NetFlow configuration on a router

logs from various sources. Correlate events to identify potential DoS attacks and automate response actions [27].

In this project, an Apache web server was built and it happened to be the Netflow collector where all traffic collected is saved and analyzed using a Netflow analyzer (Developed by SolarWind).

Netflow is a Cisco proprietary network protocol used for extracting IP traffic information on the network. From Figure 21.2, Netflow can be configured on router and switches (From catalyst 3650 switches) and it extract IP traffic information on the interface(s) where Netflow is applied, and the information will later be transferred to the Netflow collectors, which is usually a server.

Netfow configuration is shown in Figure 21.2.

From the configuration command lines above, int f0/0 is to enter the interface mode where packets are to be captured, while IP flow ingress and IP flow egress are to specify the types of packet to capture. IP flow ingress and egress are to capture the packet entering and leaving the interface respectively. IP flow-export version 9 is used to specify the version of Netflow you want to use. IP flow-cache timeout active 1 is used to specify how frequently the active traffic conversations are to be exported from the cache. The default time is 30 min but for this study we used 1 min in order to get real-time report. For example, every conversation that lasts more than 10 min will be exported every 60 sec, this gives an opportunity to get a real-time report. IP flow-cache timeout inactive 15 defines how frequently information about active traffic conversations are to be exported from the cache. IP flow-export destination 192.168.2.6 9996, this command line is used to define where the exported information goes, which is the server where the Netflow analyzer is installed and 9996 is the port that the Netflow analyzer is listening to.

21.6.2 User and entity behavior analytics (UEBA)

UEBA solutions analyze user and entity behavior to detect anomalies or suspicious activities. They can identify unusual patterns of access, data exfiltration, or unauthorized activities [28].

Network-Based Application Recognition (NBAR) is also a Cisco proprietary software built into Cisco devices. NBAR can be used to inspect and classify

```
Router(config)#int fa0/0
Router(config-if)#ip nbar protocol-discovery
```

Figure 21.3 NBAR configuration on a router

protocols and packets that flow through a device (router and switch). It is a built-in protocol analyzer that runs on a system and literally identifies particular traffic that flows through a device. NBAR has two main functions, which are:

- Quality of Service (QoS)
- Protocol Analysis.

This study focuses on the second function which is protocol Analysis. The configuration shown in Figure 21.3 was applied on the router fa0/0 interface. NBAR configuration is shown below.

21.6.3 Detection of ransomware and malware attack

In today's digital landscape, the proliferation of ransomware and malware attacks poses a significant threat to organizations and individuals worldwide. As cybercriminals continue to develop sophisticated techniques to infiltrate systems and encrypt data for extortion, the need for robust detection mechanisms has never been more critical. Detecting ransomware and malware attacks early is essential for mitigating their impact, minimizing data loss, and restoring affected systems to normal operation. By leveraging advanced threat detection technologies, proactive monitoring strategies, and security best practices, organizations can enhance their resilience against ransomware and malware threats, safeguarding their assets and preserving the integrity of their operations.

21.6.4 Malware detection with Security Onion

Security Onion is an open-source platform that integrates multiple powerful tools and technologies to provide comprehensive visibility into network traffic and detect potential security threats like malware. By combining capabilities for network security monitoring, threat detection, and analysis, Security Onion enables effective malware detection across the network environment.

21.7 Results and discussion

Data was collected from the router and Apache server on the network. The results are discussed as follows.

21.7.1 Denial of service detection

From Figure 21.4, 4692 udp datagrams with more than 31,000 packets were captured and exported into the Netflow cache.

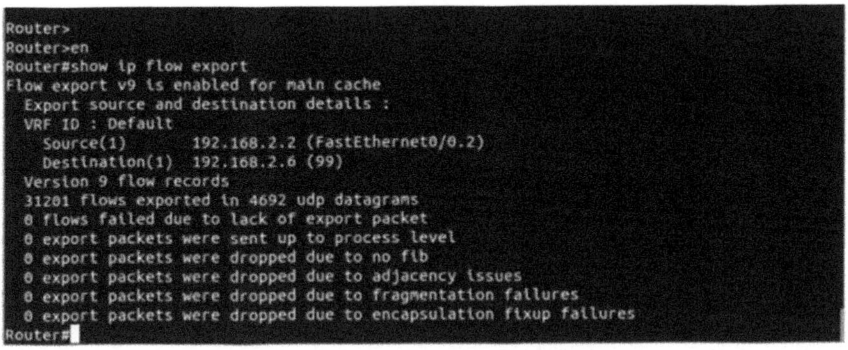

```
Router>
Router>en
Router#show ip flow export
Flow export v9 is enabled for main cache
  Export source and destination details :
  VRF ID : Default
    Source(1)       192.168.2.2 (FastEthernet0/0.2)
    Destination(1)  192.168.2.6 (99)
  Version 9 flow records
  31201 flows exported in 4692 udp datagrams
  0 flows failed due to lack of export packet
  0 export packets were sent up to process level
  0 export packets were dropped due to no fib
  0 export packets were dropped due to adjacency issues
  0 export packets were dropped due to fragmentation failures
  0 export packets were dropped due to encapsulation fixup failures
Router#
```

Figure 21.4 Netflow router output

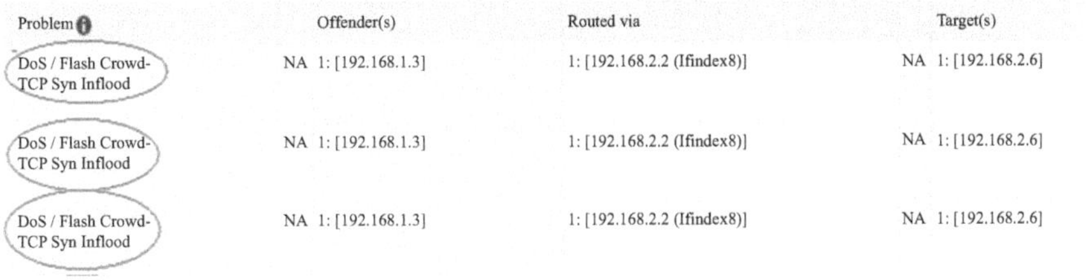

Problem	Offender(s)	Routed via	Target(s)
DoS / Flash Crowd-TCP Syn Inflood	NA 1: [192.168.1.3]	1: [192.168.2.2 (Ifindex8)]	NA 1: [192.168.2.6]
DoS / Flash Crowd-TCP Syn Inflood	NA 1: [192.168.1.3]	1: [192.168.2.2 (Ifindex8)]	NA 1: [192.168.2.6]
DoS / Flash Crowd-TCP Syn Inflood	NA 1: [192.168.1.3]	1: [192.168.2.2 (Ifindex8)]	NA 1: [192.168.2.6]

Figure 21.5 Netflow output showing the type of attack

Figure 21.5 shows an output extracted from the Netflow traffic analyzer installed on the server. NetFlow traffic analyzer is a unified solution that collects, analyses, and reports about what the network bandwidth is being used for and by whom [28].

According to SolarWinds [29,30], the developer of Netflow analyzer, one of the main functions of Netflow analyzer is to monitor network bandwidth and traffic patterns down to the interface level. From Figure 21.5, it can be seen that in less than 30–40 sec, 100 requests were sent to the server which literarily signifies a form of DoS attack. And because of these numerous requests in a short time, NetFlow analyzer was able to detect and give the form of attack that was on the way. On the far left of the screenshot, Netflow analyzer reported the type of attack which is “DoS/Flash Crowd – TCP Syn Inflood.”

The NBAR collects application and protocol statistics on the interface. The statistics collected involve the following as shown in Figure 21.6: bit rate, byte counts, and packet counts. Figure 21.6 displays the partial output of the show ip NBAR protocol discovery on the router. In less than 30 sec the maximum bit rate for DNS and ICPM packet is 1,000 bps, by this figure, one can easily deduce that there is an attack going on. The network administrator can examine the different

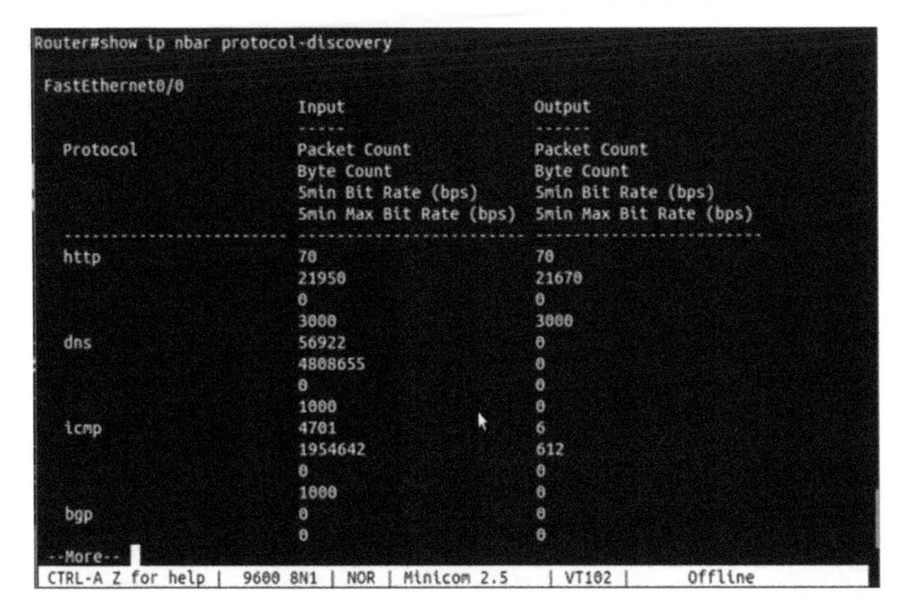

Figure 21.6 Snapshot with Nbar output

types of applications in use by the network at any given time and make a decision on how to allocate bandwidth to each application.

21.7.2 Malware and ransomware detection

"ET malware Asterope checkin"

"ET malware Asterope checkin" refers to a signature generated by the Emerging Threats (ET) rule set in Security Onion. In this context:

ET: Stands for Emerging Threats, which is a well-known provider of threat intelligence and rules for intrusion detection and prevention systems.

Malware Asterope checkin: This indicates that the signature is designed to detect network traffic associated with a specific type of malware or a specific malware family called "Asterope." The term "checkin" suggests that the signature is likely looking for patterns or behaviors indicative of malware communicating with a command and control (C2) server or performing some other form of periodic communication. Figure 21.7 gives security onion output showing malware detection.

In Security Onion, when this signature fires, it means that network traffic matching the pattern defined by the signature has been detected, potentially indicating the presence of the Asterope malware or related activity on the network. This information can then be used by security analysts to investigate further and respond appropriately.

"ET JA3 hash—possible malware—various EK"

"ET JA3 hash—possible malware—various EK" refers to a signature generated by the Emerging Threats (ET) rule set in Security Onion. Here's a breakdown:

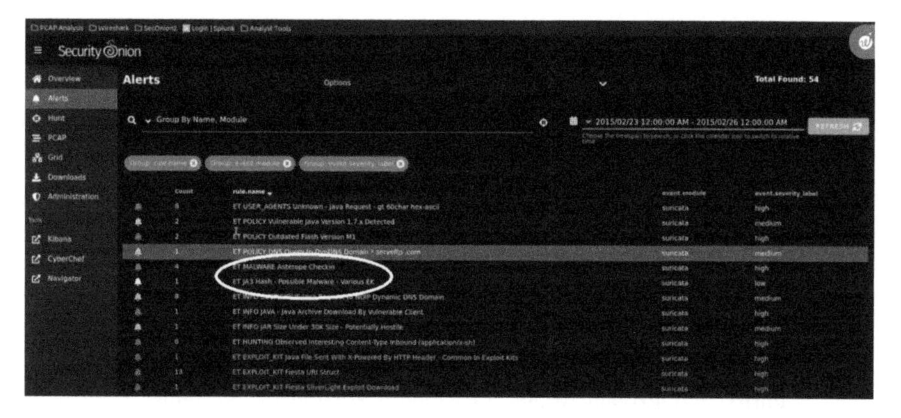

Figure 21.7 Security Onion output showing malware detection.

ET: Stands for Emerging Threats, which is a provider of threat intelligence and rules for intrusion detection and prevention systems.

JA3 hash: JA3 is a method used to fingerprint the SSL/TLS clients based on the parameters they use during the SSL/TLS handshake. It generates a unique hash value for each SSL/TLS client based on factors like supported SSL/TLS extensions, ciphersuites, and other parameters.

Possible malware: Indicates that the signature is designed to detect network traffic associated with potentially malicious activity. In this case, it's specifically looking for patterns in SSL/TLS handshakes that may indicate the presence of malware.

Various EK: "EK" commonly stands for "exploit kit." Exploit kits are tools used by attackers to exploit vulnerabilities in software, typically web browsers or plugins, to deliver malware to victims' computers. The term "various EK" suggests that the signature is looking for SSL/TLS handshake patterns associated with multiple exploit kits.

When this signature fires in Security Onion, it means that network traffic matching the JA3 hash pattern indicative of potential malware activity, particularly related to exploit kits, has been detected. This information can then be used by security analysts to investigate further and respond appropriately.

21.8 Conclusion

In conclusion, despite the array of unprecedented benefits that come with the fast integration of technology into healthcare systems, there are also emerging deadly cybersecurity threats attached to it. The chapter above has dissected, with meticulous care, the multifaceted nature of these threats ranging from malware and ransomware attacks paralyzing critical healthcare infrastructure to DoS preventing legitimate users from gaining access to networking and healthcare facilities directly risking patient safety. The seriousness of these cybersecurity challenges goes beyond cyber as evidenced by real-world incidents that interrupted healthcare operations and jeopardized patient's data and in some cases lives. In the future, it is paramount that healthcare organizations prioritize continuous detection of cyber threats using SIEM, education and training for staff, regular risk assessments, and the implementation of a proactive cybersecurity strategy and proper implementation of these security measures will further harden the security apparatus of healthcare organization.

References

[1] A. I. Newaz, A. K. Sikder, M. A. Rahman, and A. S. Uluagac. "A Survey on Security and Privacy Issues in Modern Healthcare Systems: Attacks and Defenses", *ACM Transactions on Computing for Healthcare,* 2(3), pp. 1–44. 2021.
[2] K. S. Bhosale, M. Nenova, and G. Iliev. "A Study of Cyber attacks: In the Healthcare Sector", *2021 Sixth Junior Conference on Lighting (Lighting)*, Gabrovo, Bulgaria, 2021, pp. 1–6, doi: 10.1109/Lighting49406.2021.9598947.
[3] H. Neti, and S. Parte. "Riding the Tech Wave: Exploring Tomorrow's Landscape of Information Technology", *International Journal of Innovative Research in Technology*, 10(7), 42–51. 2023.
[4] S. Suherlan, and M. O. Okombo. "Technological Innovation in Marketing and Its Effect on Consumer Behaviour", *Technology and Society Perspectives (TACIT)*, 1(2), 94–103. 2023.
[5] J. B. Awotunde, R. G. Jimoh, S. O., Folorunso, E. A. Adeniyi, K. M. Abiodun, and O. O. Banjo. "Privacy and Security Concerns in IoT-based Healthcare Systems". In *The Fusion of Internet of Things, Artificial Intelligence, and Cloud Computing in Health Care*. Cham: Springer International Publishing. pp. 105–134. 2021.
[6] E. A. Adeniyi, R. O. Ogundokun, and J. B. Awotunde. "IoMT-based Wearable Body Sensors Network Healthcare Monitoring System. *IoT in Healthcare and Ambient Assisted Living*, pp. 103–121. 2021.
[7] M. Abdulraheem, E. A. Adeniyi, J. B Awotunde, *et al.* "Artificial Intelligence of Medical Things for Medical Information Systems Privacy and Security". In *Handbook of Security and Privacy of AI-Enabled Healthcare Systems and Internet of Medical Things*. CRC Press. pp. 63–96. 2024.
[8] J. B. Awotunde, A. L. Imoize, A. E. Adeniyi, *et al.* "Explainable Machine Learning (XML) for Multimedia-Based Healthcare Systems: Opportunities, Challenges, Ethical and Future Prospects". *Explainable Machine Learning for Multimedia Based Healthcare Applications.* Springer International Publishing A&G, pp. 21–46. 2023.
[9] B. Sacks. "Safeguarding Patient Data in the Age of Healthcare Apps". https://www.linkedin.com/pulse/safeguarding-patient-data-age-healthcare-apps-brett-sacks/(accessed August 2023).

[10] J. Mohd, H. Abid, P. S. Ravi, and S. Rajiv. "Towards Insighting Cybersecurity for Healthcare Domains: A Comprehensive Review of Recent Practices and Trends", *Cyber Security and Applications*, 1, 100016, 2023, https://doi.org/10.1016/j.csa.2023.100016.

[11] H. Alami, M.P. Gagnon, M.A.A. Ahmed, and J.P. Fortin. "Digital Health: Cybersecurity Is a Value Creation Lever, Not Only a Source of Expenditure", *Health Policy Technology*, 8(4), pp. 319–321. 2019.

[12] A. Adeyemo. "Comparative Analysis of Various Denials of Service (Dos) Attack Mitigation Techniques", *International Journal of Computer Science Engineering (IJCSE)*. 8(4), pp. 162–167, 2019, doi: 10.5281/zenodo.10472128.

[13] Health and Human Services Department. (2019). *Notification of Enforcement Discretion Regarding HIPAA Civil Money Penalties*. https://www.federalregister.gov/documents/2019/04/30/2019-08530/notification-of-enforcement-discretion-regarding-hipaa-civil-money-penalties (accessed Oct. 8, 2023).

[14] M. Humayun, N. Jhanjhi, A. Alsayat, and V. Ponnusamy. "Internet of Things and Ransomware: Evolution, Mitigation and Prevention," *Egyptian Informatics Journal*, vol. 22, no. 1, pp. 105–117, 2021. doi:10.1016/j.eij.2020.05.003

[15] D.-Y. KAO, S.-C. HSIAO and R. TSO. "Analyzing WannaCry Ransomware Considering the Weapons and Exploits," *2019 21st International Conference on Advanced Communication Technology (ICACT)*, PyeongChang, Korea (South), 2019, pp. 1098–1107, 10.23919/ICACT.2019.8702049.

[16] Kaspersky, "What Is WannaCry Ransomware?," www.kaspersky.com, https://www.kaspersky.com/resource-center/threats/ransomware-wannacry (accessed Oct. 10, 2023).

[17] "What is ransomware? – Definition, prevention and more: Proofpoint us," Proofpoint, https://www.proofpoint.com/us/threat-reference/ransomware (accessed Oct. 11, 2023).

[18] E. A. Adeniyi, P. B. Falola, M. S. Maashi, M. Aljebreen, and S. Bharany. "Secure Sensitive Data Sharing Using RSA and ElGamal Cryptographic Algorithms with Hash Functions," *Information*, vol. 13, no. 10, p. 442, 2022. doi:10.3390/info13100442

[19] M. F. Prevezianou. "WannaCry as a Creeping Crisis," *Understanding the Creeping Crisis*, pp. 37–50, 2021. doi:10.1007/978-3-030-70692-0_3

[20] S. Saha. *"'WannaCry Unveiled: A Comprehensive Analysis of the Ransomware Attack That Paralyzed Global Systems,'"* 2023. *www.linkedin.com.* https://www.linkedin.com/pulse/wannacry-unveiled-comprehensive-analysis-ransomware-attack-saha/

[21] N. Scheetz and D. Strickland. "The Impact of Cyberattacks on Healthcare," CurrentWare, Apr. 06, 2022. https://www.currentware.com/blog/the-impact-of-cyberattacks-on-healthcare/#5-alarmingly-prevalent-cyber-threats-in-healthcare (accessed Nov. 16, 2023).

[22] S. T. Argaw *et al.* "Cybersecurity of Hospitals: Discussing the Challenges and Working towards Mitigating the Risks," *BMC Medical Informatics and*

Decision Making, vol. 20, no. 1, 2020, doi:https://doi.org/10.1186/s12911-020-01161-7.

[23] R. A. Ramadan, B. W. Aboshosha, J. S. Alshudukhi, A. J. Alzahrani, A. El-Sayed, and M. M. Dessouky. "Cybersecurity and Countermeasures at the Time of Pandemic," *Journal of Advanced Transportation*, vol. 2021, pp. 1–19, 2021, doi:https://doi.org/10.1155/2021/6627264.

[24] L.Freedman. "Covid-19 Vaccine Test Lab Hit by Maze Ransomware," *JD Supra*, https://www.jdsupra.com/legalnews/covid-19-vaccine-test-lab-hit-by-maze-88329/ (accessed Oct. 17, 2023).

[25] Secureworks Counter Threat Unit Threat Intelligence. "Samsam ransomware campaigns," Secureworks, https://www.secureworks.com/research/samsam-ransomware-campaigns (accessed Oct. 16, 2023).

[26] O. Hughes. "Hancock Regional Hospital Back Online after Paying Hackers $55,000," *Digital Health*, https://www.digitalhealth.net/2018/01/hancock-regional-hospital-back-online/ (accessed Oct. 16, 2023).

[27] A. Adeyemo. "Comparative Analysis of Various Denials of Service (DoS) Attack Mitigation Techniques", *International Journal of Computer Science Engineering (IJCSE).* vol. 8 no. 4, pp. 162–167, 2019, doi: 10.5281/zenodo.10472128.

[28] A. Adeyemo. "A Study of Denial of Service Attack with Its Tools and Possible Mitigation Technique", *Georgia Electronic Scientific Journals (GESJ).* vol. 57, no. 2, pp. 36–45, 2019. doi: 10.5281/zenodo.10472112

[29] Solarwind. URL: http://www.solarwinds.com/netflow-traffic-analyzer.aspx.

[30] ManageEngine. *NetFlow Analyser 9.7, User Guide*, Zoho Corp, 2010.

Chapter 22

Cybersecurity concerns and risks in emerging healthcare systems

Ozichi Nweke Emuoyibofarhe[1], Adetoye Adeyemo[2], Dauda Odunayo Olanloye[1], Abidemi Emmanuel Adeniyi[1] and Christian O. Osueke[3]

The adoption of new technologies by healthcare systems brings with it new risks related to cybersecurity and new concerns. This chapter investigates a comprehensive strategy for reducing these risks in healthcare institutions by looking into the foundation of a thorough cybersecurity strategy, which consists of risk assessments, frequent security audits, strong access controls, and data encryption. Emerging healthcare systems leverage on advanced technologies to enhance patient care, streamline operations, and improve efficiency. In addition, the study examines the cybersecurity challenges facing emerging healthcare systems, focusing on the vulnerabilities inherent in interconnected medical devices, electronic health records, and telehealth platforms. The chapter explores the potential consequences of cyberthreats, including data breaches, privacy violations, and disruptions to patient care. Furthermore, the study discusses strategies to mitigate these risks, such as implementing robust encryption protocols, adopting multi-factor authentication, and enhancing employee cybersecurity awareness through a comprehensive training. By understanding and addressing these cybersecurity concerns, emerging healthcare systems can better safeguard their patient data and maintain the integrity of their operations.

Keywords: Cybersecurity concerns; cybersecurity risks; healthcare systems; data breaches; privacy violations; encryption protocols

[1]Computer Science Programme, Bowen University, Nigeria
[2]Cybersecurity Programme, Bowen University, Nigeria
[3]Mechatronics Programme, Bowen University, Nigeria

22.1 Introduction

The healthcare business is undergoing a substantial shift, fueled by the increasing adoption of emerging technologies such as artificial intelligence (AI), the Internet of Medical Things (IoMT), and telehealth [1,2]. While these developments promise to improve patient care, efficiency, and accessibility, they also open up a new set of cybersecurity issues and hazards [3]. Remarkable case studies demonstrate how the healthcare industry has emerged as a primary target for cyberthreats. In February 2016, a disruptive ransomware attack occurred at the Lukaskrankenhaus Neuss in Germany, highlighting the vulnerability of hospital operations. High-risk procedures were postponed despite prompt offline measures, and unexpected difficulties arose during the integration of manual records into the electronic health record (EHR) system.

Similar to this, in January 2018, a highly skilled attack was launched against the regional health authority of South-eastern Norway, compromising the personal health information (PHI) of 2.9 million people. This breach, which was suspected of being planned by a foreign power, targeted patient health data as well as the health service's relationships with the armed forces [4]. The incident, which took advantage of a flaw in the antiquated Windows XP system, exposed data breaches and sparked questions about potential political motivations, underscoring the necessity of GDPR compliance [5,6]. Hancock Regional Hospital in the United States was infected with the Sam ransomware in January 2018. The attackers, who were part of a highly skilled criminal group, used a compromised administrative account and Microsoft remote desktop protocol to manipulate backup files [7]. The hospital Information Technology team had to spend days decrypting files even after they received a ransom payment of four Bitcoins or US$55,000. The deliberate and focused attack brought attention to the hospital's challenging choice to pay the ransom to maintain operational continuity, even though patient data was not compromised [8].

These case studies are clear reminders of how crucial it is for the healthcare industry to put strong cybersecurity measures in place. Safeguarding patient data and guaranteeing the continuous provision of healthcare services is more important than ever because the industry is becoming more and more dependent on digital systems and EHRs [8]. To reduce these risks, this study examines thorough security strategies, highlighting the need for preventative actions and compliance with global data protection laws [9].

The different previous reports on cybersecurity and healthcare system protection motivated this study which provides the analysis to examine cybersecurity challenges and the emerging healthcare system risks. As such, to strengthen cybersecurity and protect healthcare system data, protect patient data privacy, secure medical devices and Internet of Thing systems, compliance with regulatory requirements and conducting regular risk assessments are considered to improve data security. This research sheds light on the vulnerabilities inherent in emerging healthcare technologies and practices, offering insights into the potential risks posed by cyberthreats. Lastly, the research provides insights into future trends and emerging technologies in both healthcare and cybersecurity domains. By anticipating potential advancements and challenges, it lays the groundwork for ongoing research and innovation in mitigating cybersecurity risks in evolving healthcare systems. Cybersecurity concerns and risks in emerging healthcare systems contribute to a deeper understanding of the complex dynamics between cybersecurity and healthcare, ultimately striving to enhance the security and integrity of healthcare delivery in the digital age.

22.1.1 Chapter contribution

- The confidentiality and privacy of patient data have been greatly enhanced by the implementation of strong access controls and data encryption. Sensitive health information was kept secure by implementing encryption protocols and role-based access controls, which reduced unauthorized access.
- The timely resolution of software vulnerabilities was made possible by the methodical approach to routine patching and updates.
- Gaining outside viewpoints on the security posture of the system and receiving insightful information about new threats, which made the system to be able to stay ahead of possible problems by using the knowledge gained to drive ongoing improvement.

22.1.2 Chapter organization

The remaining parts of this chapter are structured as follows. Section 22.2 presents the related works. Section 22.3 explores the current trends of cybersecurity threats in healthcare. Section 22.4 gives the approach adopted in the study. Section 22.5 sheds light on how to mitigate data breaches and cyberattacks. Section 22.6 is on ensuring the continuity of healthcare services. Section 22.7 elaborates on securing medical devices and Internet of Things systems. Section 22.8 provides a discussion of the results, and Section 22.9 concludes the chapter.

22.2 Literature review

In this section, we provide an overview of prior research within the realm of healthcare system security, specifically focusing on cyberthreats. In [10] the researchers discussed the importance of new digital technologies in the health industry, as well as the inherent dangers that may exist, the hazards associated with digital health cybersecurity which includes data breaches, medical device vulnerabilities, phishing, insider and third-party threats, and ransomware attacks.

However, various techniques were introduced in the healthcare system from their research work since technology is advancing and changing the face of healthcare with respect to creativity and effectiveness. Some of these modern innovations which include mHealth applications, wearable, big data analytics, cloud computing, blockchain, IoMT, telemedicine, Artificial Intelligent, and machine learning are helping to revolutionize healthcare services. mHealth applications and wearable enable people to monitor their health in real time, promoting proactive healthcare management. Hence there is need to create a thorough approach to the cybersecurity framework that will perform frequent risk assessments, adaptation of strong security measures, protection of data, instruction of staff, installing a secure network division, backing up data on a regular basis, monitoring and detecting anomalies, developing an incident response plan, sharing threat intelligence, and auditing third-party vendors.

Furthermore in [11], the research aim was to assess the robustness of existing policy approaches for protecting IoMT technology which will enhance to strengthen government jurisdiction in the implementation of baseline security precautions and give regulatory guidance materials on cybersecurity in the IoMT on the legacy device management, better physical security, and breach detection. The study concluded that additional regulatory guidance is required to address hazards associated with the IoMT devices by retrofitting Information Technology infrastructures, edge-to-cloud connectivity, and off-the-shelf device components.

The challenges and the effort to mitigate the risks proposed by [12] present a practical approach to securing healthcare systems. It was suggested that a comprehensive methodology is crucial for safeguarding healthcare systems from cyberthreats. According to the research work, educating healthcare professionals about potential attack vectors empowers them to recognize and mitigate threats effectively. Also, the work emphasizes the importance of having quality information technology personnel within the foundation or enterprise. Granting appropriate administrative privileges and implementing multifactorial authentication was identified in their work which serves as an additional layer of defense. Additionally, the work advocates for the establishment of a proactive measure through a physical backup setup at the foundation, and this will serve as a contingency plan against unforeseen attacks that may occur in the future. The proposed solution combines which includes staff education, skilled information technology personnel, stringent access controls, and a proactive physical backup setup to create a robust defense against cyberthreats in healthcare systems.

The confluence of mobile health (mHealth) apps, wearable Internet of Things (WIoT) devices, and customized health improvements is transforming healthcare, but it also poses new cybersecurity threats [13]. This research paper examines the environment and possible vulnerabilities in a linked ecosystem, highlighting the importance of strong security measures to secure sensitive health data and ensure patient safety. A wide range of mHealth applications that measure exercise, monitor vital signs, manage chronic illnesses, and provide personalized health advice has been implemented and introduced to capture and retain sensitive health information [14]. Also, wearable technologies such as smartwatches, fitness trackers, and medical sensors continually gather and send health information wirelessly [15]. These gadgets, frequently with minimal security protections, are susceptible to eavesdropping, manipulation, and virus assaults. Integrating WIoT devices with medical equipment and telehealth platforms results in a complicated, linked system. Vulnerabilities in any one component can jeopardize the entire network, putting patient data and potentially physical health at risk [16,17].

The work by [18] researched on Artificial Intelligence of Medical Things (AIoMT) training, testing, and validation to address these proliferating issues but however stipulated that further research is needed to achieve efficient and effective model training, testing, and validation. In their work, they remarked that obtaining clean and quality data will help mitigate the problems with AI applications in the healthcare system since there is a continuous wide scope of artificial intelligence (AI) Artificial across many domains, such as the medical field, engineering, and others. In addition, researcher in [19] discussed about the fourth industrial revolution which was characterized by the ubiquity of cyberspace as well as its exploitation by criminal elements (hackers) that are ready to compromise cyberspace by engaging in cyberattacks. In their work various malware attacks were presented and various security measures to check the malware were proposed and also a new conceptual framework that incorporates AI and software-defined networking (SDN) was proposed, thereby providing holistic mitigation for the various threats to the artificial intelligence-enabled internet of medical things (AIoMT) system [20–27]. Finally, they had a framework that was simulated with the WUSTL-EHMS-2020 dataset to be seven machine-learning models and the extreme gradient boosting model outperformed other models with 95.02% accuracy, 98.66% F1 score, and 84.44% AUC score.

22.3 Current trends of cybersecurity threats in healthcare

The healthcare business handles some of the most sensitive data possible of our personal health information. However, as breakthrough technologies such as AI, the IoMT, and telemedicine become more widely adopted, cybercriminals attack also began to grow which necessitated the urgent implementation of effective cybersecurity measures. This research will seek to investigate the concern of cybersecurity with respect to risks in healthcare system by considering the outlining vulnerabilities, probable outcomes, and effective mitigation techniques.

22.3.1 The evolving threat in the healthcare system

- Healthcare systems are vulnerable to data breaches due to the sensitive nature of patient records, financial information, and research data.
- Hospitals and clinics are particularly vulnerable to ransomware attacks, which can interrupt crucial operations and risk patient lives. Payment for data decryption is required to restore regular functioning.
- Phishing and social engineering exploit human fallibility to deceive healthcare professionals into clicking harmful links, disclosing sensitive information, or installing malware.

- Medical Device Vulnerabilities: IoMT equipment, such as pacemakers and insulin pumps, may be hacked to collect data, change settings, or damage patients, posing a serious physical risk.

22.3.2 The consequences of cyberattacks

- Breaches of personal health information can harm trust in healthcare providers, prevent patients from seeking care, and result in identity theft and financial losses.
- Cyberattacks can disrupt healthcare delivery, causing delays in diagnostics, treatment plans, and emergency services, potentially putting lives at risk.
- Ransom payments, fines for Health Insurance Portability and Accountability Act (HIPAA) violations, and reputational harm can lead to considerable financial losses for healthcare companies, affecting their capacity to deliver excellent treatment.

22.3.3 Mitigation of the risk of cyberattacks in healthcare system

- Cybersecurity awareness and training: Educating healthcare professionals on cybersecurity risks and best practices to secure data is vital to minimize human mistakes and social engineering attacks.
- Data security best practices: Strong data security methods like as encryption, access limits, and frequent backups are critical for safeguarding sensitive information.
- Manage vulnerabilities and patch them. Keeping software and medical devices up to speed with the most recent security updates is crucial for addressing known vulnerabilities and reducing vulnerable spots.
- Plan and test incident response procedures. Having a well-defined incident response strategy in place enables a quick and effective reaction to cyber-attacks, reducing damage and delay.
- Effective coordination among healthcare companies, government agencies, and cybersecurity professionals is essential for sharing threat intelligence.

22.3.4 Emerging technology and the future of cybersecurity in healthcare system

- AI-powered cybersecurity: Using AI and machine learning for threat identification and prevention can assist healthcare institutions in proactively addressing growing cyberthreats.
- Implementing blockchain technology for secure data storage and monitoring can improve patient confidence and responsibility by creating a transparent and tamper-proof record.
- Zero-trust security: Verifying every access request can improve data security and prevent illegal access.

- Insider threats: Malicious or irresponsible workers can cause data breaches or mistakenly expose critical information.

22.4 Study approach

In this chapter, the existing protocols, systems, and best practices were combined together to address the cybersecurity issues in developing healthcare systems. The study objectives are achieved through the following current approaches and measurements:

22.4.1 Preserve the privacy of patient data current measures

In this algorithm the following steps were taken into consideration:

- Putting encryption mechanisms in place for both data at rest and in transit.
- Using access controls to limit authorized personnel access to data.
- Using data anonymization strategies in research.

Programming languages appropriate for each task were utilized where several factors were considered and patient data privacy measures were considered.

22.4.2 Implement encryption protocols component

Secure communication module programming language supports cryptographic libraries such as Python, Java, or C#. Web applications and JavaScript (Node.js) were adopted for client-side encryption. Hence the algorithm steps for the process are as stated as follows:

- Choosing a secure encryption algorithm (e.g., Advanced Encryption Standard (AES)) and implementing it using relevant libraries.
- Applying encryption to data during transmission using secure communication protocols (e.g., Transport Layer Security (TLS)/Secure Sockets Layer (SSL)).

From the above algorithm, the Python results are demonstrated in Figures 22.1 and 22.2 for patient encryption protocols.

22.4.3 Utilize access controls component

Access control system steps:

- Put in place an RBAC (role-based access control) system.
- Specify user roles (such as administrators, nurses, and physicians) and the permissions that go with them.
- Include access controls in the system, database, and application at different levels.

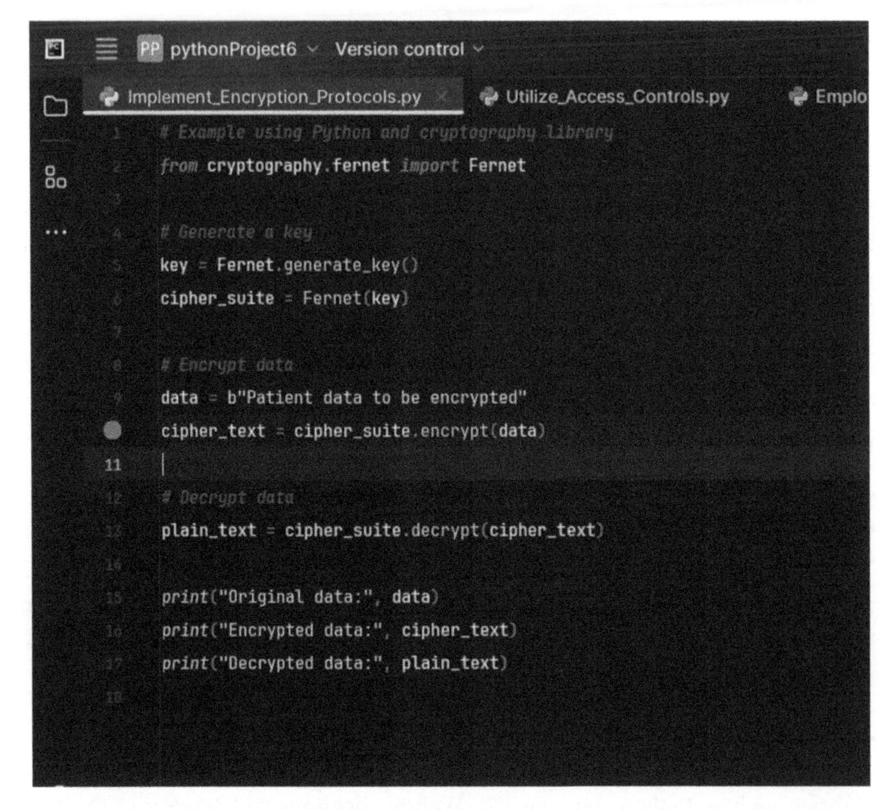

Figure 22.1 Implementation of patient encryption protocols codes 1

```
Run   Implement_Encryption_Protocols (1)
C:\Users\USER\AppData\Local\Programs\Python\Python311\python.exe C:\Users\USER\PycharmProjects\pythonProject6\Implement_Encryption_Protocols.py
Original data: b'Patient data to be encrypted'
Encrypted data: b'gAAAAABlUTv8AFPkVLm6eoBoJMFXTu8m9XsOPJav_mE850VwedJ_8452UrDj9jf2_kT1huJoJCNmpeU0lqR5lu9LUM44qL0ydqVuihVWEHJZ16VCj6FFAio='
Decrypted data: b'Patient data to be encrypted'

Process finished with exit code 0
```

Figure 22.2 Implementation of patient encryption protocols 2

The Python results for the utilized access controls component are illustrated in Figures 22.3 and 22.4 for patient encryption protocols.

Anonymization Module Programming Language such as Python, R, or any language suitable for data processing and manipulation was considered. The following algorithm steps are used:

- Determining which fields of sensitive data need to be anonymized.
- Using methods to anonymize data, such as generalization, substitution, or tokenization.

```
# Example using Python for simple RBAC
class User:
    def __init__(self, name, role):
        self.name = name
        self.role = role

def access_control(user, required_role):
    if user.role == required_role:
        print(f"Access granted for {user.name}.")
    else:
        print(f"Access denied for {user.name}.")

# Example usage
doctor = User( name: "Dr. Smith",  role: "doctor")
nurse = User( name: "Nurse Johnson",  role: "nurse")

access_control(doctor,  required_role: "doctor")
access_control(nurse,  required_role: "doctor")
```

Figure 22.3 Implementation encryption protocol code of the utilized access controls component 1

```
C:\Users\USER\AppData\Local\Programs\Python\Python311\python.exe C:\Users\USER\PycharmProjects\pythonProject6\Utilize_Access_Controls.py
Access granted for Dr. Smith.
Access denied for Nurse Johnson.
```

Figure 22.4 Results of the utilized access controls component 2

- Creating algorithms to guarantee consistent and irreversible anonymization.

The Python outcomes for simple data anonymization are displayed in Figures 22.5 and 22.6 for patient encryption protocols.

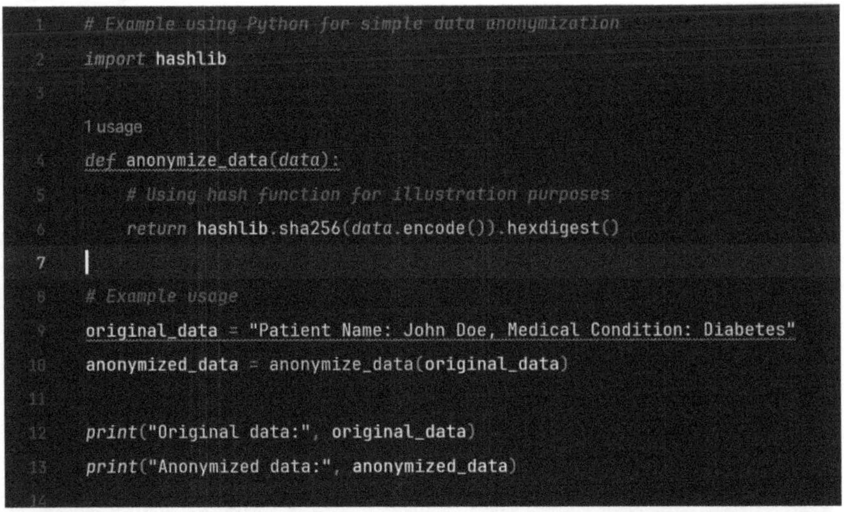

```python
# Example using Python for simple data anonymization
import hashlib

1 usage
def anonymize_data(data):
    # Using hash function for illustration purposes
    return hashlib.sha256(data.encode()).hexdigest()

# Example usage
original_data = "Patient Name: John Doe, Medical Condition: Diabetes"
anonymized_data = anonymize_data(original_data)

print("Original data:", original_data)
print("Anonymized data:", anonymized_data)
```

Figure 22.5 Implementation code of the simple data anonymization 1

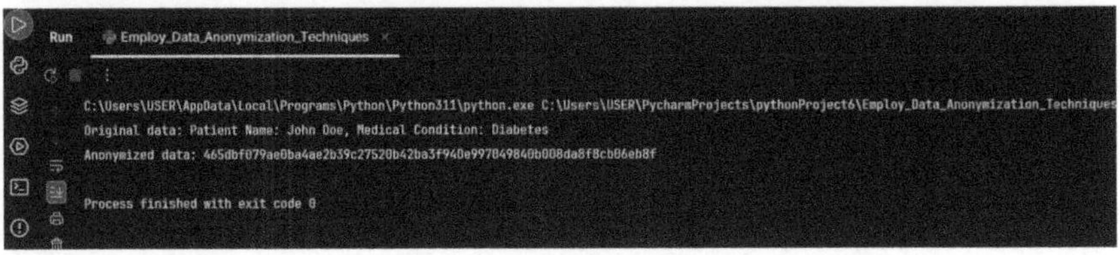

```
Run    Employ_Data_Anonymization_Techniques

C:\Users\USER\AppData\Local\Programs\Python\Python311\python.exe C:\Users\USER\PycharmProjects\pythonProject6\Employ_Data_Anonymization_Techniques
Original data: Patient Name: John Doe, Medical Condition: Diabetes
Anonymized data: 465dbf079ae0ba4ae2b39c27520b42ba3f940e997049840b008da8f8cb06eb8f

Process finished with exit code 0
```

Figure 22.6 Result of the simple data anonymization 2

22.5 Mitigate data breaches and cyber attacks

The existing measures are as follows:

- Implementing intrusion detection and prevention systems.
- Deploying firewalls to monitor and control network traffic. In this case advanced threat protection solutions were used to detect and respond to the cyberthreats attack.

22.5.1 Implement intrusion detection and prevention systems (IDPS) component

Intrusion detection and prevention module programming language such as Python, Java, or a language suitable for developing real-time monitoring and analysis components was used for the implementation.

The steps to be followed are as follows:

- Collecting and analyzing network system logs for abnormal activities.
- Implementing signature-based detection for the known attack patterns.

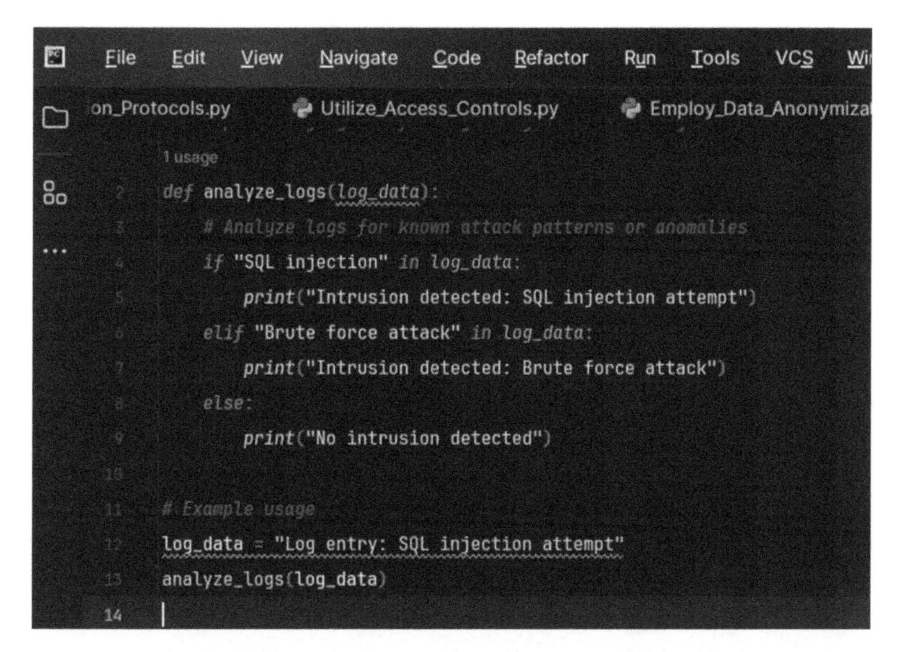

Figure 22.7 A simple example using Python programming language for the Implementation of Intrusion Detection and Prevention Systems

- Developing anomaly detection algorithms to identify unusual behaviors.

A simple example of using Python for Implement Intrusion Detection and Prevention Systems (IDPS) is shown in Figure 22.7.

22.5.2 Deploy firewalls component

Firewall configuration programming language: Firewalls are typically configured using specialized software or hardware that may not require programming. However, firewall rules can be scripted using languages like Python, PowerShell, or automation tools like Ansible.

The algorithm steps to be adopted are as stipulated below

- Defining and implementing firewall rules to control incoming and outgoing network traffic.
- Regularly updating firewall rules to adapt to emerging threats.
- Implementing rules based on the principle of least privilege.

A simple example using Python for the Deployment of Firewalls Component is illustrated in Figure 22.8.

22.5.3 Use advanced threat protection solutions component

Advanced threat protection integration programming language: Integration with advanced threat protection solutions may involve Application Programming

```
pythonProject6  Version control
ns.py   Compliance_with_Regulatory_Requirements.py   Conduct_Regular_Risk_Assessments.py
1  # Example using Python to configure firewall rules (simplified)
   1 usage
2  def configure_firewall_rules():
3      # Add rules to allow/deny specific traffic
4      print("Firewall rules configured.")
5
6  # Example usage
7  configure_firewall_rules()
8
```

Figure 22.8 A simple example using Python programming language for the Deployment of Firewalls Component

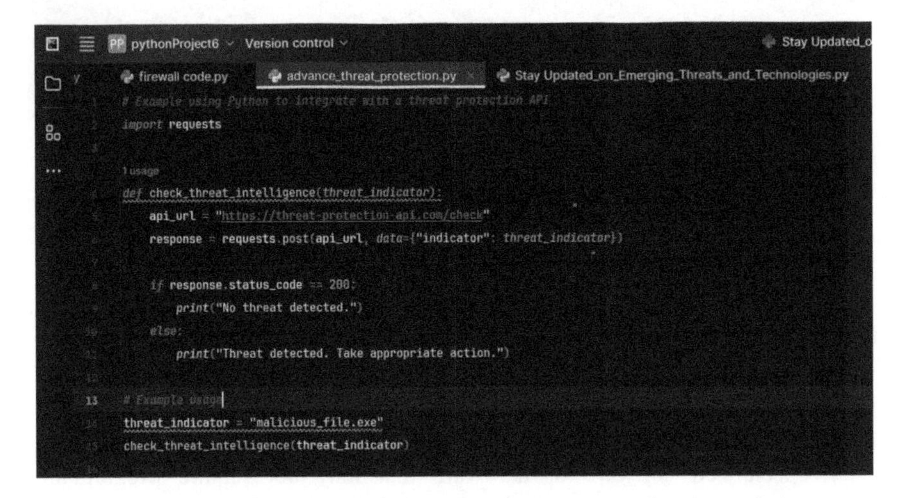

Figure 22.9 Python programming language with a hypothetical threat protection API for the integration of Advanced Threat Protection Solutions

Interface (API) usage and scripting, often in languages like Python, PowerShell, or a language supported by the solution's API.

The algorithm steps to be considered are stated below:

- Integration of threat intelligence feeds for real-time updates on known threats.
- Development of scripts to automate responses to identified threats.
- To ensure seamless communication between the system and threat protection solution.

An example using Python programming language with a hypothetical threat protection API for the integration is displayed in Figure 22.9.

22.6 Ensure continuity of healthcare services

The algorithm measures to be considered are implementation of backup and disaster recovery solutions, utilizing a redundant system measure to ensure the availability of service and the development of continuity plans for regular test business among the patients. For this to be effective the following modules have to be considered.

22.6.1 Implement backup and disaster recovery solutions component

The backup and recovery module programming language is a language used for scripting backup processes, such as Python, PowerShell, or Bash. The algorithm procedures are stated below:

- Developing a script to automate regular backups for critical data and configurations.
- Implementing versioning and secure storage for backup data.
- Establishing a disaster recovery plan outlining the process of restoring systems from backups.

An example using Python for automating the backups advance threat protection is displayed in Figure 22.10.

```
advance_threat_protection.py    backups.py    Stay Updated_on_Emerging_Th
# Example using Python for automated backups (simplified)
import shutil
import datetime

1 usage
def backup_data(source_path, backup_path):
    timestamp = datetime.datetime.now().strftime("%Y%m%d%H%M%S")
    backup_folder = f"{backup_path}/backup_{timestamp}"

    shutil.copytree(source_path, backup_folder)
    print(f"Backup created at {backup_folder}")


# Example usage
source_path = "/path/to/critical/data"
backup_path = "/path/to/backup/storage"
backup_data(source_path, backup_path)
```

Figure 22.10 An example using Python for automating the backups advance threat protection

22.7 Secure medical devices and Internet of Things systems

The existing measures to consider are to separate medical devices from another network traffic, use network segmentation, update and patch medical device software regularly, make use of authorization and authentication systems for devices, create a cybersecurity awareness culture, current measures, provide staff with regular cybersecurity training, clearly define your security policies and procedures, and encourage the reporting of security incidents without fear of retaliation.

22.7.1 Secure medical devices and IoT systems component

Security modules for medical devices programming language are based on the type of medical device and its operating system used. For embedded systems, C or C++ is used while higher-level languages like Python or Java are used for device management interfaces.

The algorithm steps considered are:

- Separating medical devices from another network traffic by using network segmentation.
- Creating scripts or using configuration tools in order to make the software easier for the medical device to be updated and patched regularly.
- Inclusion of authorization and authentication features in the firmware or software of the device.

A simplified example using Python for a device management script is shown in Figure 22.11.

```
# Example using Python for device management (simplified)
class MedicalDevice:
    def __init__(self, device_id, firmware_version):
        self.device_id = device_id
        self.firmware_version = firmware_version

    def update_firmware(self, new_version):
        print(f"Updating firmware from {self.firmware_version} to {new_version}")
        # Implement firmware update logic here
        self.firmware_version = new_version

# Example usage
device = MedicalDevice(device_id="12345", firmware_version="1.0")
device.update_firmware(new_version="1.1")
```

Figure 22.11 A simplified example using Python for a device management script

22.7.2 Collaboration with stakeholders

The measures that need to be taken include forming alliances with cybersecurity institutions through the following means: (1) disseminating threat intelligence among medical professionals, (2) working with technology suppliers to ensure secure products, adhering to regulatory mandates, (3) aligning security procedures with laws such as the General Data Protection Regulation (GDPR) and the HIPAA, and regularly auditing and evaluating compliance status, (4) creating a specialized compliance team to oversee and guarantee adherence, (5) perform continual risk evaluations, (6) conduct recurring evaluations of cybersecurity risks, (7) apply risk management models such as the National Institute of Standards and Technology (NIST) cybersecurity model, (8) determine and rank possible threats to the healthcare system, (9) remain up to date on new technologies and threats, (10) join feeds providing threat intelligence, take part in forums and conferences on cybersecurity regularly, (11) create an ongoing education program for cybersecurity teams, (12) create plans for incident response and recovery, (13) create incident response plans and record them, (14) regularly test response capabilities with tabletop exercises, and (15) make sure there are open lines of communication during incidents.

These strategies will greatly improve the cybersecurity framework of the healthcare system's capacity when implemented in order not to encounter new risks and threats. To sustain this efficacy the system requires regular updates and adaptation to changing cybersecurity environments.

22.8 Discussion of results

Here, the presented results on the Python programming language for cybersecurity and the emerging healthcare system challenges are qualitatively discussed. The outcomes and discussions of the cybersecurity measures were implemented to reduce the risks and concerns in developing healthcare systems by considering the robust access controls, data encryption, frequent security audits and risk assessments, training and awareness initiatives, frequent patching updates, and collaboration with cybersecurity specialists. Strict access controls were considered to limit data access to only those who are authorized by using role-based access control (RBAC) in assigning roles to users according to their duties in the healthcare system. This will aid in guaranteeing that every user has the right permissions for their particular role while different levels of access are granted to administrators, doctors, and nurses.

A strong data encryption system was implemented to guarantee and secure the privacy of patient data by encrypting both in transit and at rest using encryption protocols like AES, thereby making sure that all data are safe and unreadable even in the event of illegal access. This will be enhanced for both regulatory compliance and patient privacy protection. Automated tools and scripts were developed to perform periodic scans, identifying potential weaknesses in the system which will assist in regular security audits and risk assessments in order to identify the vulnerabilities and assess the overall security posture of the healthcare system. The risk assessment framework used was of the NIST which is the healthcare organization framework for cybersecurity that allows for the systematic evaluation of risks and prioritization of mitigation strategies.

A comprehensive training and awareness program was established to educate healthcare staff about cybersecurity best practices by having a regular training session which will integrate topics like recognizing phishing attempts, creating strong passwords, and understanding the importance of data security. This will not only enhance the cybersecurity knowledge of the staff but also foster a culture of vigilance and responsibility thereby enabling them to become aware of the potential threats and actively contribute to the overall security of the healthcare system. A systematic approach to regular patching and updates was implemented to address the vulnerabilities of the software systems by utilizing automated tools to monitor the latest security patches and establish a schedule for prompt application of the patches. This proactive maintenance approach ensured that every known vulnerability was patched promptly thereby reducing the risk of exploitation by cyberthreats.

In order to perform penetration testing, provide insights into emerging threats, and make suggestions for future improvements, cybersecurity professionals should be consulted and invited. Hence working together with them brings about improvement in the healthcare system's overall security posture. The cybersecurity concerns and risks in the emerging healthcare systems have been addressed by increasing the resilience against cyberattacks. Patient data will be protected, and privacy and confidentiality are guaranteed when all the strategies are implemented in the healthcare system. Furthermore, using specialized knowledge and staying ahead of emerging threats was demonstrated by the engagement with cybersecurity experts.

22.9 Conclusion and future scope

This study crucially stipulates how the dynamic landscape of emerging healthcare systems should necessitate a strong and flexible cybersecurity measures tactics that will constantly innovate and be adapted by addressing the need to protect patient data, guarantee the availability of healthcare services and reduction of ever-increasing risks posed by cyberthreats. The necessity of frequent updates, the importance of staff awareness, and the usefulness of outside expertise are among the lessons learned from the implementation of these measures. Cybersecurity measures give developing healthcare systems a strong platform on which to negotiate the ever-changing and intricate world of cyberthreats where healthcare services are given strong defense against changing risks by giving them access controls, encryption, audits, training, and cooperation. This study lays the groundwork for future advancements, adjustments to new obstacles, and a persistent dedication to protecting patient information and healthcare services in a world growing more digitally and globally connected. The confidentiality of patient information, proactive risk mitigation, and data protection support the overall integrity of healthcare services. This is achieved by developing strategies with experts through continuous training and technological measures.

References

[1] R.O. Ogundokun, J.B. Awotunde, E.A. Adeniyi and E.F. Ayo, "Crypto-Stegno based model for securing medical information on IOMT platform," *Multimedia Tools and Applications*, *80*, (pp. 31705–31727), 2021.

[2] E.A. Adeniyi, R.O. Ogundokun and J.B. Awotunde. "IoMT-based wearable body sensors network healthcare monitoring system." *IoT in Healthcare and Ambient Assisted Living* (pp. 103–121), 2021.

[3] J.B. Awotunde, M.K. Abiodun, E.A. Adeniyi, O.S. Folorunso and R.G. Jimoh. "A deep learning-based intrusion detection technique for a secured IoMT system," in *International Conference on Informatics and Intelligent Applications,* Cham: Springer International Publishing (pp. 50–62), 2021.

[4] K. Dodds, C.V. Broto, K. Detterbeck, *et al.* "The COVID-19 pandemic: Territorial, political and governance dimensions of the crisis," *Territory, Politics, Governance*, *8*(3), (pp. 289–298), 2020.

[5] A.J. Awokola, O.N. Emuoyibofarhe, A. Omotosho, O.J. Emuoyibofarhe and O.J. Mebawondu "Picture archiving and communication system," *Engineering, Technology & Applied Science Research*, *9*(5), (pp. 4859–4862), 2019.

[6] A. Funmilola, A.J. Awokola and O. Emuoyibofarhe "Development of an electronic medical record (EMR) system for a typical Nigerian hospital," *Journal of Multidisciplinary Engineering Science and Technology (JMEST)*, *2*(6), (pp. 3159–0040), 2015.

[7] O.J. Emuoyibofarhe, O.J. Adigun and O.N. Emuoyibofarhe "Development and evaluation of mobile telenursing system for drug administration," *International Journal of Information Engineering & Electronic Business*, *12*(4), (pp. 40–52), 2020.

[8] A. Kovács, "Ransomware: a comprehensive study of the exponentially increasing cybersecurity threat," *Insights into Regional Development*, *4*(2), (pp. 96–104), 2022.

[9] S. Kuamr, R. Yadav, P. Kaushik, S.B.G. Babu, R.K. Dubey and M. Subramanian. "Effective cyber security using IoT to prevent E-threats and hacking during COVID-19", *International Journal of Electrical and Electronics Research (IJEER)*, 10(2), (pp. 111–116), 2022.

[10] A. Arafa, H.A. Sheerah and S. Alsalamah, "Emerging digital technologies in healthcare with a spotlight on cybersecurity: A narrative review," *Information*, *14*(12), (p. 640), 2023.

[11] M.N. Thomasian and Y.E. Adashi. "Cybersecurity in the internet of medical things," *Health Policy and Technology*, *10*(3), (p. 100549), 2021.

[12] T.S. Argaw, R.J. Troncoso-Pastoriza, D. Lacey, *et al.* "Cybersecurity of hospitals: discussing the challenges and working towards mitigating the risks," *BMC medical informatics and decision making*, *20*, (pp. 1–10), 2020.

[13] P. Dhingra, N. Gayathri, S.R. Kumar, V. Singanamalla, C. Ramesh and B. Balamurugan, "Internet of Things–based pharmaceutics data analysis," In

Emergence of Pharmaceutical Industry Growth with Industrial IoT Approach, Academic Press (pp. 85–131), 2020.

[14] C.K. Kao and D.M. Liebovitz "Consumer mobile health apps: Current state, barriers, and future directions," *PM&R*, *9*(5), (pp. 106–115), 2017.

[15] R. Indrakumari, T. Poongodi, P. Suresh and B. Balamurugan "The growing role of Internet of Things in healthcare wearables," in *Emergence of Pharmaceutical Industry Growth with Industrial IoT Approach*, Academic Press (pp. 163–194), 2020.

[16] A.E. Adeniyi, R.G. Jimoh and J.A. Awotunde "A review on elliptic curve cryptography algorithm for Internet of Things: Categorization, application areas, and security," *Application Areas, and Security*, Computer and Electrical Engineering, Elsevier, vol. 18 (pp. 1–41), 2024.

[17] E.A. Adeniyi, J.B. Awotunde, R.O. Ogundokun, P.O. Kolawole, M.K. Abiodun and A.A. Adeniyi. "Mobile health application and COVID-19: Opportunities and challenges," *Journal of Critical Reviews*, *7*(15), (pp. 3481–3488), 2020.

[18] V.A. Iguoba and A.L. Imoize. "AIoMT training, testing, and validation," in *Handbook of Security and Privacy of AI-Enabled Healthcare Systems and Internet of Medical Things*. CRC Press (pp. 394–410), 2024.

[19] A.U. Rufai, E.P. Fasina, C.O. Uwadia, A.T. Rufai and A.L. Imoize. "Cyberattacks against artificial intelligence-enabled Internet of Medical Things," in *Handbook of Security and Privacy of AI-Enabled Healthcare Systems and Internet of Medical Things*. CRC Press (pp. 191–216), 2024.

[20] A.N. Edmund, C.A. Alabi, O.O. Tooki, A.L. Imoize and T.D. Salka. "Artificial intelligence-assisted Internet of Medical Things enabling medical image processing," in *Handbook of Security and Privacy of AI-Enabled Healthcare Systems and Internet of Medical Things*. CRC Press (pp. 309–334), 2024.

[21] M. Abdulraheem, E.A. Adeniyi, J.B. Awotunde. *et al.*, "Artificial intelligence of medical things for medical information systems privacy and security," in *Handbook of Security and Privacy of AI-Enabled Healthcare Systems and Internet of Medical Things*. CRC Press (pp. 63–96), 2024.

[22] Y. Sei, A. Ohsuga, J.A. Onesimu and A.L. Imoize. "Local differential privacy for artificial intelligence of medical things," in *Handbook of Security and Privacy of AI-Enabled Healthcare Systems and Internet of Medical Things*. CRC Press (pp. 241–270), 2024.

[23] A.L. Imoize, V.E. Balas, V.K. Solanki, C.-C. Lee and M.S. Obaidat (eds.). *Handbook of Security and Privacy of AI-Enabled Healthcare Systems and Internet of Medical Things* (1st ed.). CRC Press, 2023. https://doi.org/10.1201/9781003370321

[24] J.B. Awotunde, A.L. Imoize, Jimoh, *et al.* "AIoMT enabling real-time monitoring of healthcare systems: Security and privacy considerations," in *Handbook of Security and Privacy of AI-Enabled Healthcare Systems and Internet of Medical Things*. CRC Press (pp. 97–133), 2024.

[25] A.T. Rufai, A.U. Rufai and A.L. Imoize. "Application of AIoMT in medical robotics," in *Handbook of Security and Privacy of AI-Enabled Healthcare Systems and Internet of Medical Things*. CRC Press (pp. 335–364), 2024.

[26] S.I. Popoola, A.L. Imoize, M. Hammoudeh, B. Adebisi, O. Jogunola and A.M. Aibinu, "Federated deep learning for intrusion detection in consumer-centric Internet of Things," in *IEEE Transactions on Consumer Electronics, 70*(1), (pp. 1610–1622), 2024, doi:10.1109/TCE.2023.3347170.

[27] S.I. Olotu and A.L. Imoize, 'A review of AI-based wireless communication channels, models and protocols for telehealth systems' (Healthcare Technologies, 2023), 'Artificial Intelligence and Blockchain Technology in Modern Telehealth Systems', Chap. 3 (pp. 75–94), DOI: 10.1049/PBHE061E_ch3, IET Digital Library, https://digital-library.theiet.org/content/books/10.1049/pbhe061e_ch3

Index

Milton Keynes UK
Ingram Content Group UK Ltd.
UKHW022308260824
447373UK00001B/4